VETERINARY EMERGENCY MEDICINE SECRETS

WAYNE E. WINGFIELD, DVM, MS

Diplomate, AVECC, ACVS
Professor and Chief, Emergency and Critical Care Medicine
Department of Clinical Sciences and
Veterinary Teaching Hospital
Colorado State University
College of Veterinary Medicine and Biomedical Sciences
Fort Collins, Colorado

HANLEY & BELFUS, INC./ Philadelphia

Publisher: HANLEY & BELFUS, INC.
                    Medical Publishers
                    210 South 13th Street
                    Philadelphia, PA 19107
                    (215) 546-7293; 800-962-1892
                    FAX (215) 790-9330
                    Web site: http://www.hanleyandbelfus.com

Library of Congress Cataloging-in-Publication Data

Veterinary emergency medicine secrets / [edited by] Wayne E. Wingfield.
     p.   cm. — (The secrets series)
   Includes bibliographical references and index.
   ISBN 1-56053-215-7 (alk. paper)
   1. Dogs—Wounds and injuries—Treatment—Examinations, questions,
etc. 2. Cats—Wounds and injuries—Treatment—Examinations, questions, etc. 3. Dogs—Diseases—Treatment—Examinations, questions, etc.
4. Cats—Diseases—Treatment—Examinations, questions, etc. 5. Veterinary
emergencies—Examinations, questions, etc. 6. First aid for animals—
Examinations, questions, etc. I. Wingfield, Wayne E. II. Series.
SF991.V475   1997
636.7'0896025—dc21   97-13886
                                         CIP

VETERINARY EMERGENCY MEDICINE SECRETS   ISBN 1-56053-215-7

DEDICATION

The authors dedicate this book to our patients, past, present, and future. They inspired us to make things better, and without doubt we are improving.

> To my parents, Opal and Bud, for their lifelong love, friendship, and encouragement. To Shawna and Yvonne, the twinkles in my eyes. To Suzanne, my love, my friend.
>
> WEW

CONTENTS

III. COMMON PRIMARY COMPLAINTS
Section Editor: Tim Hackett, D.V.M., M.S.

IV. OPHTHALMIC EMERGENCIES
Section Editors: Cynthia C. Powell, D.V.M., M.S., and Steven M. Roberts, D.V.M., M.S.

V. RESPIRATORY EMERGENCIES
Section Editor: Deborah R. Van Pelt, D.V.M., M.S.

VI. CARDIOVASCULAR EMERGENCIES
Section Editor: Steven L. Marks, B.V.Sc., M.S., M.R.C.V.S.

VII. ONCOLOGIC AND HEMATOLOGIC EMERGENCIES
Section Editor: Gregory K. Ogilvie, D.V.M.

VIII. NEUROLOGIC EMERGENCIES
Section Editor: Wayne E. Wingfield, D.V.M., M.S.

IX. METABOLIC EMERGENCIES
Section Editor: Michael R. Lappin, D.V.M., Ph.D.

X. DIGESTIVE EMERGENCIES
Section Editor: Wayne E. Wingfield, D.V.M., M.S.

CONTRIBUTORS

Jonathan A. Abbott, DVM, Dip. ACVIM
Associate Professor, Department of Veterinary Internal Medicine, Western College of Veterinary Medicine, University of Saskatchewan, Saskatoon, Saskatchewan, Canada

Karin Allenspach, DMV
Emergency and Critical Care Medicine, Department of Medicine, Tufts University School of Veterinary Medicine, North Grafton, Massachusetts

Andrew William Beardow, BVM&S, MRCVS, Dip. ACVIM
Vice-President, Cardiopet, Inc., Veterinary Referral Centre, Little Falls, New Jersey

Jean M. Betkowski, VMD
Division of Cardiology, Department of Medicine, Tufts University School of Veterinary Medicine, North Grafton, Massachusetts

Terri E. Bonenberger, DVM
Associate Veterinarian, Emergency Animal Clinic, Dallas, Texas

Derek P. Burney, DVM, PhD, Dip. ACVIM
Associate Veterinarian, Gulf Coast Veterinary Internists, Gulf Coast Veterinary Specialists, Houston, Texas

Leslie J. Carter, RVT, MS, VTS
Supervisor, Critical Care Unit, Veterinary Teaching Hospital, Colorado State University, College of Veterinary Medicine and Biomedical Sciences, Fort Collins, Colorado

Kelly J. Diehl, DVM, MS, Dip. ACVIM
Staff Veterinarian, Internal Medicine Section, Veterinary Referral Center of Colorado, Denver, Colorado

Dianne Dunning, DVM, MS
Small Animal Surgery, Colorado State University, College of Veterinary Medicine and Biomedical Sciences, Fort Collins, Colorado

Teresa L. Dye, DVM
Emergency Clinician, Wheat Ridge Animal Hospital, Wheat Ridge, Colorado

Tam Garland, DVM, PhD, Dip. ABVT
Department of Physiology and Pharmacology, Texas A&M University, College of Veterinary Medicine, College Station, Texas

Kristi L. Graham, DVM
Small Animal Internal Medicine, Department of Companion Animals, Atlantic Veterinary College, University of Prince Edward Island, Charlottetown, Prince Edward Island, Canada

Timothy B. Hackett, DVM, MS, Dip. AVECC
Assistant Professor, Department of Clinical Sciences, Veterinary Teaching Hospital, Colorado State University, College of Veterinary Medicine and Biomedical Sciences, Fort Collins, Colorado

Peter W. Hellyer, DVM, MS, Dip. ACVA
Associate Professor of Anesthesiology, Colorado State University, College of Veterinary Medicine and Biomedical Sciences, Fort Collins, Colorado

Orna Kristal, DVM
Department of Medicine, Tufts University School of Veterinary Medicine, North Grafton, Massachusetts

Michael S. Lagutchik, DVM
Emergency and Critical Care Medicine, Colorado State University, College of Veterinary Medicine and Biomedical Sciences, Fort Collins, Colorado

India F. Lane, DVM, MS, Dip. ACVIM
Assistant Professor of Companion Animal Medicine, Department of Companion Animals, and Internist and Medicine Service Chief, Veterinary Teaching Hospital, Atlantic Veterinary College, University of Prince Edward Island, Charlottetown, Prince Edward Island, Canada

Michael R. Lappin, DVM, PhD, Dip. ACVIM
Associate Professor, Clinical Sciences, Colorado State University, College of Veterinary Medicine and Biomedical Sciences, Fort Collins, Colorado

Stephanie J. Lifton, DVM, Dip. ACVIM
Staff Internist, VCA West Lost Angeles Animal Hospital, Los Angeles, California

Catriona MacPhail, DVM
Small Animal Medicine and Surgery, Colorado State University, College of Veterinary Medicine and Biomedical Sciences, Fort Collins, Colorado

Dennis W. Macy, DVM, MS, Dip. ACVIM
Department of Clinical Sciences, Colorado State University, College of Veterinary Medicine and Biomedical Sciences, Fort Collins, Colorado

Steven L. Marks, BVSc, MS, MRCVS, Dip. ACVIM
Assistant Professor of Companion Animal Medicine, Department of Veterinary Clinical Sciences, Louisiana State University, School of Veterinary Medicine, Baton Rouge, Louisiana

Linda G. Martin, DVM, MS, Dip. ACVECC
Veterinary Referral Center of Colorado, Denver, Colorado

Cary L. Matwichuk, DVM, MVSc, Dip. ACVIM
Clinical Instructor, Department of Small Animal Clinical Sciences, College of Veterinary Medicine, Knoxville, Tennessee

John J. McDonnell, DVM, MS
Department of Neurology, Tufts University, School of Veterinary Medicine, North Grafton, Massachusetts

James Michael McFarland, DVM
Medical Director, Emergency Animal Clinic, Dallas, Texas

Christopher Alan McReynolds, DVM, BA
Small Animal Internal Medicine, Department of Clinical Sciences, Veterinary Teaching Hospital, Colorado State University, College of Veterinary Medicine and Biomedical Sciences, Fort Collins, Colorado

Lynda Melendez, DVM
Department of Clinical Sciences, Colorado State University College of Veterinary Medicine and Biomedical Sciences, Fort Collins, Colorado

Steven Mensack, VMD
Emergency and Critical Care, Department of Medicine, Tufts University, School of Veterinary Medicine, North Grafton, Massachusetts

Eric Monnet, DVM, PhD, Dip. ACVS, Dip. ECVS
Assistant Professor, Small Animal Surgery, Soft Tissue, Department of Clinical Sciences, Colorado State University, College of Veterinary Medicine and Biomedical Sciences, Fort Collins, Colorado

Colleen Murray, DVM
Staff Veterinarian, Emergency Animal Clinic, Dallas, Texas

Robert J. Murtaugh, DVM, MS, Dip. ACVIM, Dip. ACVECC
Professor, Department of Medicine, Tufts University, School of Veterinary Medicine, North Grafton, Massachusetts

J. Bruce Nixon, DVM
Chief of Overnight Services, Metroplex Veterinary Centre, Irvine, Texas

Maura G. O'Brien, DVM, Dip. ACVS
Staff Surgeon, VCA West Los Angeles Animal Hospital, Los Angeles, California

Gregory K. Ogilvie, DVM, Dip. ACVIM
Professor, Department of Internal Medicine/Oncology, Colorado State University, College of Veterinary Medicine and Biomedical Sciences, Fort Collins, Colorado

Donald A. Ostwald, Jr., DVM
Wheat Ridge Animal Hospital, Wheat Ridge, Colorado

Therese E. O'Toole, DVM
Small Animal Medicine, Department of Medicine, Tufts University, School of Veterinary Medicine, North Grafton, Massachusetts

Cynthia C. Powell, DVM, MS, Dip. ACVO
Assistant Professor, Department of Clinical Sciences, Colorado State University, Fort Collins, Colorado

Lisa Leigh Powell, DVM
Department of Emergency and Critical Care Medicine, Tufts University, School of Veterinary Medicine, North Grafton, Massachusetts

Jeffrey Proulx, DVM
Department of Emergency and Critical Care Medicine, Tufts University, School of Veterinary Medicine, North Grafton, Massachusetts

Adam J. Reiss, DVM
Emergency and Critical Care, Wheat Ridge Animal Hospital, Wheat Ridge, Colorado

Steven M. Roberts, DVM, MS, Dip. ACVO
Associate Professor, Department of Clinical Sciences, Colorado State University, College of Veterinary Medicine and Biomedical Sciences, Fort Collins, Colorado

Elizabeth Rozanski, DVM, Dip. AVECC
Staff Veterinarian in ICU/Emergency Medicine, Department of Medicine, Tufts University, School of Veterinary Medicine, North Grafton, Massachusetts

Howard B. Seim, III, DVM, Dip. ACVS
Associate Professor, Chief Small Animal Surgical Section, Department of Clinical Sciences, Colorado State University, College of Veterinary Medicine and Biomedical Sciences, Fort Collins, Colorado

Carolyn M. Selavka, VMD, MS
Director of Clinical Services, New Haven Central Hospital for Veterinary Medicine, New Haven, Connecticut

Cynthia J. Stubbs, DVM
Small Animal Internal Medicine, Department of Clinical Sciences, Colorado State University, College of Veterinary Medicine and Biomedical Sciences, Fort Collins, Colorado

Nancy S. Taylor, DVM
Department of Emergency and Critical Care Medicine, Tufts University, School of Veterinary Medicine and Warwick Animal Hospital, North Grafton, Massachusetts

Andrew J. Triolo, DVM, MS, Dip. ACVIM
Intern Director, VCA West Los Angeles Animal Hospital, Los Angeles, California

Deborah R. Van Pelt, DVM, MS, Dip. ACVECC
Wheat Ridge Animal Hospital, Wheat Ridge, Colorado

Ann E. Wagner, DVM, MS, Dip. ACVA
Associate Professor of Anesthesiology, Veterinary Teaching Hospital, Colorado State University, College of Veterinary Medicine and Biomedical Sciences, Fort Collins, Colorado

J. Michael Walters, DVM
Assistant Medical Director, Emergency Animal Clinic, Dallas, Texas

Ronald S. Walton, DVM
Emergency Medicine and Critical Care, Veterinary Teaching Hospital, Colorado State University, College of Veterinary Medicine and Biomedical Sciences, Fort Collins, Colorado

Suzanne G. Wingfield, RVT, VTS
Veterinary Specialist II, Veterinary Teaching Hospital, Colorado State University, College of Veterinary Medicine and Biomedical Sciences, Fort Collins, Colorado

Wayne E. Wingfield, DVM, MS, Dip. AVECC, Dip. ACVS
Professor and Chief, Emergency and Critical Care Medicine, Department of Clinical Sciences, Veterinary Teaching Hospital, Colorado State University, College of Veterinary Medicine and Biomedical Sciences, Fort Collins, Colorado

Lori A. Wise, DVM, MS, Dip. ACVIM
Wheat Ridge Animal Hospital, Wheat Ridge, Colorado

Erika Zsombor Murray, DVM
Department of Medicine, Tufts University, School of Veterinary Medicine, North Grafton, Massachusetts

PREFACE

Over the past few years, Veterinary Emergency and Critical Care Medicine has emerged as an important specialty encompassing major veterinary fields such as internal medicine, surgery, anesthesia, and oncology. Emergencies represent one of the most common reasons for the animal owner to seek veterinary care. In emergencies the art comes with the ability to evaluate, diagnose, and treat—often with minimal diagnostic data and time. Knowing the right questions and answers that routinely confront the veterinarian on the front line of medicine is the first step in surviving the chaotic atmosphere that often surrounds an emergency.

The Secrets Series® has long been a standard reference in the numerous specialties of human medicine. Now *Veterinary Emergency Medicine Secrets* joins the ranks of these specialties and introduces the veterinarian to an important resource for learning. The need for the Secrets Series® is well known to students, postdoctoral trainees, practicing veterinarians, and faculty. Too often we are faced with a requirement to read through volumes of material in an attempt to extract key information. In order to solve this problem, we have extracted the material through a series of key questions and answers often presented in emergency and critical care medicine.

Teaching students and veterinarians in practice is done by asking questions. Knowing the key question and answer is the secret for success by both. One cannot learn medicine by concentrating on only basic facts. A veterinary patient presents with a constellation of problems which must all be addressed at once. Thus, this volume encompasses a significant number of issues likely to arise in the emergency setting and later during convalescence in the critical care facility or veterinary hospital.

Like the other books in the series, *Veterinary Emergency Medicine Secrets* is not intended to be a traditional textbook. Rather, it is designed to provide factual information for the reader and to stimulate further learning and discussion. In preparing this book we have attempted to take a middle ground between oversimplification and over-complication. For the most part we have made a conscious effort to avoid the "zebras" often discussed in academic texts. Instead, we have tapped into the veterinary resources and gained the assistance of experienced clinicians, up-and-coming trainees, and, most importantly, practicing veterinarians who are truly on the front line. It is hoped that this balance will provide the reader with substance, state-of-the-art ideas, and practical information.

We are indebted to the many patients, animal owners, and students for many of these questions and answers. Our patients may not communicate in an understandable language, but simply spending time with them, observing, and learning provides us with the means to communicate and respond to their needs. To the many students who have "survived" their rotations in emergency and critical care medicine, you are extended a heartfelt "thank you" for moving us out of the dark ages and into an era for providing superior patient care. A special thanks goes to the graduating class of 1997 at Colorado State University. They tested the theory of teaching the Socratic method and passed with flying colors. To the veterinarians and veterinary technicians contributing to this text, your insights are delightful, your enthusiasm unprecedented, and your future is most bright. We hope you find the book enjoyable and educational.

Wayne E. Wingfield, DVM, MS

I. Life-threatening Emergencies

Section Editor: Wayne E. Wingfield, D.V.M., M.S.

1. DECISION MAKING IN VETERINARY EMERGENCY MEDICINE

Wayne E. Wingfield, D.V.M., M.S.

1. Why is emergency medicine so important in veterinary medicine?
Emergencies are reported to constitute up to 60% of hospital admissions in veterinary medicine.

2. How does the approach to an emergency patient differ from the conventional hospital admission?
A comprehensive medical history, physical examination, routine laboratory diagnostic studies, specialized diagnostic techniques, and the formulation of lists of written rule-outs often takes too long. The veterinarian is often faced with minimal history and a cursory physical examination that hones in on obvious injuries or illnesses—and often institutes therapy as the animal is examined.

3. What is an emergency?
An emergency is any illness or injury perceived by the person presenting the animal to the veterinarian as requiring immediate attention. Not every "emergency" is life-threatening; thus, the most important question that must be answered is, "What is the threat to the animal's life?" In an emergency, conventional approaches to the diagnosis and treatment do not ensure an expeditious answer to this question. An emergency may have significant time constraints that impede the use of conventional methods.

4. How is the life-threatened animal identified?
Three components are necessary to recognize quickly the life-threatened animal.
1. A primary complaint.
2. A complete and accurate set of vital signs.
3. An opportunity to visualize, auscultate, and touch the animal.

5. Why is the primary complaint so important?
The primary complaint helps the veterinarian to categorize the general type of problem (e.g., respiratory, cardiovascular, traumatic, urinary).

6. Why are vital signs so important in the initial management of an emergency?
Vital signs represent the first objective data available to the veterinarian. The results of vital signs, along with the primary complaint, are used to triage the vast majority of life-threatened patients.

7. What vital signs are most important in the emergency patient?
- Respiratory rate and character
- Heart rate and rhythm
- Pulse rate, rhythm, and character
- Accurate core body temperature
- Color of mucous membranes and capillary refill time

8. What are the determinants of normal vital signs?

Age, the animal's behavior, underlying physical condition, medical problems (e.g., hypertension, increased cerebrospinal fluid pressure), and current medications are important considerations in determining normal vital signs for a given animal. For example, a well-conditioned, athletic, hunting breed dog brought to the hospital after sustaining a major trauma may arrive with a pulse rate of 100. The dog probably is in shock and may have significant blood loss because the dog's normal pulse is likely 40–50 beats per minute.

9. Why do I need to visualize, auscultate, and touch the animal?

In many instances, these measures help to identify the threat to life (e.g., is it the upper airway, lower airway, or circulation?). Touching the animal helps to identify areas of tenderness. Touching the skin is important to determine whether shock is associated with vasoconstriction (traumatic, hypovolemic, or cardiogenic) or vasodilatation (septic, neurogenic, or anaphylactic). Auscultation identifies life threats associated with the lower airway (e.g., bronchoconstriction, tension pneumothorax) or circulation (mitral valvular insufficiency, aortic stenosis).

10. Once I have identified the life threat, what do I do?

Stop! Intervene to reverse the life threat. If the problem is respiratory distress due to tension pneumothorax, immediate thoracocentesis is required. If the problem is blood loss, volume restoration and control of hemorrhage (when possible) are indicated.

11. Now that I have identified and reversed the life threat, what next?

The veterinarian must develop a list of rule-outs, beginning with the most serious condition and working downward. An example is a young dog with a seriously swollen head and respiratory distress. Instead of assuming that the condition is due to trauma, the veterinarian must also consider cellulitis, anaphylaxis, or rattlesnake envenomation. If respiratory distress has been alleviated, one has time to consider the other possibilities and take appropriate action.

12. Why do rule-outs sometimes lead to problems?

The tendency is to think of the most common or statistically most probable condition to explain the animal's condition. If the veterinarian does so, he or she will be correct in most cases but may overlook the most serious, albeit usually most uncommon, problem. Therefore, the practice of veterinary emergency medicine often requires one to *react* rather than contemplate the answer. This involves considering the most serious condition possible, and, through a logical process of elimination, ruling it out and thereby arriving at the correct and generally more common diagnosis.

13. Is diagnosis a requirement during an emergency?

Of course not. Sometimes it takes hours, days, weeks, or even months to make the final diagnosis. It is unreasonable to expect that every emergency patient should have a diagnosis. The veterinarian's role in an emergency is to rule out serious or life-threatening causes for the animal's immediate condition. If you are an obsessive-compulsive personality with a need for absolute certainty before you act to stabilize an animal, emergencies are unhealthy work for you.

14. How do I decide whether to hospitalize the animal?

Tough question. Obviously several factors are important in making this decision:
- The medical/surgical condition is the first factor to consider. One crucial question must be answered: "Is there a need that can be fulfilled only by hospitalization?" For example, is oxygen, special monitoring, intensive fluid therapy, or intravenous medication required?
- Will the animal receive proper observation and treatment if discharged to the owner? Is there even an owner for the animal?
- Unfortunately, economics must be factored into the decision. If the animal's owner cannot afford hospitalization, the veterinarian is faced with two important decisions: (1) Is there

any way the animal can be treated at home without endangering survival? (2) Is the condition so severe that euthanasia is a viable option?

15. What criteria may be used for treatment of animals admitted without the owner?
- Are there any means on the animal to allow identification? Check for microchips by scanning, look for a tattoo inside the groin or pinna, check for tags on the animal's collar, ask the person admitting the animal if he or she has seen the animal before, and ask the hospital staff if they recognize the animal.
- Can the animal be made comfortable enough to be held for at least a part of the holding period required by local ordinances?
- Is the animal adoptable? Have you met a veterinarian, veterinary technician, or student who has not adopted an ill or injured animal? I doubt it.

Remember, if the animal enters your front door, you are committed to provide at least first aid care, no matter what the resources of the person admitting the animal.

16. When is euthanasia for humane reasons indicated?
First, you need to know local ordinances. If the animal cannot be made comfortable, it probably should be euthanatized. Make complete notes in the medical record and focus on terms such as pain, suffering, imminent demise, coma, severe respiratory distress, irreversible shock, uncontrollable hemorrhage, irreversible neurologic injuries, and the unlikelihood of returning the animal to a "useful purpose."

17. Any last thoughts about decision-making in emergencies?
Often the good samaritan who brings the animal to you in an emergency will go to great lengths to sway your judgment. He or she may even offer to pay (but rarely do!). Consult with colleagues and professional staff, and, ultimately, do what you think is best for the animal. By all means, keep good records.

2. CARDIOPULMONARY ARREST AND RESUSCITATION IN SMALL ANIMALS

Wayne E. Wingfield, D.V.M., M.S.

1. Define cardiopulmonary arrest and list the three phases of resuscitation.
Cardiopulmonary arrest is defined as the abrupt, unexpected cessation of spontaneous and effective ventilation and systemic perfusion (circulation). Cardiopulmonary resuscitation (CPR) provides artificial ventilation and circulation until advanced life support can be provided and spontaneous circulation and ventilation can be restored. CPR is divided into three support stages:
- Basic life support
- Advanced life support
- Prolonged life support.

2. Which animals are at risk for cardiopulmonary arrest? What are the predisposing factors?
Cardiopulmonary arrest usually results from cardiac dysrhythmia. It may be due to primary cardiac disease or diseases that affect other organs. In most animals, arrest is associated with diseases of the respiratory system (pneumonia, laryngeal paralysis, neoplasia, thoracic effusions, and aspiration pneumonitis) as a result of severe multisystem disease, trauma, and cardiac dysrhythmias.

Predisposing factors include the following: (1) cellular hypoxia, (2) vagal stimulation, (3) acid–base and electrolyte abnormalities, (4) anesthetic agents, (5) trauma, and (6) systemic and metabolic diseases.

3. What are the warning signs of cardiopulmonary arrest?
Changes in respiratory rate, depth, or pattern
Weak or irregular pulse
Bradycardia
Hypotension
Unexplained changes in the depth of anesthesia
Cyanosis
Hypothermia

4. How is cardiopulmonary arrest diagnosed?
The classical description of arrest includes the following: (1) absence of ventilation and cyanosis (respiratory arrest); (2) absence of a palpable pulse (pulse disappears when systolic pressure < 60 mmHg); (3) absence of heart sounds (heart sounds disappear when systolic pressure < 50 mmHg); and (4) dilatation of the pupils.

5. What is involved with each of the phases of cardiopulmonary resuscitation?
Basic life support
   A = Establishment of an **A**irway
   B = **B**reathing support
   C = **C**irculation support
Advanced life support
   D = **D**iagnosis and **d**rugs
   E = **E**lectrocardiography
   F = **F**ibrillation control
Prolonged life support
   G = **G**auging a patient's response
   H = **H**opeful measures for the brain
   I = **I**ntensive care
To optimize CPR, one should *assess* before initiating basic, advanced, and prolonged life support. For example, assessment → airway support, assessment → breathing support, assessment → circulation support, assessment, and so on through each phase.

6. Should I keep accurate records for each animal with cardiopulmonary arrest?
Yes. Although you are not likely to record every action during the arrest, it is important to record basic information.

BASIC LIFE SUPPORT

7. How important is basic life support?
Basic life support is the most important phase of cardiopulmonary resuscitation. It requires practice by the entire staff. It is easy to develop simulated arrests using stuffed toy animals on which you can practice the ABCs of CPR. Through such practice sessions the staff can be trained to respond rapidly to this serious emergency.

8. How do we establish an airway?
The first step is to assess and establish the unresponsiveness of the airway. Quickly check the airway for foreign materials (bones, blood clots, fractured mandible, vomitus). Position the animal in ventral recumbency in preparation for intubation with an endotracheal tube. Place the endotracheal tube accurately.

9. How do we breathe for the animal?

First, ensure that the animal is apneic and requires assisted ventilation. Once you have seen that there is no movement to the chest wall, begin to ventilate the animal with two *long* breaths (1.5–2.0 seconds each). If the animal does not begin to breathe within 5–7 seconds, begin to ventilate at a rate of 12–20 times/minute.

Use of acupuncture to stimulate respirations has been reported. Placing a needle in acupuncture joint Jen Chung (GV26) may reverse respiratory arrest under clinical conditions. The technique involves using a small (22–28 gauge, 1–1.5 inch) needle in the nasal philtrum at the ventral limit of the nares. The needle is twirled strongly and moved up and down while improvement in respiration is monitored. This simple technique can be used quickly.

10. How is circulation supported during CPR?

Assessment is necessary to determine the pulselessness of the animal before initiating external cardiac compression. Currently there are two theories to explain the mechanism of forward blood flow during CPR: (1) cardiac pump theory and (2) thoracic pump theory. The cardiac pump theory is probably more important in smaller animals (< 7 kg) and the thoracic pump in larger animals (> 7 kg). It is believed that the cardiac and thoracic pumps are interactive; each contributes to the pressure gradients responsible for blood flow during CPR.

11. What is the cardiac pump theory?

The original hypothesis suggests that blood flow to the periphery during external cardiac compression of the heart results from direct compression of the heart between the sternum and vertebrae (dorsal recumbency) or between the right and left thoracic wall (lateral recumbency) of the dog and cat. According to this concept, thoracic compression (artificial systole) is similar to internal cardiac massage and results in squeezing of blood from both ventricles into the pulmonary arteries and aorta as the pulmonary and aortic valves open. Retrograde flow of blood is prevented by closure of the left and right atrioventricular valves. During the relaxation phase of thoracic compression (artificial diastole), the ventricles recoil to their original shape and fill by a suction effect, while elevated arterial pressure closes the aortic and pulmonic valves.

12. What is the thoracic pump theory?

As pressure is applied to the animal's thorax, there is a correlation between the rise in intrathoracic pressure during compression and the apparent magnitude of carotid artery blood flow and pressure. For brain flow blood to occur during resuscitation, a carotid arterial-to-jugular pressure gradient must be present during chest compression. Experimental studies in large dogs have shown that thoracic compression during CPR results in an essentially equal rise in central venous, right atrial, pulmonary artery, aortic, esophageal, and lateral pleural space pressures with no transcardiac gradient. Aortic pressure is efficiently transmitted to the carotid arteries, but retrograde transmission of intrathoracic venous pressure into the jugular veins is prevented by valves at the thoracic inlet and possibly by venous collapse. Thus, during artificial systole a peripheral arterial venous pressure gradient appears, and blood flow results from this gradient. In such a system, there is no pressure gradient across the heart; thus, the heart acts merely as a passive conduit. Cineangiographic studies in large dogs confirm these observations by demonstrating partial right atrioventricular valve closure, collapse of the venae cavae, and opening of the pulmonary, left atrioventricular, and aortic valves during thoracic compression. When thoracic compression is released (artificial diastole), intrathoracic pressures fall toward zero, and venous flow to the right heart and lungs occurs. During artificial diastole, a modest gradient also develops between the intrathoracic aorta and the right atrium, providing coronary (myocardial) perfusion.

In small dogs receiving vigorous chest compressions, intrathoracic vascular pressures are much higher than recorded pleural pressures. The rise in vascular pressures probably results from compression of the heart during chest compression and not from rising intrathoracic pressure.

13. What are the determinants of vital organ perfusion during CPR?
Cerebral blood flow depends on the gradient between the carotid artery and intracranial pressure during systole (thoracic compression). Myocardial blood flow depends on the gradient between the aorta and right atrium during diastole (release phase of thoracic compression). During conventional CPR, cerebral and myocardial blood flow is less than 5% of prearrest values. Below the diaphragm, renal and hepatic blood flow during CPR is 1–5% of prearrest values.

14. What are the determinants of improved vital organ perfusion during CPR?
Force, rate, and duration of chest compression during CPR determine the effectiveness of organ perfusion. Regardless of the mechanism of forward blood flow during CPR, increasing the force of chest compressions increases arterial pressures. At pressures > 400 newtons (about 40 kg), bone and tissue trauma are more likely. Increasing the rate of chest compressions significantly increases the arterial pressure.

GENERAL GUIDELINES FOR CPR IN ANIMALS

15. What is the optimal position for maximizing blood flow?
Lateral recumbency (with the sternum parallel to the table top) is used for animals < 7 kg and, ideally, dorsal recumbency for animals > 7 kg. It is extremely difficult to maintain a dog in dorsal recumbency without special V-shaped troughs or other techniques. However, dorsal recumbency provides maximal changes in intrathoracic pressure and thus forward blood flow. When no peripheral pulse is felt during CPR, consider changing the animal's position and CPR technique.

16. What is the optimal compression/relaxation ratio for administering external cardiac compression?
Studies have shown the best ratio of cardiac compression to ventilation is 1:1 (simultaneous compression-ventilation) in animals. You breathe for the animal each time you compress the thoracic wall.

17. At what rate should you compress and ventilate when two persons are available to do CPR?
In animals weighing less than 7 kg the recommended rate of ventilation and compression is 120 times/minute. In animals weighing > 7 kg, the rate of compression and ventilation is 80–100 times/minute.

18. What is interposed abdominal compression?
To improve venous return and to decrease arterial run-off during external thoracic compression, have one person press on the cranial abdomen between each compression of the chest. In humans, this technique improves hospital discharge rates as much as 33%. No comparable studies are yet available in animals.

19. What if there is only one person available to do CPR?
One-person CPR in animals is highly ineffective. The ratio of ventilation to chest compression is 15:2. Give 15 chest compressions and then 2 long ventilations. Use a rate of 120 chest compressions/minute when the animal weighs < 7 kg and 80–100 times/minute when the animal weighs > 7 kg.
A recent report in experimentally induced CPR in swine has shown an excellent resuscitation rate through providing only cardiac compression. In fact, the researchers were unable to detect a difference in hemodynamics, 48-hour survival, or neurologic outcome when CPR was applied with or without ventilatory support. With this in mind, if inadequate numbers of professional staff are available, apply only cardiac compression if cardiopulmonary arrest is present.

20. When should I open the chest and do CPR?

Chest compressions raise the venous (right atrial) pressure peaks almost as high as arterial pressure peaks and increase intracranial pressure, thus causing low cerebral and myocardial perfusion pressures. Open-chest CPR does not raise atrial pressures and provides better cerebral and coronary perfusion pressures and flows than external CPR in animals. When applied promptly in operating room arrests, open-chest CPR, which was introduced in the 1880s, yields good clinical results in people. The switch from external to open-chest CPR has not yet improved outcome in human patients, probably because its initiation is too late. No comparable studies are available for clinical open-chest CPR in animals. Currently, open-chest CPR should be restricted to the operating room and in selected instances of penetrating thoracic injury.

21. How can I monitor the effectiveness of external thoracic compressions?

Traditionally, the presence of a pulse during thoracic compression has been the hallmark of effective compression. More recently, monitoring of peripheral pulses with quantitative Doppler techniques has shown that the pulse generated during compression was in fact from venous and not arterial flow. In veterinary medicine, monitoring the pulse is the most common technique of monitoring effectiveness.

Pulse oximetry provides information about hemoglobin saturation. During CPR you should see an improvement in oximetry values and mucous membrane color. End-tidal carbon dioxide monitoring has proved to be the most effective means of measuring the effectiveness of CPR. This device fits in-line with the endotracheal tube and measures carbon dioxide levels. With effective CPR you should see an *increased* end-tidal CO_2.

22. What can I do if there is no pulse or change in oximetry or end-tidal CO_2?

Consider changing the position of the animal and the force or rate of thoracic compression.

23. How can I train my staff in CPR?

Periodic training sessions in basic life support should be conducted in every veterinary practice. This is not a time-consuming activity, and the benefits are tremendous when the staff can respond quickly and efficiently. An effective means to provide training is to develop an inexpensive CPR animal. Such teaching aids were developed by taking old corrugated anesthetic tubing (trachea), an anesthetic Y-piece (tracheal bifurcation), two anesthetic rebreathing bags (lungs), and implanting them in the chest of a stuffed animal. These devices can be used to practice CPR techniques with your staff. One can place foreign materials in the mouth, practice Jen Chung maneuvers, palpate for pulses, see the thorax expand with each breath, and feel the expanding lungs as you apply chest compression. Practice sessions can be called at any time to simulate a sudden, unexpected arrest.

ADVANCED LIFE SUPPORT

24. Which drugs should I have available in the "crash cart"?

Drugs considered necessary for cardiopulmonary arrest are (1) epinephrine, (2) atropine, (3) magnesium chloride, (4) naloxone, (5) lidocaine, (6) sodium bicarbonate, (7) methoxamine, and (8) bretylium tosylate.

25. What other drugs should I have available?

Drugs that are important in the postresuscitation phase of CPR include (1) dobutamine, (2) mannitol, (3) furosemide, (4) lidocaine, (5) verapamil, (6) sodium bicarbonate, (7) dopamine, and (8) intravenous fluids.

26. What are the indications for emergency drug use during CPR?

1. To initiate electrical activity
2. To increase heart rate
3. To improve myocardial oxygenation
4. To control life-threatening dysrhythmias

27. What is the best route for administration of drugs during CPR?

Each of the four commonly used routes for drug administration during CPR has its advantages and disadvantages.

1. **Intravenous (IV)**. The preferred route for drug administration during CPR is the IV route. With central venous catheters, drugs can be rapidly delivered to their site of action via the coronary arteries. In giving IV drugs during CPR, it is important to follow each drug with a bolus of saline or water for injection to encourage the transport of the drug toward the heart because cardiopulmonary arrest usually results in hypotension, vasoconstriction, and hypovolemia. At present no conclusive data support the use of a central venous rather than a peripheral venous route.

2. **Intratracheal (IT)**. The IT route has the advantages of accessibility, close proximity to the left side of the heart via the pulmonary veins, and a large surface area for drug absorption. The disadvantages are the increased dosage required for many drugs (often 10 times the dosage given IV), decreased efficacy in the presence of pulmonary disease, and the fact that some drugs cannot be given IT (i.e., sodium bicarbonate).

3. **Intraosseous (IO) or intramedullary**. The bone marrow cavity provides extensive venous access to the cardiovascular system. Drugs normally given via the IV route may be given via the bone marrow cavity. The bone marrow cavity is most commonly accessed either through the trochanteric fossa of the femur or the distal cranial femur during CPR.

4. **Intracardiac (IC)**. Drugs can be delivered directly to the heart via the intracardiac route. The difficulty of using the IC route comes with the inability of personnel to inject drugs into the heart. Without the apex beat normally present, many find this technique to be most difficult in animals. In addition there are problems with the delivery of drugs into the myocardium instead of the ventricular chambers. Delivery into the myocardium may result in dysrhythmias and laceration of coronary arteries, and requires discontinuance of basic life support while IC injections are attempted.

28. What are the common cardiac rhythms of cardiopulmonary arrest?

The only way to distinguish the various dysrhythmias of arrest is an electrocardiogram.

1. **Ventricular asystole** is characterized by absence of both mechanical and electrical activity on the electrocardiogram (see figure below).

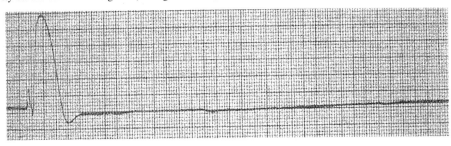

Treatment: epinephrine, atropine.

2. **Nonperfusing rhythm** (generally referred to as electromechanical dissociation [EMD]) is characterized by electrical activity without sufficient mechanical activity to cause adequate cardiac output or pulses (see figure below). The failure of contractility is probably due to depletion of myocardial oxygen stores and may be perpetuated by endogenous endorphins.

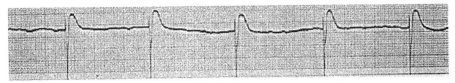

Treatment: naloxone, epinephrine, megadosage atropine.

3. **Ventricular fibrillation** is characterized by chaotic, disorganized, ectopic ventricular activity resulting in sustained ventricular systole (see figure below). Because the coronary arteries perfuse the myocardium during diastole, no perfusion takes place as long as the animal has ventricular fibrillation.

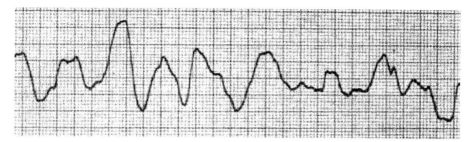

Treatment: Electrical DC countershock is the treatment of choice for ventricular fibrillation. If ventricular fibrillation is the first rhythm encountered, sequential attempts at electrical defibrillation should be performed. If ventricular fibrillation is not the first rhythm encountered or if countershock results in persistent ventricular fibrillation or another nonperfusing spontaneous cardiac rhythm, endotracheal intubation should be performed, chest compressions initiated, and an IV line established in preparation for subsequent management of the observed rhythm.

The cardiac response to countershock is largely time-dependent. If countershock can be performed within 3 minutes of the onset of ventricular fibrillation, 70–80% of patients convert to a rhythm associated with adequate perfusion (human data). After 5 minutes of ventricular fibrillation, countershock rarely results in a spontaneous perfusing rhythm; asystole, EMD, or persistent ventricular fibrillation are the usual results.

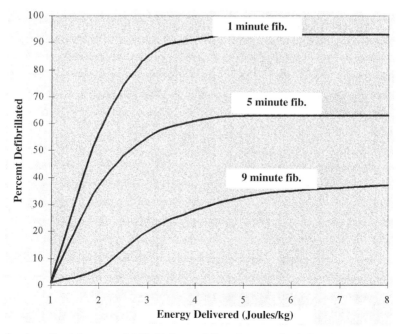

Curves showing estimated success of defibrillation vs. delivered energy after 1, 5, and 9 minutes of fibrillation in dogs receiving closed-chest cardiac massage and artificial ventilation with epinephrine. (From Yakaitis RW, Ewy GA, Otto GW, et al: Influence of time and therapy on VF in dogs. Crit Care Med 8:157, 1980; with permission.)

If countershock fails to convert the ventricular fibrillation, epinephrine should be given (IV or IT). The beneficial effects of epinephrine depend primarily on its α_1-adrenergic effects, which include arterial vasoconstriction and selective redistribution of cardiac output. Epinephrine increases the CPR diastolic aortic-to-right-atrial myocardial perfusion gradient (coronary perfusion pressure) by increasing aortic diastolic pressure and improves the cerebral perfusion gradient by increasing carotid arterial pressure. Chemical defibrillating drugs have unproven efficacy in clinical veterinary medicine. Unfortunately, many veterinarians do not have electrical defibrillators; thus, the chemical defibrillating drugs may be the only option. Drugs that may be tried in ventricular fibrillation include bretylium tosylate or magnesium chloride. These drugs have been reported to be effective in terminating ventricular fibrillation when electrical countershock has failed.

29. In using an electrical defibrillator, what important points should be kept in mind?

The electrical defibrillator is the treatment of choice for ventricular fibrillation. It is also a dangerous instrument that can cause injury to the patient and death to the veterinarian if improperly used. The optimal delivered energy to the myocardium is roughly 2–4 joules/kg. In delivering this countershock to the myocardium, it is necessary to "hit" only about 28% of the myocardial cells to defibrillate. Thus, paddle position is not as important as once believed. One should make every effort to reduce transthoracic impedance during electrical defibrillation. The following factors influence impedance:

1. Use large surface area paddles.
2. Countershocks applied close together may be most effective.
3. Use an electrode-skin interface material such as electrolyte paste or gel. Do **not** use alcohol.
4. Apply pressure to the electrodes.
5. Defibrillate during expiration.

Be careful! Always announce "all clear!," and look around to be sure that nobody is in contact with the animal, table, or instruments.

30. What is the difference between a cat and dog in ventricular fibrillation?

In normal cats, the heart is generally small enough that it may spontaneously convert from ventricular fibrillation to sinus rhythm. Unfortunately, sick cats also may have enlarged hearts. In such cases, electrical defibrillation should be attempted.

31. Which drugs should be used with caution during advanced life support?

1. Calcium enhances ventricular excitability (thus increasing myocardial oxygen requirements); it decreases sinus nodal impulse formation, reduces blood flow to the brain to nearly zero during CPR, causes coronary artery vasospasm, and is an important mediator in the formation of arachidonic acid and oxygen-free radicals. Currently, use of calcium during CPR is not routinely recommended except under conditions of hyperkalemia or hypocalcemia or when calcium channel blockers have been previously used. $CaCl_2$ results in the longest and most predictable increase in plasma ionized calcium.

2. Isoproterenol is a pure β-agonist drug. It increases myocardial oxygen demands and reduces cerebral blood flow during CPR. Currently, isoproterenol is reserved for patients with atropine-resistant bradycardias.

3. Sodium bicarbonate was once used routinely during CPR, but its empirical use is associated with:

- Increased serum osmolality (8.5% solution = 1500 mOsm).
- The metabolism of sodium bicarbonate results in the formation of increased PCO_2 ($HCO_3^- + H^+ \leftrightarrow H_2CO_3 \leftrightarrow CO_2 + H_2O$).
- With inadequate ventilation, paradoxical cerebrospinal fluid (CSF) acidosis results (HCO_3^- crosses the blood-brain barrier more slowly than CO_2).
- Sodium bicarbonate shifts the oxyhemoglobin dissociation curve to the left (decreased amounts of oxygen are released to tissues).
- Direct myocardial depression results with alkalosis (decreasing cardiac output).

- Metabolic alkalosis (pH > 7.55) predisposes to cardiac dysrhythmias that may be unresponsive to antiarrhythmic therapy.
- Before giving sodium bicarbonate, be sure the animal has adequate ventilation.
- Ideally, administration of sodium bicarbonate should be based on pH and $PaCO_2$.

Use of buffer therapy depends on the duration of arrest and CPR times. Metabolic acidemia (base deficit) should be corrected, because proper acid–base balance improves cardiovascular resuscitability and cerebral recovery in dogs. After ventricular fibrillation results in no flow for 5 minutes in dogs, metabolic acidemia is mild and transient, and early empirical $NaHCO_3$ administration is not harmful to the heart and may benefit the brain. After longer arrest or CPR times, evidence in animals of improved cardiovascular and cerebral recovery supports the recommendation to accompany epinephrine with an empirical dose of 1 mEq/kg of IV $NaHCO_3$ during CPR, to be followed by correction of monitored base deficit > 5 mEq/kg $NaHCO_3$. This may produce a transient CO_2 load that worsens the arrest-induced myocardial hypercarbia, which may depress cardiac resuscitability. This $NaHCO_3$-induced hypercarbia is usually mild, transient, correctable with hyperventilation, and harmless for the heart when epinephrine is used and apparently was not harmful to the brain.

4. Intravenous fluids are administered during CPR only when hypovolemia is the cause of arrest. Fluid-loading during CPR decreases cerebral blood flow, increases right atrial pressures (resulting in decreased coronary perfusion pressures), and therefore decreases coronary blood flow.

5. Doxapram hydrochloride is a central respiratory stimulant. Its use during CPR is not advised. Often the stimulation of the respiratory center results in transient hyperventilation followed by apnea.

32. What is the dilution of epinephrine during CPR?
Epinephrine is no longer diluted. The concentration of 1:1000, as packaged, is used with IV, IT, IO, and IC routes.

PROLONGED LIFE SUPPORT

33. What are the main complications after resuscitation?
Recurrence of either respiratory or cardiopulmonary arrest is the biggest concern after resuscitation. In most cases, arrest recurs within the first 4 hours of the first episode (see figure).

After arrest, cerebral resuscitation becomes the next most important complication. Because of the low flow state to the brain during CPR, ischemia and hypoxia lead to cerebral edema. As

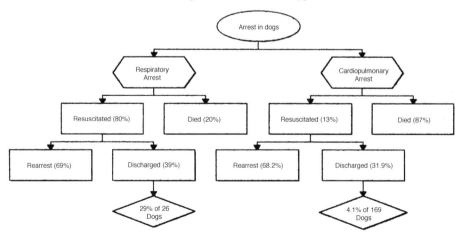

Cardiopulmonary arrest in dogs. (From Wingfield WE, Van Pelt DR: Respiratory and cardiopulmonary arrest in dogs and cats: 265 cases (1986–1991). J Am Vet Med Assoc 200:1993–1996, 1992, with permission.)

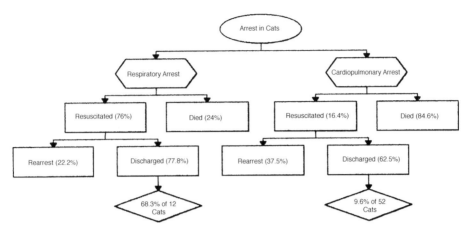

Cardiopulmonary arrest in cats. (From Wingfield WE, Van Pelt DR: Respiratory and cardiopulmonary arrest in dogs and cats: 265 cases (1986–1991). J Am Vet Med Assoc 200:1993–1996, 1992, with permission.)

the heart begins to reperfuse tissues, significant injury products may be released to the systemic circulation.

34. What cerebral complications may be expected after cardiac arrest?
In normal brain, autoregulation maintains a global cerebral brain flow of about 50 ml/100 gm brain/minute despite cerebral perfusion pressures (CPP) (i.e., mean arterial pressure minus intracranial pressure) between 50 and 150 mmHg. When CPP drops below 50 mmHg, cerebral blood flow decreases, and the viability of normal neurons seems threatened by CPP < 30 mmHg, global cerebral blood flow < 15 ml/100 gm/minute, or cerebral venous oxygen partial pressures (PO_2) < 20 mmHg. During complete cerebral ischemia, calcium shifts, brain tissue lactic acidosis, and increases in the brain free acids, osmolality and extracellular concentration of excitatory amino acids (particularly glutamate and aspartate) set the stage for reoxygenation injury.

35. What is the pathophysiology of the cerebral injury after resuscitation?
Postresuscitation cerebral injury appears to consist of four components: (1) perfusion failure (i.e., inadequate oxygen delivery, (2) reoxygenation chemical cascades to cerebral necrosis, (3) extracerebral derangements, including intoxication from postanoxic viscera, and (4) blood derangements due to stasis.

Perfusion failure seems to progress through four stages: (1) multifocal no reflow occurs immediately and seems to be readily overcome by normotensive or hypertensive reperfusion, (2) transient global "reactive" hyperemia, which lasts 15 to 30 minutes, (3) delayed, prolonged global and multifocal hypoperfusion, event from about 2 to 12 hours postarrest; global cerebral blood flow is reduced to about 50% of baseline, while global O_2 uptake returns to or above baseline levels and cerebral venous PO_2 decreases to less than 20 mmHg, reflecting mismatching of O_2 delivery to O_2 uptake, and finally (4) after 20 hours, either normal global cerebral blood flow and global oxygen uptake are restored or both remain low (with coma), or there is a secondary hyperemia, postulated to be associated with reduced O_2 uptake, followed by brain death.

Reoxygenation, while essential, also might provide chemical cascades (involving free iron, free radical, calcium shifts, acidosis, excitatory amino acids, and catecholamines) that result in lipid peroxidation of membranes.

Extracerebral derangements can worsen cerebral outcome. Studies in dogs have shown a delayed reduction in cardiac output following cardiac arrest despite controlled normotension. Pulmonary edema can be prevented by prolonged controlled ventilation.

Blood derangements include aggregates of polymorphonuclear leukocytes and macrophages that might obstruct capillaries, release free radicals, and damage endothelium.

36. How do we manage the postresuscitation patient to reduce the adverse complications of CPR?

Careful monitoring is most important during the first 4 hours after arrest. All patients require oxygen administered via oxygen cage, nasal insufflation, or facemask. If CPR was successful, one needs to support the heart during the postresuscitation phase. This support is directed to inotropic support (dobutamine or dopamine), possibly using vasodilator drugs (sodium nitroprusside), and antiarrhythmic drugs (lidocaine). These drugs help to reduce the pulmonary edema usually seen after arrest. In addition, furosemide is usually administered to reduce pulmonary edema. Cerebral hypoxia and ischemia result during CPR. The end result is cerebral edema. Treatment for cerebral edema includes mannitol and usually corticosteroids. Additional drugs that may improve cerebral resuscitation include the following:

- Calcium channel blockers reverse cerebral vasospasm and prevent lethal intracellular calcium influx.
- Barbiturates, which are mild calcium antagonists, decrease arachidonic acid and free fatty acid levels in neurons as well as metabolic demands of the brain. To date, no conclusive evidence supports the use of barbiturates. In addition, the sedation that results makes sequential neurologic assessment impossible.
- Iron-chelating drugs and free radical scavengers. Although experimental at this point, results are promising.

37. How do you know the cerebral outcome of the patient after CPR?

One should always be concerned about irreversible cerebral injury after arrest. Daily neurologic evaluations and assessment are required. Record findings each day to note the patient's progress. Clinical features to observe after arrest include the following:

- Reactivity of the pupils
- Increased responsiveness
- Breathing patterns
- Motor responses
- Motor postures

38. Are certain patients unlikely to be resuscitated?

No studies are currently available in animals, but studies in humans indicate that certain groups of patients do not survive—patients with oliguria, metastatic cancer, sepsis, pneumonia, and acute stroke. Probably animals with these conditions also will not survive.

39. When do we use do-not-resuscitate orders?

Do-not-resuscitate orders must be initiated by the owner. Good client communications are useful whenever an animal is hospitalized. It is probably wise to advise owners that arrest occurs suddenly and unexpectantly. Ask the owner how far you should go if the pet arrests. Record the response, and abide by the owner's wishes.

The decision to stop CPR must be tempered with common sense, client communication, and experience of the resuscitators. Our experience suggests that the mean duration of CPR is generally about 20 minutes.

After more than 30 years of widespread use of CPR, reevaluation of its benefits in terms of survival and quality of life shows it to be a desperate effort that helps only a limited number of patients. For most, CPR is unsuccessful.

BIBLIOGRAPHY

1. Babbs CF: Interposed abdominal compression-CPR: A case study in cardiac arrest research. Ann Emerg Med 22:24–32, 1993.
2. Babbs CF: New versus old theories of blood flow during CPR. Crit Care Med 8:191–196, 1980.
3. Babbs CF: Effect of thoracic venting on arterial pressure, and flow during external cardiopulmonary resuscitation in animals. Crit Care Med 9:785–788, 1981.
4. Berg RA, Wilcoxson D, Hilwig RW, et al: The need for ventilatory support during bystander CPR. Ann Emerg Med 26:342–350, 1995.

5. Brown SA, Hall ED: Role of oxygen-derived free radicals in the pathogenesis of shock and trauma, with focus on central nervous system injuries. J Am Vet Med Assoc 200:1849–1858, 1992.
6. Chandra NC: Mechanisms of blood flow during CPR. Ann Emerg Med 22:281–288, 1993.
7. DeBehnke DJ: Effects of vagal tone on resuscitation from experimental electromechanical dissociation. Ann Emerg Med 22:1789–1794, 1993.
8. Gonzales ER: Pharmacologic controversies in CPR. Ann Emerg Med 22:317–323, 1993.
9. Haskins SC: Internal cardiac compression. J Am Vet Med Assoc 200:1945–1946, 1992.
10. Henik RA: Basic life support and external cardiac compression in dogs and cats. J Am Vet Med Assoc 200:1925–1930, 1992.
11. Janssens L, Altman S, Rogers PAM: Respiratory and cardiac arrest under general anesthesia: Treatment by acupuncture of the nasal philtrum. Vet Rec Sep:273–276, 1979.
12. Kass PH, Haskins SC: Survival following cardiopulmonary resuscitation in dogs and cats. J Vet Emerg Crit Care 2:57–65, 1993.
13. Neimann JT, Rosborough JP, Hausknecht M, et al: Pressure synchronized cineangiography during experimental cardiopulmonary resuscitation. Circulation 64:985, 1981.
14. Neimann JT: Cardiopulmonary resuscitation. N Engl J Med 327:1075–1080, 1992.
15. Rudikoff MT, Maughan WL, Effron M, et al: Mechanisms of flow during cardiopulmonary resuscitation. Circulation 61:345–351, 1980.
16. Safer P: Cerebral resuscitation after cardiac arrest: Research initiatives and future directions. Ann Emerg Med 22:324–349, 1993.
17. Van Pelt DR, Wingfield WE: Controversial issues in drug treatment during cardiopulmonary resuscitation. J Am Vet Med Assoc 200:1938–1944, 1992.
18. Ward KR, Sullivan RJ, Zelenak RR, et al: A comparison of interposed abdominal compression CPR and standard CPR by monitoring end-tidal CO_2. Ann Emerg Med 18:831–837, 1989.
19. Wingfield WE, Van Pelt DR: Respiratory and cardiopulmonary arrest in dogs and cats: 265 cases (1986–1991). J Am Vet Med Assoc 200:1993–1996, 1992.
20. Wingfield WE: Cardiopulmonary arrest and resuscitation in small animals. Part I: Basic life support. Emerg Sci Technol 2:21–26, 1996.
21. Wingfield WE: Cardiopulmonary arrest and resuscitation in small animals. Part II: Advanced and prolonged life support. Emerg Sci Technol 2:21–31, 1996.
22. Yakaitis RW, Ewy GA, Otto CW, et al: Influence of time and therapy on VF in dogs. Crit Care Med 8:157, 1980.

3. RESPIRATORY DISTRESS

Michael S. Lagutchik, D.V.M.

1. Define respiratory distress, dyspnea, tachypnea, orthopnea, hyperventilation, hypoventilation, and apnea.

Respiratory distress—outwardly evident, physically labored ventilation or respiratory efforts; clinically evident inability to ventilate and/or oxygenate adequately. This is currently the preferred term for veterinary patients who present with severe respiratory difficulty.

Dyspnea—conscious perception of "air hunger" or a sense of "shortness of breath," subjective in nature. This term is not ideal to use in reference to veterinary patients, because they cannot relay the perception of respiratory difficulty.

Tachypnea—greater than normal respiratory rate.

Orthopnea—increased respiratory distress when the patient is lying down or the chest is compressed.

Hyperventilation—ventilation that exceeds metabolic demands; defined as ventilation causing a reduction in $PaCO_2$ < 35 mmHg (hypocapnia).

Hypoventilation—ventilation that does not meet metabolic demands; by definition, ventilation that results in a $PaCO_2$ > 45 mmHg (hypercapnia, hypercarbia, ventilatory failure).

Apnea—cessation of breathing for an indeterminate period.

2. What is acute hypercapnic respiratory failure?

Hypercapnic respiratory failure is defined as acute respiratory distress resulting in an arterial partial pressure of carbon dioxide ($PaCO_2$) > 45 mmHg. Typically, it involves abnormalities with central nervous system control of respiration, peripheral nervous system interaction with the respiratory apparatus, chest wall/bellows apparatus, and/or airways involved with gas transport. Hypercapnic respiratory failure is thus often called *respiratory pump failure* or *ventilatory failure*.

3. What is acute hypoxemic respiratory failure?

Hypoxemic respiratory failure is defined as acute respiratory distress resulting in a PaO_2 < 60 mmHg despite addition of supplemental oxygen of at least 60%. Typically, it involves the alveoli component of the pulmonary system. Hypoxemic respiratory failure is also called *lung failure* or *oxygenation failure*. Causes include (1) decreased inspired oxygen content [F_IO_2] (e.g., high altitude ascent or reduction in the F_IO_2 setting on a mechanical ventilator); (2) hypoventilation (e.g., respiratory paralysis, airway obstruction, or atelectasis); (3) diffusion impairment (e.g., severe pneumonia, interstitial fibrosis, or interstitial pulmonary edema); (4) ventilation-perfusion (V/Q) mismatch (e.g., emphysema, alveolar pulmonary edema, pneumothorax, atelectasis); and (5) intra- and extrapulmonary shunting (technically the most severe form of V/Q mismatch; e.g., lung consolidation, atelectasis).

4. What are the initial treatment priorities in any patient with respiratory distress?

Reestablishment of adequate arterial oxygen tension and removal of excessive CO_2 are the overriding aims of the immediate treatment of patients with severe respiratory distress. The major ways in which to achieve this aim, regardless of the underlying cause, are establishing a patent airway, instituting or assisting ventilation, and maintaining adequate oxygen tension by administration of supplemental oxygen to maximize oxygen delivery.

5. What are the most useful diagnostic tools in evaluating patients with respiratory distress?

The simplest and often most useful tools are a good history, detailed physical exam, and careful chest auscultation. Other useful tools include arterial blood gas analysis, pulse oximetry, capnography, thoracic radiography, and lung perfusion scans (not usually in emergent patients, however).

6. Describe measures that allow differentiation of the various causes of hypoxemia in emergency patients with respiratory distress.

Hypoxemia is diagnosed by the presence of SpO_2 < 90% or arterial blood gas (ABG) analysis that reveals PaO_2 < 60 mmHg. ABG analysis is essential for proper interpretation of causes of hypoxemia. Alternatively, pulse oximetry and capnography can be useful in diagnosis. Hypoxemia with hypercapnia defines hypoventilation as the underlying cause. Hypoxemia with normocapnia implies diffusion impairment, ventilation/perfusion imbalance (V/Q mismatch), or shunt as underlying causes. In veterinary patients, diffusion impairment is rarely severe enough to cause hypoxemia in and of itself. Response to oxygen supplementation usually allows differentiation between V/Q mismatch and shunting. The typical patient with V/Q mismatch demonstrates marked response (i.e., improved PaO_2) with supplemental oxygen, whereas the patient with shunt shows only minimal if any, improvement in PaO_2 (i.e., by definition, refractory hypoxemia with < 10 mmHg increase with at least 40% oxygen administration).

7. How do I recognize a patient with severe respiratory distress?

Usually, such patients are not hard to recognize. Abnormal sounds (stridor, wheezes), abnormal posture (orthopnea, head and neck extended, elbows abducted, sternal recumbency), abnormal mucous membrane color (cyanosis or pale), tachypnea, weakness and exhaustion, altered respiratory effort (shallow and rapid, or labored and forceful, or absent), and vigorous resistance to restraint are the typical signs in animals with respiratory distress. However, pets may have significant respiratory compromise and yet outwardly show minimal clinical signs of distress. Cats are more likely to have this type of presentation. Careful and quiet examination is essential to avoid sending the patient into stress-induced overt distress or respiratory arrest.

8. What physical exam findings may help to differentiate the cause or location of the primary respiratory problem?

Patients with a rapid, shallow respiratory pattern frequently have pleural space disease (pleural effusion, hemothorax, pneumothorax). Patients with end-expiratory effort and wheezes on chest auscultation frequently have small airway obstructive disease (asthma). Patients with deep, labored chest movements frequently have pulmonary parenchymal disease (pulmonary edema, pulmonary contusions, space-occupying masses). Patients with obvious stridor, minimal air movement at the nares or mouth, and marked inspiratory effort typically have upper airway obstruction (laryngeal edema or paralysis, foreign body aspiration). These patterns are hardly exclusive: Often patients have multiple problems, and some patients may have serious underlying respiratory problems and yet appear clinically normal.

9. Define cyanosis, its causes, and significance and treatment of an emergent patient with cyanosis.

Cyanosis develops (1) when blood is insufficiently oxygenated in the lungs; (2) when hemoglobin is unable to carry oxygen; and (3) when blood stagnates in peripheral capillary beds. To be detected clinically, unoxygenated hemoglobin concentration must be > 5 gm/dl of blood. At this level, significant hypoxemia may already be present ($\leq$ 50 mmHg), thus reinforcing the significance of cyanosis in a critical patient with respiratory distress. In addition, anemic patients may not demonstrate cyanosis. Cyanosis is centrally mediated (right-to-left cardiovascular shunts, hypoventilation, airway obstruction, V/Q mismatching, methemoglobinemia) or peripherally mediated (arterial thromboembolism, venous obstruction, arteriolar constriction, low cardiac output heart failure, shock). Emergency treatment consists of provision of supplemental oxygen and rapid identification and correction of the underlying cause.

10. What nonrespiratory conditions may mimic acute respiratory distress?

Numerous disorders cause tachypnea, orthopnea, and other signs referable to the respiratory system in the absence of true respiratory disease. These disorders can confuse the clinician. Examples include hyperthermia, shock, metabolic acidosis and alkalosis, hyperthyroidism, fear or anxiety, pericardial tamponade, anemia, abdominal organ enlargement or ascites, and abnormalities with central control of respiration from drugs and metabolic or organic central nervous system disease.

11. What are the two broad categories of traumatic respiratory emergencies in dogs and cats?

Blunt thoracic trauma (e.g., vehicular trauma, falls from height) and penetrating trauma (e.g., bullets, arrows, bite wounds, penetrating foreign bodies).

12. Categorize the location and most common types of traumatic respiratory emergencies in small animals.

Larynx and major extrathoracic airways. Commonly caused by collars, bite wounds, and gun shot injury; airway obstruction may occur from blood clots, edema, foreign debris, tissue debris, and secretions. Typical signs include labored inspiration, stridor, and cyanosis; aspiration pneumonia may be present.

Chest wall. Rib fractures (including flail chest segments) and open (sucking) chest wounds are not infrequent in patients suffering thoracic trauma.

Pleural space. Pneumothorax and hemothorax are the most common complications seen after chest trauma. Diaphragmatic hernias are infrequent and can be difficult to diagnose.

Pulmonary parenchyma and major intrathoracic airways. Pulmonary contusions are seen in about 45% of blunt trauma cases. Lung lacerations and pulmonary hematomas are uncommon. Intrabronchial hemorrhage carries a grave prognosis and is seen in major chest trauma cases fairly commonly. Rupture or disruption of intrathoracic airways probably occurs frequently, because many cases of pneumothorax have no outward source of air leakage. Blatant disruption of major airways from the parenchyma likely leads to rapid death.

13. What are the three goals of supplemental oxygen therapy in treating hypoxemic patients? When should supplemental oxygen be administered?

The goals are (1) to treat the hypoxemia, (2) to decrease the work of breathing, and (3) to decrease myocardial work. Supplemental oxygen therapy is indicated for virtually any patient with respiratory embarrassment. With conventional delivery methods (see next question), it is not possible to harm a patient with additional oxygen, and it may mean the difference between life and death.

14. Describe the ways in which supplemental oxygen therapy can be administered, listing the advantages and disadvantages of each.

Four methods are commonly used to provide supplemental oxygen: (1) face mask, (2) nasal oxygen insufflation, (3) oxygen cage, and (4) intratracheal oxygen administration.

Method	Advantages	Disadvantages
Face mask	Simple Inexpensive Readily available Provides F_IO_2 of 40–60%	Requires high O_2 flow rates Patient may not tolerate mask Patient must be attended at all times
Nasal Oxygen	More freedom of movement for patient	F_IO_2 is not known (24–44%?) Excessive flow may cause gastric dilatation
Oxygen Cage	Noninvasive Provides known F_IO_2 in humidity- and temperature-controlled environment Less stressful to patient	Patient is physically separated from caregivers Opening doors drops F_IO_2 Maximum F_IO_2 is 40–50% at economic rates
Intratracheal	Can place transtracheal catheter during emergencies F_IO_2 from 40–80%, depending on whether catheter or endotracheal tube is used	Endotracheal tube placement may require sedation or anesthesia Tracheostomy tube may be required Requires continuous monitoring

15. List the common causes of airway obstruction in dogs and cats.

Trauma

Infections involving the nasal passages, pharynx, and larynx

Obstruction with foreign material

Localized or systemic anaphylaxis with edema formation and bronchoconstriction

Compressive tumors of the airways and surrounding soft tissues

Brachycephalic syndrome components (stenotic nares, elongated soft palate, laryngeal malformation, everted laryngeal saccules, hypoplastic [collapsing] trachea)

Laryngeal paralysis

Tracheal stenosis

16. List the common pulmonary parenchymal disorders that cause respiratory distress, and briefly describe findings that may aid in diagnosis in the acute setting.

Pneumonia (acute fulminant bronchopneumonia, aspiration pneumonia, and smoke inhalation pneumonia), pulmonary contusions, pulmonary edema, asthma (in cats), and pulmonary thromboembolism are the common parenchymal disorders causing respiratory distress. Patients with pneumonia are usually depressed, anorectic, and febrile and may or may not have a deep, moist, productive cough. Abnormal lung sounds (crackles) may suggest bronchopneumonia. Patients with contusions invariably have a history of trauma, and areas of the chest on auscultation, especially adjacent to rib fractures or skin bruising, may be quiet, reflecting alveolar and small airway filling with blood and edema. Patients with pulmonary edema usually have fine or coarse crackles on auscultation and may have cardiac or other exam findings to suggest either cardiac or noncardiac causes of the edema in addition to historical information suggesting an underlying cause (e.g., congestive heart failure, electric cord shock). Cats with asthma typically have a supporting history and usually have wheezes on chest auscultation and a characteristic end-expiratory effort caused by forcing air in the small airways against partial or complete small airway closure. Patients with pulmonary thromboembolism (PTE) frequently have another significant medical problem that predisposes them to embolize (hyperadrenocorticism, diabetes mellitus, trauma, disseminated intravascular coagulation). The hallmark findings in patients with PTE are acute, severe respiratory distress and minimal radiographic changes and marked response to oxygen supplementation in the absence of signs suggesting another cause.

17. How do I recognize and manage a patient with a pleural space disorder presenting with respiratory distress?

Patients with pleural cavity disease or disruption of the integrity of the chest wall tend to present with characteristic restrictive respiratory pattern (rapid, shallow breathing with other attendant signs of distress). Chest auscultation usually demonstrates generalized loss of lung sounds (muffled). Common causes of pleural space disease include open chest wounds, flail chest, pneumothorax, pleural effusions, hemothorax, and diaphragmatic hernia. Management depends on the cause, but in general, rapid careful thoracentesis is required for pneumothorax, hemothorax, and severe pleural effusions. Cautious handling until definitive surgery is possible is required for patients with diaphragmatic hernias. Chest wall trauma is managed by appropriate wound care with local anesthetic blocks at sites of rib fractures.

18. How do I manage the patient with fulminant pulmonary edema?

Management depends on the pathophysiologic mechanism responsible for the edema formation. Acute cardiogenic edema is managed by (1) minimizing cardiac work (cage rest, sedation, inotropic support); (2) improving oxygenation (supplemental oxygen, bronchodilators, airway suctioning, mechanical ventilation); (3) resolving pulmonary edema (diuretics, vasodilators, phlebotomy); and (4) improving cardiac performance (inotropic support). Management of noncardiogenic edema (due to increased capillary permeability) is more challenging, because the underlying cause is not often found. Oxygen supplementation is the key tool, and mechanical ventilation with positive end-expiratory pressure may be required. Cautious fluid therapy is essential, and diuretics and vasodilators are recommended only if the patient is normovolemic. Cardiovascular support is important, including inotropic support and blood transfusions to maintain oxygen delivery.

19. What are the indications for placement of an indwelling thoracotomy tube (chest tube)?

Indications include intractable persistence of air in the chest due to continued leakage, large volumes of air accumulating in a short time (e.g., tension pneumothorax), or accumulation of fluid (blood, chyle, pus) in significant quantities in the pleural space. Good clinical judgment is required in deciding on placement of an indwelling tube. Tubes are not without potentially serious complications, increase client costs and patient discomfort, and mandate continuous observation. Exact guidelines are impossible, but the author usually places a tube immediately if tension pneumothorax develops and as soon as practicable when large volumes of air or fluid are repeatedly removed from the chest over a period of 6–8 hours, or sooner if the patient is clinically affected.

20. What are the indications for performing a tracheotomy in emergent patients with respiratory distress?

The most common indications are emergency management of extrathoracic airway obstruction and hypoventilation due to CNS and neuromuscular diseases and severe hypoxemia requiring ventilatory support due to underlying pulmonary disease.

21. What are the indications for mechanical ventilation in patients with respiratory distress?

Mechanical ventilation is indicated for patients with ventilatory failure or severe hypoxemia unresponsive to supplemental oxygen administration by face mask, nasal cannula, or oxygen cage. Specific indications in ventilatory failure are (1) apnea, (2) administration of paralyzing agents, and (3) ineffective respiratory efforts with progressive hypercarbia and acidosis (usually defined as a $PaCO_2 > 60$ mmHg and arterial pH < 7.30), regardless of cause. Specific indications for treating hypoxemic patients include (1) presence of an arterial $PO_2 < 50$–60 mmHg on a test of 100% oxygen and (2) inability to maintain a PaO_2 above 50–60 mmHg with a nontoxic level of oxygen supplementation (< 60% O_2).

22. What is the emergency treatment for acute small airway disease (asthma) in cats?

The mainstays of emergency treatment include oxygen administration, corticosteroids (prednisolone sodium succinate, 10–20 mg/kg IV), and bronchodilators (aminophylline, 2–4 mg/kg IM or slowly IV). If these agents fail to resolve the crisis in 5–15 minutes, additional agents may be necessary, including epinephrine (0.5 to 1.0 ml of 1:10,000 dilution IM or SQ), beta-adrenergic agonists (terbutaline, 1.25–2.5 mg PO), and parasympatholytics (atropine, 0.04 mg/kg SC or IM).

23. What is the alveolar-arterial oxygen difference? How is it useful in managing a patient with respiratory distress?

The alveolar-arterial oxygen tension difference (A-a gradient) is a calculation that allows the clinician to estimate adequacy of oxygen transfer from the alveolus to pulmonary capillary blood. In the ideal alveolus, every bit of oxygen inspired rapidly crosses over into the capillary blood, with an A-a gradient of 0. In physiologic systems, with normal shunting of some blood, the A-a gradient may be as high as 10 mmHg. In certain pathologic conditions (diffusion impairment, V/Q mismatching, and shunt), the A-a gradient increases, reflecting inadequacy of oxygen transfer. The alveolar component of the equation is calculated by using the alveolar gas equation:

$$P_AO_2 = (\text{barometric pressure} - 47)F_IO_2 - (PaCO_2/0.8),$$

where P_AO_2 is the expected alveolar partial pressure of oxygen, 47 is the vapor pressure of water, F_IO_2 is the inspired oxygen concentration (21% or 0.21 for room air), and 0.8 is the respiratory quotient. Once P_AO_2 is determined, subtract the measured arterial partial pressure of oxygen (PaO_2) from the P_AO_2 to yield the A-a gradient. Example: The patient has a PaO_2 of 50 mmHg breathing room air and a $PaCO_2$ of 50 mmHg; the barometric pressure is 760 mmHg. The estimated alveolar O_2 tension, from the formula above, is 87 mmHg. Subtract the actual PaO_2 (87 – 50) to give the A-a gradient, in this case 37 mmHg.

A gradient of 0–10 mmHg is considered normal; 10–20 is considered mild impairment of oxygen exchange; 20–30 is considered moderate impairment; and > 30 is considered severe gas exchange abnormality. Clinically, the A-a gradient may be used to assess gas exchange function over time and is thus useful in monitoring patients with certain types of respiratory distress.

When supplemental oxygen is administered, the A-a gradient, as calculated above, is not accurate. Dividing the measured PaO_2 by the fraction of inspired oxygen yields the PaO_2/F_IO_2 ratio, which is accurate. Normal values for this ratio are > 200–250 mmHg; patients with severe respiratory failure have values < 200. Example: a patient with a PaO_2 of 50 mmHg breathing 50% oxygen will have a PaO_2/F_IO_2 ratio of 100 (50/.50), indicating severe respiratory failure.

24. What is the adult respiratory distress syndrome (ARDS)? Does it occur in dogs and cats?

ARDS is a life-threatening form of respiratory failure due to acute lung injury. Numerous causes are described in people, and despite recent advances, the mortality rate remains high. Recently, Parent et al. reported a syndrome similar to human ARDS in dogs. Human diagnostic criteria that were applicable in this study include severe respiratory distress, severe hypoxemia refractory to supplemental oxygen, bilateral alveolar infiltrates on thoracic radiography, decreased lung compliance, and near-normal cardiac function. These findings reflect the severe pulmonary edema and profound pulmonary inflammatory response characteristic of ARDS. Treatment is nonspecific, aimed at correcting the underlying condition and the hypoxemia (which frequently requires mechanical ventilation with positive end-expiratory pressure), fluid and nutritional therapy, and prevention of secondary infection.

25. What are the most common immediately reversible acute respiratory causes of cardiopulmonary arrest (CPA)?

Clinicians should be alert for tension pneumothorax and obstructive asphyxia. These rapidly developing conditions are immediately reversible and carry a grave prognosis if not corrected immediately. Tension pneumothorax is typically seen in trauma patients or mechanically ventilated patients; it is characterized by rapid-onset hypotension, hypoxia, high airflow resistance (in ventilated patients), subcutaneous emphysema, and reduced lung sounds. Obstructive asphyxia is typically seen after foreign body aspiration, laryngeal paralysis, retropharyngeal abscessation, or cervicofacial trauma.

BIBLIOGRAPHY

1. Crowe DT Jr: Managing respiration in the critical patient. Vet Med 1:55–76, 1989.
2. Drobatz KJ, Concannon K: Noncardiogenic pulmonary edema. Comp Cont Educ Pract Vet 16:333–345, 1994.
3. Frevert CW, Warner AE: Respiratory distress resulting from acute lung injury in the veterinary patient. J Vet Intern Med 6:154–165, 1992.
4. Hackner SG: Emergency management of traumatic pulmonary contusions. Comp Cont Educ Pract Vet 17:677–686, 1995.
5. Harpster N: Pulmonary edema. In Kirk RW, Bonagura JD (eds): Current Veterinary Therapy, 10th ed. Philadelphia, W.B. Saunders, 1989, pp 385–392.
6. Keyes ML, Rush JE, Knowles KE: Pulmonary thromboembolism in dogs. J Vet Emerg Crit Care 3:23–32, 1993.
7. Kovacic JP: Management of life-threatening trauma. Vet Clin North Am: Small Anim Pract 24: 1057–1094, 1994.
8. Lanken PN: Respiratory failure: An overview. In Carlson RW, Geheb MA (eds): Principles and Practice of Medical Intensive Care. Philadelphia, W.B. Saunders, 1993, pp 754–762.
9. Murtaugh RJ, Spaulding GL: Initial management of respiratory emergencies. In Kirk RW, Bonagura JD (eds): Current Veterinary Therapy, 10th ed. Philadelphia, W.B. Saunders, 1989, pp 195–201.
10. Parent C, King LG, Van Winkle TJ, Walker LM: Respiratory function and treatment in dogs with acute respiratory distress syndrome: 19 cases (1985–1993). J Am Vet Med Assoc 208:1428–1433, 1996.
11. Taboada J, Hoskins JD, Morgan RV: Respiratory emergencies. In Emergency Medicine and Critical Care in Practice. Trenton, VLS Books, 1996, pp 227–247.
12. Tams TR, Sherding RG: Smoke inhalation injury. In Emergency Medicine and Critical Care in Practice. Trenton, VLS Books, 1992, pp 42–49.
13. Van Pelt DR, Wingfield WE, Hackett TB, Martin LG: Application of airway pressure therapy in veterinary critical care. Part I: Respiratory mechanics and hypoxemia. J Vet Emerg Crit Care 3:63–70, 1993.

---

4. PATHOPHYSIOLOGY OF CONGESTIVE HEART FAILURE

Wayne E. Wingfield, D.V.M., M.S.

---

1. What is heart failure?

Heart failure in the small animal results from the combined effects of chronic cardiac insufficiency and attempts by the neurohumeral system to compensate. Peripheral venous congestion (i.e., pulmonary edema) results when the left ventricle begins to fail, systemic venous congestion (i.e., ascites, hepatic congestion, and rarely, peripheral edema) occurs when the right ventricle begins to fail, and generalized heart failure results when both right and left ventricles fail.

2. What are the four common mechanisms accounting for heart failure in small animals? List common causes for each.
1. Pressure or volume overload (mitral valvular insufficiency, systemic hypertension)
2. Myocardial failure (dilated cardiomyopathy)
3. Diastolic failure (hypertrophic cardiomyopathy)
4. Cardiac dysrhythmias (atrial fibrillation, ventricular fibrillation)

3. Define the relationship between pressure and flow as they relate to vascular resistance.
The heart generates pressure and flow. Both must be maintained within certain limits to produce viable organ function. Thus the relationship between pressure and flow is defined by vascular resistance.

$$\text{Vascular resistance} = \frac{\text{Pressure}}{\text{Flow}}$$

4. How can I use the relationship between vascular resistance, pressure, and flow in the clinical use of cardiac drugs?
Arterial vasoconstriction improves blood pressure, but it also decreases blood flow and possibly tissue perfusion. Arterial vasodilation decreases blood pressure but improves blood flow and tissue perfusion.

5. What is cardiac output? What are its determinants?
Cardiac output is the total forward blood flow coming from the heart and is the product of stroke volume and heart rate. The three determinants of stroke volume are (1) preload, (2) afterload, and (3) contractility.

6. What is preload?
The stretch or load placed on a myocardial fiber before contraction is termed preload. Within limits, this load or stretch increases myocardial fiber shortening and stroke volume. Atrial pressure is a clinical measure of the amount of preload. The Frank-Starling (cardiac output) curve describes this relationship.

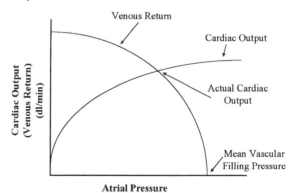

The actual cardiac output is determined by the intersection of the cardiac output and the venous return curve. Cardiac output changes when either the cardiac output or the venous return (preload) curve begins to shift.

7. What two extracardiac factors affect venous return to the heart? What are the determinants of these two factors?
Peripheral vascular resistance, determined by arterial vascular tone and blood viscosity, and mean vascular filling pressure, determined by vascular volume and venous vascular tone.

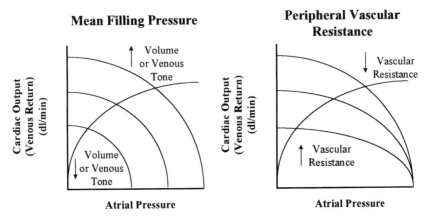

Changes in preload as a response to changes in venous return.

8. What is afterload?

Afterload is the peak load or stress developed in the ventricular wall during systole. The myocardial fibers must develop tension equal and opposite to afterload for myocardial fiber shortening to occur. The total amount of work by the myocardium is related directly to the amount of afterload that it develops and the degree of myocardial fiber shortening or cardiac stroke volume. For any given amount of myocardial work, there is an inverse relationship between afterload and stroke volume. As myocardial afterload increases, stroke volume and cardiac output decrease, and vice versa.

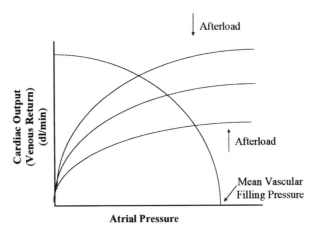

An increase in afterload results in a downward shift of the cardiac output curve, whereas a decrease in afterload increases cardiac output.

9. What factors determine cardiac afterload?

The LaPlace relation determines cardiac afterload. This relation predicts that wall stress in a sphere is directly proportional to pressure and radius of the sphere and inversely proportional to wall thickness. Thus, afterload is largely a function of systolic pressure. A decrease in systolic pressure increases cardiac output. In addition, systolic pressure is affected by aortic impedance (i.e., wall stiffness) and peripheral vascular resistance (see figure at top of next page).

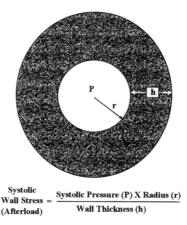

$$\text{Systolic Wall Stress (Afterload)} = \frac{\text{Systolic Pressure (P) X Radius (r)}}{\text{Wall Thickness (h)}}$$

Afterload is equal to ventricular wall stress during systole and is determined by the systolic pressure (P), ventricular radius (r), and wall thickness (h).

10. What is contractility? How is it influenced?

Contractility is the intrinsic property of cardiac muscle that allows it to change myocardial fiber shortening and stroke volume independently of cardiac loading (i.e., afterload and preload). Changes in contractility are reflected in changes in cardiac output.

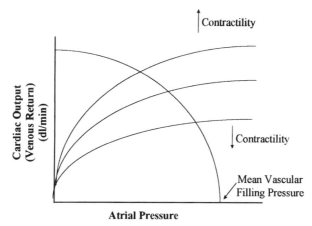

Changes in contractility shift the cardiac output curve.

11. How is myocardial contractility modulated?

Sympathetic tone to the heart modulates contractility. This tone is mediated by the β_1 receptors that alter calcium influx during myocardial contraction. Inotropic drugs change myocardial contractility by altering the amount of calcium available for contraction. Cardiac hypertrophy also modulates cardiac contractility to a point. Loss of myocardial mass decreases contractility, and myocardial hypertrophy increases contractility.

12. What happens to the Frank-Starling (cardiac output) curve in congestive heart failure?

Pathologic changes in the myocardium result in a downward, rightward shift in the cardiac output curve (low-output heart failure) or downward, leftward changes in the venous return curve (hypovolemic shock) (see figure in question 6).

13. What are the three neurohumeral phases in heart failure?
1. Cardiac injury or insufficiency
2. Activation of neurohumeral responses to injury or insufficiency
3. Neurohumeral overcompensation

14. What happens during cardiac injury or insufficiency?
The injury or insufficiency, which may be either congenital or acquired, primary or secondary, ultimately results in hemodynamic overload on the heart. The two types of hemodynamic overload are (1) pressure overload (stenotic heart valves or systemic hypertension) and (2) volume overload (valvular insufficiencies, patent ductus arteriosus, ventricular septal defects. In most cases this neurohumeral response goes unnoticed clinically.

15. How does the body activate the neurohumeral responses to injury or insufficiency? List some of the effects of each.
Many responses are activated in response to myocardial injury or insufficiency:
• Renin-angiotensin (vasoconstriction to increase blood pressure and cardiac output)
• Aldosterone (volume expansion via retention of sodium and thus water)
• Sympathetic nervous system (vasoconstriction, increased heart rate, increased contractility)
• Vasopressin (ADH) (water retention to expand volume)
• Atrial natriuretic peptide (ANP) (vasodilation, decreased venous congestion)
• Myocardial hypertrophy (increased myocardial mass, increased chamber dilation to increase contractility)

16. How does overcompensation adversely affect animals in heart failure?
High venous filling pressures in the atria result in venous pooling in the lungs (left atrium) or peripheral venous system (right atrium). In addition, arterial vasoconstriction impairs tissue perfusion. This state is called congestive heart failure (CHF).

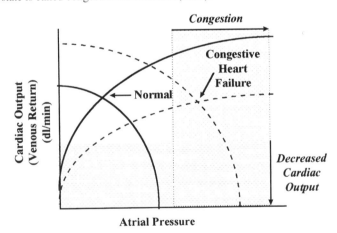

Congestive heart failure results from chronic myocardial insufficiency or injury and neurohumeral responses.

17. What strategies are used in treating animals with CHF?
Optimize cardiac performance by manipulating the four determinants of cardiac output:
• Reduce venous congestion (preload).
• Improve cardiac output (preload, afterload, and contractility).
• Normalize heart rate and rhythm (heart rate).
• Slow progression of the disease (preload, afterload, contractility, and heart rate).

18. How is venous congestion reduced?

Venous congestion is reduced by decreasing preload, which decreases atrial pressures and thus pulmonary and/or systemic venous congestion. Decreasing preload also may reduce cardiac output. There are two means to reduce preload: (1) decrease vascular volume (diuretics, salt-restriction) and (2) decrease venous tone (venous or mixed vasodilator drugs). Both strategies result in a leftward shift in venous return curve (see figure in question 6).

19. How can cardiac output be improved?

Cardiac output can be improved by reducing preload, increasing contractility, or decreasing afterload. Preload is reduced as mentioned in question 18. Contractility is increased with positive inotropic drugs, which shift the cardiac output curve upward and leftward (see figure in question 16). Positive inotropic drugs are especially indicated with evidence of systolic dysfunction. Arterial and mixed vasodilator drugs reduce afterload and result in an upward shift of the cardiac output curve.

20. How does one normalize heart rate and rhythm?

One should make every effort to identify the cause of dysrhythmia and treat the cause. Treating the dysrhythmia does not alleviate the cause. Slowing tachyarrhythmias with digitalis or antiarrhythmics may be required in some cases. In addition, third-degree atrioventricular (AV), severe second-degree AV, and sick sinus rhythms may require implantation of a pacemaker.

21. Describe the clinical classification of patients with heart failure.

Of the many schemes to describe the degree of heart failure in animals, the one that has withstood the test of time and experience is the clinical classification of the New York Heart Association, which is taken from human medicine but helps the clinician to decide the severity and therapeutic needs of animals in heart failure. Of interest, most new heart failure schemes relate to the New York Heart Association scheme. The classification is as follows:

Class I: No obvious exercise limitations.

Class II: Slight exercise limitation or coughing with routine physical activity.

Class III: Comfortable at rest but clinical signs develop during minimal physical activity.

Class IV: Clinical signs of heart failure are evident at rest and any exercise is severely limited.

22. How can one slow progression of heart failure?

Neurohumeral responses to CHF drive the progression of failure. To slow progression, one must minimize neurohumeral responses. Little clinical evidence is currently available in animals, but angiotensin-converting-enzyme (ACE) inhibitors and beta antagonists, as well as digoxin, improve survival in humans.

BIBLIOGRAPHY

1. Atkins CE: Cardiovascular disease seminar. Proceedings of the 55th Annual Conference of Veterinarians, Colorado State Univ., January 8–11, 1994, pp 185–213.
2. Francis GS: Neuroendocrine manifestations of congestive heart failure. Am J Cardiol 62:9A–13A, 1991.
3. Gheorghiade M, Ferguson D: Digoxin: A neurohumeral modulator in heart failure? Circulation 84:2181–2186, 1991.
4. Kittleson MD: Myocardial function in small animals with chronic mitral regurgitation and severe congestive heart failure. J Am Vet Med Assoc 184:455–459, 1984.
5. Mancini DM, LeJemtel TH, Factor S, et al: Central and peripheral components of cardiac failure. Am J Med 80:2–13, 1986.
6. Massie BM, Swedberg K, Cohn JN: Is neurohormonal activation deleterious to the long-term outcome of patients with congestive heart failure? J Am Coll Cardiol 12:547–558, 1988.
7. Moe GW, Grima EA, Angus C, et al: Response of atrial naturetic factor to acute and chronic increases of atrial pressures in experimental heart failure in dogs. Circulation 83:1780–1787, 1991.
8. Packer M, Bristow MR, Cohn JN, et al: The effect of carvedilol on morbidity and mortality in patients with chronic heart failure. N Engl J Med 334:1349–1355; 1396–1397, 1996.
9. Wall RE: Congestive heart failure: Pathogenesis and treatment. Proceedings of the 10th ACVIM Forum, San Diego, May, 1992, pp 19–24.

10. Ware WA, Lund DD, Subieta AR, et al: Sympathetic activation in dogs with congestive heart failure caused by chronic mitral valve disease and dilated cardiomyopathy. J Am Vet Med Assoc 197: 1475–1481, 1990.
11. Zells R: Sympathetic nervous system, angiotensin and other hormones in CHF. Proceedings of the 10th ACVIM Forum, San Diego, May, 1992, pp 586–588.

5. SHOCK

Ronald S. Walton, D.V.M.

1. Define shock in small animals.

Shock is a critical imbalance between the delivery of oxygen and nutrients to the cell and utilization of oxygen and nutrients by the cell. Shock may be any syndrome, disease state, or injury that results in a critical decrease in effective blood flow. Lack of effective blood flow leads to derangement in cellular metabolism and ultimately cell death. When left unchecked, shock leads to multiple organ dysfunction and failure, culminating with death.

2. What are the immediate concerns for a patient in shock?

The three most important concepts in dealing with shock are summarized in the acronym **VIP**:
V = **V**entilation to ensure a patent airway and maximize oxygenation and oxygen carrying capacity of the blood.
I = **I**nfusion of fluids to restore vascular volume.
P = Maintenance of myocardial **p**umping function to restore cardiac output and blood flow.

3. Name the four pathophysiologic classifications of shock.

(1) Hypovolemic, (2) cardiogenic, (3) distributive, and (4) obstructive.

4. Give an example of each of the four classifications of shock.

Blood volume, vascular resistance, vascular capacitance, and pump function determine the pattern of blood flow. Each of the four pathophysiologic classifications can be related to one or more of these determinants.

Hypovolemic shock is the most common form of shock in small animals. A typical patient has volume loss due to hemorrhage, severe volume loss due to third spacing of fluids, or volume loss due to diuresis, as in severe diabetic ketoacidosis.

Cardiogenic shock is a form of shock seen in heart failure characterized by pump failure and high central venous pressures. Pump failure may be related to cardiomyopathy, arrhythmias, and valvular abnormalities.

Distributive shock is a form of vasogenic shock seen with sepsis, anaphylaxis, trauma, neurogenic causes, and adverse pharmacologic reactions.

Obstructive shock in many classification schemes is grouped with cardiogenic causes; however, obstructive shock involves obstruction of flow, not necessarily pump dysfunction. Severe heartworm disease, pericardial tamponade, intracardiac tumors, and pulmonary or aortic thromboembolism are classified as obstructive shock.

5. During the course of the physical examination, how do you determine the classification of shock?

A patient with hypovolemic, cardiogenic, or obstructive shock typically has cool extremities, pallor of the mucous membranes, hypotension, and tachycardia. A patient with distributive shock also may present in this manner during the late stages. Typically, a patient with distributive shock has warm extremities, hyperemic mucous membranes, normotension to hypertension, and tachycardia.

6. What is central venous pressure? How is it measured?

Central venous pressure (CVP) is the measure of the luminal blood pressure in the intrathoracic jugular vein as it enters the right atrium. The CVP represents a measure of the relative ability of the heart to pump the venous return. Measurement of CVP can be expressed in centimeters of water (cm H_2O) or millimeters of mercury (mmHg). Typically CVP is measured with a water column manometer in veterinary patients. An imaginary line is drawn from the estimated region of the right atrium and the manometer to serve as the zero reference mark. The difference between the meniscus of the water column and the zero point is the measured CVP (cm H_2O). However, a standard mechanical pressure transducer can be applied to the central venous catheter to measure the CVP directly (mmHg). Most published values in dogs and cats are expressed as cm of H_2O. To convert mmHg to cm H_2O, multiply the value by 1.36. *Note:* In cats, caudal vena caval pressures can serve as an accurate indicator of CVP when a jugular catheter cannot be placed.

7. What is normal CVP in dogs and cats?

The normal CVP for dogs and cats ranges from 0–10 cm H_2O. Values < 0 cm H_2O indicate relative hypovolemia and values > 10 cm H_2O indicate relative hypervolemia.

8. What are the four determinants of CVP?

Intrathoracic pressure, intravascular volume, right ventricular function, and venous tone.

9. What are the body's initial hemodynamic responses to volume loss?

The loss of effective circulating volume leads to a decrease in cardiac output. Reflex tachycardia ensues in an attempt to maintain blood pressure. In response to decreasing cardiac output, baroreceptor-mediated initiation of the sympathoadrenal reflex occurs. This reflex initiates the release of norepinephrine, epinephrine, and cortisol from the adrenal gland, leading to increased cardiac output. Increased contractility, heart rate, and venous tone are responsible for the initial increase in cardiac output. Arteriolar vasoconstriction in the skin, muscle, kidney, and gastrointestinal tract allows blood to be shunted centrally to the heart and brain. Decreased renal blood flow secondary to activation of the renin-angiotensin-aldosterone system reduces urinary output and fluid loss and increases retention of sodium and water. The release of antidiuretic hormone and aldosterone also promotes volume conservation. Cortisol and catecholamines promote release, mobilization, and conversion of energy substrates to help meet metabolic demands. The diagram below illustrates these initial steps.

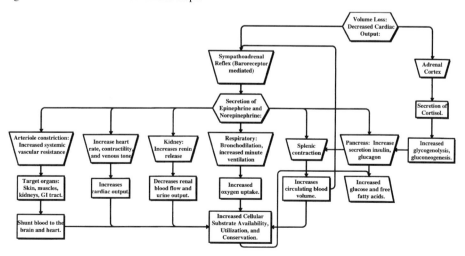

Compensatory responses to volume loss.

10. Define sepsis.

Sepsis is usually defined as the systemic response to generalized infection. Others have defined sepsis as the body's response to the presence of pathogenic organisms or their toxins in blood. Typically sepsis is due to a gram-negative bacterial infection or toxin but may be caused by gram-positive bacterial, fungal, viral, or parasitic infections.

11. Define systemic inflammatory response syndrome (SIRS).

The systemic inflammatory response is a generalized inflammatory response to a variety of severe systemic insults. Current defining criteria for SIRS include two or more of the following criteria:

1. Temperature > 103.5°F or < 100.0°F
2. Heart rate > 160 bpm (dog) or > 250 bpm (cat)
3. Respiratory rate > 20 bpm or $PaCO_2$ < 32 mmHg
4. White blood cell count > 12,000 or < 4,000 cells or > 10% nucleated cells band neutrophils.

12. When should you suspect septicemia or septic shock?

When patients present with tachycardia, hypotension, hypovolemia, fever or hypothermia, high or low white blood cell count, and signs of multiple organ involvement.

13. What is septic shock?

Septic shock is a form of vasogenic shock secondary to sepsis. The characteristic findings are hypotension and perfusion abnormalities that persist despite adequate fluid therapy.

14. What are the classic changes in systemic vascular resistance (SVR) and cardiac output in early septic shock?

In the early presentation of septic shock (hyperdynamic phase) SVR is decreased and cardiac output is increased. The increase in cardiac output is a compensatory response to the falling SVR.

15. What is cardiogenic shock?

Cardiogenic shock is secondary to pump failure. The key features of cardiogenic shock are systemic hypotension, elevated heart rate, increased central venous pressure, increased oxygen extraction, and decreased cardiac output. The pump failure may be related to valvular and/or myocardial incompetence. In some classifications obstructive forms of shock, such as heartworm disease, pericardial tamponade, and pulmonary thromboembolism, are also classified as cardiogenic shock because of a general failure of forward blood flow.

16. How can septic shock and cardiogenic shock appear similar?

In the hypodynamic (late) phases of septic shock, cardiac output is depressed by a decreased cardiac index and increased pulmonary capillary resistance. Combined, these factors can markedly decrease cardiac output and increase CVP, appearing quite similar to right heart failure. Patients typically have cool extremities due to decreased perfusion and tachycardia. The prognosis for late-stage (hypodynamic) septic shock is poor.

17. What are the primary goals of treatment for septic shock?

The primary goals are to maximize tissue oxygen delivery because of the increased oxygen demand. You must improve the hemodynamic status and correct the underlying metabolic abnormalities. Then you must aggressively seek and eliminate the source of infection.

18. What are the primary goals of treating hemorrhagic shock?

Stop continued loss, restore volume, and restore oxygen-carrying capacity.

19. What is neurogenic shock?

Neurogenic shock results from acute loss of sympathetic vascular tone, which leads to arteriolar and venous dilatation. Neurogenic shock may result from spinal cord injury and even excessive administration of general anesthetics. This form of vasogenic or distributive shock may be refractory to standard fluid therapy. An α-agonist may be needed to treat refractory hypotension.

20. What type of shock is pericardial tamponade?

Obstructive, pericardial tamponade physically compresses the heart within the pericardial sac. This compression limits the amount of blood that can enter the heart during diastole and subsequently limits the stroke volume, leading to a decrease in cardiac output.

21. What clinical signs suggest pericardial tamponade? How do you confirm the diagnosis?

No single sign is pathognomonic for pericardial tamponade. The typical patient with cardiac tamponade presents with a history of acute collapse. Abnormal physical parameters include increased central venous pressure, tachycardia, jugular pulsation, peripheral vascular distention, and muffled heart sounds. Electrocardiographic findings of a decreased amplitude QRS complex and electrical alternans are supportive. Echocardiography is considered the gold standard for diagnosis of pericardial effusion and tamponade.

22. What is the emergency treatment for pericardial tamponade?

Pericardiocentesis. The patient can be positioned in left lateral or sternal recumbency. Pericardiocentesis is typically performed at the right fifth intercostal space, approximately at the midpoint of the thoracic wall, with a long over-the-needle catheter. Often removal of a small amount of fluid is adequate to relieve the signs of tamponade. The act of penetrating the pericardial sac creates a small hole that will continue to drain after the needle catheter is removed into the pleural space.

23. What is the fluid of choice for treating patients in shock?

Fluid administration is the cornerstone of effective therapy for patients with noncardiogenic shock. Although the exact fluid may be controversial, depending on the author, the basic principle is the same. Crystalloids (containing sodium) are the preferred initial fluid of choice. The crystalloid fluids are easy to administer, readily available, inexpensive, and effective. Shock initially should be treated aggressively with fluid containing an adequate amount of sodium because of the relatively high concentration of sodium in extracellular fluid. Isotonic solutions readily available and commonly used are 0.9% sodium chloride, lactated Ringer's solution, Plasmalyte, and Normosol-R.

24. Why is Plasmalyte or Normosol-R preferred over lactated Ringer's for patients in shock?

Lactated Ringer's solution uses lactate as its primary buffer, which depends on active hepatic metabolism for conversion to bicarbonate. In the shock patient hepatic metabolism is markedly impaired. Normosol-R and Plasmalyte contain acetate and gluconate as their primary buffers. Acetate and gluconate are metabolized primarily by the skeletal muscle to bicarbonate. While blood cell flow is decreased to skeletal muscle in shock, acetate and gluconate can be converted to bicarbonate easily as circulation is restored. As the circulatory system and peripheral perfusion are reestablished, the liver is presented with an excess of lactate to metabolize (lactic acidosis) and may not be able to metabolize the excessive lactate adequately.

25. What is hypertonic saline? When is it used?

Hypertonic saline is a crystalloid fluid with a supraphysiologic amount of sodium. The typical sodium concentration is 3–7%. A dose of 4–5 ml/kg of 7% hypertonic saline has been shown to be an effective acute volume expander in dogs. It acts by drawing water from the intracellular and interstitial spaces into the vascular compartment. These changes cause a rapid but transient increase in intravascular volume. When combined with a synthetic colloid such as dextran 70, the volume-expanding effects can be prolonged. The contraindications for hypertonic saline are hypernatremia, hyperosmolality, cardiogenic shock, and renal failure. Hypertonic saline is used only for the rapid emergency restoration of volume and *must* be followed with definitive treatment, because the effects of hypertonic saline are only temporary.

26. What volume of crystalloid fluid is used to resuscitate a shock patient?

The volumes for cats and dogs are different in the published literature. In dogs, shock volumes of fluid are reported at 50–90 ml/kg/hr or up to complete blood volume per hour. In cats, volumes are reported at 40–60 ml/kg/hr or approximately complete plasma volume per hour. The difference between cat and dog resuscitation volume is unclear in the literature. Typically these volumes should be regarded as indicators to be prepared to deliver volume in an hour, but treatment should be titrated to the volume needed by the individual patient. A highly effective method is to deliver shock fluid volumes in one-fourth shock volume increments. One-fourth of the calculated shock volume is delivered every 15 minutes with monitoring of the deviation from the baseline packed cell volume and total protein. Few patients require 90 ml/kg/hr using this method, and volume overload is unlikely.

27. What is a standard volume of infusion for a synthetic colloid solution in patients in shock?

The standard volume of colloid, whether synthetic or natural, is generally 10–20 ml/kg/day. This volume is typically given over 4–6 hours but may be given faster if needed. Often the infusion of a synthetic colloid in the fluid therapy program allows a reduction in the crystalloid fluid requirement by 40–60%.

BIBLIOGRAPHY

1. Astiz ME, Rackow EC, Weil MH: Pathophysiology and treatment of circulatory shock. Crit Care Clin 9:183–203, 1993.
2. Crystal MA, Cotter SM: Acute hemorrhage: A hematologic emergency in dogs. Compend Cont Educ Pract Vet 14: 1992.
3. Falk JL, Rackow EC, Astiz M, et al: Fluid resuscitation in shock. J Cardiothoracic Anesth 2:33–38, 1988.
4. Ford SL, Schaer M: Shock syndrome in cats. Compend Cont Educ Pract Vet 15:120–125, 1993.
5. Kirby R: Septic shock. In Kirk RW (ed): Current Veterinary Therapy, vol XII. Philadelphia, W.B. Saunders, 1995, pp 139–146.
6. Muir WW: Overview of Shock. 14th Annual Kal Kan Waltham Symposium, 7–13, 1990.
7. Rackow EC, Astiz ME: Mechanisms and management of septic shock. Crit Care Clin 9:219–237, 1993.
8. Schertel ER, Muir WW: Shock: Pathophysiology, monitoring, and therapy. In Kirk RW (ed): Current Veterinary Therapy, vol X. Philadelphia, W.B. Saunders, 1989, pp 316–330.
9. Ware WA: Shock. In Murtaugh RJ, Kaplan PM (eds): Veterinary Emergency and Critical Care Medicine. Chicago, Mosby-Year Book, 1992, pp 163–175.

6. ACUTE GASTRIC DILATATION-VOLVULUS

Wayne E. Wingfield, D.V.M., M.S.

1. What characterizes the dog with acute gastric dilatation-volvulus (GDV)?

The dog with acute GDV is characterized by varying degrees of malposition of the stomach, rapid accumulation of gas within the stomach, increased intragastric pressure, shock, and often death.

2. Is "bloat" the same thing as GDV?

Dog owners frequently refer to GDV as "bloat." The name may be slightly misleading to veterinarians, most of whom consider bloat a problem of ruminants with a frothy, fermentation etiology. Frothy bloat is not seen in dogs or cats.

3. Which animals are more prone to GDV?

Large and giant breed dogs, especially purebreds, seem to be at higher risk for GDV. The frequency of GDV appears to range from 2.9–6.8 per 1000 dogs. The most common breeds with

GDV include the Great Dane, weimaraner, Saint Bernard, Gordon setter, Irish setter, and standard poodle. Domestic cats and nonhuman primates are also reported to develop GDV.

4. Describe what is known about risk factors for GDV in dogs.

Increasing adult weight of the breed, based on breed standards, is a significant risk factor; that is, body weight (e.g., obesity) is less important than breed weight as a risk factor for GDV. The pattern of risk suggests that body conformation, particularly a narrow and deep thoracic cavity, also influences the risk of GDV for specific breeds.

5. How is diet related to the cause of GDV?

To date, there is no conclusive evidence that diet causes GDV. No specific diets or feeding practices have been shown to increase the occurrence of GDV in dogs.

6. What is the cause of GDV?

The cause is unknown. Researchers have implicated locally active peptides such as gastrin, gastric myoelectric dysfunction, and abnormal esophageal sphincter function. It is certainly not a gastric bacterial disease (e.g., *Clostridium perfringens*) that leads to rapid accumulation of gas.

7. What is the composition of the gas in the stomach of a dog with GDV?

Air collected from the stomach of dogs with GDV is most consistent with room air. The gas is apparently accumulated through aerophagia.

8. Describe the physical examination findings which most likely point to the diagnosis of GDV.
- Cranial abdominal distention with tympany.
- Retching with inability to vomit.
- Inability to pass an orogastric (stomach) tube. This criterion is often misinterpreted. Inability to pass a stomach tube suggests a diagnosis of GDV, but if the tube is passed and gas is relieved, this does not rule out GDV. One should consider passing of the orogastric tube more of a therapeutic than a diagnostic procedure.

9. How should you initiate treatment for GDV?

There are two important initial treatments for GDV:
- Decompress the stomach.
- Begin treatment for shock (see chapter 5).

10. Describe how you pass the stomach tube in dogs with GDV.

Do not stress the dog unnecessarily. Use a moderately large, flexible tube (e.g., foal stomach tube). Measure the distance from the tip of the nose to the last rib, and place a piece of tape on the tube to indicate how far to pass the tube. Place the dog in a sternal position, insert a mouth gag (e.g., a full roll of 2-inch tape), lubricate the tube, and slowly and gently pass the tube. You will see the dog swallow the tube, and as the tube is advanced, you can palpate the trachea and the tube as it extends down the esophagus. At the gastroesophageal junction, resistance may be encountered. *Do not force the tube into the stomach.* Try twisting the tube as you advance it through the junction. If you apply too much force, you may rupture either the esophagus or the stomach. Once the tube is in the stomach, place one end of the tube into a bucket of warm tap water, and gas will be seen escaping. Have an assistant gently press on the cranial abdomen and evacuate as much gas as possible. Attach a stomach pump to the tube, and lavage the stomach until all contents are removed and the effluent is clear. As you prepare to remove the tube, kink the tube. Slowly remove the tube and then the mouth gag.

11. What should you do if you cannot pass the orogastric tube?

Gastric decompression is a mandatory part of GDV treatment. The simplest means to decompress is to trocarize the stomach. Percuss the cranial abdomen until you detect a resonant area, which is generally located on the right lateral abdominal wall. Clip the hair from the area, apply a quick surgical preparation of the skin, and insert a 14–16 gauge, 1- or 1.5-inch needle. Gas should evacuate through the trocar. Most commonly you will now be able to pass the orogastric tube and thoroughly evacuate and then lavage the stomach.

12. Which gastropexy technique should be used at the time of surgery?

Numerous gastropexy techniques are described in the veterinary literature, but the two most favored techniques at this time are the circumcostal and belt-loop gastropexy. Both have relatively low recurrence rates (< 6.9%). Use of the tube gastrostomy is reported to have a higher morbidity rate associated with premature tube removal, development of cellulitis around the tube, and alteration of gastric myoelectric activity. The most critical factors in the success rate are probably the surgeon's familiarity with the technique and the ability to perform it proficiently with minimal anesthesia time.

13. Should pyloric surgery be performed to prevent recurrence and to accelerate gastric emptying?

No. Studies in normal dogs have shown that neither pyloroplasty nor pyloromyotomy significantly alters gastric emptying; in fact, both may delay emptying. In addition, there is no evidence, to date, that delayed gastric emptying or pyloric lesions are factors in the disease. These findings strongly suggest that pyloric surgery in GDV is contraindicated, unless gastric outflow obstruction can be demonstrated.

14. What should you do when you find evidence of gastric ischemia or necrosis?

Gastrectomy of nonvital tissue must be performed. The area most frequently involved is on the greater curvature where the short gastric arteries attach to the spleen. The experience of most surgeons suggests that when a gastrectomy is required, the mortality rate is increased, probably because of prolonged shock, anesthesia time, and delay in seeking professional assistance by the dog owner.

15. Will splenectomy prevent recurrence of GDV in dogs?

No. Removal of the spleen does not prevent recurrence of GDV. At the time of surgery, partial or total splenectomy may be indicated in dogs with evidence of splenic infarcts.

16. What are the most common postoperative complications in dogs with GDV?

- Shock
- Pain management
- Surgical complications
- Cardiac dysrhythmias
- Hypokalemia

17. What are the most common cardiac dysrhythmias after GDV surgery?

Premature ventricular contractions and ventricular tachycardia are the most common dysrhythmias. They are often difficult to control unless shock is first resolved. In most cases, lidocaine and procainamide are used to control these dysrhythmias. Occasionally a dog may go into atrial fibrillation postoperatively. In this case, there may be an underlying etiology (e.g., dilated cardiomyopathy). Atrial fibrillation sometimes converts to a sinus rhythm when shock is resolved or through administration of calcium channel blockers, adenosine, or, rarely, quinidine.

18. Outline precautions that the owner should take to reduce future risk of bloat.

- Feed several smaller meals each day rather than one large meal.
- Minimize exercise and excitement before and after feeding.
- Know how to identify the clinical signs of bloat, and have an emergency number for a veterinarian immediately available.
- Owners of high-risk dogs should be encouraged to discuss the pros and cons of prophylactic gastropexy.

CONTROVERSY

19. Should you radiograph the dog's abdomen before proceeding to surgery?

For: Radiography confirms the diagnosis and possibly suggests other complications that may be encountered in surgery. Gastrocentesis may lead to accumulation of free air within the abdomen and should not be regarded as a ruptured stomach.

Against: Radiography is expensive, time-consuming, and stressful to the dog with GDV. Given certain breed characteristics, risk factors, and positive findings on physical examination, the dog should be taken to surgery.

BIBLIOGRAPHY

1. Glickman LT, Glickman NW, Perez CM, et al: Analysis of risk factors for gastric dilatation-volvulus in dogs. J Am Vet Assoc 204:1465–1471, 1994.
2. Greenfield CI, Walshaw R, Thomas MW: Significance of the Heineke-Mikulicz pyloroplasty in the treatment of gastric dilatation-volvulus: A prospective clinical study. Vet Surg 18:22–26, 1989.
3. Hall JA, Twedt DC, Curtis CR: Relationship of plasma gastrin immunoreactivity and gastroesophageal sphincter pressure in normal dogs and dogs with previous gastric dilatation-volvulus. Am J Vet Res 50:1228–1232, 1989.
4. Hosgood G: Gastric dilatation-volvulus in dogs. J Am Vet Assoc 204:1742–1747, 1994.
5. Leib MS, Wingfield WE, Twedt DC, et al: Plasma gastrin immunoreactivity in dogs with gastric dilatation-volvulus. J Am Vet Assoc 185:205–208, 1984.
6. Leib MS, Konde LJ, Wingfield WE, et al: Circumcostal gastropexy for preventing recurrence of gastric dilatation-volvulus in the dog: An evaluation of 30 cases. J Am Vet Assoc 187:245–248, 1985.
7. van Sluijs FJ, van den Brom WE: Gastric emptying of a radionucleotide-labeled test meal after surgical correction of gastric dilatation-volvulus in dogs. Am J Vet Res 50:433–435, 1989.
8. van Sluijs FJ: Gastric dilatation-volvulus in the dog: Current views and a retrospective study in 160 patients. Tijdscher Diergereeskd 116:112–120, 1991.
9. Whitney WO, Scavelli TD, Matthiesen DT, et al: Belt-loop gastropexy technique and surgical results in 20 dogs. J Am Anim Hosp Assoc 25:75–83, 1989.

7. ANAPHYLAXIS

Michael S. Lagutchik, D.V.M.

1. Define systemic anaphylaxis.

Systemic anaphylaxis is an acute, life-threatening reaction resulting from generation and release of endogenous chemical mediators and the effects of these mediators on various organ systems (primarily the cardiovascular and pulmonary systems).

2. What are the various forms of anaphylaxis? Which is most important in the emergent patient?

Anaphylaxis may occur systemically or locally. The term *anaphylaxis* is commonly used to describe three separate clinical entities: systemic anaphylaxis, urticaria, and angioedema. Systemic anaphylaxis results from generalized massive release of mast cell mediators and is the most severe form. Urticaria and angioedema are localized variants of immediate hypersensitivity. Urticaria is characterized by wheal or "hive" formation involving superficial dermal blood vessels with varying degrees of pruritus. Angioedema involves deeper vessels in the skin with edema formation in the deeper layers of the skin and subcutaneous tissues. Although not common, urticaria and angioedema may progress to systemic anaphylaxis.

3. What basic mechanisms lead to anaphylaxis?

Two general mechanisms result in mast cell and basophil activation and hence anaphylaxis. Anaphylaxis is most commonly immune-mediated. Less frequently, nonimmune interactions induce anaphylaxis. The latter syndrome is termed *anaphylactoid reaction*. Essentially, there is no difference in patient management, but recognizing the difference allows more complete understanding of potential causes and aids in more rapid recognition of the condition.

4. What is the pathophysiologic mechanism of immune-mediated (classic) anaphylaxis?

On first exposure to an antigen in susceptible individuals, immunoglobulin E (IgE) is produced and binds to surface receptors of effector cells (mast cells, basophils). On second exposure to the antigen, the subsequent antigen–antibody complex triggers calcium influx into the effector cell with initiation of an intracellular cascade of events that ultimately results in degranulation of preformed chemical mediators and generation of newly formed mediators. These mediators are responsible for the pathophysiologic events in anaphylaxis.

5. What is the pathophysiologic mechanism of nonimmune-mediated anaphylaxis?

Anaphylactoid reactions are caused by two separate mechanisms. The more common is direct activation of mast cells and basophils by drugs and other chemicals (i.e., idiosyncratic pharmacologic or drug reactions). Further effects are similar to the classic anaphylaxis described above. Prior exposure is not required for this form of anaphylaxis. Less commonly, activation of the complement cascade results in the generation of anaphylatoxins (C3a, C5a). These anaphylatoxins cause degranulation of mast cells with release of histamine, enhance smooth muscle contraction, and aid in release of hydrolytic enzymes from polymorphonuclear leukocytes.

6. Describe the mediators responsible for the pathophysiologic events in anaphylaxis.

The mediators of anaphylaxis are (1) primary (preformed) and (2) secondary. Primary mediators include histamine (vasodilatation; increased vascular permeability; and bronchial, gastrointestinal, and coronary artery smooth muscle constriction); heparin (anticoagulation; possibly bronchospasm, urticaria, fever, and anticomplement activity); eosinophil and neutrophil chemotactic factors (chemotactic for eosinophils and neutrophils); proteolytic enzymes (generation of kinins, initiation of disseminated intravascular coagulation; activation of complement cascade); serotonin (vasoactive events); and adenosine (bronchospasm, regulation of mast cell degranulation).

Secondary mediators are generated by eosinophils and neutrophils and other mechanisms after activation by primary mediators. The major secondary mediators are metabolites of arachidonic acid (prostaglandins and leukotrienes) and platelet-activating factor. These mediators include prostaglandins E_2, D_2, and I_2 (prostacyclin); leukotrienes B_4, C_4, D_4, and E_4; thromboxane A_2, and platelet-activating factor. The majority of these mediators induce vasodilatation; increase vascular permeability; potentiate generation of histamine, bradykinin, leukotrienes, and chemotactic factors; cause bronchoconstriction; promote platelet aggregation; stimulate chemotaxis of eosinophils and neutrophils; induce cardiodepression; increase airway mucus production; induce platelet release; and increase release of granules from polymorphonuclear cells. Some (prostaglandin D_2, prostaglandin I_2, and products of eosinophils) function to limit the hypersensitivity response.

7. Describe common causes of anaphylaxis in dogs and cats.

Immune-mediated anaphylaxis

Bites of venomous insects and reptiles (bees, spiders, snakes)

Vaccines

Hormones (insulin, vasopressin, corticotropin, betamethasone, triamcinolone)

Antibiotics (penicillin derivatives, chloramphenicol, gentamicin, tetracycline, trimethoprim-sulfonamide combinations, cephalosporins, many others)

Anesthetic agents (acepromazine, ketamine, barbiturates, lidocaine, opiate narcotics, diazepam)

Parasiticides (piperazine, diethylcarbamazine, thiacetarsamide, ivermectin)

Other commonly used drugs (aminophylline, L-asparaginase, dextrans, allergen extracts, amphotericin B)
   Blood and blood components
   Anaphylactoid reactions
   Iodinated radiocontrast agents
   Nonsteroidal antiinflammatory drugs (aspirin, ibuprofen)
   Opiate narcotics
   Mannitol
   Dextrans

8. What are the target organs of an anaphylactic response in both cats and dogs?

Major target organs depend on the type of anaphylaxis. Local anaphylaxis (urticaria and angioedema) generally elicits cutaneous and gastrointestinal responses. The most common cutaneous signs are pruritus, edema, erythema, and the typical wheal and flare reaction. The most common GI signs are nausea, vomiting, tenesmus, and diarrhea. The major target organs in systemic anaphylaxis are the liver in dogs and the respiratory and gastrointestinal tracts in cats.

9. How do I recognize clinical systemic anaphylaxis in dogs and cats?

The clinical manifestations of systemic anaphylaxis differ significantly in dogs and cats.

In **dogs**, the earliest signs of anaphylaxis are often initial excitement, with vomiting, defecation, and urination frequently reported. As anaphylaxis progresses, respiratory depression or distress and collapse related to muscle weakness and cardiovascular collapse develop. Death may occur rapidly (i.e., within 1 hour). As the liver is the major target organ in dogs, severe hepatic congestion with portal hypertension is a common finding on necropsy. There is seldom time to evaluate the liver appropriately before death for these findings to be helpful.

In **cats**, the earliest reported sign of anaphylaxis is severe pruritus, especially of the face and head. As bronchoconstriction and pulmonary edema are the typical sequelae in cats, severe respiratory distress is the most common sign. Other signs include laryngeal edema and upper airway obstruction, profuse salivation, vomiting and incoordination. Ultimately, severe respiratory and cardiac involvement leads to collapse and death.

10. What is anaphylactic shock?

Anaphylactic shock is the terminal phase of anaphylaxis, due to a combination of vaculogenic, neurogenic, and endotoxic changes involving multiple organ systems, especially the cardiovascular and pulmonary systems. Primary and secondary mediators induce microcirculatory vascular changes that lead to peripheral pooling of 60–80% of the blood volume. Also critical in anaphylaxis is increased vascular permeability with leakage of intravascular volume. These mediators also cause hypovolemia, dysrhythmias, depressed myocardial contractility, and pulmonary hypotension, which eventually lead to tissue hypoxia, metabolic acidosis, and cell death. Clinical signs of anaphylactic shock are not pathognomonic; they resemble signs from any cause of severe cardiopulmonary collapse.

11. How soon does anaphylaxis develop?

Anaphylaxis usually occurs almost immediately after or within a few minutes of exposure to the inducing agent. However, it may be delayed for several hours. In people, anaphylaxis is reported to reach peak severity in 5–30 minutes.

12. How do you diagnose systemic anaphylaxis?

Diagnosis is based on history, physical exam, and clinical signs. Maintaining a high index of suspicion is essential for rapid identification and initiation of treatment. The key point in diagnosis of systemic anaphylaxis is rapid progression of clinical signs related to the target organ system in each species, usually with a history of recent exposure to a known inducer of anaphylaxis.

13. If immediate recognition and treatment are the hallmarks of successful management of anaphylaxis, what other differential diagnoses must be ruled out quickly?

Conditions that must be ruled out rapidly in patients presenting with severe signs consistent with systemic anaphylaxis include acute pulmonary events (asthma attack, pulmonary edema, pulmonary embolus, spontaneous pneumothorax, foreign body aspiration, and laryngeal paralysis), and acute cardiac events (supraventricular and ventricular tachyarrhythmias, septic and cardiogenic shock).

14. What is the initial treatment for systemic anaphylaxis?

The immediate therapy for anaphylaxis includes establishment of a patent airway and vascular access, aggressive fluid therapy, and administration of epinephrine. Depending on severity, airway management ranges from providing supplemental oxygen by face mask to orotracheal intubation; tracheostomy may be necessary. Mechanical ventilation may be required in severely affected patients with compromised (edematous) airways, pulmonary edema, and bronchoconstriction. Vascular access, preferably central venous, is critical for administration of fluid therapy and drugs. Aggressive fluid therapy should be predicated on the extent of shock, but the clinician should be prepared to administer shock doses of isotonic crystalloid solutions and possibly colloids. Epinephrine is the cornerstone of therapy for anaphylaxis, because it relieves bronchoconstriction, supports arterial blood pressure, inhibits further mast cell degranulation, improves cardiac contractility and heart rate, and improves coronary artery blood flow. The recommended dose is 0.01–0.02 mg/kg given intravenously. This is equivalent to 0.01–0.02 ml/kg of 1:1,000 epinephrine hydrochloride. If vascular access is not available, this dose can be doubled and given intratracheally. In severe cases with refractory hypotension and bronchoconstriction, the dose can be repeated every 5–10 minutes, or a constant-rate infusion can be established at a rate of 1–4 µg/kg/min.

15. What are adjunct therapies for management of systemic anaphylaxis?

Adjunctive therapy for anaphylaxis includes use of antihistamines, glucocorticoids, and additional supportive measures, as needed, for hypotension, pulmonary edema, bronchoconstriction, and arrhythmias. Although antihistamines and glucocorticoids are too slow to be helpful in the initial management, they play an important role in preventing late-phase reactions and complications caused by secondary mediators. Diphenhydramine (5–50 mg/kg slowly IV 2 times/day) is the most commonly used antihistamine. Some authors recommend concurrent use of H_2 antagonists (e.g., cimetidine, 5–10 mg/kg orally every 8 hr). Dexamethasone sodium phosphate (1–4 mg/kg IV) and prednisolone sodium succinate (10–25 mg/kg IV) are the most commonly used glucocorticoids. Dopamine (2–10 µg/kg/min) is often needed for cardiac or pressor support. Aminophylline (5–10 mg/kg IM or slowly IV) is recommended in patients with persistent bronchoconstriction.

16. If the initial treatment for systemic anaphylaxis is successful, is the patient "out of the woods"?

By no means is it safe to send the patient home. Late-phase reactions are common in patients recovering from the immediate effects of systemic anaphylaxis. These effects, mediated by late-developing events induced by secondary mediators, may occur 6–12 hours after the initial attack. Meticulous attention to patient monitoring, aggressive treatment for shock and pulmonary complications, and use of antihistamines and glucocorticoids are usually recommended to prevent this potentially fatal complication. It is advised to hospitalize the patient for at least 24 hours and monitor aggressively for signs of impending complications.

BIBLIOGRAPHY

1. Cohen RD: Systemic anaphylaxis. In Bonagura JD (ed): Current Veterinary Therapy, vol XII. Philadelphia, W.B. Saunders, 1995, pp 150–152.
2. Haupt MT: Anaphylaxis and anaphylactic shock. In Parrillo JE, Bone RC (eds): Critical Care Medicine: Principles of Diagnosis and Management. St. Louis, Mosby, 1995, pp 433–447.

3. Markovchick V: Anaphylaxis. In Parsons PE, Wiener-Kronish JP (eds): Critical Care Secrets. Philadelphia, Hanley & Belfus, 1992, pp 407–409.
4. Mueller DL, Noxon JO: Anaphylaxis: Pathophysiology and treatment. Comp Cont Educ Pract Vet 12:157–170, 1990.
5. Noxon JO: Anaphylaxis, urticaria, and angioedema. Semin Vet Med Surg (Sm Anim) 6:265–272, 1991.
6. Ware WA: Shock. In Murtaugh RJ, Kaplan PM (eds): Veterinary Emergency and Critical Care Medicine. St. Louis, Mosby, 1992, pp 163–175.

8. HYPOTHERMIA

Ronald S. Walton, D.V.M.

1. Define hypothermia in small animals.
Hypothermia is defined as a subnormal body temperature in a homeothermic animal. The normal body temperature should be > 99.5°F (37.5°C) for dogs and 100.0°F (37.8°C) for cats.

2. How is the severity of hypothermia graded?
• Mild: 90–99°F (32.3–37.2°C)
• Moderate: 82–90°F (27.8–37.5°C)
• Severe: core temperature < 82°F (27.8°C).

3. Name the four primary mechanisms by which heat is lost from the body.
• Convection   • Radiation
• Conduction   • Evaporation

4. Of the four primary mechanisms for heat loss, which is most common in small animals?
Radiation accounts for the majority of heat loss under normal conditions. Radiation is the exchange of heat between objects in the environment that are not in direct contact with the skin. Relative temperature determines the direction of heat transfer.

5. How is body temperature maintained in normal dogs and cats?
Body temperature is regulated by the central nervous system, more specifically the hypothalamus. Decreasing body temperature causes behavioral and physiologic responses in dogs and cats. The common behavioral responses are heat-seeking and minimizing body surface area by curling up. Physiologic responses to decreasing body temperature start with piloerection and peripheral vasoconstriction. These responses attempt to conserve body heat by shifting blood flow centrally. Shivering thermogenesis and increased metabolic rate are the next efforts to increase temperature. When these methods fail, heat is lost and core body temperature falls.

6. How can thermoregulation be impaired?
The thermoregulatory system can be impaired by four primary mechanisms: metabolic, peripheral, local, and pharmacologic. Altered plasma osmolality combined with metabolic derangement such as diabetic ketoacidosis and uremia may lead to centrally mediated hypothermia. Hypothalamic function can be affected by various CNS processes (traumatic, degenerative, neoplastic, and congenital) and induce a hypothermic state. Pharmacologic agents (e.g., phenothiazines and barbiturates) can induce hypothermia by impairment of central thermoregulation.

7. Define core body temperature. How is it measured?
Core body temperature is a measure of central body temperature unaffected by the vasoconstrictor effect of peripheral vasculature. Core body temperature can be measured rectally,

esophageally, tympanically, or from a central intravenous catheter equipped with a thermistor. Rectal temperature may be falsely low if the thermometer is in cold feces.

8. What factors predispose an animal to hypothermia?

Factors that decrease heat production or increase heat loss predispose to hypothermia. Factors involved in decreased heat production include age (neonates), trauma, immobility, anesthesia, cardiac disease, impaired central thermoregulation, endocrine disorders (hypothyroidism, hypoadrenocorticism, hypoglycemia, and hypopituitarism), and neuromuscular disorders. Factors that predispose to increased heat loss are trauma, burn injury, immobility, environmental exposure, anesthesia, surgery, contact with cold surfaces, and exposure to chemical agents (e.g., barbiturates, alcohol, phenothiazines, ethylene glycol).

9. What clinical findings are commonly seen in hypothermic patients?

The hypothermic patient may present with various clinical signs, depending on the degree and length of exposure. Common clinical signs include obtundation, weak-to-absent pulse, slow or undetectable heart rate, muscle stiffness, and shallow and infrequent respiration. Bowel sounds may be decreased or absent. Shivering may be observed in mild cases but is absent at body temperatures < 31°C. Normal cerebral functions are impaired at < 32°C. Cardiac arrhythmias are seen at < 30°C. Peripheral reflexes are lost at < 27°C. At body temperatures < 26°C dogs have absent pupillary light reflexes and loss of consciousness.

10. What is the key decision in deciding how to rewarm a patient?

The primary decision is whether to rewarm the patient passively or actively. Passive rewarming is noninvasive and involves simply covering the patient in a warm environment. Active rewarming often requires specialized equipment or facilities. The flow chart below provides a guideline to rewarming options in small animals.

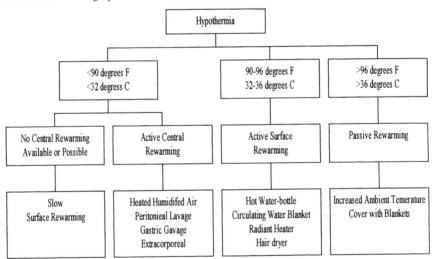

Management of hypothermia. (Adapted from Haskins SC: Thermoregulation, hypothermia, hyperthermia. In Ettinger SJ, Feldman EC (eds): Textbook of Small Animal Medicine. Philadelphia, W.B. Saunders, 1995, p 28.)

11. Discuss active rewarming and guidelines for its use.

Active rewarming delivers heat directly to the core of the body. The current options for active rewarming include extracorporeal rewarming, heated intravenous fluids, warm peritoneal lavage, and warm gastrointestinal irrigation. Active rewarming becomes necessary when cardiovascular instability is present or the core body temperature is below 92°F (33.3°C).

12. Discuss passive rewarming and guidelines for its use.

Passive rewarming is suitable for mild cases of hypothermia in a previously healthy patient. Passive rewarming consists simply of increasing the ambient temperature and covering the patient with a blanket.

13. What common clinical pathologic changes are associated with hypothermia?

- **Glucose**. Hyperglycemia is seen early because of increased cortisol release and increased sympathetic activity. When hypothermia persists, hyperglycemia is due to insulin resistance, which occurs at temperatures of < 30°C. Prolonged hypothermia results in hypoglycemia due to impaired gluconeogenesis, and hepatic glycogen depletion.
- **Electrolyte abnormalities**. Electrolyte changes are unpredictable and vary from patient to patient. Prolonged hypothermia tends to lead to hyponatremia and hyperkalemia, probably because of decreased function in the cell membrane sodium–potassium ATPase pump. If this is the case, total body levels of sodium and potassium are close to normal.
- **Acid–base status**. Decreased tissue perfusion and increased use of muscle tissue during shivering leads to accumulation of lactic acid and subsequent metabolic acidosis. Hepatic metabolism of lactate also is decreased. In mild cases of hypothermia, the patient may exhibit a mixed metabolic acidosis and respiratory alkalosis. If hypothermia persists, consciousness is depressed and results in reduction of respiratory rate, which may lead to development of respiratory acidosis.
- **Coagulation abnormalities**. The effects of hypothermia on blood coagulation are complex. Experimentally hypothermia has produced variable alterations in functional clotting factors in dogs. Hypothermia has been shown to prolong both activated partial thromboplastin time (APTT) and prothrombin time (PT) in humans. Hypothermia also causes reversible platelet dysfunction. Severe hypothermia may even lead to development of disseminated intravascular coagulation (DIC). DIC usually occurs secondary to rewarming with increased fibrinolytic activity, vascular endothelium damage, and decreased factor and platelet function.

14. What are the common electrocardiographic abnormalities associated with hypothermia?

Early in the course of hypothermia atrial arrhythmias are common. Ventricular arrhythmias occur in cases of prolonged hypothermia. Common ventricular arrhythmias are premature ventricular contractions (PVCs) and ventricular tachycardia. In severe cases of hypothermia, when core temperature drops below 28°C, ventricular fibrillation is common. Ventricular fibrillation secondary to hypothermia is often refractory to electrical defibrillation.

15. What common complications are seen during and after active rewarming?

When a moderately-to-severely hypothermic patient is rewarmed actively, many systemic complications are possible. The patient should be closely monitored for the following:

- **Temperature afterdrop**. The core temperature continues to drop after the patient is removed from the cold environment, possibly because of the return of cold peripheral blood to the heart and continued conductance of heat from the warmer core region to the cooler peripheral tissue.
- **Rewarming shock**. Many factors are involved in this phenomenon. Metabolic factors include lactic acidosis due to decreased perfusion. Electrolyte abnormalities (hyponatremia and hyperkalemia) due to cold diuresis may be a feature of reperfusion injury. Coagulation abnormalities range from prolongation of clotting times to DIC. Cardiac dysrhythmias such as PVCs and ventricular fibrillation are seen in severe cases. Pulmonary complications, such as pneumonia secondary to increased viscosity of pulmonary secretions and capillary leakage, are common. Other systemic derangements include increased intracranial pressure due to cerebral edema, pancreatitis, rhabdomyolysis, and acute renal tubular necrosis. Sepsis may result from bacterial translocation across ischemia-damaged barriers such as skin and gastrointestinal tract. Combined with decreases in phagocytic and migratory function of polymorphonuclear cells is a marked decrease in clearing of translocated organisms.

BIBLIOGRAPHY

1. Dhupa N: Hypothermia in dogs and cats. Cont Educ Pract Vet 17:61–66, 1995.
2. Haskins SC: Hypothermia and its prevention during general anesthesia in cats. Am J Vet Res 42:856–861, 1981.
3. Haskins SC: Thermoregulation, hypothermia, hyperthermia. In Ettinger SJ, Feldman EC (eds): Textbook of Small Animal Internal Medicine. Philadelphia, W.B. Saunders, 1995, pp 26–29.
4. Moon PF: Surface induced hypothermia in dogs. J Am Vet Med Assoc 202:856–861, 1993.
5. Smith M: Hypothermia. Comp Cont Educ Pract Vet 7:321–326, 1985.

9. HEAT STROKE

Tim Hackett, D.V.M., M.S.

1. What is heat stroke?

Heatstroke is a severe pyrexia (104.9–109.4°F [40.5–43.0°C]) after exposure to elevated ambient temperatures. Heat stroke is most commonly caused when animals are confined in overheated automobiles or kept outdoors on hot, sunny days without adequate shelter. Exertional heatstroke is less common but may occur when animals are exercised in hot, humid weather or have an impaired ability to dissipate heat.

2. How is normal temperature maintained?

Thermal homeostasis is a balance between heat-gaining and heat-dissipating mechanisms controlled by the thermoregulatory center in the hypothalamus. Heat gain is a function of environmental temperature and metabolic heat. Heat is lost through behavioral mechanisms, changes in circulation, evaporative cooling, and radiation. With increasing body temperature, radiation and convection from the skin are facilitated by peripheral vasodilatation and increased cutaneous circulation. Animals seek shelter and assume body postures to maximize radiant and conductive heat loss. Lacking significant sweat production for evaporative cooling, dogs and cats rely heavily on panting for heat loss. Panting increases dead space ventilation and thus evaporative heat loss in the upper respiratory passages without changing alveolar ventilation.

3. What factors are associated with increased risk of heat stroke?

Various conditions can impair the animal's ability to dissipate heat. Respiratory evaporative heat loss is reduced by humid conditions or upper airway obstruction. Animals with brachycephalic conformation, laryngeal paralysis, tracheal collapse, or mass lesions obstructing airflow may not be able to dissipate heat. Conditions causing hypovolemia or decreased cardiac output decrease cutaneous circulation and convective heat loss from the skin. Obesity also impairs convection and decreases heat loss.

4. What differential diagnoses should be considered in an animal with a temperature above 40.5°C?

In most cases, clinical signs and a history of confinement, forced exercise, and extreme temperatures or humidity are sufficient to diagnose heat stroke. Inflammatory diseases such as meningitis and encephalitis may cause extreme hyperthermia. Space-occupying lesions involving the hypothalamus and thermoregulatory center also should be considered. Malignant hyperthermia is uncommon in dogs but may be associated with exposure to inhalation anesthetics such as halothane. Unwitnessed seizure activity and muscle tremors associated with poisons such as strychnine or metaldehyde also may cause severe hyperthermia.

5. What are the presenting clinical signs of heatstroke?

The initial signs are rapid panting, tachycardia, hyperdynamic arterial pulses, and hyperemic and dry mucous membranes. These findings correspond with increased cardiac output as blood is shunted to the periphery in an attempt to increase convective heat loss. Rectal temperatures are usually between 40.5–43.0°C (104.9–109.4°F). Later, as heat stroke worsens, signs include profound CNS depression and circulatory shock. Weak pulse, gray mucous membranes, vomiting, and diarrhea signal impending organ failure. Marked respiratory effort may lead to shallow respirations, seizures, coma, and death.

6. What laboratory abnormalities are expected in patients with heat stroke?

Biochemical profiles may reflect major organ damage. Elevated levels of blood urea nitrogen (BUN) and creatinine are seen with acute renal tubular necrosis. Hepatic injury causes elevations in aspartate transaminase (AST), alanine transaminase (ALT), and serum bilirubin. Thermal injury to muscles may cause rhabdomyolysis with marked increase in serum creatinine phosphokinase (CK) and AST. Blood glucose is often very low and may require supplementation.

Packed cell volume and total solids are often elevated because of dehydration. Thrombocytopenia, increased fibrin degradation products (FDPs), and prolonged prothrombin (PT) and partial thromboplastin times (PPT) indicate disseminated intravascular coagulation (DIC).

Blood gas analysis is variable. Early in heat stress, animals may pant without affecting alveolar ventilation. As heat stress progresses to heat stroke, respiratory effort may become more forceful and respiratory alkalosis may develop. As the hyperdynamic phase of heat stroke progresses to vasomotor collapse, metabolic acidosis results from increased lactic acid production.

The presence of renal casts or glucosuria in the face of normal-to-low serum glucose may suggest significant tubular damage. Myoglobinuria suggests rhabdomyolysis and exacerbates acute tubular necrosis.

7. What is the most important initial therapy in stabilizing a heat stroke patient?

Lowering the core body temperature. The animal should be taken out of the heat and moved into the shade or indoors to a cool area. Soaking the coat with cool water and providing a fan maximizes evaporative cooling. Placing cool compresses near the axillary and femoral vessels also helps. It is imperative that first responders not overcool the animal. Cooling attempts should be discontinued when the core temperature reaches 39.5°C (103°F). The goal is to decrease the core temperature to 39°C (102°F) in 30–60 minutes.

8. Discuss other ways to lower body temperature.

Massaging the animal helps to increase peripheral blood flow, vasodilation, and cooling. Chilled intravenous fluids, iced gastric lavage, and cold water enemas have been described as ways to lower core body temperature without causing peripheral vasoconstriction. One study concluded that cold peritoneal lavage was more effective at lowering body temperature than evaporative cooling techniques. Another study demonstrated that evaporative cooling was more effective than iced gastric lavage. Peritoneal and gastric lavage are more difficult to perform in conscious animals than evaporative cooling and should be reserved for cases when core temperature does not respond to less invasive cooling techniques.

9. Why stop cooling the animal when the temperature reaches 39.5°C (103°F)?

When the body temperature drops below 39°C (102°F), the animal may begin to shiver, thus producing more heat. Rapid external cooling also may cause peripheral vasoconstriction, making convective heat loss less efficient. Cerebral edema and thermal damage to the hypothalamus make it difficult to maintain thermal homeostasis. Continuous monitoring of core temperature is imperative to guide therapy and to prevent iatrogenic hypothermia.

10. Should a rapid infusion of intravenous fluids be started immediately?

Early in heat stress and heat stroke actual fluid deficits may be relatively minor. With increased cardiac output and peripheral vasodilation, additional fluids may lead to fluid overload and pulmonary or cerebral edema. Hypotension may improve with cooling alone, because peripheral vasoconstriction increases circulating blood volume. Because of the wide range of potential presentations and complications, fluid needs should be assessed individually. Factors such as overall hydration, central venous pressure, electrolyte balance, and urine output should be assessed.

11. How about the use of antiinflammatory drugs? Corticosteroids?

No. Heat stroke is a form of nonpyrogenic hyperthermia; as such, the hypothalamic temperature set point is normal. The use of antipyretics such as dipyrone, aspirin, and flunixin meglumine is contraindicated. These drugs act on the hypothalamic set point and may contribute to iatrogenic hypothermia. They also may worsen gastrointestinal ulceration and ischemic damage to the kidneys.

Corticosteroid use is unproven, although its use for specific complications such as cerebral edema may be warranted.

12. What complications should be anticipated in animals with heat stroke?

Core temperatures at or above 43°C (109°F) may result in irreparable organ damage. Oxidative phosphorylation is uncoupled, cellular membrane function is impaired, and enzymes are denatured. Kidney damage is common because of direct thermal injury to the renal tubular epithelium, decreased renal flow, and hypotension and thrombosis associated with DIC. Clinically BUN and creatinine levels are increased, and renal tubular casts are seen in the urine. Oliguria and anuria may develop.

Hypotension and thermal injury also affect the gastrointestinal tract, causing gastric and intestinal ulceration. Disruption of the normal mucosal barrier may lead to bacteremia and sepsis. Liver damage, as evidenced by increased levels of AST, ALT and serum bilirubin, may result from thermal injury or prolonged splanchnic hypotension.

Disseminated intravascular coagulation is a common sequela of heat stroke. Endothelial cell damage from the heat and widespread cell necrosis lead to inactivation and consumption of platelets and coagulation factors. Thrombocytopenia, increased fibrin degradation products, and prolonged prothrombin and partial thromboplastin times also are seen.

Nerve tissue is susceptible to thermal injury. With direct effects of the heat on endothelium, thermal injury may cause brain hemorrhage and edema as well as thrombosis and infarction of cerebral tissue. Prolonged exposure to high temperatures leads to neuron death and permanent brain damage.

13. How long after successful cooling can the above complications be a problem?

Clinical signs related to the above complications may develop 3–5 days after apparent recovery. Changes in mental status, oliguria, vomiting, bloody diarrhea, icterus, dyspnea, and petechiation should alert the clinician to the possibility of significant complications. Continuous monitoring well past resolution of the hyperthermia is mandatory.

14. How should complications be managed?

Acute renal failure should be aggressively treated with intravenous fluids to restore hydration and to improve glomerular filtration rate. Central venous pressure and urine output should be followed regularly in all patients with heat stroke. If oliguric renal failure is present, intravenous furosemide and a constant rate infusion of dopamine may be given to improve urine output.

Patients with signs of liver failure or gastrointestinal damage should receive supportive care to maintain fluid and electrolyte balance. Because of the risk of bacterial translocation across damaged tissues, broad-spectrum, nonnephrotoxic antibiotics should be started.

Fresh frozen plasma should be used to replace clotting factors in patients with DIC. Subcutaneous injections of heparin may be indicated to prevent microvascular thrombosis associated with DIC.

Seizures are initially treated with intravenous diazepam. Coma or other signs of cerebral edema may be managed with intravenous dexamethasone.

15. Discuss ways to prevent heat stroke.

Heat stroke is most likely to occur when animals are confined in a hot environment. Owners should be educated about the risks of keeping animals in cars or under the sun without adequate shade or water. Animals with preexisting airway problems or obesity should be exercised carefully, preferably not during the hottest times of the day. When possible, underlying problems such as laryngeal paralysis and obesity should be corrected.

BIBLIOGRAPHY

1. Bouchama A, Hammami M, Haq A, Jackson J: Evidence for endothelial cell activation/injury in heat-stroke. Crit Care Med 24:1173–1178, 1996.
2. Drobatz KJ: Heat-induced illness in dogs. Proceedings of the Fourth International Veterinary Emergency and Critical Care Symposium. 1994, pp 361–364.
3. Holloway SA: Heatstroke in dogs. Comp Contin Educ Pract Vet 14:1598–1604, 1992.
4. Lee-Parritz DE, Pavletic MM: Physical and chemical injuries: Heatstroke, hypothermia, burns, and frostbite. In Murtaugh RJ (ed): Veterinary Emergency and Critical Care Medicine. St. Louis, Mosby, 1992, pp 194–196.
5. Ruslander D: Heat stroke. In Kirk RW (ed): Kirk's Current Veterinary Therapy, vol XI. Philadelphia, W.B. Saunders, 1992, pp 143–146.

II. Trauma

Section Editor: Wayne E. Wingfield, D.V.M., M.S.

10. TREATMENT PRIORITIES IN TRAUMA

Wayne E. Wingfield, D.V.M., M.S.

1. Define trauma.

Trauma is any insult to the body. Obviously, the variety of insults is tremendous. Encounters with automobiles, animal fights, leghold traps, burns, weapons such as guns or arrows, and abuse are common traumatic injuries seen by veterinarians.

2. Why is trauma such an important topic?

Trauma is the leading cause of death of small animals. Experience in veterinary emergency and critical care facilities has shown that many deaths can be prevented through an organized approach to care. A well-defined systematic approach includes appropriate triage by body systems, careful evaluation of the animal, prompt and aggressive resuscitation, definitive treatment, and a team-oriented approach between the veterinarian and veterinary technician.

3. Define triage.

Triage, derived from the French word *trier*, means to pick or cull and originally described how French traders sorted wool into various categories according to quality. In veterinary medicine, triage is used to treat the most severely injured patients first and to define the most life-threatening injury. In other words, given an animal with severe respiratory distress and an open fracture to the femur, the respiratory distress is more life-threatening and must be treated immediately.

4. What is the "golden hour"?

At the moment the trauma insult is delivered, the clock begins ticking. The golden hour is the first hour after injury. Ideally, all traumas are evaluated systematically, and life-threatening injuries are identified, and treatment is instituted. In veterinary medicine there are three intervals in which death results from trauma:

- The first interval occurs within minutes of the trauma. Rarely are such animals seen in the veterinary hospital.
- The second interval occurs within the first 3–4 hours of trauma. This is the most common presentation in the veterinary hospital. Prompt, aggressive treatment can make a difference in survival.
- The third interval is after 3–5 days. With attention to detail, recognition of hidden injuries, and appropriate monitoring, the veterinarian can prevent unnecessary deaths in this group.

5. Define mechanism of injury.

The mechanism of injury refers to the events and conditions that lead to both known and unknown traumatic injuries. Significant mechanism of injury is associated with a higher likelihood of multiple trauma.

Significant Mechanisms of Injury

BLUNT TRAUMA	PENETRATING TRAUMA
Hit by an automobile	Gunshot wounds
Kicked by a horse	Arrow penetration
Animal abuse	Foreign body penetration
Falling from a moving vehicle	Animal bite wounds

6. What is multiple trauma?

Multiple trauma refers to significant injuries to more than one major body system. Most animals with significant mechanisms of injury also have multiple trauma. No matter how good the animal looks on presentation after a major mechanism of injury, a high index of suspicion for multiple injury is critical.

7. What are the initial steps in managing the traumatized animal?

- Alert the veterinarian(s) and veterinary technician(s) that an animal is on its way or has arrived at the hospital.
- Quickly obtain a history of the incident, including mechanism of injury.
- If possible, have the receptionist, veterinary technician, trained paraprofessional, or veterinary student stay with the owner of the animal. The owner is also feeling traumatized and needs attention.
- Transfer the animal to a specific area of the hospital designated and equipped to diagnose and treat the trauma patient.
- Assess the ABCDs (see next question) and intervene as necessary.
- Collect the vital signs as quickly as possible (see chapter 1).
- Collect blood and urine samples for the emergency minimum database and baseline laboratory testing.

8. What are the ABCDs of trauma?

- **A = Airway**. Airway patency is evaluated by listening for vocalizations and looking in the mouth for signs of obstruction (blood, emesis, or foreign debris). Fortunately, airway obstructions are not common in small animals. For all trauma animals, supplemental oxygen is continuously administered if it does not unduly stress the animal. The means by which oxygen is administered ranges from face mask to nasal insufflation, oxygen tent, or just blowing oxygen by the nares if the animal does not tolerate other means.
- **B = Breathing**. Ventilation is assessed by observing for symmetric rise and fall of the thoracic walls and by auscultating for bilateral breath sounds. The thoracic walls should be gently palpated for evidence of subcutaneous emphysema or fractured ribs. If possible, oxygen saturation as assessed by pulse oximetry is useful in determining the need for thoracocentesis.
- **C = Circulation**. Circulatory function is assessed by noting the animal's mental status, mucous membrane color and character (cool and clammy vs. warm and dry), vital signs, and presence, character, and rhythm of the femoral arterial pulses. If possible, electrocardiographic monitoring should be started, and vascular access is established to begin volume resuscitation.
- **D = Disabilities**. The animal's neurologic status should be assessed and recorded. Especially important is an evaluation of the cranial nerves for evidence of brain trauma and peripheral reflexes for evidence of spinal or peripheral nerve injury. At this stage also note any abnormal motor postures (e.g., decerebrate rigidity, decerebellate or Schiff-Sherrington posture).

9. Describe the type of intravenous access you should establish in an animal with major trauma.

Use a large-bore (16-gauge or greater) intravenous catheter. Often more than one catheter may be required. The cephalic veins, recurrent tarsal (lateral saphenous) vein in dogs, or medial saphenous (femoral) vein in cats is most commonly chosen for catheterization. Jugular venous catheterization is useful for administering hypertonic solutions and for measuring the central venous pressure but may be too stressful for most animals when first presented to the hospital.

10. What is an adequate minimum database in the trauma patient?

Each hospital should establish its own minimal database. We use the following baseline parameters in each emergency patient: Packed cell volume, total solids (protein), blood glucose, activated clotting time, and, if at all possible, urine specific gravity. These parameters are monitored for changes during therapy.

11. Are other laboratory parameters useful?

Not really. Although samples from most trauma victims should be sent to the laboratory for complete blood count and biochemical profile, baseline packed cell volume should determine preexisting anemia, urinalysis may detect preexisting renal disease and hematuria, and blood glucose showing hypoglycemia may alert the veterinarian to sepsis. No laboratory test defines injury, and initial laboratory studies rarely influence management or disposition.

12. List, in order of priority, the body systems important in trauma.

- **Arterial bleeding**. Realistically, if the animal has arrived at the hospital, the degree of arterial bleeding probably is not significant. More likely you will see evidence of bleeding in the area of a fracture, but arterial bleeding may not become evident until you begin fluid therapy and raise the blood pressure.
- **Respiratory system**. Undoubtedly the respiratory system is the most important body system in trauma. The variety of injuries includes pneumothorax, pulmonary contusions, hemothorax, flail chest, and diaphragmatic hernia. Usually there are multiple injuries to the respiratory system (e.g., pneumothorax with pulmonary contusions).
- **Cardiovascular system**. Two components of the cardiovascular system need attention in the trauma patient: (1) the pump and (2) volume. If the pump is abnormal (e.g., significant arrhythmias or valvular disease), it may not be capable of handling the volume administered for shock.
- **Hemorrhage and transfusion**. Definitive control of venous and/or arterial hemorrhage is accomplished. Packed cell volume and total solids are reassessed to avoid excessive hemodilution. If necessary, a transfusion is administered.
- **Neurologic system**. Three components of the neurologic system are evaluated: (1) brain, (2) spinal cord, and (3) peripheral nerves.
- **Musculoskeletal system**. Fractures are not emergencies. The blood loss and tissue injury surrounding a fracture are more likely to lead to the demise of the animal than the broken bone(s). Occasionally you encounter luxations that cause extreme pain (e.g., elbow luxation) and may prevent alleviation of shock until the luxation is reduced. If a splint can be correctly applied using the principle of immobilizing the joint above and below the fracture, the fracture can be immobilized at this stage.
- **Other injuries**. The veterinarian is faced with identifying and deciding the approach to abdominal injuries (e.g., ruptured liver, kidney, spleen, or urologic injuries). Clues to the existence of such injuries are associated with abdominal pain, and often such animals are difficult to stabilize.

13. Should a thoracic radiograph be taken as soon as possible to rule out pneumothorax or diaphragmatic hernia?

No. Radiography can be stressful to the animal as it is held in place. Thoraco- or abdominocentesis can determine the presence of abnormal substances in the two major cavities.

Early radiography may provide a false sense of security if no evidence of pulmonary contusions are seen. It may be 12–24 hours before radiographic evidence of these contusions is seen.

14. How is tissue perfusion assessed clinically?

Organ perfusion is not democratic. Blood is preferentially distributed to coronary and carotid arteries. If cardiac output is adequate, blood is then delivered to the liver, kidneys, mesenteric organs, and finally the skin. Evidence of urine output is evidence of adequate renal perfusion, and warming of extremities usually suggests adequate perfusion to the skin.

15. What fluids should be used for initial resuscitation?

The mainstay of fluid resuscitation is rapid crystalloid infusion. Colloid solutions (e.g., dextrans, hetastarch) are costly and have not proven advantageous in reducing mortality. Hypertonic saline solutions may lead to prompt rises in blood pressure and may even raise the cardiac output, but their duration is apparently less than 24 hours. Whole blood and, eventually, recombinant hemoglobin, serve to temporize patients with massive blood loss.

CONTROVERSIES

16. Should fluid resuscitation be withheld to minimize bleeding in the trauma patient?

Only one report currently recommends delaying fluid resuscitation until major vascular injuries have been controlled. This study of humans with penetrating thoracic injuries argued that the increase in perfusion pressure dislodges clots and overcomes hemostatic mechanisms, allowing uncontrolled hemorrhage. Numerous letters to the editor have disputed these findings by noting the excessive times in the emergency department and the lack of patient stratification by degree of shock. No clinical veterinary studies are available at present. Because most veterinarians do not do emergency thoracic and abdominal surgery, low-volume resuscitation cannot be recommended.

17. What is the role of pneumatic antishock garments or wrapping extremities to increase venous return during shock?

The pneumatic antishock garment was once believed to autotransfuse blood from the extremities to the central circulation. The use of these garments and wraps to increase blood flow appears also to increase peripheral vascular resistance and may be detrimental with major thoracoabdominal injuries. These techniques have no role in veterinary emergencies.

18. What is a secondary survey?

The secondary survey involves a detailed evaluation of potential life-threatening injuries. The secondary survey includes a head-to-toe physical examination, possible radiographs, further laboratory testing, and special diagnostic tests.

19. What is a tertiary survey?

A complete reevaluation of the animal is completed after 12–24 hours. The purpose is to identify hidden, previously diagnosed injuries and to note the progress of the animal since admission to the hospital.

BIBLIOGRAPHY

1. Bickell WH, Wall MJ Jr, Pepe PE, et al: Immediate versus delayed fluid resuscitation for hypotensive patients with penetrating torso injuries. N Engl J Med 331:1105–1109, 1994.
2. Eisenberg MS, Copass MK: Trauma. In Emergency Medical Therapy. Philadelphia, W.B. Saunders, 1988, pp 403–503.
3. McAnulty JF, Smith GK: Circumferential external counterpressure by abdominal wrapping and its effect on simulated intra-abdominal hemorrhage. Vet Surg 15:270–274, 1986.
4. Spackman GJA, Laywood DD, Feeney DA, et al: Thoracic wall and pulmonary trauma in dogs sustaining fractures as a result of motor vehicle accidents. J Am Vet Med Assoc 185:975–977, 1984.
5. Wingfield WE, Henik RA: Treatment priorities in multiple trauma. Semin Vet Med Surg 3(3):193–201, 1988.

11. ARTERIAL BLEEDING

Wayne E. Wingfield, D.V.M., M.S.

1. By what mechanisms does arterial bleeding occur?

Blunt trauma   Orthopedic injuries
Penetrating trauma   Surgical trauma
Iatrogenic trauma

2. What is the kinetic energy of a bullet? Why is it important in penetrating injuries?

The kinetic energy (K) of a bullet is determined by the following equation:

$$K = \frac{1}{2} MV^2$$

where M = mass and V = velocity. The tissue energy is related to the square of the velocity. Thus, a high-velocity bullet causes more damage and requires more extensive debridement than a bullet of smaller mass and lower velocity.

3. When is arterial bleeding seen in animals hit by a car?

Any animal experiencing trauma is at risk for arterial bleeding. If the bleeding is severe, the animal will not survive to arrival at the veterinary hospital. Most arterial bleeding is usually noted when intravenous fluids are administered and the blood pressure is rising. In most cases, the arterial bleeding is noted with open fractures of the distal radius or ulna, tibia or fibula.

4. How do you recognize arterial bleeding?

Arterial blood usually has a brighter red color than venous blood. In addition, arterial bleeding usually spurts with each heartbeat, whereas venous bleeding usually oozes from the wound.

5. What is the first response to managing arterial bleeding of a distal extremity?

Arterial bleeding of a distal extremity is best managed by applying pressure to the wound site. Blind clamping should be avoided to prevent unnecessary soft tissue or nerve injury. In trauma this is usually done by applying a 4 × 4 gauze sponge over the wound and applying tape and gauze around the extremity. Surgical ligation of the artery is usually unnecessary at this stage of triage. It is more important to assess respiratory and cardiovascular function and to begin intravenous fluid resuscitation before considering definitive control of bleeding.

6. Which arterial injury bleeds more—a complete transection or an incomplete transection? Why?

The incomplete transection bleeds more because, unlike the complete transection, it does not have the ability to undergo retraction, vasoconstriction, and thrombosis.

7. What are the three anatomic layers of an artery?

Tunica intima, tunica media, and tunica adventitia.

8. What is the mechanism of arterial injury from blunt trauma?

As the arterial wall is stretched, the elastic adventitial and muscular layers remain intact as the tunica intima fractures. Blood dissects beneath the intima, resulting in an intimal flap that occludes the lumen.

9. Should a tourniquet be used to control arterial hemorrhage?

If at all possible, avoid placement of a tourniquet. The tourniquet occludes collateral circulation, making distal ischemia worse. If improperly applied, it may allow arterial inflow and impede venous return, thus making the bleeding worse.

10. Should you ligate or repair an injured artery surgically?

Tough question. In a perfect world, surgical repair makes good sense. In the real world, veterinarians generally are not trained in the surgical repair of vessels. Repairs must be precise, involve use of very small suture material, and require magnification of the surgical site. Surgical skill is mandatory. For most arterial bleeding from extremity fractures, surgical ligation is done. Fortunately, collateral circulation is usually more than adequate to prevent distal ischemia. Obviously, if you are in surgery and have damaged an artery, you must combine surgical judgment with skill to make this decision.

11. If you are going to attempt surgical repair, what are the initial steps?

Using specialized vascular clamps, obtain proximal and distal control of the injured vessel.

12. What are the surgical steps in arterial repair?

Debridement, removal of thrombi, careful arterial reconstruction, and soft-tissue coverage.

13. What is the most common intraabdominal arterial injury in veterinary patients?

Who knows? No reports in the veterinary literature detail this information. Anecdotal experience suggests that the most common arterial injury is probably to smaller intrahepatic or intrasplenic arteries. Occasionally an avulsed kidney may be identified at surgery (but probably more often at necropsy).

14. Define compartment syndrome.

With serious injury to the upper fore- or hindlimb, edema often results from ischemia or massive soft tissue trauma. The increased pressure decreases capillary blood flow and may lead to tissue necrosis. In this syndrome, neurologic injury occurs first, because nerves are most sensitive to ischemia. Systemic manifestations of the compartment syndrome include hyperkalemia, myoglobinuria, and sepsis.

15. If you suspect compartment syndrome, what is the initial treatment?

Prompt fasciotomy.

16. Which injury is most likely to show compartment syndrome?

Anecdotally, rattlesnake envenomations are most likely to show compartment syndrome.

17. Can Doppler signals over an artery be used to rule out an arterial injury?

No. Doppler signals are not reliable for arterial injury or adequate perfusion.

18. What is the most likely injury resulting in arterial bleeding in the thorax?

No data are available to answer this question in veterinary medicine. If there is a severe blunt or penetrating trauma, the injury causing death is most likely to the aorta or pulmonary arteries. The surgical procedure that seems most likely to result in arterial bleeding is surgical repair of a patent ductus arteriosus.

19. Significant swelling in the early postoperative period is suggestive of what complication?

Venous thrombosis.

BIBLIOGRAPHY

1. Eisenberg MS, Copass MK: Emergency Medical Therapy. Philadelphia, W.B. Saunders, 1988, pp 403–503.
2. McAnulty JF, Smith GK: Circumferential external counterpressure by abdominal wrapping and its effect on simulated intra-abdominal hemorrhage. Vet Surg 15:270–274, 1986.
3. Wingfield WE, Henik RA: Treatment priorities in multiple trauma. Semin Vet Med Surg 3(3):193–201, 1988.

12. RESPIRATORY EMERGENCIES

Deborah R. Van Pelt, D.V.M., M.S.

1. What are the most common respiratory injuries associated with thoracic trauma?
- Pulmonary contusions
- Rib fractures
- Pneumothorax
- Diaphragmatic hernia

2. What is a tension pneumothorax?
A tension pneumothorax results from blunt or penetrating injury of the lung that creates a one-way valve. Air leaks from the lung into the pleural space and is unable to escape, resulting in increased intrapleural pressure. Intrapleural pressure eventually increases to the point that it interferes with venous return, resulting in blood pooling in capacitance vessels with ensuing cardiovascular collapse and shock.

3. What are the radiographic signs of tension pneumothorax?
- Hyperlucent, overly expanded hemithorax
- Mediastinal shift to the opposite side
- Radiographic signs of pneumothorax—heart elevated from the sternum, lung lobes retracted from the thoracic wall

4. How should tension pneumothorax be treated?
The most immediate goal in the treatment of tension pneumothorax is to alleviate the increased intrapleural pressure. This goal is accomplished most quickly by performing thoracocentesis with a 20-gauge needle in the 7th or 8th intercostal space. If pneumothorax recurs or persists once the pleural space has been evacuated, a tube thoracostomy should be performed.

5. What is a flail chest?
A flail chest occurs when a segment of the thoracic wall becomes detached from the rest of the chest wall. In the most typical scenario, ribs that are fractured in two places allow the flail segment of the thoracic wall to float independently. Flail chest also may occur when ribs are fractured proximally in conjunction with distal disarticulation of costochondral cartilages. In young animals in whom the costal cartilages are quite flexible, a flail chest may occur when several ribs are fractured proximally and the costal cartilages allow the segment to move independently of the rest of the chest wall.

6. How should a flail chest be treated?
Treatment of flail chest is dictated by the clinical condition and degree of respiratory distress. Local block of the affected ribs (bupivacaine instillation caudal to the affected ribs at the rib origin) decreases the patient's pain. If the flail segment impairs gas exchange or contributes to hypoxemia, it should be supported by a firm chest wrap; laying the patient with the flail segment downward against the exam table provides temporary support. Support prevents the flail segment from moving out paradoxically during expiration. Oxygen supplementation may be necessary, depending on the underlying lung pathology. Surgical stabilization of the flail segment is rarely necessary.

7. Discuss the use of oxygen supplementation and diuretics in the treatment of pulmonary contusions.
Supplemental oxygen. Microscopic hemorrhage into the pulmonary interstitium and alveoli results in hypoxemia secondary to diffusion impairment and ventilation/perfusion mismatch,

both of which are responsive to oxygen supplementation. Oxygen supplementation can be administered by oxygen mask, nasal oxygen cannula, oxygen cage, or, in severe cases, intubation and positive pressure ventilation.

Diuretics. In a hypovolemic patient with pulmonary contusions, diuretics complicate hypovolemia and thereby further decrease tissue oxygen delivery and precipitate cardiovascular collapse. In a patient with severe pulmonary contusions in whom cardiovascular status is stable, diuretics may decrease the rate of pulmonary edema formation. However, diuretics do not alter the underlying degree of alveolar capillary damage and therefore should not be used routinely in the treatment of pulmonary contusions.

8. Discuss the controversial use of steroids in the treatment of pulmonary contusions.

Corticosteroids have not been documented to be beneficial in the management of patients with pulmonary contusions. In fact, by contributing to immunosuppression, corticosteroids may predispose the patient to the development of bacterial pneumonia.

9. Describe the concerns related to use of fluid therapy in patients with pulmonary contusions.

Progression of pulmonary contusions is often related to aggressive administration of fluid volume during resuscitation of trauma patients. Overly aggressive crystalloid administration may result in pulmonary edema, which complicates pulmonary contusions. Cautious crystalloid administration during resuscitation is necessary to support the cardiovascular system; pulmonary contusions may be worsened by overzealous fluid administration. Colloid administration may decrease the amount of lung water that accumulates during resuscitation.

10. When should thoracic radiographs be performed in a patient with suspected pneumothorax?

The initial presumptive diagnosis of pneumothorax should be based on physical findings of respiratory distress, tachypnea, and muffled heart and lung sounds on thoracic auscultation. Thoracic radiographs should be performed only after the immediate respiratory distress has been alleviated and the patient is relatively stable. Thoracocentesis should be performed before chest radiographs and based on physical findings. Thoracocentesis is both diagnostic (confirming suspicions of pneumothorax) and therapeutic (relieving the pneumothorax).

11. Describe the etiologies of respiratory distress in patients with diaphragmatic hernia.

- Abdominal organ herniation into the thorax results in compression of thoracic viscera and pulmonary atelectasis.
- Atelectasis and potential pleural effusion result in loss of functional lung capacity.
- Concurrent thoracic injury may cause pulmonary contusions and subsequent hypoxemia.
- Herniation of the stomach may result in gastric tympany with compression of thoracic viscera and decreased lung capacity and cardiovascular collapse.

BIBLIOGRAPHY

1. Coalson JJ: Pathophysiologic features of infant and adult respiratory distress syndrome. In Shoemaker WC, Ayres S, Grenvik A, et al (eds): Textbook of Critical Care. Philadelphia, W.B. Saunders, 1989, pp 464–478.
2. Crowe DT: Traumatic pulmonary contusions, hematomas, pseudocysts, and acute respiratory distress syndrome: An update. Comp Cont Educ Pract Vet 5:396–407, 1983.
3. Hackner SG: Emergency management of traumatic pulmonary contusions. Comp Cont Educ 17:677–686, 1995.
4. Hudson LD, Milberg JA, Anardi D, Maunder RJ: Clinical risks for development of the acute respiratory distress syndrome: 1983–1993. JAMA 273:306–309, 1995.
5. Kirby R, Crowe DT: Emergency medicine. Vet Clin North Am Small Animal Prac 24:997–1274, 1994.
6. Kramek BA, Caywood DD: Pneumothorax. Vet Clin North Am Small Animal Prac 17:285–300, 1987.

7. Orton EC: Management of thoracic trauma. Proceedings of Respiratory and Pulmonary Conditions: A refresher course for veterinarians. Sydney, University of Sydney, 1993, pp 181–202.
8. Schaer M: Dyspnea in the cat—an update. Proceedings in Veterinary Continuing Education. Taupo, Australia, 1993, pp 91–99.
9. Wingfield WE, Henik RA: Treatment priorities in cases of multiple trauma. Semin Vet Med Surg Small Animal 3:193–201, 1988.

13. TRAUMATIC MYOCARDITIS

Steven L. Marks, B.VSc., M.S., M.R.C.V.S.

1. Define traumatic myocarditis. What is the suspected pathophysiology?

Traumatic myocarditis is a generic term used to describe cardiac arrhythmias after blunt trauma. A combination of processes affecting the myocardium leads to the arrhythmias. The cause of the arrhythmias is unknown but may be multifactorial, including reperfusion, shock, neurologic injury, and sympathetic stimulation. Myocarditis is not usually present; necrosis or contusion is more common and often results from multiple forces to the heart after blunt trauma.

2. What forces to the heart may cause arrhythmias?

- Unidirectional
- Compression
- Indirect
- Decelerative
- Concussive

3. When should myocardial trauma be suspected?

Myocardial trauma should be suspected after any blunt trauma or thoracic injury, including blunt trauma leading to pulmonary contusions, pneumothorax, hemothorax, chylothorax, or diaphragmatic hernia. Penetrating thoracic injuries also may lead to myocardial changes. Traumatic myocarditis is seen more commonly in dogs, and arrhythmias may not occur until 24–48 hours after injury.

4. What is the clinical evidence of traumatic myocarditis in dogs and cats?

Often no clinical signs are present with traumatic myocarditis. Clinical signs may be related to chest trauma, but they are not specific for myocardial damage. Arrhythmias may be associated with pulse deficits, lethargy, and hypotension.

5. What adjunctive diagnostic testing should be performed?

Additional diagnostics should be considered only after thorough physical examination and triage of the patient. Thoracic radiographs and electrocardiography should be considered after thoracic trauma. Other diagnostic testing should be considered as dictated by clinical condition, including thoracocentesis, blood gas analysis, electrolytes, echocardiography, and pulse oximetry.

6. What is the role of the electrocardiogram (ECG) in traumatic myocarditis?

The ECG is a valuable tool for both the diagnosis and monitoring of cardiac arrhythmias. Supraventricular tachyarrhythmias, ventricular arrhythmias, and bradyarrhythmias have been documented in posttraumatic cases. Reported arrhythmias include ventricular tachycardia, accelerated idioventricular rhythms, ventricular premature complexes, atrial fibrillation, sinus rhythm with bundle branch blocks, and atrioventricular block.

7. What are the most common arrhythmias after trauma?

Ventricular tachycardia and accelerated idioventricular rhythms.

8. What is an accelerated idioventricular rhythm?

An accelerated idioventricular rhythm is one of the most common posttraumatic cardiac arrhythmias in dogs and may occur within 48 hours of injury. The mechanism is unknown but may be related to autonomic disturbance or reperfusion injury. An abnormal automaticity may explain why an underlying ventricular rhythm overtakes the normal pacemaker. Generally the rate of this rhythm is < 150 beats/minute; it is often preceded by a pause in the sinus rate. Accelerated idioventricular rhythm is often misdiagnosed as ventricular tachycardia and treated with antiarrhythmic agents. This rhythm does not lead to hemodynamic instability; it is self-limiting and requires no treatment.

9. Describe treatment criteria for arrhythmias associated with traumatic myocarditis.

Treatment for arrhythmias is a common dilemma facing the emergency clinician. Treatment of arrhythmias should be based on clinical assessment of the patient. Basing therapy solely on the ECG rather than on the patient is a mistake. Antiarrhythmic agents are not without complications and may be arrhythmogenic. All antiarrhythmic agents can also cause myocardial depression. Therapy, therefore, should be based on clinical signs, perfusion, and blood pressure. Underlying problems, such as hypovolemia, electrolyte disturbances, acid-base disorders, or pain should be addressed before considering antiarrhythmic agents. If clinical signs of supraventricular tachycardias are present, calcium channel blockers or beta-blockers may be considered. If ventricular tachycardia is suspected, treatment criteria include rate (> 150 beats/minute), multifocal morphology, and presence of R on T phenomenon.

10. Which antiarrhythmic agents may be used for trauma-induced arrhythmias?

Tachycardia	*Bradycardia*
Supraventricular	Atropine
Propranolol	Glycopyrrolate
Esmolol	Dopamine
Diltiazem	Isoproterenol
Procainamide	Theophylline
Ventricular	Aminophylline
Lidocaine	Terbutaline
Procainamide	
Mexiletine	
Magnesium sulfate	
Esmolol	
Propranolol	

11. Can animals with traumatic myocarditis be anesthetized?

The evaluation for anesthesia should be based on thorough physical examination. Anesthesia should not be considered until the patient is stable and malignant arrhythmias are controlled. The classification adopted by the American Society of Anesthesiologists can be applied to animals with traumatic injuries:

Class I: Normal patient with no systemic disease.
Class II: Patient with mild systemic disease.
Class III: Patient with severe systemic disease that limits activity.
Class IV: Patient with incapacitating systemic disease that is a threat to life.
Class V: Moribund patient not expected to survive 24 hours.

In young and otherwise healthy animals a minimal database of packed cell volume, total protein, and glucose is suggested. In animals older than 5 years, a more extensive database, including biochemical profile, may be indicated. In trauma patients, electrocardiography and thoracic radiographs should be considered. Other specific diagnostic tools for cardiopulmonary trauma may include blood pressure evaluation, blood gas analysis, and pulse oximetry.

Choice of anesthetic agents should be based on clinical evaluation of the patient. All anesthetic agents can change the electrophysiologic properties of the heart and should be used cautiously. The use of inhalant anesthetics has the advantage of concurrently providing oxygen. Of these agents, halothane has the greatest potential for being arrhythmogenic via catecholamine sensitization of the myocardium. Injectable agents that are known to be arrhythmogenic, such as xylazine, should be avoided. The benzodiazepines and opioids may be the safest injectable induction agents. Low dosages of thiobarbiturates also may be tolerated.

12. How should patients be monitored?

Patient monitoring should be based on clinical condition. Continuous ECG monitoring is valuable to assess the progression of arrhythmias. Other parameters such as blood pressure, blood gas analysis, central venous pressure, packed cell volume, and total protein should be monitored as needed.

BIBLIOGRAPHY

1. Abbott JA: Traumatic myocarditis. In Bonagura JD (ed): Kirks Current Veterinary Therapy XII: Small Animal Practice. Philadelphia, W.B. Saunders, 1995, pp 846–850.
2. Abbott JA, King RR: Third degree atrioventricular block following non-penetrating chest trauma in a dog. J Small Animal Pract 34:377–380, 1993.
3. Alexander JW, Bolton GR, Koslow GL: Electrocardiographic changes in nonpenetrating trauma to the chest. J Am Animal Hosp Assoc 11:160–166, 1975.
4. Macintire DK, Snider TG III: Cardiac arrhythmias associated with multiple trauma in dogs. J Am Vet Med Assoc 184:541–545, 1984.
5. Muir WW, Mason D: Cardiovascular System. Baltimore, Williams & Wilkins, 1996, pp 62–113.
6. Murtaugh RJ, Ross JN: Cardiac arrhythmias: Pathogenesis and treatment in the trauma patient. Compend Cont Educ Pract Vet 10:332–339, 1988.
7. Roy LM, Short CE: Anesthetic consideration in dogs with traumatic myocarditis. Cornell Vet 76:175–187, 1986.
8. Thurmon JC, Tranquilli WJ, Benson GJ (eds): Lumb and Jones Veterinary Anesthesia. Baltimore, Williams & Wilkins, 1996, pp 5–34.

14. FLUID SELECTION IN TRAUMA

Wayne E. Wingfield, D.V.M., M.S.

1. Where is water located in the body?

Most water is located in the intracellular compartment (~ 66%). The extracellular compartment contains about 34% of the body's water. The extracellular compartment is further subdivided into the intravascular (~ 25%) and interstitial (~ 75%) spaces.

2. What governs the distribution of water in the body?

The semipermeable membranes between the fluid compartments allow rapid equilibrium of free water and low-molecular-weight solutes (< ~ 40,000 Da). The particles (solutes) that are unable to pass through this semipermeable membrane generate oncotic pressure. This relative difference in oncotic pressure governs fluid distribution between compartments.

3. What happens when free water is infused into the intravascular space?

When dextrose in water (D5W) is infused, the dextrose is metabolized, leaving free water. When infused into the intravascular space, free water equilibrates with the extracellular and intracellular compartments in proportion to their relative water volumes. In other words, most water moves to the intracellular compartment (~ 75%) and relatively little remains in the intravascular space of the extracellular compartment.

4. Should D5W be used as a resuscitation fluid in shock?

No. As mentioned above, most water quickly moves to the intracellular space. In shock, the goal is to expand the intravascular space to provide volume for improving cellular perfusion and metabolism.

5. What is "third-spacing" of fluids?

The "third space" refers to the extracellular fluid that is nonfunctional, i.e., it does not participate in the transport of nutrients to nor waste products from the body cells. With burn injuries, crushing of tissue, severe soft tissue infections, postoperative wounds, pyometra, peritonitis, and hemorrhagic (traumatic) shock, significant amounts of extracellular fluid are sequestered, resulting in significant decreases in interstitial and plasma volume. Attempts to restore extracellular and intracellular compartments with intravenous fluids result in further sequestration of additional fluid in the nonfunctional third space. The end result is often massive weight gain. In acute injury, resolution of third-spacing begins 48–72 hours after the insult. This resolution is associated with resorption, diuresis, and weight loss, often leading to cardiovascular and/or pulmonary complications.

6. What are crystalloid fluids?

Crystalloid fluids contain sodium chloride and other physiologically active solutes. Sodium is the major component, and the distribution of sodium determines the distribution of the infused crystalloid.

7. How are crystalloid fluids redistributed when administered intravenously?

Because there is no difference in osmolality between the infused crystalloid and body fluids, there is no driving force to cause water to diffuse into the intracellular compartment. The intact membrane between the interstitial space and the intravascular space is permeable to ions and small particles. The membrane surrounding the intracellular space is relatively impermeable to ions and small particles. Consequently, the extracellular space is the distribution space for isotonic crystalloids. In healthy adult humans, only one-fourth of the crystalloid volume infused remains in the intravascular space after 1 hour. In critically ill or injured humans, only one-fifth or less may remain in the circulation 1–2 hours after infusion.

8. What happens to the packed cell volume (hematocrit) in shock?

Acute blood loss leads to a progressive fall in the packed cell volume (PCV) because of redistribution of interstitial and intracellular volumes to expand the intravascular volume. By 2 hours, 14–36% of the ultimate PCV change has occurred; in 8 hours, 36–50%; and in 24 hours, 63–77%. With redistribution of resuscitation crystalloids, the PCV again rises. The total serum protein levels show similar changes. Depleted intravascular volume is restored through movement of interstitial fluid to the intravascular space. Catecholamines stimulate arteriolar vasoconstriction, which diminishes capillary bed hydrostatic pressure and favors influx of interstitial fluid into the vascular tree distal to the arteriolar vasoconstriction. Subsequently, lymphatic flow returns plasma proteins to the intravascular space. This increase in lymphatic flow is enhanced when crystalloid fluids move to the interstitial space, thus increasing interstitial pressure. In addition, increased albumin synthesis and spontaneous diuresis secondary to volume expansion aid in the expansion of intravascular volume.

9. When crystalloids are used for shock resuscitation, how much volume is required?

The volume of crystalloid required to attain adequate volume replacement varies from 3–5 to 12 times the blood volume lost.

10. How are the so-called "shock volumes" determined for dogs and cats?

The answer is controversial. Traditionally, the shock volume for dogs is said to be 90 ml/kg/hr. The shock volume for cats is said to be 44 ml/kg/hr. However, to determine these values, whole blood volume is used in dogs and plasma volume in cats. Anecdotal experience has shown the dog's traditional shock volume (90 ml/kg/hour) is rarely required for resuscitation. More than likely consideration should be given to recommending plasma volume (50 ml/kg/hour) as the shock volume for dogs.

Estimates of Volumes in Dogs and Cats

	DOGS	CATS
Total body water	717 ± 17 ml/kg	596 ± 50.5 ml/kg
Red blood cell volume	36.9 ± 6 ml/kg	17 ± 3.2 ml/kg
Plasma volume	50.7 ± 4.3 ml/kg	44.3 ± 5 ml/kg
Whole blood volume	88.7 ± 8.3 ml/kg	60.1 ± 9.3 ml/kg

11. What are the most commonly used crystalloids?

If a survey were completed, Ringer's lactate would likely be the most commonly used crystalloid in veterinary practices. As a balanced electrolyte solution it probably is not the best choice. With only 130 mEq/L of sodium, Ringer's lactate is hyponatremic and hypotonic (osmolality = 273) to small animals. A more balanced solution for small animals is Normosol-R (Abbott Laboratories). The table below lists the crystalloid solutions and their composition.

Electrolyte Composition (mEq/L) of Plasma vs. Commonly Used Crystalloid Fluids

	PLASMA	0.9% SALINE	RINGER'S LACTATE	NORMOSOL-R
Sodium	145	154	130	140
Chloride	110	154	109	98
Potassium	4–5	—	4	5
Calcium and magnesium	5/2	—	3/0	0/3
Osmolality	300	308	273	295
pH	7.386	5.7	6.7	7.4
Buffer	NaHCO$_3$ 20–22	—	Lactate 28	Acetate 27 gluconate 23

12. What are the buffers in crystalloid fluids? Why are they there?

The buffers in Ringer's lactate and Normosol-R are precursors to bicarbonate. Thus, as they are metabolized, bicarbonate is formed and helps to resolve metabolic acidosis. Lactate is metabolized predominantly by the hepatic circulation, whereas acetate and gluconate are metabolized by skeletal muscle and peripheral tissues. In shock, hepatic blood flow is reduced; thus lactate may not be adequately metabolized. Evidence in lymphosarcoma dogs suggests that this lactate may be converted to lactic acid and complicate the acid-base status. Studies are underway to see if such is the case in critically ill dogs.

13. What are the major pitfalls in crystalloid resuscitation?

One must avoid inadequate fluid administration and excessive hemodilution. In addition, crystalloid fluids must be carefully administered when the animal has either pulmonary injury (i.e., contusions) or brain trauma.

14. What is meant by excessive hemodilution?

As mentioned above, when crystalloids are used in shock resuscitation, they contribute to the dilution of red blood cells and plasma proteins. This dilution can affect tissue oxygenation and obviously may lead to interstitial edema. Currently, packed cell volumes in shock patients should be maintained above 20%, and total protein values are kept at least at the level of 50% of the starting value. In other words, do not allow the PCV to fall below 20% or the total protein below 50% of its initial value.

15. Is hemodilution detrimental to cardiac output and tissue oxygenation?
Within limits, hemodilution improves cardiac output and increases tissue oxygenation.

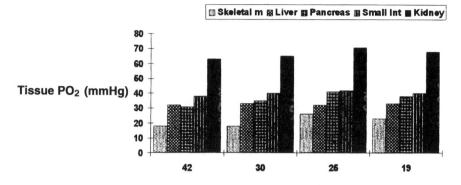

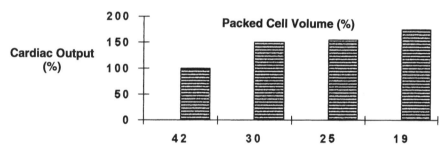

Effects of hemodilution on cardiac output and tissue oxygenation.

16. What is hypertonic saline? How is it used for shock resuscitation in small animals?
Concentrated (> 0.9%) crystalloid solutions containing sodium and chloride are called hypertonic saline. They are useful because they require smaller volumes of fluid for resuscitation, have decreased risks of edema, and improve the ability to deliver effective volume resuscitation in nonhospitalized patients. In animal studies and human clinical trials of hemorrhagic shock, hypertonic saline has proved effective.

17. List the advantages and disadvantages for hypertonic saline in shock resuscitation.

Advantages	*Disadvantages*
Significantly improved hemodynamics	Induces hypernatremia
Increases cardiac output	
Improves peripheral blood flow and distribution	
Increases oxygen delivery	
Improves coronary, mesenteric, and renal artery blood flow	
Promotes urine production	Induces hyperchloremia
Lowers intracranial pressure	Hyperosmolar (7.5% = 2400 mOsm)
Reduces peripheral and central nervous system edema	Induces hypokalemia
Has a more sustained hemodynamic effect	May produce a non-respiratory acidosis
	(hyperchloremic acidosis)
Reduces initial and subsequent fluid volumes	Cardiac dysrhythmias are reported
Corrects metabolic abnormalities	Increased risk of bleeding
Improves survival	Anaphylaxis
	Impaired renal function may be worsened

18. What are colloids?
Colloids are high-molecular-weight substances that, because of their size, do not readily cross capillary walls. They are retained in the vascular space and exert an osmotic force (colloid osmotic force or colloid oncotic force) that helps to retain fluid in the intravascular space.

19. What are the two main types of colloids? Give examples of each.

Hematogenous colloids	Synthetic colloids
Whole blood	Dextrans
Plasma	Hydroxyethyl starch
Packed red blood cells	Pentastarch
	Albumin

20. What is the rationale for use of colloids in shock?
Colloids are more effective than crystalloids for increasing intravascular volume.

21. Are only synthetic colloids administered for shock resuscitation?
No. When the synthetic colloids are administered, water is drawn from the interstitial and intracellular spaces, which need to be rehydrated. Thus a combination of colloids and crystalloids is usually given.

22. What are dextrans?
The dextrans are high-molecular-weight polysaccharides originally obtained from the juice of sugar beets. The two most commonly used products are dextran-70 (average molecular weight [AMW] = 70,000 Da) and dextran-40 (AMW = 40,000 Da). Because albumin has an AMW of 69,000 Da, dextran-70 appears to be an ideal substitute based on size. However, a more useful measure of size is the number average molecular weight (NAMW), which for dextran-70 may be as low as 39,000 Da.

23. What is hydroxyethyl starch?
Hydroxyethyl starch (Hetastarch) is a synthetic starch with an AMW of 480,000 Da and an NAMW of 69,000 Da. In a review of nine studies, hydroxyethyl starch increased plasma volume by 70–200% of the volume infused, with a mean expansion of 141%.

24. What is the duration of clinical effects of the various synthetic colloids?
- Plasma half-life of dextran-70 is 25.5 hr, and duration of clinical effect is approximately 24 hr.
- Plasma half-life of dextran-40 is 2.5 hr; duration of clinical effect ranges from 20 min (particle sizes of 18,000–23,000) to 12 hr (particle sizes of 55,000–69,000).
- Plasma half-life of hydroxyethyl starch is 25.5 hr, and duration of clinical effect is 12–48 hr.

25. What adverse effects are associated with synthetic colloids?
- The use of dextrans and hydroxyethyl starch is associated with increased risk of bleeding in animals and people. At present, the degree of bleeding abnormalities appears to be related to dosage; such abnormalities are readily reversible. Animals at risk for bleeding include those with thrombocytopenia, abnormal platelet function, von Willebrand factor deficiency, and factor VIII:c deficiency.
- The incidence of anaphylactic reactions (skin erythema, hypotension, respiratory distress, cardiac arrest) to hydroxyethyl starch in humans is estimated at 0.007%. The incidence of dextran anaphylactic reactions in humans varies from 0.03–4.7%. No reports are found in available veterinary literature.
- Dextran-40 is associated with acute renal failure in humans.
- Serum amylase levels in humans rise 2–4 times normal during hydroxyethyl starch infusion and may persist for 5 days. Hyperamylasemia is a normal response to degrade the

product and does not indicate that the animal has pancreatitis. One must use serum lipase to diagnose and follow pancreatitis in animals after administration of hydroxyethyl starch.
• Synthetic colloids are contraindicated in animals with congestive heart failure because of the potential for profound volume expansion and edema formation.

26. Can a refractometer be used after administration of synthetic colloids to estimate total protein concentration?

Estimation of oncotic pressure using the refractometer may not be accurate. Direct measurement of colloid oncotic pressure with an oncometer is the method of choice to guide colloidal fluid therapy.

CONTROVERSY

27. Which fluid should be used to treat shock—crystalloid or colloid?

The appropriate resuscitation fluid is more than a topic of debate; it is a passionately fought war. The table below provides a brief summary of the salient arguments. As in all wars, the truth is likely somewhere in the middle.

The Colloids vs. Crystalloids War

	CRYSTALLOIDS	SYNTHETIC COLLOIDS
Hemodynamic effects	Require larger volumes	Direct intravascular volume expansion Smaller volumes required Improve cardiac output Improve oxygen transport
Risk for pulmonary edema	Small risk with excessive hemodilution May cause more edema if capillaries are leaky	Theoretically may leak from the capillaries and promote increased edema Cause no more edema than crystalloids
Clinical outcome	No advantage over colloids in survival (humans)	No advantage over crystalloids in survival (humans)
Expense	Much less expensive than colloids	Significantly more expensive than crystalloids
Conclusions	If the goal is to expand the whole extracellular space, use crystalloids.	If the goal is to expand the intravascular volume, use colloids.

BIBLIOGRAPHY

1. Carey JS, Scharschmidt BF, Culliford AT: Hemodynamic effectiveness of colloid and electrolyte solutions for replacement of simulated operative blood loss. Surg Gynecol Obstet 131:679–686, 1970.
2. Concannon KT: Colloid oncotic pressure and the clinical use of colloidal solutions. J Vet Emerg Crit Care 3:49–62, 1995.
3. Ebert RV, Stead EA Jr, Gibson JG: Response of normal subjects to acute blood loss with special reference to the mechanism of restoration of blood volume. Arch Intern Med 68:578–590, 1941.
4. Hauser CJ, Shoemaker WC, Turpin I: Oxygen transport responses to colloids and crystalloids in critically ill surgical patients. Surg Gynecol Obstet 150:811–816, 1980.
5. Hulse JD, Yacobi A: Hetastarch: An overview of the colloid and its metabolism. Drug Intell Clin Pharmacol 17:334–341, 1983.
6. Lowe RJ, Moss GS, Jilek J, et al: Crystalloid versus colloid in the etiology of pulmonary failure after trauma: A randomized trial in man. Surgery 81:676–683, 1977.
7. Lewis RT: Albumin: Role and discriminative use in surgery. Can J Surg 23:322–328, 1980.

8. Mishler JM: Pharmacology of Hydroxyethyl Starch. Use in Therapy and Blood Banking. New York, Oxford University Press, 1982, pp 1–53.
9. Moss GS, Lower RJ, Jilek J, et al: Colloid or crystalloid in the resuscitation of shock. A controlled clinical trial. Surgery 89:434–438, 1981.
10. Weil MH, Morissette M, Michaels S, et al: Routine plasma colloid osmotic pressure measurements. Crit Care Med 2:229–234, 1974.

15. BLOOD TRANSFUSIONS

Michael S. Lagutchik, D.V.M.

1. What are the immediate treatment priorities in patients with major hemorrhagic shock?

Rapid restoration of intravascular pressures, cardiac output, and oxygen content of blood are the immediate priorities in resuscitation from hemorrhagic shock. Administration of blood or blood products is effective in all three areas.

2. What are the alternatives to increase oxygen-carrying capacity of the blood?

Current alternatives include homologous and autologous blood transfusions. A third alternative soon to be available is use of red blood cell substitutes (see question 21).

3. What are common causes of blood loss anemia in critically ill dogs and cats?

- Trauma
- Coagulopathies (congenital, anticoagulants, liver disease)
- Platelet disorders (thrombocytopenia, von Willebrand's disease, drugs, thrombopathias)
- Splenic rupture (trauma, neoplasia, torsion)
- Gastrointestinal hemorrhage (ulceration, neoplasia, endoparasites, foreign bodies, hemostatic disorders)
- Epistaxis (neoplasia, infection, hemostatic disorders)

4. What are the general indications for blood transfusions in critically ill or injured patients?

Red cell transfusion is indicated whenever the oxygen-carrying capacity is insufficient to meet metabolic requirements. Insufficiency may be due to loss of red cells, decreased hemoglobin concentration, or poor tissue perfusion from numerous causes. General indications include acute and chronic blood loss, hemolytic anemias, decreased red cell production, and refractory shock.

5. At what packed cell volume (PCV) should a transfusion of whole blood or packed red blood cells be considered?

Do not succumb to the habit of transfusing at a cut-off PCV. The need for transfusion is determined by the time to onset of anemia (acute or chronic), cause and degree of anemia, potential for further loss of blood, response to other supportive therapies, and cardiac, pulmonary, and renal status of the patient.

6. What hematocrit value should cause concern about the patient's ability to transport oxygen effectively?

Although somewhat controversial, most authors agree that serious abnormalities related to oxygen transport develop below a PCV of 20% and may be irreversible if allowed to continue uncorrected. Many recommend a cut-off of 20–30%. When the hematocrit is < 30%, ventricular function is depressed, but oxygen extraction and central venous PO_2 remain normal until the hematocrit reaches 20%, perhaps even lower. In trauma cases especially, it may be better to transfuse earlier rather than later to avoid a serious game of catch-up.

7. What is a good target hematocrit value when transfusing blood?

For the same reasons, see the preceding question. It is seldom necessary, and some argue that it may be detrimental, to transfuse a patient to the mid-range of the normal PCV. As the hematocrit increases, blood viscosity also increases. Increased blood viscosity may not be desirable in a patient with poor tissue perfusion due to shock or acute hemorrhage.

8. List specific parameters that suggest the need for blood transfusion in dogs and cats with acute blood loss.
- Acute loss of > 30% of blood volume (30 ml/kg)
- Packed cell volume (hematocrit) < 20%
- Plasma protein concentration < 3.5 g/dl
- Ongoing blood loss unresponsive to crystalloid/colloid therapy
- Conditions noted in hypovolemic shock without loss of oxygen-carrying capacity, but, if persistent and unresponsive to therapy, may respond to blood administration
  Pale mucous membranes
  Prolonged capillary refill time (> 2.0 sec)
  Increased heart rate (> 180 bpm)
  Increased respiratory rate (> 60 bpm)
  Decreased arterial blood pressure (MAP < 80 mmHg)
  Decreased central venous pressure (≤ 0 cm H_2O)

9. What are the current recommendations concerning the need for blood transfusions in people? Are they applicable to veterinary patients?

According to the National Institute of Health Consensus Conference on Perioperative Red Cell Transfusions, attitudes have changed concerning the need for red cell transfusions in people:
- If the hemoglobin is > 10 g/dl, transfusion is rarely necessary.
- If the hemoglobin is < 7 g/dl, transfusion is usually indicated.
- If the hemoglobin is > 7 g/dl, but < 10 g/dl, use clinical status, mixed venous oxygen tension, and extraction ratio to determine transfusion need.

Although these recommendations probably can be extrapolated to veterinary patients, the criteria described in questions 4–8 are recommended for dogs and cats. For the most part, the state-of-the-art of monitoring in veterinary medicine is not as high as in human critical care facilities (e.g., routine use of pulmonary artery catheters, cardiac output determination).

10. Assuming whole blood transfusion is needed, how do I calculate how much blood to give?

How much do you want to raise the hematocrit? (See questions 5–8.) Once the answer is known, several formulas are available to help decide what volume to administer:
- A quick and reliable method is the "rule of 1's:" 1 ml of transfused blood per 1 pound of body weight (BW) should raise the PCV by 1%. This is about the same as 2.2 ml blood/kg BW raises the PCV 1%. Another quick estimation is that a transfusion of 20 ml/kg BW of whole blood or 10 ml/kg of packed red cells should raise the hematocrit 10%.
- Volume of blood to transfuse (ml) $= \dfrac{BW\ (kg) \times \text{desired increase in Hb} \times 70}{\text{donor Hb}}$
- BW (kg) $\times$ 90 ml/kg $\times \dfrac{\text{Desired PCV} - \text{Patient PCV}}{\text{Donor PCV}}$

The disadvantage of the second and third formulas is that the donor PCV and/or hemoglobin (Hb) concentration must be known.

11. What are the rates of blood administration in critically ill patients?

The rate depends on the need for speed. Patients in profound hemorrhagic shock with ongoing losses unresponsive to crystalloid and synthetic colloid fluids need blood *now!* Blood administration should be as fast as possible, using pressure infusors and multiple catheters if necessary.

The risks of rapid administration are certainly outweighed by the life-saving benefits. Autotransfusion is an option in addition to blood replacement therapy.

In more routine situations in which blood transfusion is to replace losses that occurred over a longer period, the recommended rate of infusion for whole blood or blood products is 10–22 ml/kg/hr.

12. How is acute hemorrhage managed during surgery?

The first step is to quantify the amount of blood lost (use suction canisters, or estimate that 1 4×4 gauze sponge contains about 5–10 ml of blood when soaked). Then decide if it is necessary to replace the lost blood. Many healthy animals can safely lose 10% of blood volume acutely, and some authors suggest they may be able to lose 40–50%. Sick animals, however, certainly cannot tolerate such a loss. Initially, treat blood loss with crystalloid volume replacement, recognizing that it takes 3 times as much crystalloid to replace 1 unit of blood. Monitor for hemodilution. If the hematocrit remains above 20%, total protein (albumin) remains above 3.5 gm/dl (1.5 gm/dl), and blood pressure is adequate, blood transfusion is usually not indicated. If these parameters fall below the above levels, or if cardiovascular function deteriorates and is unresponsive to conventional therapy, transfuse with whole blood.

13. What is autotransfusion? How is it done?

Autotransfusion, or autologous transfusion, is the collection and reinfusion of a patient's own blood. Although it has numerous indications and uses, in the emergent patient its use is limited to acute replacement of blood losses into a major body cavity (chest or abdominal cavities). Such use may gain time and save life while more appropriate measures are instituted. The usual methods of collection include centrifuge-based cell salvage, passive canister collection, and direct aspiration and reinfusion. Three components are essential: appropriate suction that does not damage red cells, filtration of blood to minimize contamination, and anticoagulation. Complications include coagulopathies, sepsis, microembolism, air embolism, and dissemination of malignancy. These risks must be weighed against the potential benefits (i.e., life) in each patient.

14. What are the risks of blood transfusions?

Risks of blood transfusions include acute and delayed hemolytic reactions, localized or systemic anaphylaxis, transmission of infectious agents, citrate toxicity (hypocalcemia), and circulatory overload.

15. What hemolytic transfusion reactions may occur? How do I recognize and treat them?

Acute hemolytic reactions (intravascular hemolysis) to donated blood occur within minutes to hours from the start of the transfusion. Signs include fever, tachycardia, restlessness, vomiting, salivation, tremors, weakness, respiratory distress, acute collapse, hypotension, and seizures. Stop the transfusion immediately, and begin aggressive fluid therapy to maintain blood pressure and renal perfusion.

Delayed hemolytic reactions (extravascular hemolysis) occur from 3 days to 3 weeks after transfusion. Signs include fever, anorexia, and icterus. Laboratory abnormalities include hyperbilirubinemia, hyperbilirubinuria, and anemia. Most delayed reactions are mild, and specific therapy is not required. The anemia that led to the initial transfusion obviously has redeveloped.

16. What immune-mediated (nonhemolytic) reactions may occur? How do I recognize and treat them?

Acute hypersensitivity reactions (anaphylaxis) usually occur almost immediately, up to 45 minutes after a transfusion is started. Signs may include urticaria, pruritus, erythema, emesis, respiratory distress, hypotension, bronchoconstriction, and severe shock, increasing in severity as anaphylaxis develops. Usually, in mild reactions, stopping the transfusion is all that is necessary to alleviate signs. Administration of diphenhydramine or glucocorticoids may help to prevent further complications.

17. Can transfusion reactions be prevented?

The risk can be reduced greatly by following these recommendations:

1. Use universal donors whenever possible.
2. Cross-match all donors with recipients, even universal donors.
3. Store and administer blood and blood products properly.

Some authors advise prophylactic treatment of high-risk patients with diphenhydramine (2–4 mg/kg SC or IM) or glucocorticoids, 15–20 minutes before transfusion. No evidence supports the prophylactic nature of this therapy, but the risks are minimal.

18. What are the blood types of dogs? Which are the most immunogenic?

Canine blood types are as follows:

- DEA 1.1
- *DEA 1.2
- *DEA 3
- DEA 4
- DEA 5
- DEA 6
- *DEA 7
- DEA 8

Types with an asterisk are most immunogenic.

19. What type is the universal canine donor?

Canine universal donors are DEA 1.1 negative and preferably DEA 1.2 negative and DEA 7 negative. Blood that is DEA 1.1 positive should be given only to DEA 1.1 positive recipients.

20. What are the blood types in cats? Which is most common?

Feline blood types are A, B, and AB. A is the most common.

21. What new treatment modalities may help to manage patients with blood loss?

The most promising new developments, soon to be available for veterinary use, are hemoglobin-based oxygen carriers (artificial blood), most of which are polymerized bovine hemoglobin solutions. These solutions have excellent oxygen-carrying capacity, provide excellent colloid osmotic pressure, and thus are effective plasma volume expanders. They also have long shelf lives and low viscosity and are minimally antigenic.

BIBLIOGRAPHY

1. Callan MB, Oakley DA, Shofer FS, Giger U: Canine red blood cell transfusion practice. J Am Animal Hosp Assoc 32:303–311, 1996.
2. Consensus Conference: Perioperative red blood cell transfusion. JAMA 260:2700, 1988.
3. Cotter SM: Practical transfusion medicine. Proceedings of the 20th Annual Waltham/OSU Symposium for the Treatment of Small Animal Diseases, 1996, pp 95–98.
4. Crowe DT, Devey JJ: Assessment and management of the hemorrhaging patient. Vet Clin North Am (Sm Anim Pract) 24:1095–1122, 1994.
5. Crystal MA, Cotter SM: Acute hemorrhage: A hematologic emergency in dogs. Comp Cont Educ Pract Vet 14:60–67, 1992.
6. Giger U, Bucheler J: Transfusion of type-A and type-B blood to cats. J Am Vet Med Assoc 198:411–418, 1991.
7. Gould SA, Lakshman R, Sehgal R, et al: Hypovolemic shock. Crit Care Clin 9:239–259, 1996.
8. Kerl ME, Hohenhaus AE: Packed red blood cell transfusions in dogs: 131 cases. J Am Vet Med Assoc 202:1495–1499, 1993.
9. Kirby R: Transfusion therapy in emergency and critical care medicine. Vet Clin North Am (Sm Anim Pract) 25:1365–1386, 1995.
10. Norsworthy GD: Clinical aspects of feline blood transfusions. Comp Cont Educ Pract Vet 14:469–475, 1992.
11. Purvis D: Autotransfusion in the emergency patient. Vet Clin North Am (Sm Anim Pract) 25:1291–1304, 1995.
12. Rudloff E, Kirby R: Hypovolemic shock and resuscitation. Vet Clin North Am (Sm Anim Pract) 24:1015–1039, 1994.
13. Van Pelt DR, Miller E, Martin LG, Hackett TB: Hematologic emergencies. Vet Clin North Am (Sm Anim Pract) 24:1139–1172, 1994.
14. Wagner AE, Dunlop CI: Anesthetic and medical management of acute hemorrhage during surgery. J Am Vet Med Assoc 203:40–45, 1993.

16. BRAIN INJURIES

Wayne E. Wingfield, D.V.M., M.S.

1. What are some of the common causes of brain injury in dogs and cats?
- Cardiopulmonary arrest
- Severe hypotension
- Status epilepticus
- Trauma
- Cerebral vascular injury (stroke)
- Thromboembolism

2. What are the intracranial components? Why are they important in discussing brain injuries?
The intracranial components are brain tissue (86%), cerebrospinal fluid (CSF) (10%), and blood (4%). An increase in any one component results in a decrease in cranial vault volume, an increase in intracranial pressure, or both.

3. What is the significance of primary vs. secondary head injury?
Primary injury is direct disruption of brain tissue at the moment of impact. Primary injury may result in contusion, hemorrhage, and/or laceration. In humans, primary injuries account for approximately 50% of deaths due to head injuries. There is no treatment for the sudden mechanical disruption of brain tissue.

Secondary injury refers to delayed insults, both systemic and intracranial. Delayed intracranial hematomas (subdural, epidural, and parenchymal) as well as generalized cerebral edema that results in elevated intracranial pressure. Secondary systemic complications generally result from hypoxemia, increased intracranial pressure, and hypotension leading to decreased perfusion and thus brain ischemia, brain swelling, and possible herniation.

4. What is cerebral perfusion pressure?
Cerebral blood flow is regulated by neuronal stimulation, $PaCO_2$, PaO_2, and pressure autoregulation. Through autoregulation, cerebral blood flow is maintained over a range of mean arterial pressures of 50–150 mmHg. Below and above this range, cerebral blood flow is linearly related to blood pressure. Cerebral perfusion pressure (CPP) is the difference between mean arterial pressure (MAP) and intracranial pressure (ICP).

$$CPP = MAP - ICP$$

An increase in ICP may result in significant changes in CPP. Even temporary occlusion of the jugular vein raises the intracranial pressure. Thus, you should probably avoid inserting a jugular catheter in such animals.

5. What are the mechanisms by which brain injury elevates intracranial pressure?
- Increased CSF volume secondary to obstruction to flow by edema or clot formation
- Increased brain tissue secondary to diffuse or localized edema
- Increased mass secondary to intracranial hematoma formation
- Increased blood volume secondary to loss of autoregulation

6. How are levels of consciousness described in head injuries?
Levels of consciousness vary from awake to mental depression, delirium, stupor (unconsciousness but responsive to noxious stimuli), and coma (unresponsive loss of consciousness).

7. How can respiratory patterns help to localize the brain lesion?
Cheyne-Stokes respiratory patterns are rhythmic waxing and waning in ventilatory depth and rate. Severe and diffuse cerebral and diencephalic lesions result in this pattern of respiration

in dogs. Hyperventilation is seen with injuries of the midbrain or pons. Obviously, hyperventilation also may result when the animal is in pain, a state of excitement, metabolic acidosis, or respiratory alkalosis. Apneustic (irregular) breathing (often accompanied by bradycardia) is associated with injury to the brainstem.

8. Describe the motor response of a decerebrate animal.

Extensor rigidity is present in both fore- and rearlimbs. The head is thrown back in opisthotonus. The prognosis is extremely grave.

9. What does an animal with decerebellate motor posturing look like?

The forelimbs are extended, the rearlimbs are flexed, and the head is thrown back into opisthotonus.

10. In animals with opisthotonus, extensor rigidity of the forelimbs, and flaccid paralysis of the rearlimbs, where is the lesion?

Trick question! This animal probably has a spinal cord lesion between T3 and L3.

11. If seizures immediately follow trauma, what does it mean?

First, you need to get a good history from the animal's owner. It is possible that the animal has a history of seizures and may well even be treated for seizures. Ask about a history of seizures before you begin to relate the seizures with head injury. Epileptiform seizures associated with head injury usually develop weeks to months (even years) after the trauma. Epileptiform seizures occurring soon after trauma suggest the presence of intraparenchymal cerebral hemorrhage.

12. Describe pupil size, reactivity, and prognosis in head trauma.

Severity	Pupil Size	Reactivity	Prognosis
Least severe	Normal (midrange)	Normal	Good
	Bilateral miosis	Poor to nonresponsive	Guarded (variable, depending on other signs)
	Unilateral mydriasis	Poor to nonresponsive (mydriatic side)	Guarded to poor
	Unilateral mydriasis with ventromedial strabismus	Nonresponsive	Guarded to poor
	Normal (midrange)	Nonresponsive	Poor to grave
Most severe	Bilateral mydriasis	Poor to nonresponsive	Poor to grave

13. What is the small animal coma score for evaluating head trauma victims?

The small animal coma score is a modification of the Glasgow coma scale used to monitor human head trauma victims. It is an attempt to standardize the assessment of the depth and duration of impaired consciousness and coma.

The Small Animal Coma Scale for Evaluating Head Trauma Victims

CATEGORY DESCRIPTION	SCORE
Motor activity	
Normal gait; normal spinal reflexes	6
Hemiparesis, tetraparesis, or decerebrate activity	5
Recumbent; intermittent extensor rigidity	4
Recumbent; constant extensor rigidity	3
Recumbent; constant extensor rigidity with opisthotonus	2
Recumbent; hypotonia of muscles; depressed or absent spinal reflexes	1

Table continued on next page.

The Small Animal Coma Scale for Evaluating Head Trauma Victims (Continued)

CATEGORY DESCRIPTION	SCORE
Brainstem reflexes	
Normal pupillary light responses and oculocephalic reflexes	6
Slow pupillary light reflexes; normal-to-reduced oculocephalic reflexes	5
Bilateral unresponsive miosis; normal-to-reduced oculocephalic reflexes	4
Pinpoint pupils; reduced-to-absent oculocephalic reflexes	3
Unilateral, unresponsive mydriasis; reduced-to-absent oculocephalic reflexes	2
Bilateral, unresponsive mydriasis; reduced-to-absent oculocephalic reflexes	1
Level of consciousness	
Occasional periods of alertness and responsive to environment	6
Depression or delirium; capable of responding to environment	5
Semicomatose; responsive to visual stimuli	4
Semicomatose; responsive to auditory stimuli	3
Semicomatose; responsive to noxious stimuli	2
Comatose; unresponsive to repeated noxious stimuli	1

Total score	Likely Prognosis
3–8	Grave
9–14	Poor to guarded
15–18	Good

From Shores A: Treatment and prognosis of head trauma. Proceedings of 13th Kal Kan Symp 29–36, 1990, with permission.

14. How are leaks of the cerebrospinal fluid detected?

CSF leaks through tears in the dura. CSF leaks can be distinguished from blood by the presence of a double-ring sign when applied to filter paper. CSF migrates further than blood, forming a target shape with blood in the center and blood-tinged CSF forming a ring outside the clot. CSF rhinorrhea can be detected by checking the glucose content of the fluid with a Dextrostix or glucometer. CSF contains approximately 60% of serum levels of glucose; nasal mucus does not contain glucose. No data are available to assess the sensitivity or specificity of these tests in dogs or cats.

15. List the cranial nerves, how to test for each, and clinical signs of deficits and abnormal neurologic signs for each.

Examination of the Cranial Nerve Responses in Brain Trauma

CRANIAL NERVE	CLINICAL TEST	NORMAL RESPONSE	CLINICAL SIGNS OF DEFICITS	ABNORMAL NEUROLOGIC SIGNS
I. Olfactory	Smell food or nonirritating, volatile substance	Interest in food Recoil or lick nose in response to the volatile substance	Decreased or no ability to smell	No reaction
II. Optic	Obstacle test	Avoidance of obstacles	Visual impairment and hesitancy in walking	Bumping into objects No reaction
	Visual placing	Visual placing of limbs		
	Menace reaction	Eye blink		No reaction
	Following movement test	Eyes follow objects		No reaction

Table continued on next page.

Examination of the Cranial Nerve Responses in Brain Trauma (Continued)

CRANIAL NERVE	CLINICAL TEST	NORMAL RESPONSE	CLINICAL SIGNS OF DEFICITS	ABNORMAL NEUROLOGIC SIGNS
II. Optic (*cont.*)	Point source of light in each eye	Direct and consensual pupillary light reflexes	Dilated pupil (mydriasis)	On affected side, direct pupillary reflex is absent, consensual reflex is present; on normal side, direct pupillary reflex is present, consensual reflex is absent
III. Oculomotor	Ocular movements in horizontal and vertical planes	Normal ocular excursion	Ventrolateral strabismus Paralysis of upper eyelid (Ptsosis)	Impaired movements of affected eye
	Point source of light in each eye	Direct and consensual pupillary light reflexes	Mydriasis	On affected side direct pupillary reflex is absent, consensual reflex is present; on normal side, direct pupillary reflex is present, consensual reflex is absent
IV. Trochlear			Usually not noted	
V. Trigeminal (motor and sensory)	Jaw tone—palpate and observe masticatory muscles	Resistance to opening the jaws; normal muscle contour to skull	Atrophy of masticatory muscles Inability to close jaws with impaired prehension	Lack of resistance; atrophy of muscles
	Palpebral reflex	Eye blink		No reaction
	Corneal reflex	Globe retraction		No reaction
	Probe nasal mucosa	Recoil from nasal probe		No reaction
	Touch face	No reaction to touching face		Intense discomfort to touching the face
VI. Abducent	Ocular movements in horizontal plane	Normal ocular excursion	Medial strabismus	Impaired lateral movement of affected eye
VII. Facial	Palpebral reflex	Eye blink	Asymmetry of facial expression	No reaction
	Corneal reflex	Eye blink	Inability to close eyelids	No reaction
	Menace reaction	Eye blink		No reaction
	Tickle ear	Ear flick	Lip commissure paralysis Ear paralysis	No reaction

Table continued on next page.

Examination of the Cranial Nerve Responses in Brain Trauma (Continued)

CRANIAL NERVE	CLINICAL TEST	NORMAL RESPONSE	CLINICAL SIGNS OF DEFICITS	ABNORMAL NEUROLOGIC SIGNS
VIII. Vestibulo-cochlear				
Vestibular	Ocular movements in horizontal or vertical plane	Physiologically induced nystagmus (post-rotatory nystagmus)	Nystagmus, head tilt	No reaction, spontaneous positional nystagmus, strabismus (ventrolateral with dorsal head extension)
	Caloric or rotatory test	Physiologically induced nystagmus (post-rotatory nystagmus)	Circling	Same as above
	Righting reactions	Normal righting	Righting reflexes	Same as above
Cochlear	Handclap over ear	Startle reaction; blink; ear contraction	Deafness	No reaction
IX. Glosso-pharyngeal	Gag reflex	Swallow	Dysphagia	No reaction
X. Vagus	Gag reflex	Swallow	Dysphagia	No reaction
	Laryngeal reflex	Cough	Abnormal vocalizing	No reaction
	Oculocardiac reflex	Bradycardia	Inspiratory distress	No reaction
XI. Spinal accessory	Palpation of of cervical musculature	Normal cervical contour and muscle tone	Usually not noted but may see dorsolateral cervical muscle atrophy; torticollis	Muscle atrophy or hypotonia
XII. Hypoglossal	Tongue stretch	Retraction	Deviation of tongue	No reaction
	Rub nose	Lip response		No reaction

16. Do skull radiographs help in the evaluation and treatment of animals with head trauma?

Unfortunately, radiographs provide no evaluation of soft tissue structures within the cranial vault, but they do indicate the presence and severity of skull fractures. Computed tomography (CT) is considered the best means to assess skull fractures and magnetic resonance tomography (MRI) is the best method for visualizing detail of brain parenchymal injury.

17. Describe the essentials of management of head-injured animals.

- Management and protection of the airway
- Controlled ventilation to maintain normal or low $PaCO_2$
- Maintenance of cerebral blood flow
- Treatment of elevated intracranial pressure
- Evaluation and treatment of secondary systemic complications:

    Gastrointestinal bleeding   Neurogenic pulmonary edema

    Disseminated intravascular   Hypotension secondary to blood loss or spinal shock

      coagulopathy   Hypoxemia secondary to thoracic trauma or aspiration

18. What is involved in the initial emergency management of a dog or cat with head trauma?

Follow the system-based priorities. Arterial bleeding, respiratory compromise, cardiovascular function, and hemorrhage and transfusion should be managed before definitive treatment for brain injury. Because hypoxemia and hypovolemia are extremely detrimental to an already compromised brain, oxygen delivery and cardiovascular support are immediate therapeutic requirements.

19. What is known about emergency fluid therapy in animals with brain injury?

The goal of fluid therapy is to administer the minimal amount of fluid necessary to maintain hydration and autoregulatory blood pressure values (50–150 mmHg). The decision to use crystalloid, hypertonic saline, or synthetic colloidal fluids remains extremely controversial. If large volumes of crystalloids (i.e., 90 ml/kg/hr in dogs) are administered, brain edema worsens and results in further increases in intracranial pressure. Hypertonic saline administration in hypotensive small animals increases myocardial contractility and cardiac output, improves peripheral perfusion, increases urine output, and improves mesenteric and coronary blood flow. These effects are transient (15–60 min). Obviously, hypertonic saline is not used in dehydrated animals, animals with uncontrolled hemorrhage or hypernatremia, hyperosmolar animals, or animals with hypothermia, congestive heart failure, or oliguric renal failure. Evidence of ongoing intracranial hemorrhage should raise concern. Concerns over the use of synthetic colloids are directed mainly to leakage from the vessels of the brain. Although hypertonic saline and Hetastarch reduce or prevent brain edema and elevations in intracranial pressure, they fail to increase oxygen delivery and perfusion to damaged brain tissue.

20. So what is the answer? Which and how much fluid should you use in brain trauma?

Intravenous crystalloid fluids are administered at an initial volume not to exceed 20 ml/kg/hr. After this initial bolus of fluids, fluid rates are given using the following formula to provide basal water requirements:

$$\text{ml crystalloid fluids/day} = (\text{body weight [kg]} \times 30) + 70$$

Monitor blood pressure, if possible, and monitor for negative changes in neurologic status during intravenous fluid administration.

21. How do you hyperoxygenate an animal with head trauma?

Methods for supplemental oxygen administration include oxygen cages, nasal oxygen insufflation catheters, and tracheal intubation. Although often mistrusted, the oxygen cage provides a constant concentration of oxygen, the least amount of stress, and the least invasive means of delivery. Nasal insufflation catheters provide oxygen levels of approximately 40% oxygen with flow rates of 50 ml/kg/min. The disadvantages are that the animal often will not tolerate the cannula, patient movement is restricted, and nasal drying and hemorrhage are common.

22. When is ventilator therapy used to reduce intracranial pressure?

Tough decision, with little information in the veterinary literature. Generally speaking, positive pressure ventilation is used whenever an animal cannot ventilate or oxygenate or works excessively to maintain ventilation and oxygenation. Reliable guidelines can be gained only from arterial blood gas values. Hypoventilation is defined as a $PaCO_2 > 60$ mmHg. Inadequate oxygenation is defined as a $PaO_2 < 60$ mmHg. Hyperventilation reduces cerebral blood volume as much as 36%, whereas hypoventilation increases cerebral blood volume as much as 170%. The goal is to maintain the $PaCO_2$ near 25 mmHg, which has been determined to be the optimal $PaCO_2$ for producing cerebrovascular vasoconstriction while still maintaining adequate perfusion to the brain. This effect is mediated through acute alterations in cerebral interstitial fluid pH; therefore, it generally becomes less effective after 48–72 hours. Humidify all oxygen when ventilating an animal. While the animal is ventilated, the head should be at approximately 30° to ensure adequate venous return of blood from the head.

23. How does mannitol decrease the intracranial pressure?

Brain tissue has a slightly greater osmolarity than blood. A gradient of approximately 3 mOsm/L is maintained by the blood–brain barrier. Mannitol is an osmotically active drug that reverses this osmotic gradient and shifts water from the brain to the blood. An increase of osmolarity by 10 mOsm/L removes 100–150 ml of water from the brain. In humans, it is reported that hyperosmolar treatment of elevated intracranial pressure increases the normal serum osmolarity of 290 to a value of 300–315 mOsm/L. An osmolarity < 300 is ineffective; an osmolarity > 315 results in renal and neurologic dysfunction. Such data are not available for dogs or cats.

24. Should mannitol be administered to head-injured dogs and cats?

Administration of mannitol is controversial and may pose inherent risks. The controversy centers largely on the safety of administration of mannitol when intracranial hemorrhage may be undetectable. There are several pitfalls in this scenario:
- Extravascular hemorrhage may increase.
- Increased blood flow may exacerbate hemorrhage.
- More room may be available for extravasation of epidural or subdural hemorrhage.

Of interest, these theoretical contraindications have not been confirmed through experimentation. Focal neurologic deficits may suggest hemorrhage, and mannitol is usually not administered. More commonly, diffuse deficits are noted, suggesting edema; thus, mannitol is given at a dosage of 0.25 gm/kg by slow intravenous injection.

25. Should furosemide be given in head trauma?

In humans with head trauma, furosemide reduces intracranial pressure and improves neurologic outcome. Presumably it exerts its effects by causing diuresis, decreasing cerebrospinal fluid production, and reducing astroglial swelling. Some suggest that mannitol and furosemide have a synergistic effect in reducing intracranial pressure.

26. Should corticosteroids be used in head trauma?

Old habits are hard to break. The primary rationale for glucocorticoid administration is to reduce brain swelling. Unfortunately, glucocorticoids have consistently failed to show any significant beneficial (clinical or experimental) effects on the outcome of animals with brain trauma. In humans, glucocorticoid therapy does not reduce intracranial pressure or cerebral edema or improve overall outcome. Will it do harm? Probably not. If you need an excuse for administering glucocorticoids in head trauma, remember the old adage, "No animal should die without the benefit of corticosteroids."

27. What is the role of barbiturates in the treatment of increased intracranial pressure?

Barbiturates decrease cerebral metabolic rate and cerebral blood flow. Theoretically, they should lower intracranial pressure. To date, their use is controversial.

28. Is dimethyl sulfoxide (DMSO) useful in treating head trauma?

DMSO has been effective in reducing intracranial pressure and improving the outcome of brain injury, both experimentally and clinically. It reportedly exerts a neuroprotective effect by reducing oxygen and glucose requirements of brain tissue, scavenges oxygen free radical species, stabilizes lysosomal membranes, directly decreases brain edema by stabilizing capillary endothelial cells, and indirectly reduces brain edema through antiinflammatory and diuretic properties. DMSO is given at a dosage of 0.5–1.0 gm/kg by slow (30–45 min) intravenous injection every 8–12 hours. Detrimental effects from DMSO include intravascular hemolysis and prolonged bleeding times. If you use DMSO, use it soon after injury and be prepared for its obnoxious smell.

29. What factors are useful in establishing a prognosis for brain-injured animals?

Factors such as level of consciousness, brainstem reflexes, motor ability, respiratory patterns, and presence of other injuries help the veterinarian to establish a prognosis. Such signs as coma persisting more than 48 hours despite therapy, decerebrate rigidity, and ataxic or apneustic respiratory patterns in comatose patients usually culminate in permanent dysfunction or death.

BIBLIOGRAPHY

1. Braund KG: Idiopathic and exogenous causes of neuropathies in dogs and cats. Vet Med 91:755–769, 1996.
2. Cottrell JE, Marlin AE: Furosemide and human head injury. J Trauma 21:805–806, 1981.
3. Dewey CW, Budsberg SC, Oliver JE Jr: Principles of head trauma management in dogs and cats—Part I. Comp Vet Cont Educ 14:199–207, 1992.
4. Dewey CW, Budsberg SC, Oliver JE Jr: Principles of head trauma management in dogs and cats—Part II. Comp Vet Cont Educ 15:177–193, 1993.
5. Poole GV, Johnson JC, Prough DS, et al: Cerebral hemodynamics after hemorrhagic shock: Effects of the type of resuscitation fluid. Crit Care Med 14:629–633, 1986.
6. Prough DS, Johnson JC, Poole GV, et al: Effects on intracranial pressure of resuscitation from hemorrhagic shock with hypertonic saline versus lactated Ringer's solution. Crit Care Med 13:407–411, 1985.

17. ACUTE SPINAL CORD INJURIES

Wayne E. Wingfield, D.V.M., M.S.

1. List the common causes of spinal cord trauma in small animals.
- Exogenous causes
  Automobile trauma
  Falls
  Falling objects
  Projectile wounds
- Endogenous causes
  Intervertebral disc extrusion
  Fibrocartilagenous infarct

2. Explain the mechanism of spinal cord trauma.

The spinal cord is encircled by a rigid, inelastic bony encasement (vertebrae). If the spinal canal diameter decreases due to displacement of vertebrae, hemorrhage, or edema, the spinal cord is easily displaced and intraspinal pressure increases. Pressure changes lead to ischemia, further hemorrhage, or edema, all of which lead to a self-perpetuating process of spinal cord damage that often was present with the initial mechanical injury (second injury theory).

3. What are some of the endogenous mediators of the second injury theory in spinal cord trauma?
- Excitatory amino acid neurotransmitters
- Endorphins
- Catecholamines
- Eicosanoids
- Unstable oxygen-free radicals

4. Why are endogenous mediators important?

Most current therapeutic efforts are directed at counterbalancing or neutralizing endogenous mediators of cell injury.

5. What is Schiff-Sherrington syndrome?

Schiff-Sherrington syndrome is characterized by thoracic limb hyperextension and paraplegia of the rear limbs due to injury to the thoracolumbar spinal cord (T3–L3). The mechanism is based on neurons located in the lumbar spinal cord that are responsible for tonic inhibition of extensor muscle alpha motorneurons in the cervical intumescence. These inhibitory neurons are called border cells, and their cell bodies are located on the dorsolateral border of the ventral grey column from L1 through L7 with a maximal population from L2 through L4. Their axons cross to the contralateral fasciculus proprius of the lateral funiculus, where they ascend to the cervical intumescence. Acute spinal injuries cranial to border cell neurons and caudal to the cervical intumescence result in sudden deprivation of tonic inhibition of cervical intumescence neurons and cause their release. This release results in the extensor hypertonia observed in the thoracic limbs; there are no abnormalities cranial to C5. This posture is usually seen with severe spinal cord injuries.

6. How do you know if you are dealing with a Schiff-Sherrington lesion or a lesion to the cervical spine?

Provide minimal manipulation to the paw of the forelimbs with a pin or mild pressure with forceps to determine whether pain and voluntary motion are present. In the Schiff-Sherrington syndrome, pain and voluntary motion are present in the thoracic limbs and absent in the pelvic limbs. With cervical cord injuries, tone and deficit in pain and voluntary movement are more nearly equal in all four limbs.

7. What is spinal shock?

Spinal shock is a temporary concussive-like condition in which cord-mediated reflexes are absent. It results in complete suppression of all spinal segmental reflexes below the level of a lesion affecting the upper motor neuron (UMN) because of separation from higher centers and from functional disturbances caused by sudden disorganization in the dendritic zone and cell body of the general somatic efferent motor neuron. Spinal shock in domestic animals is of little clinical significance because spinal reflexes are present caudal to the lesion by the time the animal is presented to the veterinarian. Spinal shock appears to last only about 30–60 minutes. This fact is important when the animal presents shortly after the injury. Be sure to reexamine the animal 1–2 hours later to determine the location and extent of the lesion.

8. What parameters should be assessed on physical examination?

The key parameters are the spine itself and the neurologic examination. The spine is carefully palpated to assess tenderness, deformity, and muscle spasm. Because the veterinarian is palpating only one side of the vertebrae, a fracture may still be present even in the absence of tenderness or displacement. During the neurologic evaluation allowances must be made for the fact that the animal may have an unstable vertebral fracture and normal manipulations may be detrimental. Begin the examination in whichever position the animal arrives at the hospital (usually lateral recumbency). First note motor responses that may suggest the presence of decerebrate, decerebellate, or Schiff-Sherrington syndrome. The cranial nerves usually can be assessed accurately but the head must be manipulated with caution because cervical injury is possible. Reflex function of the thoracic and pelvic upside is assessed in the recumbent animal. Check for a panniculus response (cutaneous trunci reflex) and evidence of hyperesthesia. Check for superficial and deep pain responses last. If a spinal cord trauma is suspected at this point, the animal should be stabilized (taped) to a rigid surface (sheet of plexiglass) before further manipulation. Radiographs should be taken as soon as possible to assess for instability, compression, or other injuries to the vertebrae.

9. What neurologic findings suggest complete spinal cord compression along the various vertebral segments?

Neurologic Findings Suggesting Complete Spinal Cord Compression

SEGMENT OF THE SPINAL CORD	MOTOR	SENSORY	AUTONOMIC
C1–C4	UMN tetraplegia	Anesthesia	Apnea, no micturition
C5–C6	UMN tetraplegia, LMN suprascapular nerve	Anesthesia, hyperesthesia-midcervical	Apnea-phrenic nerve, LMN, no micturition
C7–T2	Tetraplegia or UMN paraplegia, LMN brachial plexus	Anesthesia, hyperesthesia-brachial plexus	Diaphragmatic breathing only, no micturition
T3–L3	UMN paraplegia, Schiff-Sherrington syndrome	Anesthesia	Diaphragmatic breathing, some intercostal and abdominal respiration (depending upon the level of the lesion), no micturition
L4–S1	Paraplegia with LMN lumbosacral plexus	Anesthesia, segmental hyperesthesia	No micturition, with an S1 lesion the anal sphincter tone may be atonic
S1–S3	Knuckling of the hind foot, paralysis of the tail	Anesthesia, segmental hyperesthesia	No micturition, atonic sphincters
Cy1–Cy5	Paralysis of the tail	Anesthesia, segmental hyperesthesia	None

C = cervical, T = thoracic, L = lumbar, S = sacral, Cy = coccygeal, UMN = upper motor neuron, LMN = lower motor neuron.

10. What radiographs should be taken of a suspected spinal cord injury?

Two views are mandatory. With the animal taped to a solid surface, such as a sheet of plexiglass, the lateral radiograph is easily obtained without manipulating the animal. If at all possible, the ventrodorsal view should be taken using a horizontal beam from the radiographic machine.

11. Does the radiographic appearance of the vertebral column help with prognosis?

No. The radiograph is a static record of the lesion at the time of the study. It does not assess the degree of displacement of the vertebrae at the time of the injury or before the radiograph was taken. The paraspinal musculature is extremely strong and often can pull displaced vertebrae back to near-normal position before the radiograph is taken.

12. What are the ABCS of interpreting the lateral radiograph of the vertebrae?

A = **A**lignment
B = **B**ones
C = **C**artilage (intervertebral joint spaces and facet joints)
S = **S**oft tissue

13. What initial resuscitative efforts do you administer to an animal with a spinal cord injury?

Spinal immobilization is important to prevent worsening the injury. Airway management is important but is usually not faced by most veterinarians. The animal with a cervical fracture sufficient to paralyze the phrenic nerve often does not arrive at the hospital. Undoubtedly airway management is the most immediate threat to patients with injury to the spinal cord. This threat comes from hypoxemia (hypoventilation) and aspiration pneumonitis. Animals that are mildly hypoxemic may respond to supplemental, nasally administered oxygen. If the lesion is above C5, the animal requires early intubation and assisted ventilation. Fortunately, emergency tracheostomy is rarely required. Pulse oximetry should be used for continuous assessment of the adequacy of arterial oxygen saturation, and arterial blood gases are used to monitor the partial pressure of oxygen and carbon dioxide.

14. What are the cardiovascular consequences of a cervical spinal cord injury?
Loss of systemic sympathetic vasomotor tone after a cervical injury may result in vasodilation, increased venous capacity, and hypotension. The associated bradycardia should distinguish this reaction from shock due to hemorrhage. Careful administration of crystalloids is usually adequate to correct this relative hypovolemia.

15. How do you decide whether to administer medical or surgical therapy?
Tough question. First it depends on the surgical skills of the veterinarian or the availability of a surgical specialist. Second, there is little objective guidance in the available literature to help make this decision. Most of the veterinary data is derived from anecdotal experiences or extrapolated from research animals or human medicine. The table below summarizes the 1996 guidelines devised by Bagley.

Scoring of Severity of Spinal Cord Injury

SCORE	CLINICAL STATUS	SEVERITY	THERAPY
10	Normal	Least severe	
8	Pain only		Candidate for
6	Paresis (walking)		medical therapy
5	Paresis (not walking)		Candidate for a
4	Plegia (micturition, pain intact)		combination of
3	Plegia (micturition absent, deep pain intact)		medical and
2	Plegia (deep pain absent < 48 hr)		surgical therapies
1	Plegia (deep pain absent > 48 hr)		Extremely poor
0	Myelomalacia	Most severe	prognosis

16. Are corticosteroids indicated in spinal cord injury?
No clinical data are available for veterinary patients. Most recommendations follow published results of the Second National Acute Spinal Cord Injury Study (in humans), which indicate improved neurologic outcome when methylprednisolone is given in a bolus dosage of 30 mg/kg, followed by 5.4 mg/kg/hr for 23 hours. Patients were not cured but demonstrated greater preservation of neurologic function. Veterinarians have modified this approach and give 2 additional dosages of methylprednisolone instead of the constant-rate infusion at a rate of 15 mg/kg IV at 2 and 6 hours. No data are available to note the effectiveness.

17. What are the absolute indications for surgery?
Spinal instability and spinal cord compression.

18. What other therapies may be tried?
Many drugs, including dimethyl sulfoxide, thyrotropin-releasing hormone (TRH), naloxone, and other corticosteroids have been tried. No results have proved to be effective in reversing the second injury of spinal cord trauma.

BIBLIOGRAPHY

1. Anderson DK, Hall ED: Pathophysiology of spinal cord trauma. Ann Emerg Med 22:987–992, 1993.
2. Bagley RS: Treatment of spinal cord trauma in companion animals. Proceedings of the Annual Conference of Veterinarians. Washington State University, 1996, pp 243–247.
3. Bracken MB, Shepard MJ, Collins WF Jr, et al: A randomized, controlled trial of methylprednisolone or naloxone in the treatment of acute spinal cord injury: Results of the second National Acute Spinal Cord Study. N Engl J Med 322:1405–1411, 1990.
4. Bracken MB, Shepard MJ, Collins WF Jr, et al: Methylprednisolone or naloxone treatment after acute spinal cord injury: 1-year follow-up data: Results of the second National Acute Spinal Cord Injury Study. J Neurosurg 76:23–31, 1992.
5. Brown SA, Hall ED: Role of oxygen-derived free radicals in the pathogenesis of shock and trauma, with focus on central nervous system injuries. J Am Vet Med Assoc 200:1849–1858, 1992.
6. De Lahunta A: Small animal spinal cord disease. In Veterinary Neuroanatomy and Clinical Neurology, 2nd ed. Philadelphia, W.B. Saunders, pp 175–214.
7. Hall ED: Lipid antioxidants in acute central nervous system injury. Ann Emerg Med 22:1022–1027, 1993.
8. Shell LG: Differential diagnosis for acute-onset paraparesis. Vet Med 91:230–239, 1996.

18. PERIPHERAL NERVE TRAUMA

Wayne E. Wingfield, D.V.M., M.S.

1. What is the most common cause of neuropathies in animals?

Trauma is the most common cause of neuropathy to peripheral, cranial, and spinal nerves in animals.

2. What are some of the causes of nerve injury?
- Projectiles
- Fractures
- Pressure
- Stretching (see brachial plexus below)
- Mechanical blows
- Iatrogenic causes
  Surgery
  Casts and splints
  Injections

3. Numerous terms are associated with injuries to nerves. For each of the following, provide a working definition in terms of structural damage:
- **Neuropraxia**
  An interruption in the function and conduction of a nerve, without structural damage.
- **Wallerian degeneration**
  Axonal necrosis and myelin fragmentation.
- **Neurotmesis**
  Complete severing of all nerve structures with Wallerian degeneration of the distal nerve stump.
- **Axonotmesis**
  Damage to the nerve fibers results in degeneration, but the endoneurial and Schwann cell sheaths remain intact and provide a framework for axonal regeneration.

4. What two fractures are most commonly associated with neuropathy in small animals?
- Humerus: radial nerve
- Acetabulum: ischiatic (sciatic) nerve

5. Identify the nerves, spinal cord origin, muscles innervated, and clinical signs of injury for each of the thoracic limbs.

Thoracic Limb Nerves and Associated Origin, Muscles Innervated, and Clinical Signs of Injury

NERVE	SPINAL CORD ORIGIN	MUSCLES INNERVATED	CLINICAL SIGNS OF INJURY
Suprascapular	C6–C7	Supraspinatus Infraspinatus	Loss of shoulder extension Muscle atrophy with prominent scapular spine
Axillary	C7–C8	Deltoideus Teres minor Teres major	Reduced shoulder flexion Deltoid atrophy Reduced sensation over lateral shoulder surface
Musculocutaneous	C6–C8	Biceps brachii Brachialis Coracobrachialis	Reduced elbow flexion Loss of bicipital reflex Reduced sensation over medial forearm surface
Radial	C7–T2	Triceps brachii Extensor carpi radialis Lateral digital extensor Common digital extensor	Reduced extension of elbow, carpus, and digits Loss of extensor postural thrust and limb support Loss of triceps reflex Reduced sensation over dorsal paw and craniolateral forearm surface
Median	C8–T2	Flexor carpi radialis Superficial digital extensor	Reduced flexion of carpus and digits Reduced sensation over palmar paw surface
Ulnar	C8–T2	Flexor carpi ulnaris Deep digital flexor	Reduced flexion of carpus and digits Reduced sensation over caudal forearm surface

6. Which nerves make up the brachial plexus of the thoracic limb?

The brachial plexus is made up of the ventral branches of the sixth, seventh, and eighth cervical and first two thoracic spinal nerves.

7. What is the proposed mechanism of injury leading to brachial plexus root avulsion?

It is speculated that the thoracic limb is abducted severely from the body or the entire shoulder mechanism is driven away from its normal position. This force puts a tremendous tension on the nerve roots, and injury is due to stretching and tearing of the roots within the spinal canal. Nerve roots lack a perineurium and thus are susceptible to stretch injuries. The avulsion is usually intradural, and degenerative changes are characterized by axonal necrosis, myelin fragmentation, and loss of myelinated fibers. Many fibers are damaged where they penetrate the leptomeninges, resulting in neuroma formation.

8. What clinical signs are associated with a brachial nerve root avulsion?

Clinical signs of brachial nerve root avulsion include various gait abnormalities, depending on the site and extent of damage, and Horner's syndrome due to damage to the sympathetic nerves at their exit point from the spinal canal at the cranial thoracic vertebrae.

9. How do you differentiate brachial nerve root avulsion from radial nerve paralysis?

	Brachial Nerve Root Avulsion	*Radial Nerve Paralysis*
Location of lesion	Sixth, seventh, eighth cervical and first two thoracic nerves	Seventh, eighth cervical and first two thoracic nerves
Loss of sensation	Any sensory dermatome on thoracic limb	Craniolateral forearm and dorsum of paw
Panniculus reflex	May be absent ipsilaterally	Present
Horner's syndrome	May be present (often only partial)	Absent
Presence of muscle atrophy	Any thoracic limb muscle	Triceps brachii, carpal extensors

10. What is the likelihood of return of function in a thoracic limb with brachial plexus avulsion?

The prognosis should be considered guarded to poor. In one study, 28% (8 of 29 dogs) regained reasonable return of function of the affected limb 4 or more months after injury.

11. What is the treatment for brachial nerve root avulsion?

There is no practical means to affect return of function. Assuming no evidence of infection, self-mutilation, or limb trauma, it is reasonable to wait 4–6 months before considering amputation. Some may choose transposition of the bicipital tendon and carpal fusion as alternatives to amputation, but long-term studies are unavailable to review expected results.

12. Identify the nerves, spinal cord origin, muscles innervated, and clinical signs of injury for each of the pelvic limbs.

Pelvic Limb Nerves and Associated Origin, Muscles Innervated, and Clinical Signs of Injury

NERVE	SPINAL CORD ORIGIN	MUSCLES INNERVATED	CLINICAL SIGNS OF INJURY
Femoral	L4–L6	Iliopsoas	Inability to extend the stifle or bear weight
		Quadriceps	Loss of patellar reflex
		Sartorius	Reduced sensation over medial paw, hock, stifle, and thigh surface
Obturator	L5–L6	External obturator	Inability to adduct hip or thigh (animal does splits on smooth surface)
		Pectineous	
		Gracilis	
Sciatic	L4–S1	Biceps femoris	Inability to flex the stifle
		Semimembranosus	Loss of flexor reflex
		Semitendinosus	
Tibial	L6 or 7–S1	Gastrocnemius	Inability to extend the hock or flex digits
		Popliteus	Reduced sensation over plantar paw surface
		Deep digital flexor	Loss of gastrocnemius reflex
		Superficial digital flexor	
Common peroneal	L6-7–S1	Peroneus longus	Inability to flex hock or extend digits
		Lateral digital extensor	Knuckling of dorsal paw
		Cranial tibial	Reduced sensation over craniodorsal paw, hock, and stifle surface
Pudendal	S1–S3	External anal sphincter	Loss of anal reflex and bulbocavernosus reflex (males)
		Striated urethral muscle	Reduced sensation to perineum
Pelvic plexus (parasympathetic)	S1–S3	Smooth muscle of rectum and bladder	Urinary incontinence

13. What determines a nerve's regenerative ability? If it occurs, at what rate does the nerve grow?

The ability of a nerve to regenerate is directly proportional to the continuity of its connective-tissue structures. In neuropraxic and axonotmestic lesions, in which the endoneurial connective tissue and Schwann cells remain intact, the potential for axonal regeneration is good. In neurotmesis, axonal regeneration is thwarted by lack of connective-tissue tubes and scar tissue. Once the axon has grown past the point of injury and penetrates a Schwann tube in the distal nerve stump, remyelination occurs. Axonal regeneration occurs at a rate of 1–4 mm/day.

14. How can a diagnosis of neuropathy be confirmed? When should this diagnostic test be run?

Electrodiagnostic testing is most helpful in evaluating the integrity and severity of nerve injury. Increased insertional activity, positive sharp waves, and fibrillation potentials are detected at 5–7 days after injury.

15. What is the treatment for peripheral nerve injury?

Realistically, little can be done by most veterinarians. Surgical anastomosis of a severed nerve is an extremely difficult procedure, and few veterinary surgeons have the necessary skill. Most animals with peripheral nerve injuries are monitored for infection, self-mutilation, and complications of injury. Ultimately, amputation is often the treatment provided.

16. What immunosuppressive drug shows promise in accelerating nerve regeneration?

Cyclosporin A.

BIBLIOGRAPHY

1. Braund KG: Idiopathic and exogenous causes of neuropathies in dogs and cats. Vet Med 91:755–769, 1996.
2. Duncan ID: Peripheral neuropathy in the dog and cat. Prog Vet Neurol 2:111–128, 1991.
3. Gibson KL, Daniloff JK: Peripheral nerve repair. Comp Vet Cont Educ 11:938–944, 1989.
4. Gilmore DR: Sciatic nerve injury in twenty-nine dogs. J Am Animal Hosp Assoc 20:403–407, 1984.
5. Steinberg SH: Brachial plexus injuries and dysfunctions. Vet Clin North Am (Sm Animal Pract) 18:565–580, 1988.
6. Wheeler SJ, Clayton Jones DG, Wright JA: The diagnosis of brachial plexus disorders in dogs: A review of 22 cases. J Small Animal Pract 27:147, 1986.

19. EXTREMITY TRAUMA

Wayne E. Wingfield, D.V.M., M.S.

1. What are the immediate treatment priorities in an open fracture?

Open fractures are considered orthopedic emergencies. If you find a break in the skin, it should be assumed to communicate with the fracture until proved otherwise. Immediate care includes the following:

- Application of a sterile pressure dressing to control hemorrhage, if necessary
- Assessment for neurovascular damage
- Management of pain
- Careful removal of hair surrounding the open fracture
- Debridement of foreign debris and dead tissue at the fracture site
- Thorough irrigation of the site with copious volumes of sterile saline
- Culture of the wound site

- Application of Betadine dressing to cover the wound
- Application of splint, if possible
- Institution of intravenous antibiotics (cephalosporins)
- Consultation with a surgical specialist

2. What rule should be applied in splinting a fracture?
Immobilize the joint above and the joint below the fracture.

3. Which fractures are more likely to be open fractures in dogs and cats?
The radius/ulna and tibia/fibula are the long bones most likely to have an open fracture. Because of their proximity to the skin, with any break in the skin overlying the fracture you should treat the fracture as if it were open to the air.

4. What neurologic deficit is most likely to be seen with a humeral shaft fracture?
The radial nerve may be stretched (neuropraxia) or lacerated. If so, the patient cannot extend the carpus and forefoot. The dorsum of the paw is anesthetic, and self-mutilation often ensues. In checking for superficial pain via the superficial radial nerve, it is imperative to avoid dermatomes innervated by the ulnar and median nerves.

5. What is a Monteggia fracture?
A fracture of the proximal one-third of the ulna with radial head dislocation, usually anterior, constitutes a Monteggia fracture.

6. What are the major complications in pelvic fracture?
Urologic injuries	Osteoarthritis when fractures involve the acetabulum
Hemorrhage	Urinary incontinence with sacroiliac fractures
Narrowing of pelvic canal	

7. What is a greenstick fracture?
A greenstick fracture is caused by an angular force applied to a long bone with bowing of one side of the cortex and fracture of the other. They are sometimes called incomplete fractures and are more likely in younger animals because of their more elastic bones.

8. What is the Salter-Harris classification of fractures?
The Salter-Harris (SH) classification is a method of classifying epiphyseal injuries. Any epiphyseal injury may result in growth disturbances, and the animal's owner should be so informed. The following descriptions are used in the SH classification:

Salter-Harris Classification of Epiphyseal Injuries

TYPE	DESCRIPTION
I	Fracture extends through the epiphyseal plate, resulting in displacement of the epiphysis.
II	As in type I, with the additional fracture of a triangular segment of metaphysis.
III	Fracture line runs from the joint surface through the epiphyseal plate and epiphysis.
IV	Fracture line, as seen in type III, passes through the adjacent metaphysis.
V	Crush injury of the epiphysis; may be difficult to determine with radiographic examination. Look for significantly narrowed epiphyseal space, using the opposite leg for comparison.

9. How do you initially manage fractures of the metacarpal/metatarsal or phalangeal bones?
All have the potential of being open fractures. Pain relief and splinting are important initial treatments, followed by careful assessment for evidence of tendon injuries.

10. How do you initially manage carpal or tarsal fractures?

Open fractures are managed as described above. With closed fractures, splinting and consultation with an orthopedic specialist are the best strategies.

11. With coxofemoral luxation, in which direction do the femoral head and neck normally move?

In a cranial and dorsal direction.

12. When do you attempt closed reduction of coxofemoral luxation?

If you expect to have success in replacing a coxofemoral luxation via closed reduction, the procedure should be done within the first 24 hours after trauma. The animal also should be stable enough to withstand general anesthesia.

13. What is a Velpeau sling?

The Velpeau sling is used to hold a coxofemoral luxation in place after reduction.

14. Why take postreduction radiographs in luxations of the coxofemoral or elbow?

You need confirmation that the reduction was successful. Reduced joints may luxate again.

15. Why do you usually replace an elbow luxation earlier than a coxofemoral luxation?

Pain seems to be a bigger problem with elbow luxations. Unless you can reduce the fracture, it is sometimes difficult to resolve the clinical signs of shock.

16. Are shoulder luxations common? How are they usually managed?

Luxations of the scapulohumeral joint are not common in dogs and cats. Management includes a thorough neurologic assessment followed by surgical repair.

17. Do pelvic fractures require surgical repair?

Surgery is indicated for the following reasons in pelvic fractures:
• Fractures of the acetabulum involving weight-bearing surfaces of the acetabulum
• Instability of the sacroiliac joint(s)
• Narrowing of the pelvic canal, as seen with multiple pelvic fractures
• Fractures of the ischium resulting in loss of hamstring muscle function

18. How do you manage a patient with a fractured head or neck of the femur?

Controversial issue. Ideally one would surgically repair the fracture to restore the functional coxofemoral joint. Unfortunately, most animals also lose the blood supply to the capital epiphysis; thus, avascular necrosis results. If surgical reduction is not successful, one can always resort to a femoral neck ostectomy or, more rarely, consider insertion of a prosthetic device.

19. How would one manage a gunshot wound to a joint?

Generally treatment of all open joint injuries should include broad-spectrum antibiotics before, during, and after arthrotomy, surgical debridement and irrigation, and primary closure of the wound, whenever possible. All retained intrasynovial shot or fragments should be removed. Not only do they cause mechanical dysfunction, but the lead is dissolved by the synovial fluid and becomes deposited in subsynovial tissues, causing subsequent periarticular fibrosis. The toxic action of lead on joint cartilage may also cause chondrolysis and, eventually, severe arthritis.

20. What are the complications of flail chest? How is it treated?

Rib fractures are reported in 25% of trauma patients. When rib fractures are found, internal thoracic damage should be assumed. Isolated rib fractures are rarely of concern. Flail chest occurs when multiple adjacent ribs are fractured in two places, creating a free-floating section of chest wall. Severe respiratory signs result from paradoxical motion of the unstable segment, underlying thoracic trauma, and marked hypoventilation due to pain. Treatment should be directed at resolving the underlying pulmonary contusions and draining air or fluid. Conservative treatment of the flail segment consists of local intercostal nerve blocks and pain management. Fixation is rarely used to stabilize the flail segment.

21. In birds, is immediate surgical repair of a fracture necessary?
Many birds that present with fractures have been ill and in a catabolic state for some time. Presurgical conditioning tremendously increases surgical success rates. Temporary splinting of fractures followed by cage rest, fluid therapy, and possibly tube feeding for 24 hours before fracture repair may be indicated. The goals of presurgical treatment are to maintain or improve cardiovascular and renal output, to revitalize diseased or damaged organs, to treat microbial infections, to ensure proper oxygen transport throughout the body, and to minimize the risk of any problems during surgery.

BIBLIOGRAPHY

1. Aron DN: Management of open musculoskeletal injuries. Semin Vet Med Surg (Small Animal) 3:290–301, 1988.
2. Cockshutt J: Management of fracture-associated thoracic trauma. Vet Clin North Am 25:1031–1046, 1995.
3. Eisenberg MS, Copass MK: Trauma. In Emergency Medical Therapy. Philadelphia, W.B. Saunders, 1988, pp 403–503.
4. McCluggage DM: Surgical principles and common procedures in the avian patient. Proceedings of the 54th Annual Conference Veterinarians, Fort Collins, CO, 1993, pp 221–237.
5. Tillson D: Open fracture management. Vet Clin North Am 25:1093–1110, 1995.
6. Wingfield WE, Henik RA: Treatment priorities in multiple trauma. Semin Vet Med Surg 3(3):193–201, 1988.

20. ABDOMINAL INJURIES

Wayne E. Wingfield, D.V.M., M.S.

1. What are the two major traumatic abdominal injuries?
• Blunt trauma
• Penetrating trauma

2. What is the pathophysiology of blunt abdominal injuries?
Blunt trauma involves a combination of crushing, stretching, and shearing forces. The magnitude of these forces is proportional to the mass of the objects, rate of change of velocity (deceleration vs. acceleration), direction of impact, and elasticity of the tissues. Blunt trauma results when the sum of the forces exceeds the cohesive strength and mobility of the tissues and organs in the abdomen. When high energy is transferred to the abdomen, a pronounced rise in intraabdominal pressure may result in rupture of hollow organs or produce solid-organ burst injuries. In addition, organs may be trapped between the thoracic cage or vertebral column, thus resulting in crush injuries. Some organs may be avulsed from their vascular pedicles with abrupt shearing forces.

3. Describe the pathophysiology of penetrating abdominal injuries.
When the abdomen is penetrated, energy is dissipated along the path of the penetrating object. Firearm injuries are especially prone to energy transmission because the kinetic energy is proportional to the mass (m) and velocity (v):

$$KE = MV^2/2$$

An increase in mass of a given missile by a factor of 2 doubles the kinetic energy, whereas doubling the velocity of the bullet quadruples the kinetic energy. In addition, the physical characteristics of the bullet determine the efficiency of energy dissipation. Soft lead or hollow-point bullets mushroom, fragment, and tumble, whereas jacketed bullets tend only to spiral. Low-velocity projectiles directly crush and tear, whereas high-velocity bullets induce variable tissue cavitation as well. The extent of cavitation is governed by the rate of energy dissipation and the physical characteristics of the tissues. Solid, inelastic organs such as the liver, spleen, and kidney are more susceptible to cavitation than more pliant tissues such as the lung or skeletal muscle. Shotgun wounds involve a group of pellets of varying sizes and number. The pellets disperse as a function of distance and length of taper of the gun barrel. Because of their spherical shape, pellets rapidly disperse their velocity over distance. Unless the shotgun is fired at close range, most pellets do minimal injury.

4. Should abdominal and thoracic injuries be considered separately?

No. The diaphragm permits significant transmission of force between the abdomen and thorax. Multiple organ system injury is most likely with blunt abdominal trauma.

5. What are the most common physical findings associated with blunt abdominal injury?

Abdominal tenderness and guarding, abdominal bruising, hemodynamic instability, and increasing girth dimensions are characteristic of abdominal injuries. In human adults, each inch of increase in girth may represent 500–1000 ml of blood. Other reports in humans suggest that abdominal distention is not a sensitive indicator of hemoperitoneum. No information is available for veterinary patients. Of interest, 20–40% of human patients with abdominal injury are said to be asymptomatic. This is true in veterinary patients as well. Considering the forces of injury in proportion to body size, the occurrence of abdominal injuries may be even higher.

6. Which abdominal organs are most commonly injured in blunt abdominal trauma?

No information is currently available in veterinary patients. In humans, the spleen is reported to be most commonly injured. However, because CT scans are more commonly used for evaluation of humans, the liver appears to be more frequently injured but requires operative intervention less often.

7. Which diagnostic tools are most useful for the initial evaluation of blunt trauma?

Abdominocentesis is one means for confirming abdominal injury. A four-quadrant tap is performed, and from the fluid obtained packed-cell volume, total solids, cytology, blood urea nitrogen (or creatinine), and perhaps total bilirubin should be requested.

Diagnostic peritoneal irrigation is useful when the abdominocentesis has been unfruitful and the index of suspicion for blunt abdominal injury is high.

Abdominal radiography is rarely fruitful in blunt abdominal injuries. If fluid is present, you still need abdominocentesis for a diagnosis. In addition, radiography should *always* precede abdominocentesis or irrigation. These invasive procedures may introduce atmospheric air and thus complicate diagnosis of a ruptured hollow organ.

Ultrasonography is becoming more popular for initial evaluation of blunt abdominal trauma. In humans, ultrasonography is about 95% sensitive to significant hemoperitoneum. The procedure is safe, noninvasive, and nonionizing. Unfortunately, ultrasonography cannot reliably stage solid-organ injuries or reliably assess hollow-organ perforations. Ultrasonography will probably supplant diagnostic lavage in certain instances.

Computed tomography (CT) in humans currently is an important diagnostic adjunct in early evaluation of abdominal injuries. CT has unquestioned specificity for organ injuries. The obvious limitation to use of CT in veterinary medicine is lack of available instruments. As CT instruments become more widely available, especially in large metropolitan areas, CT will assume a larger role in the diagnosis of abdominal trauma.

8. What constitutes a positive test for blood during abdominocentesis or irrigation?

When the packed cell volume (PCV) of the blood from centesis exceeds the packed cell volume from a peripheral vascular sample, the injury usually involves the liver, spleen, and, rarely, kidney. Centesis PCV is higher than peripheral vascular samples because of the higher PCV in splenic tissue and the fact that when whole blood is spilled into the abdomen, the peritoneal surface resorbs water and electrolytes immediately, whereas the red blood cells may require up to 2 weeks to be absorbed.

In observing for blood from irrigation procedures, one subjective criterion has been the ability to read newsprint through intravenous (IV) tubing containing the fluid. Others believe that a quantitative red blood cell count of 100,000/mm³ or a white blood cell count of 500/mm³ is positive for significant abdominal hemorrhage. In humans, lavage levels of amylase and alkaline phosphatase are reported to have a 95% specificity for small bowel perforation.

Criteria in Humans for a Positive Diagnostic Peritoneal Lavage

SAMPLE	POSITIVE	EQUIVOCAL
Abdominocentesis		
Blood	> 10 ml	—
Fluid	Enteric contents	—
Abdominal irrigation		
Red blood cells	> 100,000/mm³	> 20,000/mm³
White blood cells	—	> 500/mm³
Enzyme	Amylase > 20 IU and alkaline phosphatase > 3 IU	Alkaline phosphatase < 3 IU
Bile	Confirmed biochemically	—

9. How do you diagnose urologic trauma with abdominocentesis or irrigation?

The traditional confirmation of urine in the abdominal cavity is an elevated creatinine level. Urea nitrogen is as accurate as creatinine for diagnosis of acute urologic injury.

10. Which other diagnostic tests are useful in urologic injury?

Contrast studies of the urologic system are required before surgical exploration. A complete evaluation includes the following radiographic assessment:

- Excretory urograms assess the kidneys and ureter, and contrast material empties into the bladder as well.
- Positive contrast urethragrams in male dogs or cats are advised if a ruptured urethra is suspected. One needs to consider mixing the contrast agent with an agent such as K-Y jelly to increase adherence of the material to the urethral mucosa.
- Positive and/or negative cystograms are used to assess the urinary bladder.

11. Does passing a urinary catheter rule out a ruptured urethra?

No. In fact, passing a urinary catheter in a ruptured urethra may lead to either complete separation of the torn urethra or passage of the catheter into cavernosum tissue and the possibility of air embolism if air is injected.

12. Does passing a urinary catheter and retrieving urine rule out a ruptured bladder?

No. Most ruptures are on the cranial-dorsal portion of the bladder. A catheter can easily be inserted into the bladder where urine may still reside. Aspiration of urine tells nothing about whether the bladder is intact.

13. How do you manage a patient with a positive centesis and penetrating abdominal injury?

Surgical laparotomy

14. Describe the management of an animal with a penetrating wound when abdominocentesis and lavage are negative.

If abdominal radiographs taken before centesis show free air within the peritoneal cavity, surgical laparotomy is indicated. If the abdominal fluid collected via centesis has few white blood cells, repeat the abdominocentesis about 4 hours later. If the white count is still elevated or has risen, surgical exploration is indicated. Penetrating wounds into the peritoneal cavity have the potential of significant organ injury. Such animals should be hospitalized for observation.

15. How are urologic injuries managed?

During the first 12–24 hours, if the abdominal cavity is drained of urine, the animal may be a more respectable anesthetic risk. Ultimately, surgery is the treatment of choice.

16. Which abdominal injury may escape diagnosis until several weeks after the insult?

We probably miss many abdominal injuries. The one that is often overlooked is injury to the common or major bile duct. In such cases, bile continues to effuse into the peritoneal space, and it may be 3–4 weeks before icterus is identified clinically. To avoid the embarrassment of missing this diagnosis, run a bilirubin test on any blood from abdominocentesis or lavage. If the total bilirubin of the centesis fluid is greater than the peripheral blood bilirubin, suspect an injury to the biliary tree. Surgery is not considered an emergency but should be done soon after diagnosis. It is often technically difficult, and one should consider referring this animal to a surgical specialist.

CONTROVERSY

17. Should you use a surgical or conservative approach in animals with hemoabdomen secondary to trauma?

Surgeons, of course, want to explore any animal with hemoabdomen. Unfortunately, once the surgeon takes the animal, which is at high risk for anesthetic complications, to the operating table and opens the abdomen, often the only result is confirmation of hemoabdomen. Some surgeons remove a damaged spleen, but most traumatized spleens have already clotted by the time of surgery. Suturing of the liver is an inexact, frustrating experience. Again, the bleeding is generally well controlled before surgery. Without doubt, if a kidney is avulsed from the aorta, surgery may be life-saving.

Conservative management of the hemoabdomen appears anecdotally to be more successful than surgery. Crystalloids, occasionally colloids, and whole blood transfusions are administered to stabilize the animal hemodynamically. In addition, if there is no evidence of severe thoracic injury or diaphragmatic hernia, a circumferential compression bandage is applied to the abdomen. The idea behind this approach is simply to compress the abdominal organs and thus control hemorrhage. Currently, abdominal compression bandaging and intensive fluid therapy are the only techniques used for hemoabdomen secondary to trauma.

BIBLIOGRAPHY

1. Alyono D, Perry JF Jr: Value of quantitative cell count and amylase activity of peritoneal lavage fluid. J Trauma 21:345–348, 1981.
2. Burrows CF, Bovee KC: Metabolic changes due to experimentally induced rupture of the canine urinary bladder. Am J Vet Res 35:1083–1088, 1974.
3. Crowe DT, Crane SW: Diagnostic abdominal paracentesis and lavage in evaluation of abdominal injuries in dogs and cats: Clinical and experimental investigations. J Am Vet Med Assoc 168:700–708, 1976.
4. McAnulty JF, Smith GK: Circumferential external counterpressure by abdominal wrapping and its effect on simulated intra-abdominal hemorrhage. Vet Surg 15:270–274, 1986.
5. Powell DC, Bivens BA, Bell RM: Diagnostic peritoneal lavage. Surg Gynecol Obstet 155:257–264, 1982.
6. Rubin MJ, Blahd WH, Stanisic TH, et al: Diagnosis of intraperitoneal extravasation of urine by peritoneal lavage. Ann Emerg Med 14:433–437, 1985.

7. Shaw PM, Kim KH, Ramirez-Schon G, et al: Elevated blood urea nitrogen: An aid to the diagnosis of in-traperitoneal rupture of the bladder. J Urol 122:741–743, 1979.
8. Wilson RF: Trauma. In Shoemaker WC, Thompson WL, Holbrook PR (eds): Textbook of Critical Care. Philadelphia, W.B. Saunders, 1984, pp 877–914.

21. PAIN MANAGEMENT IN EMERGENCIES

Peter W. Hellyer, D.V.M., M.S., and Ann E. Wagner, D.V.M., M.S.

1. What are the benefits of effective pain management in emergency patients?

Improving patient comfort after trauma or surgery has important benefits. Unrelieved pain may induce a state of distress in which the animal diverts an excessive amount of energy away from healing simply to cope with the pain. Effective pain management reduces anxiety, decreases the stress response with its associated hormonal and metabolic derangements, and allows the patient to get the rest needed for more rapid recovery. The benefits of effective pain management on recovery after trauma or surgery have been well documented in human medicine, and anecdotal observations support a similar beneficial effect in veterinary patients. Shortened stays in the intensive care unit and a more rapid return to normal function provide evidence that effective pain management may have economic as well as medical benefits in people. Although not documented, similar benefits may occur with animals.

2. Should pain management be considered of secondary importance to treating the primary emergency problem(s)?

There is no question that pain management must be considered in the context of overall patient management. In many emergency situations, stabilizing the cardiopulmonary systems to ensure adequate oxygen delivery and to prevent organ failure or cardiovascular collapse is the highest priority. Similarly, careful physical examination and a minimal database are essential to formulating an initial differential diagnosis. Nevertheless, the judicious use of analgesics should be incorporated into the initial care plan for animals in pain. All too often pain relief is not considered until long (hours or days) after the animal may have benefited most from alleviation of pain.

3. Under what circumstances are analgesics contraindicated in emergency patients?

Analgesic therapy is contraindicated during the initial phases of resuscitation in an animal with cardiovascular collapse. Once the animal is stabilized, appropriate analgesic therapy can be instituted. There may be contraindications to the use of specific drugs, depending on the animal's underlying condition and health status. For example, most of the currently available nonsteroidal antiinflammatory drugs are contraindicated in animals with concurrent renal disease, gastrointestinal bleeding, or coagulopathy. Similarly, opioid use may be contraindicated in patients at risk of brainstem herniation secondary to increased intracranial pressure.

4. What are the reasons for withholding analgesia from an animal in pain?

In many cases, concern for patient health is the main reason for withholding analgesia, particularly in emergency situations in which the animal has not been stabilized. All of the analgesic drugs have potential adverse effects that must be taken into account before administration to compromised animals. Inexperience with analgesic use and an overstated incidence of adverse side effects (particularly with the opioids) often lead to excessive caution. Traditional beliefs that relieving pain leads to excessive activity in an animal are also cited as a reason to withhold analgesia. Unfortunately, the inability of caregivers to recognize the clinical signs of pain and to appreciate the importance of pain to the patient are also primary reasons why analgesic therapy may be withheld in both human and veterinary medicine. The actual or perceived increase in drug costs is another reason.

5. Do veterinarians routinely provide aggressive analgesic therapy to traumatized and suffering animals?

To date, no comprehensive studies have evaluated the prevalence of use of analgesics in private veterinary practice. Over the past decade veterinarians have increasingly recognized that alleviation of pain is an important therapeutic goal. Still there remains an entire spectrum of views among veterinarians and veterinary staff about the necessity of alleviating pain. Considering the well-documented and widespread practice of either withholding or grossly underdosing analgesic therapy in humans, it is not surprising that veterinarians do not have a uniform appreciation for the importance of pain management.

6. Providing emergency therapy for animals is already expensive. Does analgesic therapy greatly increase the cost?

Selection of the specific analgesic drug and/or technique largely influences the costs of analgesic therapy. For example, oxymorphone costs approximately 28 times more than morphine although morphine is equally efficacious. Furthermore, anecdotal reports indicate that many clients are willing to pay extra to ensure that their pet receives adequate pain relief during hospitalization.

7. What are the clinical signs of acute pain in dogs?

Vocalization may indicate pain in dogs; however, it is an insensitive and nonspecific indicator. Pain is frequently associated with abnormal activity, which may appear as either an increase or a decrease in activity. Dogs may appear restless, agitated, or even delirious; or they may be lethargic, withdrawn, dull, or depressed. Such dogs may not pay attention to environmental stimuli. The normal sleep/wake cycle may be disrupted, so that less sleep than normal is obtained. Normal activity such as grooming or eating may decrease or stop. Dogs may bite, lick, chew, or shake painful areas.

Dogs may adopt abnormal body postures in an attempt to relieve or cope with pain in a given area. For example, dogs with abdominal pain may assume a posture with a rigid torso and arched back. Dogs with thoracic pain may be reluctant to lie down despite obvious exhaustion. Disuse or guarding of a painful area is a fairly reliable indicator of pain. The dog's gait may be abnormal, or the dog may appear much more rigid than normal.

Interactive behaviors are frequently changed in painful animals. Dogs may become more aggressive and resist handling or palpation. In contrast, they may become more timid and seek increased contact with caregivers. Although dogs do not have the same degree of motor control over their facial muscles as primates, changes in facial expression can be used in some dogs to detect pain. The dog may hold its ears back or in a downward position. The eyes may be wide open with dilated pupils or partially closed with a dull appearance. Many dogs display a fixed stare into space, apparently oblivious to their surroundings. Some dogs may display an uncharacteristic grimace.

Tachypnea, tachycardia, hypertension, dilated pupils, and salivation are physiologic signs suggestive of pain. Tachypnea, tachycardia, and hypertension are less likely to be observed in conscious patients than in patients under inadequate general anesthesia.

8. If a dog is not vocalizing, does it mean that the dog is not in pain?

No. Vocalization is neither a specific nor sensitive indicator of pain. Stoic dogs that do not routinely vocalize may have severe pain without making any sound. Vocalization has been shown to be the number one clinical sign in dogs that prompts administration of analgesic drugs in the postoperative period. Thus, animals that do not vocalize are much more likely to receive inadequate or no pain relief, regardless of degree of pain.

9. Are the clinical signs of acute pain different in cats and dogs?

Although dogs and cats may express similar clinical signs, it is often more difficult to evaluate the degree of pain in cats. Vocalization is much less common in cats than dogs. The clinical signs of pain in cats are frequently subtle and may be characterized as a lack of activity. The cat may sit in the back of the cage and avoid interaction with caregivers. At the other end of the behavioral spectrum, some painful cats thrash around the cage violently. This response to pain probably occurs more commonly in young healthy cats that have undergone a painful procedure (e.g., declawing).

10. Are the outwardly recognizable clinical signs of pain ever obtunded by the underlying disease process?

Yes. Trauma, major surgery, and metabolic derangements may blunt an animal's behavioral response to pain. Lack of overt signs of pain (e.g., vocalizing, thrashing) does not confirm that the animal is not in pain. On the contrary, some animals with severe pain and depression become much more alert and interactive once effective analgesia has been administered.

11. Does the routine use of analgesics mask clinical signs that may indicate deterioration in the animal's health?

The likelihood that analgesic therapy will mask deterioration of health status in dogs and cats is probably small, particularly if the animals are closely monitored. However, it is certainly possible that analgesics may mask some clinical signs that signal the need to alter the current course of therapy. The most common situation is the administration of potent analgesics to horses with colic. The degree and duration of abdominal pain are often used as a guide to determine whether the horse requires an exploratory laparotomy. A similar situation may occur in small animals with a painful abdomen. Small animals that sleep after administration of an analgesic may be easier for a busy nursing staff to overlook. Caregivers may assume that the animal is comfortable and stable, whereas in fact the animal's medical condition is deteriorating.

12. What are some of the most painful injuries or procedures that require analgesic treatment?

Trauma (particularly with extensive musculoskeletal injuries), pancreatitis, peritonitis, and intervertebral disc disease are a few of the conditions that often result in distressing levels of pain in animals. Numerous surgical procedures also induce severe pain, particularly amputations, proximal limb and pelvic orthopedic procedures, thoracotomies, surgeries of the cervical spine, and auricular and perianal surgeries.

13. What classes of drugs are available to treat acute pain in emergency patients?

Opioids (morphine, oxymorphone, fentanyl), alpha-2 agonists (xylazine, medetomidine), local anesthetics (lidocaine, bupivacaine), and nonsteroidal antiinflammatory drugs (banamine, ketoprofen, carprofen) may be used to treat acute pain in dogs and cats.

14. Describe the potential adverse effects of alpha-2 agonists used to treat pain in emergency patients.

The alpha-2 agonists may elicit marked cardiopulmonary effects in compromised animals, particularly when administered intravenously. Bradycardia, atrioventricular blocks, and decreases in myocardial contractility contribute to significant decreases in cardiac output. The IV administration of alpha-2 agonists may cause arterial constriction, transiently increasing arterial pressure at the expense of forward flow (perfusion). This initial increase in arterial pressure may be followed by a sustained period of hypotension. Alpha-2 agonists predispose the myocardium to ventricular dysrhythmias in small animals, particularly in the presence of hypoxemia, acid-base disturbance, and electrolyte abnormalities. Depression of CNS respiratory centers may lead to hypoventilation, hypercapnia, and hypoxemia.

15. Should nonsteroidal antiinflammatory drugs (NSAIDs) be routinely used in traumatized or emergency patients in pain?

The currently available NSAIDs are only effective in the treatment of mild-to-moderate pain; therefore they have limited utility in animals with severe trauma or pain. The well-established side effects of gastrointestinal ulceration, decreases in renal blood flow, and coagulopathies are due to inhibition of prostaglandin synthesis. Newer NSAIDs (e.g., carprofen) are weak inhibitors of cyclooxygenase; however, their utility in emergency patients has yet to be established. The effects of NSAIDs on renal blood flow may be particularly detrimental in hypovolemic emergency patients. Accordingly, NSAIDs should be used only after the animal is stabilized and the possibility of renal impairment, GI ulceration, and coagulopathies has been ruled out.

16. Why should I consider using opioids in my clinic?

Opioids have been shown to be the most effective and useful analgesics available for the management of acute severe pain in people and small animals.

17. Considering all the record-keeping hassles mandated by the Drug Enforcement Agency (DEA), how can I afford to keep controlled substances in my clinic?

Without a doubt, the record-keeping requirements mandated by the DEA for administering scheduled drugs (e.g., opioids) increase the amount of paperwork. The myth in veterinary medicine is that these requirements are so onerous that they preclude the use of opioids. In fact, the amount of additional work is minimal in comparison with the benefits that the drugs can provide for patient comfort.

18. Are any good analgesics not controlled substances?

Butorphanol is an opioid agonist-antagonist that is not controlled in most states. Although butorphanol is not as efficacious as the opioid agonists, it may be effective in treatment of mild-to-moderate pain. Local anesthetics, alpha-2 agonists, and NSAIDs are not controlled drugs and may be useful in controlling pain if used cautiously in emergency patients.

19. What specific opioids are clinically used to control pain in dogs and cats?

Morphine, oxymorphone, fentanyl, butorphanol, and buprenorphine.

20. How should I choose an appropriate opioid analgesic?

The choice of opioid is usually based on availability, cost, efficacy, and duration of action. Opioid agonists (e.g., morphine, oxymorphone, fentanyl) are much more effective in the treatment of moderate-to-severe pain than the agonist-antagonists (e.g., buprenorphine, butorphanol, nalbuphine). The duration of action varies markedly and depends on the specific drug, route of administration, species treated, and individual variability (dose and frequency depend on the amount of pain).

21. Is a more potent opioid a better choice for the treatment of severe pain than a less potent opioid?

A more potent opioid is not necessarily more effective than an opioid of lesser potency. Opioids are compared according to analgesic potency, with morphine arbitrarily assigned a potency of 1. In practical terms, analgesic potency determines the dose that must be administered to achieve the desired effect. For example, both morphine and oxymorphone are opioid agonists, but oxymorphone is approximately 10–15 times more potent than morphine. As a result of these differences in potency, an equianalgesic dose of morphine (0.5–1.0 mg/kg) is 10 times the dose of oxymorphone (0.05–0.1 mg/kg). Although fentanyl is approximately 100 times more potent than morphine, it is generally a poor choice for sustained analgesia because of its short duration of action (approximately 15–30 minutes). Fentanyl can be highly effective, however, if it is delivered as a constant-rate IV infusion or in the form of a transdermal patch. In contrast to the opioid agonists, butorphanol and buprenorphine are agonist-antagonists and are approximately 5 and 30 times more potent than morphine, respectively. Although these drugs are more potent than morphine, neither is as efficacious at controlling pain (agonist-antagonists have a ceiling effect on analgesia).

22. What are effective doses and approximate duration of effect of the commonly used opioids?

Drugs Used for Analgesia in Dogs and Cats

DRUG	ANALGESIC POTENCY	DOSAGE (MG/KG)	SPECIES	ROUTE OF ADMINI-STRATION	DURATION OF EFFECT (HR)	INDICATIONS (TYPES OF PAIN)
Opioid Agonists						
Morphine	1	0.05–1.0	Canine	IV	1–2	Mild to severe
		0.2–2.0	Canine	IM, SQ	2–6	
		0.05–0.2	Feline	IV	1–2	
		0.1–0.5	Feline	IM, SQ	2–6	
Oxymorphone	5–10	0.02–0.1	Canine	IV	1–2	Mild to severe
		0.05–0.2	Canine	IM, SQ	2–4	
		0.02–0.05	Feline	IV	1–2	
		0.05–0.1	Feline	IM, SQ	2–4	
Fentanyl	75–125	0.001–0.004 (mg/kg/hr CRI)	Canine	IV	Constant-rate infusion (CRI)	Moderate to severe
		0.001–0.002 (mg/kg/hr CRI)	Feline	IV	CRI	
Agonists-Antagonists						
Butorphanol	5	0.2–0.5	Canine	IV	1–2	Mild to moderate
		0.2–0.8	Canine	IM, SQ	2–4	
		0.1–0.2	Feline	IV	1–2	
		0.1–0.4	Feline	IM, SQ	2–4	
Buprenorphine	30	0.005–0.02	Canine	IV, IM	4–12	Mild
		0.005–0.01	Feline	IV, IM	4–12	

IV = intravenous, IM = intramuscular, SQ = subcutaneous

23. Is morphine a dated drug that is not as effective as oxymorphone?
No. Both morphine and oxymorphone are opioid agonists that may induce the same degree of analgesia if the appropriate dose is administered. The primary disadvantage of morphine compared with oxymorphone is that morphine may cause histamine release in dogs and presumably in cats. Histamine release may cause peripheral vasodilation and hypotension, which may be particularly problematic in anesthetized or compromised animals. IM, SQ, or slow IV administration of morphine minimizes the incidence of histamine release. Vomiting may be more frequent in ambulatory animals who receive morphine rather than oxymorphone. On the other hand, morphine has a slightly longer duration of action than oxymorphone and is much less expensive.

24. Are opioid analgesics contraindicated in cats?
No. The opioids are excellent analgesics for cats. Cats are more sensitive to the excitatory effects of opioids, but administering lower doses (¼ to ½ of the dog dose) often prevents opioid-induced excitement. As in dogs, the concurrent administration of low doses of acepromazine usually eliminates unwanted excitation.

25. Is respiratory depression a potentially life-threatening side effect of opioids in compromised animals?

Opioids are clearly respiratory depressants; however, the importance of opioid-induced respiratory depression is often overstated in veterinary medicine. Opioids act centrally to decrease the responsiveness of the ventilatory centers to carbon dioxide and interfere with regulation of respiratory rhythm by the pontine and medullary ventilatory centers. The clinical significance of opioid-induced respiratory depression appears to be much more important in people than in animals. Administering opioids in small incremental doses, to effect, greatly decreases the likelihood of depressing ventilation. Greater care, coupled with vigilant monitoring, should be used for administering opioids to animals with preexisting respiratory disease or increased intracranial pressure (e.g., head trauma, intracranial tumor).

26. What should I do if the animal sleeps for long periods after administration of an opioid analgesic?

Effective analgesic doses of opioids frequently cause animals to sleep. The animal should be monitored periodically, with particular attention to pulse (rate and strength), color of mucous membranes, capillary refill time, and respiratory rate. As long as vital signs are stable, the animal is probably benefiting from the rest. If the amount of sleep appears excessive or if the vital signs are in question, the dose and frequency of opioid administration may be reduced. Alternatively, the opioid agonists (morphine, oxymorphone, fentanyl) may be partially antagonized with an agonist-antagonist (butorphanol, nalbuphine) to decrease sedation without completely removing analgesia.

27. What should I do if an animal becomes agitated or disoriented after receiving an opioid?

Administering either a low dose of acepromazine (0.01–0.05 mg/kg SQ or IV) or a benzodiazepine (diazepam or midazolam, 0.1–0.2 mg/kg IM or IV) sedates most animals that are agitated or disoriented. Alternatively, the opioids can be either partially reversed with an opioid agonist-antagonist or completely reversed with naloxone. Naloxone is only rarely administered because the acute awareness of pain and subsequent autonomic effects may induce ventricular dysrhythmias in compromised animals.

28. What if I have given what I think is an appropriate dose of an opioid and the animal remains agitated? How can I tell if the animal is still in pain, anxious, or dysphoric?

Differentiating pain from anxiety and/or opioid-induced dysphoria is difficult and represents a significant challenge clinically. Careful observation of the dog's clinical signs may shed some light on the root problem. Determining whether the dog responds to attention and interaction with caregivers may help to determine if anxiety has a significant role. Assessing the level of consciousness is important in differentiating pain from dysphoria. Some dogs receiving opioids vocalize continually, although otherwise they appear sedate and comfortable. Administering a test dose of additional analgesic may help to determine if the dog is still in pain. Alternatively, partial or complete reversal of the opioid with either an opioid agonist-antagonist or antagonist, respectively, can be used to rule out dysphoria. Unfortunately, if the dog is truly in pain, administering an antagonist only worsens the situation. Of importance, the clinician needs to consider the extent of the animal's injuries and to determine how likely it is to be still in pain. Many animals require relatively high doses of opioids initially to control pain. Beginning therapy with low doses of opioids and adding additional doses at preset intervals is a safe and effective method to control pain while minimizing adverse effects.

29. Are there any advantages to administering drugs in the epidural space rather than systemically?

Epidural administration of drugs allows a greater response (analgesia) with a much lower dose than systemic administration. The lower doses used in the epidural space are associated with a reduced incidence of side effects. The epidural administration of drugs also may provide longer duration of analgesia. For example, epidural morphine may provide analgesia for 12 hours or more in comparison with 4 hours when administered systemically. Opioids and local anesthetics are most commonly administered in the epidural space in dogs and cats.

30. How do I know if I overdosed an animal with opioids, alpha-2 agonists, or NSAIDs?
Overdosages of opioids and alpha-2 agonists result in excessive cardiopulmonary depression as evidenced by bradycardia, decrease in pulse quality, slowed capillary refill time, and pale or cyanotic mucous membranes. Overdosage with NSAIDs may not be immediately apparent but may manifest as gastrointestinal bleeding, azotemia, or prolonged bleeding times.

31. What are some means to provide analgesia besides systemic analgesics?
Ensuring that the animal is in a comfortable position, appropriate use of splints or bandages, attention to the needs of the animal (e.g., does the animal need to urinate, defecate), and interacting with the animal frequently to decrease stress and anxiety may increase comfort and tolerance of pain.

BIBLIOGRAPHY

 1. Bridenbaugh PO: Preemptive analgesia—is it clinically relevant? Anesth Analg 78:203–204, 1994.
 2. Hansen BD: Analgesic therapy. Comp Cont Educ 16:868–875, 1994.
 3. Hansen B, Hardie E: Prescription and use of analgesics in dogs and cats in a veterinary teaching hospital: 258 cases (1983–1989). J Am Vet Med Assoc 202:1485–1494, 1993.
 4. Kehlet H: Surgical stress: The role of pain and analgesia. Br J Anaesth 63:189–195, 1989.
 5. Kehlet H, Dahl JB: The value of "multimodal" or "balanced analgesia" in postoperative pain treatment. Anesth Analg 77:1048–1056, 1993.
 6. Kyles AE, Papich M, Hardie EM: Disposition of transdermally administered fentanyl in dogs. Am J Vet Res 57:715–719, 1996.
 7. Lees P, May SA, McKellar QA: Pharmacology and therapeutics of non-steroidal anti-inflammatory drugs in the dog and cat. I: General pharmacology. J Small Animal Pract 32:183–193, 1991.
 8. Lin HC, Benson GJ, Thurmon JC, et al: Influence of anesthetic regimens on the perioperative catecholamine response associated with onychectomy in cats. Am J Vet Res 54:1721–1724, 1993.
 9. McKellar QA, May SA, Lees P: Pharmacology and therapeutics of non-steroidal anti-inflammatory drugs in the dog and cat. 2: Individual agents. J Small Animal Pract 32:225–235, 1991.
10. Pascoe PJ, Dyson DH: Analgesia after lateral thoracotomy in dogs: Epidural morphine vs. intercostal bupivacaine. Vet Surg 22:141–147, 1993.
11. Quandt JE, Rawlings CR: Reducing postoperative pain for dogs: Local anesthetic and analgesic techniques. Comp Cont Educ 18:101–111, 1996.
12. Sackman JE: Pain. Part II: Control of pain in animals. Comp Cont Educ 13:181–187, 190–192, 1991.
13. The DEA: Following its "10 commandments." J Am Vet Med Assoc 205:1371, 1994.
14. Thurmon JC, Tranquilli WJ, Benson GJ: Perioperative pain and distress. In Thurmon JC, Tranquilli WJ, Benson GJ (eds): Lumb and Jones' Veterinary Anesthesia, 3rd ed. Baltimore, Williams & Wilkins, 1996, pp 40–60.

III. Common Primary Complaints

Section Editor: Tim Hackett, D.V.M., M.S.

22. VOMITING

Tim Hackett, D.V.M., M.S.

1. What is the difference between vomiting and regurgitation?

Vomiting is the forceful ejection of gastric and occasionally proximal small intestinal contents through the mouth. Sustained contraction of abdominal muscles, elevation and opening of the cardia, and contraction of the pylorus result in the movement of gastric contents out of the stomach. **Regurgitation** is the passive, retrograde movement of ingested material, usually before it has reached the stomach. Regurgitation may occur immediately after ingestion of food or water or be delayed for hours.

2. How can vomiting and regurgitation be differentiated?

Question witnesses carefully about the timing and nature of the event. Tubular, undigested food passed without effort is most likely regurgitation. Vomiting is accompanied by retching, nausea, ptyalism, and forceful contractions. By measuring the pH of the material recovered, vomitus may be differentiated from regurgitated ingesta. Vomitus usually contains hydrochloric acid and has a pH less than 4.

3. Describe the neural pathways involved in vomiting.

Two functionally and anatomically separate regions are responsible for emesis: the **chemoreceptor trigger zone** (CTZ) in the floor of the fourth ventricle and the **vomiting center** in the reticular formation of the medulla oblongata. All stimuli pass through the vomiting center, which integrates afferent information and coordinates the patterned response of nausea, retching, and vomiting. Afferent input includes stimuli from other neural centers (psychogenic, vestibular, CTZ) and the gastrointestinal (GI) tract. The CTZ acts in response to chemical substances in the blood. Examples of chemical stimuli include anesthetic agents, cardiac glycosides, chemotherapeutic agents, and emetic agents such as apomorphine.

4. What are the common causes of regurgitation?

Causes of Regurgitation

Cleft palate	Esophageal disorders
Pharyngeal disorders	Esophagitis
Foreign bodies	Esophageal diverticula
Neoplasia	Esophageal stricture
Retropharyngeal lymphadenopathy	Foreign bodies
Rabies	Hiatal hernia
Botulism	Neoplasia: esophageal, mediastinal
Cricopharyngeal achalasia	Vascular ring anomalies
Myasthenia gravis	Periesophageal masses
	Granulomas
	Congenital and acquired megaesophagus
	Hypomotility

5. What electrolyte and acid–base changes may be seen with vomiting?

Vomiting may result in profound dehydration. Loss of sodium, chloride, and potassium varies with the cause. Serum sodium is often low. Hypokalemia is often due to lack of intake, loss in vomitus, and increased loss due to alkalemia. Serum chloride levels depend on the source of fluid loss. Loss of gastric secretions in patients with pyloric or duodenal obstruction may result in loss of hydrochloric acid, profound hypochloremia, and metabolic alkalosis. Total plasma bicarbonate (TCO_2) may be increased, normal, or decreased depending on the type of fluid lost and underlying systemic disease. Metabolic alkalosis may progress to a mixed acid–base disorder if volume loss and hypovolemia lead to decreased oxygen delivery to the tissues.

6. What is the initial management of intractable vomiting?

Careful assessment of vital functions includes evaluation of airway patency, adequacy of respirations, and cardiovascular status. Vomiting and especially regurgitation may predispose an animal to aspiration pneumonia. Respiratory distress, tracheal sensitivity, or harsh airway sounds may indicate respiratory complications. Supplemental oxygen, thoracic radiographs, and arterial blood gas analysis may be indicated. Protracted vomiting may cause significant dehydration and signs of hypovolemic shock. Intravenous fluid replacement is indicated in any clinically dehydrated, vomiting animal. Enteral fluid replacement should be withheld until vomiting has ceased. The estimated fluid deficit should be replaced along with maintenance fluid volumes and any further losses. Approximately 80% of the deficit is replaced in the first 24 hours along with maintenance fluids. Ongoing volume losses are estimated and replaced in a 6–8 hour period.

7. What is the diagnostic approach to the vomiting patient?

Thorough history and physical examination help to identify the likelihood of an ingested foreign body or other dietary indiscretion. Young animals without obvious signs of distress may be treated conservatively by withholding food and water for 24 hours. Animals still vomiting or animals presenting in obvious distress should have a blood chemistry panel, complete blood count, and abdominal radiographs. Young animals should be screened for viral enteritis. Electrolyte changes may suggest hypoadrenocorticism, whereas pancreatic enzymes are elevated in cases of pancreatitis. Metabolic diseases causing vomiting secondarily should be identified through screening blood tests. If plain radiographs are not diagnostic, contrast radiographs may be performed to evaluate GI motility and patency. Endoscopic examination may be used to visualize the esophagus, stomach, and proximal bowel, to obtain diagnostic samples, and to remove gastric foreign bodies.

8. What common gastrointestinal diseases cause vomiting in dogs and cats?

Common primary GI complaints include gastroenteritis, pancreatitis, gastric and intestinal foreign bodies, and enteric viral diseases such as canine parvovirus.

Causes of Vomiting

PRIMARY GASTROINTESTINAL DISORDERS	SECONDARY CAUSES
Adverse reactions to food	**Other primary organ disorders**
Dietary indiscretions	Pancreatitis
Food hypersensitivity or allergies	Peritonitis
Obstructions	Pyometra
Delayed gastric emptying	Renal failure
Ileus	Hepatic failure
Foreign bodies	Congestive heart failure
Intussusception	**Neurologic diseases**
Torsions	Central nervous system disease (neoplasia,
Pyloric hypertrophy	trauma, meningitis)
Neoplasia	Central or peripheral vestibular disease
Granuloma	Dysautonomia
Strictures	*Table continued on next page.*

Causes of Vomiting (Continued)

PRIMARY GASTROINTESTINAL DISORDERS	SECONDARY CAUSES
Inflammatory diseases	**Systemic disorders**
Primary gastritis	Uremia
Inflammatory bowel disease	Metastatic neoplasia
Diffuse neoplasia	Acid–base or electrolyte imbalance
Hemorrhagic gastroenteritis	**Endocrine diseases**
Ulcerative gastroenteritis	Hypoadrenocorticism
Lymphangiectasia	Diabetic ketoacidosis
Infectious enteritis	Gastrinoma
Viral	Hyperthyroidism
Bacterial	Hyperparathyroidism
Fungal	**Drugs, chemical, poisons**
Gastrointestinal parasites	Apomorphine, narcotics
	Chemotherapeutic agents
	Anesthetics
	Digitalis
	Thiacetarsamide
	Lead

9. What radiographic signs suggest small bowel obstruction?

Some foreign objects are visualized directly either because they are radiopaque or because they are surrounded by a gas interface. Obstruction of the stomach or bowel may be seen as gas or fluid distention, delayed transit of contrast material, fixation or displacement of loops of bowel, and luminal filling defects.

10. Discuss the common antiemetic drugs, including their mechanism of action and contraindications to their use.

D_2-dopaminergic antagonists such as metoclopramide act centrally at the chemoreceptor trigger zone. Metoclopramide is also a 5-HT_3 serotonergic antagonist. Because metoclopramide enhances gastric emptying and intestinal motility, it should not be used when intestinal obstruction is suspected. **M_1-cholinergic antagonists** such as chlorpromazine and scopolamine also act on the chemoreceptor trigger zone, emetic center, and vestibular apparatus. Because chlorpromazine is a potent α-adrenergic antagonist, it should not be used in hypotensive patients. **Newer, more potent centrally acting antiemetics** include ondansetron and granisetron, 5-HT_3 serotonergic antagonists that work at the emetic center, chemoreceptor trigger zone, and afferent nerves from the gut.

11. How can nutrition be addressed in a vomiting patient?

Enteral nutrition can be given to a vomiting patient only through a jejunostomy feeding tube. Nasogastric, pharyngostomy, esophagostomy, and gastrostomy feeding tubes aggravate vomiting by stimulating gastric secretions and motility. Feeding tubes also may become dislodged during vomiting and aspirated down the trachea. Radiographic confirmation of tube position is mandatory after emesis to prevent iatrogenic aspiration pneumonia. Parenteral nutrition is another means of providing calories while bypassing the GI tract.

12. What is the significance of nonproductive vomiting?

Nonproductive vomiting is a symptom of gastric dilatation volvulus (GDV). GDV primarily affects large-breed dogs and results in abdominal distention and circulatory shock.

13. A client telephones about her vomiting dog. What is your first concern?

In talking to clients over the telephone, it is imperative to rule out possible GDV before suggesting conservative management of the vomiting dog. When the stomach twists on its axis, it may cut off blood supply to the gastric walls and spleen. The sooner the animal is treated for shock and the GDV surgically corrected, the better the prognosis for recovery.

BIBLIOGRAPHY

1. Guilford WG: Strombek's Small Animal Gastroenterology, 3rd ed. Philadelphia, W.B. Saunders, 1996, pp 58–62.
2. Kirby R, Jones B: Gastrointestinal emergencies: Acute vomiting. Semin Vet Med Surg 3:256–264, 1988.
3. Washabau RJ: Anti-emetic strategies. Proceedings of the ACVIM Forum. 1995, pp 82–84.

23. DIARRHEA

Tim Hackett, D.V.M., M.S.

1. What life-threatening problems are associated with diarrhea?

Diarrhea may result in dramatic loss of fluids. Patients often present with severe dehydration. Primary gastrointestinal disease may result in loss of electrolytes and inability to absorb nutrients, especially proteins. Many causes of diarrhea damage the mucosal integrity of the bowel, allowing normal intestinal flora to cross into the bloodstream. Animals with diarrhea may present in shock from blood loss, fluid loss, and sepsis.

2. What is the most important treatment for patients with severe diarrhea?

Patients with diarrhea may be unable to maintain hydration. Common causes of diarrhea leave the patient weak and anorectic. Even if an animal drinks, intestinal pathology may prevent adequate absorption of water. Parenteral fluid therapy is necessary to prevent dehydration and to support the patient until normal intestinal function is restored. Hospitalized patients receiving intravenous fluids may become dehydrated if gastrointestinal losses of fluid are not quantified and returned to the patient. Fluid volumes should be based on maintenance volumes plus dehydration plus ongoing losses. Daily body weight can be used to determine precisely whether fluid therapy is adequate.

3. What are the common causes of acute diarrhea?

Acute diarrhea may result from a change in diet, dietary indiscretion, or intolerance to a type of food or medicine. Dietary indiscretions include overeating and ingestion of spoiled garbage, decomposing carrion, and abrasive or other nondigestible foreign material. Intestinal parasites, viruses, bacteria, and rickettsia are potential causes of infectious diarrhea. New sources of stress or metabolic disturbances also may cause acute diarrhea.

4. How should an animal presenting with diarrhea be managed?

All diarrhea, acute or chronic, should be considered infectious until proved otherwise. Young animals, debilitated animals, and animals from shelters or kennels are most likely to have infectious diarrhea. Hospital staff should plan to isolate such animals immediately. If possible, they should be treated as outpatients. Systemically ill and dehydrated patients should be hospitalized away from other animals. Feces should be removed and kept away from other animals. Personnel should wear protective clothing and wash hands, stethoscopes, and thermometers before handling other patients.

5. What steps should be taken to identify the cause of acute diarrhea?

The diarrhea should be classified as either small bowel or large bowel. Clients should be questioned about duration of signs, possible exposure to other animals, travel history, vaccination status, and new stress in the animal's life. A complete physical exam should be followed by fecal examination to look for parasites and, when indicated, to test for canine parvovirus. Animals with signs of systemic illness should be checked for other primary problems. A minimal database includes complete blood count, electrolytes, and serum chemistries. Fecal cultures for *Salmonella* spp., *Campylobacter jejuni, Yersinia enterocolitica,* and *Shigella* spp. are indicated when an infectious cause is strongly suggested.

6. Describe the various pathophysiologic mechanisms of diarrhea.

Intestinal disease may cause diarrhea through decreased absorption, hypersecretion, increased permeability, and abnormal motility. Poor absorption (osmotic diarrhea) results in accumulation of nonabsorbable solutes in the gut. These solutes draw water into the lumen of the gut and result in bulky, fluid diarrhea. Secretory diarrhea occurs when the mucosal lining of the bowel is stimulated to secrete fluid and electrolytes without compensatory changes in absorption, permeability, or osmotic gradients. Increased permeability (exudative diarrhea) is usually accompanied by increased transmural hydrostastic pressure. The result is loss of protein-rich fluid into the intestinal lumen.

7. How is diarrhea classified?

Diarrhea is often classified as either small bowel or large bowel. Small-bowel diarrhea is characterized by a large volume of stool usually without increased frequency or urgency. Small-bowel diarrhea results from small intestine dysfunction due either to primary gastrointestinal disease or diseases of other digestive organs such as the liver and pancreas. Large-bowel diarrhea refers to cecal, colonic, or rectal etiologies. Large-bowel diarrhea is characteristically small in volume, is associated with blood and mucus, and usually presents with signs of tenesmus.

8. What are the common infectious causes of diarrhea?

When confronted with a young animal with diarrhea, viral enteritis is usually a top differential. Coronavirus, parvovirus, rotavirus, and astrovirus are among the agents identified in the stools of diarrhetic dogs and cats. Bacterial pathogens include enteropathogenic *Escherichia coli, Clostridium* spp., *Salmonella* spp., *Yersinia enterocolitica, Campylobacter jejuni,* and *Bacillus piliformis* (Tyzzer's disease). Systemic mycoses such as *Histoplasma capsulatum, Aspergillus* spp., and *Candida albicans* may affect gastrointestinal function and result in diarrhea.

9. What are the potential zoonotic causes of diarrhea in small animals?

Several important bacterial and parasitic zoonoses are seen in small animals with diarrhea. The enteric bacteria of zoonotic significance include *Salmonella* spp., *Campylobacter jejuni, Shigella* spp., and *Yersinia enterocolitica. Giardia* spp., *Toxoplasma gondii, Cryptosporidium parvum, Toxocara canis, Toxascaris leonina, Uncinaria stenocephala, Ancylostoma caninum, Strongyloides stercoralis, Echinococcus multilocularis,* and *Echinococcus granulosa* are the most significant enteric parasite zoonoses in small animals and often cause clinical disease.

10. What are the common iatrogenic causes of diarrhea?

Sudden changes in an animal's diet may cause diarrhea. A gradual transition in diet is recommended to prevent this problem. Osmotic diarrhea is a common complication of enteral feeding in critically ill patients with esophagostomy, gastrostomy, or jejunostomy feeding tubes. Many drugs may cause acute intestinal upset resulting in diarrhea.

11. How does the presence of blood in the stool affect medical management?

With any injury to intestinal mucosa, hemorrhage and melena are often noted. The presence of blood, either fresh or digested, implies damage to the lining of the bowel. Normal enteric bacteria may become pathogenic if allowed to cross the mucosal barrier and enter the circulation. Antibiotic therapy is indicated.

12. Discuss symptomatic treatments for diarrhea.

Acute diarrhea may be managed conservatively by withholding food for 12–24 hours to allow the GI tract time to heal. Small, bland, low-fat meals are then started. Fluid and electrolyte homeostasis should be monitored closely. Parenteral fluid replacement and oral supplementation with glucose-electrolyte solutions may be used to maintain hydration. Drugs that alter intestinal motility include the opiates (diphenoxylate, loperamide, and paragoric) and anticholinergic-anti-spasmodics. Examples of intraluminal absorbents and protectants include kaolin-pectin, bismuth, and barium sulfate. Bismuth subsalicylate is a protectant and also has antisecretory and antiendo-toxin effects. It should be used with caution in patients sensitive to salicylates. Antibiotics are indicated only for bacterial diarrhea and animals with significant disruption of intestinal mucosa.

13. When should a detailed diagnostic work-up be recommended?

Any animal that does not respond to routine supportive care and whose condition is deteriorating should be evaluated more completely. Intestinal biopsy is usually required for diagnosis in animals with chronic, unresponsive diarrhea. Increasing clinical signs and owner frustration may result from prolonged symptomatic care. Infiltrative and inflammatory diseases of the bowel should be pursued when a patient continues to have diarrhea despite dietary and medical intervention.

BIBLIOGRAPHY

1. Guilford WG: Strombek's Small Animal Gastroenterology, 3rd ed. Philadelphia, W.B. Saunders, 1996, pp 62–70.
2. Murphy MJ: Toxin exposures in dogs and cats: Pesticides and biotoxins. J Am Vet Med Assoc 205:414–421, 1994.
3. Tams TR: Gastrointestinal symptoms. In Tams TR (ed): Handbook of Small Animal Gastroenterology. Philadelphia, W.B. Saunders, 1996, pp 40–62.

24. SYNCOPE VS. SEIZURES

Andrew J. Triolo, D.V.M., M.S.

1. Syncope or seizure—which is it?

At times it is difficult to tell the difference. A systematic diagnostic approach is vital in distinguishing between the two.

2. What is syncope?

Syncope is loss of consciousness caused by inadequate glucose or oxygen to the brain. The causes tend to be neurogenic or cardiovascular.

Common Causes of Syncope

Brain	Metabolic disorders
Thromboembolic disease	Causes of hypoglycemia
Neoplasia	Insulin-secreting tumors
Trauma	Glycogen storage diseases
Cardiovascular system	Starvation (especially in small breeds)
Arrhythmias	Iatrogenic causes
Thromboembolic disease	Insulin overdose
Blood loss	Digitalis intoxication
Congenital or acquired heart disease	
Low blood pressure	

3. What is a seizure?

Seizure is one of the clinical signs of abnormal brain function. Although the causes of seizure are many, the underlying process causes a similar outcome—a favorable balance toward neuron excitation.

4. How do I approach a patient with syncope or seizures?

The basics are the same. Evaluate the patient for immediate life-threatening diseases such as arterial blood loss and hyperthermia. Once the most immediate concerns are evaluated and addressed, one can resume solving the mystery of the cause.

5. What diagnostic tests are recommended to distinguish among the many causes of syncope and seizures?

Always start with a minimum database (complete blood count, biochemistries, urinalysis), which should help to rule in or out major causes of both. Additional diagnostics may be needed, including an electrocardiogram, radiographs, CT or MRI, and cerebrospinal fluid tap.

6. What should you do when the client cannot afford a full work-up?

You have to make choices about which diagnostic tests to pursue. Start with tests for readily treatable conditions. Performing an MRI on a patient whose owner cannot afford follow-up care (e.g., chemotherapy or radiation) is probably not the wisest way to begin.

7. How do you treat a patient with syncope?

Treating the underlying cause will most likely suppress the syncopal episode. At times the cause cannot be found, and you must treat symptomatically. Many animals do not have another episode (especially while boarded in your hospital!).

8. How is a seizuring patient treated?

A patient in status epilepticus is a medical emergency. The drug of choice is intravenous diazepam. At times patients may be refractory to diazepam, and you may need to administer phenobarbital or pentobarbital intravenously.

Drug	Dose
Diazepam	0.5–1 mg/kg IV, repeated as needed up to 3 doses
Phenobarbital	2–4 mg/kg IM, IV, or constant-rate infusion at 3–16 mg/hr
Pentobarbital	3–15 mg/kg IV to effect

9. What else do you monitor in a seizuring patient?

Seizuring patients may become hyperthermic and need immediate cooling. If the seizure has been prolonged, central nervous system edema may have developed and may require treatment with osmotic or antiinflammatory agents such as mannitol or Solu-Medrol.

10. What medications are used for diagnosed epileptics?

Phenobarbital is probably the drug of choice. Begin treatment with a dose of 2 mg/kg twice daily. If a dose of 8 mg/kg is required to control seizures, add potassium bromide at 30 mg/kg/day to start, and try to reduce the dose of phenobarbital. Other drugs include primadone or phenytoin, which, in the author's opinion should not be used in small animals except as a last resort.

11. What are the side effects of phenobarbital?

Initial side effects may include sedation or polyphagia. These effects tend to resolve in 5–7 days in normal animals. Chronic therapy may lead to hepatic toxicosis and clinical signs similar to liver disease.

12. What are the side effects of potassium bromide?

The primary side effect is gastroenteritis, although central nervous system depression or behavioral changes also may be seen with overdosage. Potassium bromide is eliminated by the kidneys and therefore may be used in patients suspected to have liver disease due to phenobarbital.

BIBLIOGRAPHY

1. Dyer KR, Shell LG: Anticonvulsant therapy: A practical guide to medical management of epilepsy in pets. Vet Med July:647–653, 1993.
2. Ettinger SJ, Barrett KA: Weakness and syncope. In Textbook of Veterinary Internal Medicine, 4th ed. Philadelphia, W.B. Saunders, 1995, pp 50–57.
3. Forrester SD, Boothe DM, Troy GS: Current concepts in the management of canine epilepsy. Comp Cont Educ Small Animals 11:811–820, 1989.
4. O'Brien D: New approaches to the management of epilepsy. Proceedings of the 13th Kal Kan Symposium, pp 37–42.
5. Podell M, Fenner WR: Use of bromide as an antiepileptic drug in dogs. Comp Cont Educ Small Animals 15:767–774, 1994.

25. ATAXIA

Tim Hackett, D.V.M., M.S.

1. What is ataxia?

Ataxia is failure of muscular coordination or irregularity of muscle action associated with various anatomic lesions within the nervous system. Ataxia is incoordination without paresis or spastic, involuntary movements. Disorders of the cerebellum, vestibular system, and spinal cord sensory pathways are the most common causes of ataxia.

2. What systems are involved in ataxia?

Conscious and unconscious proprioception
Cerebellum
Vestibular system

3. Discuss specific causes of ataxia.

Proprioceptive ataxia is caused by spinal cord disease. Examples include intervertebral disk disease, neoplasia, degenerative myelopathy, and trauma. Vestibular ataxia may be idiopathic or due to otitis media and interna, vascular accidents, granulomatous meningioencephalitis, ototoxins, neoplasia, and trauma. Cerebellar ataxia may result from cerebellar abiotrophy, globoid leukodystrophy, congenital hypoplasia, canine distemper, rabies, toxoplasmosis, trauma, toxins, or neoplasia.

4. Describe the diagnostic plan for patients with ataxia.

Signalment and a thorough history help to differentiate congenital, infectious, and traumatic causes of ataxia. Physical examination should include a complete neurologic examination and close attention to the external ear canal and tympanic membrane. In addition to a complete blood count and serum chemistries, a coagulation profile also should be performed. Skull radiographs may be useful to evaluate the tympanic bullae. Analysis of cerebrospinal fluid and advanced imaging with CT or MR scans may be necessary to identify intracranial disease.

5. What is the most serious common toxin causing ataxia in small animals?

Ethylene glycol intoxication may cause a drunken presentation. Because of the urgency of treatment, patients presenting with ataxia of unknown cause should be carefully evaluated for possible ethylene glycol ingestion. Commercial serum test kits are available. If they are unavailable, a high anion gap metabolic acidosis and calcium oxalate crystalluria are highly suggestive. Treatment with either 4-methylpyrazole or 20% ethanol and intravenous fluids should be initiated immediately.

6. What antibiotic and antiparasitic drugs may cause ataxia?

The most common antibiotic causing ataxia is metronidazole. Patients usually have received metronidazole for weeks or longer and quickly recover after discontinuation of the drug. Aminoglycosides, polymyxin B, erythromycin, and vancomycin may cause ototoxicity and ataxia; unfortunately, they also may cause permanent damage. Ivermectin toxicity often causes severe neurologic disease, including ataxia. Treatment is supportive, and it may take days to weeks to see improvement. Amitraz also has been implicated in ataxia after overdosage. Treatment includes yohimbine and supportive care.

7. What are the most common causes of otitis interna and media?

The most common causes of otitis interna and media are bacterial infections, foreign bodies, and parasites. The common bacteria involved are *Staphylococcus* spp., *Proteus* spp., *Pseudomonas* spp., *Escherichia coli, Streptococcus* spp., and *Enterococcus* spp. The most common aural parasite is the Otodectes mite. The grass-awn remains one of the most common foreign bodies found in animals' ears.

8. Describe the diagnosis and treatment of otitis interna and media.

Clinical signs of otitis externa include head tilt, head shaking, aural pain, inflammatory discharge, torticollis, circling, ataxia, positional ventral strabismus, and nystagmus. The patient may have unilateral facial nerve paralysis. If the middle ear is involved, the patient may have Horner's syndrome. Diagnosis is based on clinical signs and otoscopic exam. If the tympanic membrane cannot be visualized, debris should be removed from the ear canal with a gentle lavage of warm saline. Cytology and culture of the debris should reveal causes of otitis externa. Radiographs of the tympanic bullae show fluid density with otitis interna. Myringotomy or bulla osteotomy may provide drainage and an etiologic diagnosis. Bacterial infections are treated over the long term with an antibiotic selected on the basis of culture and sensitivity testing. Empirical treatment may begin with cephalosporins or chloramphenicol.

9. What if there does not appear to be an underlying cause for the ataxia?

Both dogs and cats may develop idiopathic vestibular disease. Clinically, such patients usually show multiple vestibular signs, including ataxia, circling, head tilt, and nystagmus. The onset is usually acute and unilateral. Although they are usually older animals, they are generally in good health. Spontaneous recovery usually begins within 72 hours, and most are normal in several weeks. Symptomatic treatment may provide some relief. Meclizine and dramamine are antiemetic, antimotion sickness drugs for symptomatic relief of idiopathic vestibular disease.

BIBLIOGRAPHY

1. Luttgen PJ: Diseases of the nervous system in older dogs. Part I: Central nervous system. Comp Cont Educ Vet 12:933–937, 1990.
2. Mansfield PD: Ototoxicity in dogs and cats. Comp Cont Educ Vet 12:331–334, 1990.
3. Schunk KL: Disorders of the vestibular system. Vet Clin North Am Small Animals 18:641–645, 1988.

26. ANOREXIA

Tim Hackett, D.V.M., M.S.

1. How is food intake regulated in normal animals?

Food intake is regulated by neurologic, metabolic, humoral, nutritional, and alimentary mechanisms. Gastric distention, enteric hormones such as insulin and cholecystokinin, and oxidation of energy-rich metabolites by the liver combine to effect the change from hunger to satiety. Neural mechanisms include nuclei located in the lateral hypothalamus. Stimulation of these nuclei initiates a psychic drive to search for and ingest food. The ventromedial nuclei of the hypothalamus contain a satiety center that, when stimulated, inhibits feeding behavior. Higher centers in the amygdala closely coupled with the olfactory nervous system can stimulate and inhibit feeding and may serve in food discrimination.

Increased blood levels of glucose and amino acids reduce feeding, whereas reduced levels stimulate feeding. Adipose stores within the body inversely affect feeding through concentration of free fatty acids and fat metabolites in the blood. As the amount of adipose tissue in the body decreases, the concentration of fat metabolites in the blood increases.

Alimentary mechanisms are important in the short-term control of feeding behavior. Mechanoreceptors in the walls of the stomach and intestines stimulate the ventromedial nuclei of the hypothalamus, inhibiting feeding. Related activities, such as salivation, mastication, tasting, and swallowing, are collectively termed cephalic regulation and inhibit the feeding center after a meal.

2. What is anorexia?

Anorexia is the lack of hunger. It is a disinterest in ingestion of food, generally associated with illness. Anorexia may be complete or partial, sometimes reflecting the severity of disease. Anorexia is associated with many pathologic processes that may directly inhibit appetite by suppressing the hunger center or stimulating the satiety center.

3. How is anorexia classified?

Anorexia is categorized as primary, secondary, or pseudoanorexia. Primary anorexia results from diseases affecting the appetite centers of the hypothalamus or other psychological disorders that directly affect neural regulation of feeding behavior. Secondary anorexia is caused by diseases outside the brain that affect the neural and endocrine control of hunger. Secondary anorexia is the most common cause of anorexia in animals. Pseudoanorexia encompasses diseases that affect the animal's ability to prehend, masticate, or swallow food. Such patients often are very hungry but physically unable to eat.

4. If an animal is not eating enough, what steps should be taken to determine the cause?

Pseudoanorexia should be ruled by observing the animal when presented with a meal. Is the animal interested in food? Can it prehend and masticate food? Is the animal acting as if in pain? A thorough oral examination should then be conducted. Many causes of primary and secondary anorexia can be identified by a complete physical examination, evaluation of serum chemistries, complete blood count, urinalysis, and chest and abdominal radiographs.

5. What are the metabolic consequences of anorexia?

Tissues prefer carbohydrates for energy over fat and protein. Carbohydrates, stored as glycogen, are limited, and less than 1 day after the last meal the body begins depleting fat and protein reserves. Fat depletion occurs steadily but cannot supply the brain with needed glucose. Protein is rapidly depleted early in starvation. Through hepatic gluconeogenesis, protein is converted to glucose, supplying the brain with most of its energy. When the readily mobilizable protein is depleted, gluconeogenesis slows. With decreased availability of glucose, alternative energy sources are exploited. Ketone bodies formed by hepatic conversion of fatty acids readily cross the blood–brain barrier for energy. When all fat stores have been depleted, the body returns to the remaining protein for energy. These proteins are essential for maintenance of cellular functions, and death occurs shortly after their depletion.

6. Describe methods of supplementing nutrition.

Animals can be force-fed or supplemented through various tube-feeding strategies. Force-feeding meatballs or a liquid diet may be effective in the short term but difficult for long-term management. Nasogastric, pharyngostomy, esophagostomy, gastrostomy, and jejunostomy tubes are used in veterinary medicine. Jejunostomy tubes require abdominal surgery for placement and a liquid diet. Because it enters beyond the stomach, the jejunostomy tube can be used in vomiting patients. Gastrostomy tubes can be placed surgically, endoscopically, or blindly. Because of their larger size, various gruel diets can be prepared from canned foods and water. Incorporated into a bandage, gastrostomy tubes can easily be maintained for months by the owner. Esophagostomy and pharyngostomy tubes can be placed with minimal equipment and provide large-bore feeding for short periods. Nasogastric tubes are uncomfortable and require a liquid diet but may provide short-term nutritional support.

7. What risks are associated with tube feeding?

Endotracheal placement of any feeding tube results in serious iatrogenic aspiration pneumonia. Feeding tubes that pass near the larynx should be checked radiographically before feeding. Nasogastric, pharyngostomy, and esophagostomy tubes may become dislodged and inhaled. If an animal vomits, the placement of the tube should again be confirmed before feeding is resumed. It is also a good idea to inject a small amount of water before each feeding while listening for a cough or sounds suggesting intratracheal placement.

8. Define TPN and PPN.

TPN or total parenteral nutrition is the delivery of essential nutrients directly into the bloodstream. The nutrients bypass intestinal absorption and the portal venous system and are available to the intermediary metabolic pathways. The standard TPN formula includes dextrose, an amino acid source, and a lipid. Additional B vitamins and potassium are also added. TPN is hyperosmolar and must be given through a central venous catheter.

PPN or partial parenteral nutrition also has been called protein-sparing fluid therapy and uses a 3% amino acid solution with electrolytes. Because the amino acid solutions are not as hyperosmolar as TPN, PPN may be given through peripheral veins. Theoretically the amino acids are used for gluconeogenesis instead of the patient's protein stores.

9. What are the risks and complications associated with TPN?

Complications of TPN include sepsis, metabolic acidosis, hyperphosphatemia, hyperglycemia, and hyperammonemia. Patients with hyperlipidemia or pancreatitis should not receive lipid-containing solutions. TPN requires the placement of a sterile, central catheter and close attention to aseptic technique during handling of related equipment. Recent clinical and experimental evidence suggest that TPN may impair host immune defenses and intestinal barrier function. Experiments comparing enterally fed animals with parenterally fed animals documented better antibacterial host defenses and improved survival against an infectious challenge in the enterally fed group. Randomized clinical trials of TPN in humans have documented an increased incidence of infectious complications in patients receiving TPN.

10. Should anorexia be anticipated in any specific group of patients?

Yes. Any debilitated, stressed patient may develop anorexia. It is most common after painful surgical procedures or abdominal surgery and with some medications. Critically ill surgical patients anticipating days of hospitalization should receive some sort of enteral feeding tube at the time of surgery. Animals with cancer or renal disease commonly develop anorexia. Strategies to treat the primary disease should be coupled with supportive measures to improve appetite and encourage caloric intake.

11. What diseases or conditions result in anorexia?

Causes of Anorexia

PRIMARY ANOREXIA	SECONDARY ANOREXIA	PSEUDOANOREXIA
Neurologic disease	Pain	Disorders of oral cavity
Increased intracranial pressure	Abdominal	Gingivitis, stomatitis
Cerebral edema	Thoracic	Pharyngitis, tonsillitis
Hydrocephalus	Musculoskeletal	Tooth root abscess
Intracranial pain	Urogenital	Broken teeth
Hypothalamic disorders	Organomegaly	Foreign bodies
Neoplasia	Inflammation	Neurologic disease
Infection	Toxic agents	Hypoglossal paralysis
Trauma	Exogenous	Mandibular paralysis
Psychologic disorders	Drugs	Tetanus
Unpalatable diet	Poisons	Blindness
Stress	Endogenous	Trauma
Sudden changes in	Metabolic wastes	Maxillary or mandibular fractures
environment	Inflammatory mediators	Temporomandibular dislocation
	Neoplasia	Retrobulbar abscess or neoplasia
	Infectious disease	Esophagitis
	Miscellaneous	
	Cardiac failure	
	Ketosis	
	Motion sickness	
	High ambient temperature	
	Autoimmune disease	

12. What is the diagnostic plan for anorectic patients?

Anorexia is a common sign of many different primary diseases. Pseudoanorexia may be eliminated by thorough physical examination and careful observation of the animal when presented with food. The animal may reveal pain when the jaws are open. Oral examination for dental disease, foreign bodies, or inflammatory lesions within the mouth may explain lack of appetite. If nothing abnormal is discovered, a complete polysystemic evaluation should be performed to uncover causes of secondary anorexia.

13. Are there any symptomatic treatments for anorectic patients?

The definitive treatment of decreased appetite is to find and correct the underlying problem. Environmental stimuli may affect appetite. Timid animals may not eat in a noisy room or around strangers. Palatability of food may be enhanced by experimenting with new diets, textures, and odors. Food can be heated to enhance olfaction. Flavoring agents such as animal fat, garlic, cheese, bouillon, clam juice, and butter also may increase palatability. Pharmacologic agents reported to stimulate appetite include anabolic steroids, corticosteroids, benzodiazepine derivatives, and cyproheptadine hydrochloride.

BIBLIOGRAPHY

1. Barrett RE: Indications for TPN vs. gastrostomy tube feeding. Proceedings of the 13th ACVIM Forum, 1995, pp 169–171.
2. Crowe DT: Nutritional support for the hospitalized patient: An introduction to tube feeding. Comp Cont Educ Vet 12:1711–1720, 1990.
3. Jeejeebhoy KN: Nutrition in critical illness. In Shoemaker WC (ed): Textbook of Critical Care. Philadelphia, W.B. Saunders, 1995, pp 1106–1115.
4. Osborne CA, Lulich JP, Sanderson SL, et al: Treatment of uremic anorexia. In Bonagura JD (ed): Current Veterinary Therapy, vol. XII. Philadelphia, W.B. Saunders, 1995, pp 966–971.

27. FEVER

Derek P. Burney, D.V.M.

1. What is fever?

Fever is an increased core body temperature due to resetting of the hypothalamic thermoregulatory center to a higher temperature.

2. How is fever defined in companion animals?

A core body temperature > 102.5° F (39.1° C) is elevated in dogs and cats. The elevated temperature may be due to fever or hyperthermia.

3. What is the physiologic basis of fever?

Fever results when white blood cells, especially neutrophils and monocytes, are activated. Activated leukocytes release **endogenous pyrogens**, such as interleukin 1, tumor necrosis factor, and certain interferons, that cause the thermoregulatory center in the hypothalamus to be reset to a higher temperature. Leukocytes are activated after exposure to antigens, called exogenous pyrogens. Endogenous pyrogens raise the thermoregulatory set point by direct stimulation of the anterior hypothalamus or stimulation of prostaglandin or cyclic adenosine monophosphate production. The set point also may be altered by intracranial diseases such as trauma or neoplasia or drugs such as tetracycline.

Antigens associated with bacteria, viruses, fungal infections, parasites, neoplasia, tissue necrosis, and immune-mediated disorders are considered to be **exogenous pyrogens**. Exogenous pyrogens have a large molecular mass and cannot cross the blood–brain barrier; therefore, they do not stimulate the hypothalamus directly.

4. Where is most body heat produced?

Most of the heat generated internally by the body is due to oxidative reactions in the liver. Of course, muscle activity can rapidly generate a tremendous quantity of heat.

5. What is the difference between hyperthermia and fever?

In hyperthermia, the hypothalamic thermoregulatory set point is not changed. Hyperthermia may result from high environmental temperature, increased metabolic rate, or increased muscle activity. Hyperthermia occurs because heat loss mechanisms are overwhelmed or poorly functioning. Hyperthermia does not result from pyrogens. Fever is due to resetting of the thermoregulatory set point in the hypothalamus by endogenous pyrogens.

6. How can you determine the difference between fever and hyperthermia?

A good history and physical examination are the most important skills to differentiate fever from hyperthermia. Examples of causes of hyperthermia from increased muscle activity include exercise, seizures, or nervousness. Heat stroke may result when a patient is left in a car on a warm day, even if only for a few minutes. Heat stroke also may result when an animal is confined to an area with no shelter or water on a hot day. Clients are often surprised when a dog gets heat stroke after a day at the beach with no water or shelter. Animals recovering from anesthesia and left on a heating pad unsupervised may become hyperthermic.

7. What major disease categories should be considered in evaluating a patient with elevated body temperature?

First, fever must be differentiated from hyperthermia. Fever may be drug-induced or caused by immune-mediated disease, neoplasia, infection, or inflammatory disorders.

8. At what body temperature is therapy necessary?

Fevers above 106° F (41.1° C) are potentially harmful to cellular metabolism and should be treated. A fever > 106° F (41.1° C) is considered a medical emergency. Prolonged exposure to body temperatures > 106.5° F (41.4° C) may result in brain damage or heat stroke.

9. How is fever treated?

Although it is controversial, fevers > 106° F (41.1° C) should be treated. Antiprostaglandin antipyretics are the first choice of therapy, beginning with aspirin (acetylsalicylic acid). Phenothiazines are also effective because they use central and peripheral vasodilatory effects to decrease body temperature. Whole body cooling (e.g., ice water baths and enemas, fans) should not be used; physical removal of heat increases metabolic stress because the body tries to meet the temperature set by the hypothalamus.

Nonsteroidal Antiinflammatory Drugs for Treatment of Fevers > 106° F (41.1 ° C)

DRUG	DOSE FOR DOGS	DOSE FOR CATS
Acetylsalicylic acid (aspirin)	25–35 mg/kg orally every 8 hr	12.5–25 mg/kg orally every 24 hr*
Sodium salicylate	10 mg/kg IV every 8 hr	10 mg/kg IV every 24 hr
Dipyrone†	25 mg/kg SQ, IM, IV, or orally every 8 hr	25 mg/kg SQ, IM, IV, or orally every 8 hr

* Do not exceed this dose.
† Should be limited to short-term use because of potential agranulocytosis and leukopenia.

10. How should hyperthermia be treated?

Hyperthermia should be treated aggressively by eliminating the cause of heat stress. The body should be cooled by use of ice water baths and enemas, alcohol baths, and fans. To avoid hypothermia, cooling procedures should be stopped when the temperature has been decreased to 103° F (39.4° C). Patients with hyperthermia should be observed closely for signs of cerebral edema and disseminated intravascular coagulation.

11. Does fever have beneficial effects?

There is no conclusive evidence that fever is beneficial. It has been suggested that fever may inhibit bacterial and viral proliferation. Proteolytic enzymes, which are easily released from lysosomes during fever, can be destructive to viruses. Fever reduces the ability of bacteria to trap and chelate iron, and exogenous pyrogens probably cause iron sequestration in hosts, making iron stores less available to bacteria. Fever may enhance interferon production, which adversely affects viral growth. Leukocyte mobility, phagocytic activity, and bactericidal effects may be enhanced by fever. Fever also has been suggested to enhance lymphocyte transformation.

12. What are the detrimental effects of fever?

Fever > 106° F interferes with cellular processes, and prolonged high fevers may result in brain damage or heat stroke. Fever also causes anorexia, which can be metabolically detrimental to an animal suffering from disease.

13. What is FUO?

FUO is a commonly used abbreviation for fever of unknown origin. FUO is a fever of unknown etiology that has persisted for 10–14 days in the face of aggressive diagnostic tests, including complete blood count, biochemical profile, urinalysis, and chest and abdominal radiographs.

14. What happens to metabolism with fever?

Data from humans and rats have estimated that metabolism increases 13.6% for each degree Celsius that the body temperature is above normal. Based on these data, an animal with fever may need to have caloric intake increased by 7 kcal/kg body weight for each degree Celsius that the temperature is above normal.

BIBLIOGRAPHY

1. Greene CE: Fever: In Infectious Diseases of the Dog and Cat, 2nd ed. Philadelphia, W.B. Saunders, 1990, pp 64–71.
2. Haupt KH: Fever of unknown origin. In Quick Reference to Veterinary Medicine, 2nd ed. Philadelphia, J.B. Lippincott, 1991, pp 23–24.
3. Lappin MR: Fever, sepsis and principles of antimicrobial therapy. In Practical Small Animal Internal Medicine. Philadelphia, W.B. Saunders, 1997, pp 829–836.
4. Lorenz MD: Pyrexia (fever). In Small Animal Medical Diagnosis, 2nd ed. Philadelphia, J.B. Lippincott, 1993, pp 15–22.

28. STRANGURIA

Stephanie J. Lifton, D.V.M.

1. What is the first thing to do for an animal with a primary complaint of stranguria?

The first thing to do is to determine whether the animal has a urinary obstruction. Palpate the abdomen for a hard, distended bladder, and do a quick but thorough physical examination. If the animal has been obstructed for some time, hyperkalemia may be a life-threatening complication, necessitating immediate supportive therapy as well as alleviation of the obstruction before further diagnostics are collected. Because of the smaller diameter and longer urethra of male dogs and cats, males tend to obstruct more often than females.

2. What are the primary differential diagnoses of an animal with stranguria?

In general, stranguria is associated with lower urinary tract disease. Possible diagnoses include the following:

- Urinary tract infection (UTI)
- Cystic and/or urethral calculi
- Neoplasia
- Idiopathic sterile hemorrhagic cystitis (idiopathic feline lower urinary tract disease [FLUTD])
- Prostatic disease
- Granulomatous urethritis
- Neurologic disease
- Urethral stricture
- Congenital anomaly

3. What other historical questions should you ask the client?

Ask clients about presence of pigmenturia, pollakiuria, polyuria, and polydipsia and whether they have noticed the animal urinating at all.

4. How should you relieve an obstruction?

There are many techniques for relieving an obstruction. In male cats with FLUTD, the obstruction is sometimes close to the tip of the penis, and simply massaging the end of the penis relieves the obstruction. More often, grit and calculi in the urethra need to be gently flushed back into the bladder before a catheter can be passed. This process is sometimes facilitated by using a small amount of lidocaine in the lubricant to decrease urethral spasms. In addition, using a syringeful of KY jelly, diluted with some saline, may relieve the obstruction when saline alone has been unsuccessful. If these techniques are ineffective, cystocentesis should be performed. Cystocentesis temporarily alleviates the adverse effects of the obstruction and provides a sample for urinalysis and culture. In addition, decompression of an overdistended bladder may relax the urethral sphincter and allow retrograde flushing of the plug back into the bladder. It is imperative not to forget the importance of intravenous fluids and treatment for hyperkalemia while attempting to relieve the obstruction.

5. What are the important parameters to monitor once the obstruction has been relieved?
Postobstructive diuresis may result in higher than expected fluid requirements. In addition, levels of potassium and other electrolytes often drop precipitously as a result of diuresis. It is also important to monitor blood urea nitrogen (BUN) and serum creatinine for evidence of permanent renal compromise.

6. What diagnostic tests should be done?
The most important piece of information to obtain is urinalysis with culture. Do not forget to include a rectal exam as part of the physical examination in dogs. Rectal exam allows assessment of the prostate and masses in the urethra or neck of the bladder. Other tests to consider include a complete blood panel (complete blood count and serum biochemistries), abdominal radiographs, abdominal ultrasound, and/or contrast radiographs as well as a prostatic wash in dogs.

7. If you find ammonium biurate crystals or calculi, what other tests should you consider?
In animals other than Dalmatians, ammonium biurate crystals may be associated with hepatic disease, especially portosystemic shunts. Therefore, further investigation of potential liver disease (e.g., serum bile acids, ammonia levels) is warranted.

8. Which types of calculi are radiopaque, and which are radiolucent? What are the most common types of uroliths?
Uroliths composed of magnesium ammonium phosphate, calcium oxalate, calcium phosphate, silica, and cystine are often radiodense; those composed of urate salts are often radiolucent. Magnesium ammonium phosphate uroliths are the most common uroliths in dogs. These calculi are often secondary to chronic bacterial cystitis. In cats, the incidence of calcium oxalate uroliths appears to be increasing, and the number of struvite uroliths is decreasing. Consumption of a diet designed to prevent formation of struvite crystals is one of the risk factors associated with development of calcium oxalate uroliths.

9. Which bacteria are most commonly cultured from the urine of dogs?
Gram-negative coliforms are the most common pathogens found in the urine of dogs and cats, with *Escherichia coli, Proteus mirabilis,* and *Klebsiella pneumoniae* accounting for most cases. Other common bacteria include *Pseudomonas* and *Enterobacter* spp., *Staphylococcus intermedius, Streptococcus* and *Enterococcus* spp., and *Pasteurella* spp. In approximately 15–20% of cases, infections are due to multiple bacteria. Less than 3% of cats with signs of lower urinary tract disease have bacterial infections.

10. Which antibiotic is best to start before culture results are available?
Many antibiotics are concentrated in urine and therefore reach levels effective against pathogens that otherwise they may not be able to treat. Almost 80% of *E. coli* infections respond to trimethoprim-sulfonimide; 80% of *Proteus* infections respond to ampicillin; 80% of *Pseudomonas* infections respond to tetracycline; 90% of *Klebsiella* infections respond to cephalexin; and almost 100% of staphylococcal and streptococcal infections respond to penicillins. Many urinary pathogens, especially *E. coli*, are most likely sensitive to the combination of amoxicillin and clavulinic acid. The fluoroquinolones are also concentrated in the urine and have a broad spectrum of activity, especially against gram-negative bacteria. The fluoroquinolones also reach good levels in the prostate; however, they probably should be reserved for more resistant infections to prevent emergence of resistant strains. A simple UTI should be treated for 10–14 days, whereas recurrent or chronic infections may need 4–6 weeks of antibiotic therapy.

11. What type of neoplasm is most common in the lower urinary tract of dogs? Of cats? What treatments are available?

Tumors of the bladder comprise only 1% of all cancers in dogs and are even less common in cats. In cats, mesenchymal tumors are almost as common as epithelial tumors, whereas epithelial tumors are much more common in dogs. The most common tumor, in both dogs and cats, is transitional cell carcinoma (87% of bladder tumors in dogs, 30% in cats). Other tumors include adenocarcinoma, squamous cell carcinoma, rhabdomyosarcoma, benign mesenchymal tumors (cats), leiomyosarcoma/leiomyoma, and lymphosarcoma.

The best treatment is surgical excision. Unfortunately, many bladder neoplasms are not discovered until surgical resection is impossible. Response of transitional cell carcinoma to traditional chemotherapy with cisplatin or carboplatin has been disappointing. Recently, treatment with piroxicam, a nonsteroidal anti-inflammatory drug, has shown promise. The mechanism of action of the antitumor activity of piroxicam is still unknown, but it appears to alleviate the clinical signs of stranguria, dysuria, and hematuria in many dogs and even induces remission in some patients. The most severe side effect of piroxicam is gastric irritation and ulceration. Animals with bladder neoplasms often have concurrent UTIs.

12. What types of prostatic disease may cause stranguria? How can you differentiate them?

The prostatic diseases commonly associated with stranguria include a large abscess, cyst, or neoplasm. Other possibilities include acute or chronic prostatitis or benign prostatic hyperplasia. Palpation of the prostate for symmetry, size, and pain is extremely important. Other diagnostic tools include radiographs (in addition to prostate size, evaluate sublumbar lymph nodes and the caudal spine for evidence of metastases), ultrasonography, and evaluation of prostatic fluid (obtained by prostatic massage or ejaculate). Ultimately, a biopsy may be necessary to distinguish among chronic prostatitis, benign prostatic hyperplasia, and neoplasm. Acute bacterial prostatitis and prostatic abscesses are contraindications to percutaneous biopsy.

13. What are the treatments for the various prostatic diseases?

The best treatment for benign prostatic hyperplasia is castration. Medical treatments (synthetic estrogens, dihydrotestosterone receptor blockers, and synthetic progestins) also have been used. Large paraprostatic cysts often require resection and marsupialization. Bacterial prostatitis requires antibiotic therapy based on culture and sensitivity testing of urine or prostatic fluid. In patients with acute prostatitis, the blood–prostate barrier is often disrupted so that most antimicrobial drugs reach the site of infection. Treatment should be continued for 3–4 weeks. In cases of chronic prostatitis, the blood–prostate barrier is often intact, necessitating the use of antibiotics with high lipid solubility. In addition, antimicrobials with a higher pK_a cross the prostatic epithelium and become ionized in the more acidic environment; thus they are "trapped" within the prostate, ensuring adequate antimicrobial concentrations. In chronic cases, treatment should continue for at least 4–6 weeks. Prostatic abscesses may require surgical marsupialization or drain placement. The most common prostatic neoplasms in dogs are adenocarcinoma and transitional cell carcinoma. In general, treatment of neoplasms has been unrewarding. Possible therapeutic options include prostatectomy, intraoperative radiation therapy, chemotherapy, and piroxicam.

14. What is feline lower urinary tract disease?

FLUTD is an umbrella term referring to a cluster of signs of lower urinary tract disease due to any number of causes. Once infection, urolithiasis, crystalluria, and neoplasms have been ruled out, the disease is diagnosed as idiopathic FLUTD. Some evidence suggests that FLUTD may be similar to interstitial cystitis in humans. Interstitial cystitis is characterized by difficult, painful, and frequent urination in the absence of an obvious etiology. On cystoscopy, some cats with idiopathic FLUTD have lesions identical to those seen in humans with interstitial cystitis. At this time, there is no effective treatment for interstitial cystitis in humans.

15. What treatments may be used for idiopathic FLUTD in cats that are not obstructed?

The signs associated with idiopathic FLUTD in cats are often self-limiting and may recur intermittently. Therefore, many people do not believe in treatment. If struvite crystals are seen in the urine, together with an alkaline pH, a diet designed to dissolve and/or prevent struvite uroliths may be recommended. Although dietary manipulations are effective at preventing signs of FLUTD in some cats, some evidence suggests that such diets may predispose cats to calcium oxalate uroliths. Phenoxybenzamine and diazepam have been used to decrease the suspected urethral spasms associated with idiopathic FLUTD. Their efficacy has not been well established. Studies have shown no benefit to treatment with glucocorticoids or dimethyl sulfide compared with placebo. Glucocorticoids are contraindicated in cats with UTIs or urethral obstruction, especially those requiring urethral catheterization. Ongoing studies may further elucidate the cause of this syndrome and lead to more successful therapeutic options. Until that time, FLUTD will continue to be a frustrating disease for both pet owners and veterinarians.

BIBLIOGRAPHY

1. Bamberg-Thalen B, Linde-Forsberg C: Treatment of canine benign prostatic hyperplasia with medroxy-progesterone acetate. J Am Animal Hosp Assoc 29:221–226, 1993.
2. Barsanti JA, Finco DP: Medical management of canine prostatic hyperplasia. In Bonagura JD (ed): Current Veterinary Therapy XII. Philadelphia, W.B. Saunders, 1995, pp 1033–1034.
3. Barsanti JA, Finco DP, Brown SA: Feline urethral obstruction: Medical management. In Kirk RW, Bonagura JD (eds): Current Veterinary Therapy XI. Philadelphia, W.B. Saunders, 1992, pp 883–885.
4. Barsanti JA, Finco DR, Brown SA: The role of dimethyl sulfoxide and glucocorticoids in lower urinary tract diseases. In Bonagura JD (ed): Current Veterinary Therapy XII. Philadelphia, W.B. Saunders, 1995, pp 1011–1013.
5. Buffington CAT, Chew DJ: Does interstitial cystitis occur in cats? In Bonagura JD (ed): Current Veterinary Therapy XII. Philadelphia, W.B. Saunders, 1995, pp 1009–1011.
6. Buffington CAT, et al: Clinical evaluation of cats with nonobstructive urinary tract diseases. J Am Vet Med Assoc 210:46–50, 1997.
7. Chun R, et al: Cisplatin treatment of transitional cell carcinoma of the urinary bladder in dogs: 18 cases (1983–1993). J Am Vet Med Assoc 209:1588–1591, 1996.
8. Dorfman M, Barsanti JA: CVT Update: Treatment of canine bacterial prostatitis. In Bonagura JD (ed): Current Veterinary Therapy XII. Philadelphia, W.B. Saunders, 1995, pp 1029–1032.
9. Dorfman M, Barsanti J: Diseases of the canine prostate gland. Comp Vet Cont Educ Small Animals 17:791–810, 1995.
10. Dorfman M, Barsanti J, Budsberg SC: Enrofloxacin concentrations in dogs with normal prostate and dogs with chronic bacterial prostatitis. Am J Vet Res 56:386–390, 1995.
11. Hammer AS, LaRue S: Tumors of the urinary tract. In Ettinger SJ, Feldman ED (eds): Textbook of Veterinary Internal Medicine, 4th ed. Philadelphia, W.B. Saunders, 1995, pp 1788–1796.
12. Kirk CA, et al: Evaluation of factors associated with development of calcium oxalate urolithiasis in cats. J Am Vet Med Assoc 207:1429–1434, 1995.
13. Knapp DW: Medical therapy of canine transitional cell carcinoma of the urinary bladder. In Bonagura JD (ed): Current Veterinary Therapy XII. Philadelphia, W.B. Saunders, 1995, pp 1016–1018.
14. Knapp DW, et al: Piroxicam therapy in 34 dogs with transitional cell carcinoma of the urinary bladder. J Vet Intern Med 8:273–278, 1994.
15. Krawiec DR: Canine prostatic disease. J Am Vet Med Assoc 204:1561–1564, 1994.
16. Lees GE, Forrester SD: Update: Bacterial urinary tract infections. In Kirk RW, Bonagura JD (eds): Current Veterinary Therapy XI. Philadelphia, W.B. Saunders, 1992, pp 909–914.
17. Lulich JP, Osborne CA: Bacterial infections of the urinary tract. In Ettinger SJ, Feldman EC (eds): Textbook of Veterinary Internal Medicine, 4th ed. Philadelphia, W.B. Saunders, 1995, pp 1775–1788.
18. Lulich JP, et al: Canine lower urinary tract disease. In Ettinger SJ, Feldman EC (eds): Textbook of Veterinary Internal Medicine, 4th ed. Philadelphia, W.B. Saunders, 1995, pp 1833–1861.
19. Osborne CA, et al: Feline lower urinary tract disease. In Ettinger SJ, Feldman EC (eds): Textbook of Veterinary Internal Medicine, 4th ed. Philadelphia, W.B. Saunders, 1995, pp 1805–1832.
20. Thumchai R, et al: Epizootiologic evalution of urolithiasis in cats: 3,948 cases (1982–1992). J Am Vet Med Assoc 208:547–551, 1996.

29. OBSTIPATION AND CONSTIPATION

Andrew J. Triolo, D.V.M., M.S.

1. Are constipation and obstipation common problems in small animals?
Absolutely. Although occasionally seen in dogs, they are more common in cats.

2. Define constipation and obstipation.
Constipation is the difficult passage of feces. Obstipation is more severe constipation with fecal impaction. Obstipated animals usually cannot eliminate feces on their own.

3. How are constipation and obstipation diagnosed?
Most cases can be diagnosed with a complete history and physical examination. In extremely large or obese animals, radiographs also may be helpful.

4. What causes constipation and obstipation?
Although there are many causes, any disease state that encourages fecal stasis and/or colonic water absorption may lead to constipation or obstipation.

Common Causes of Constipation and Obstipation

Diet	Environment
Bones	Decreased exercise
Grass	Dirty litter box
Rocks	Neurologic disease
Low fiber	Idiopathic megacolon
Drugs	L4–S3 spinal disease
Anticholinergics	Obstructions
Antihistamines	Foreign bodies
Anticonvulsants	Neoplasia and strictures
Barium sulfate	Pelvic fractures
Endocrine or metabolic disease	Perianal hernias
Hypothyroidism	Perirectal disease
Hyperparathyroidism	Anal gland disease
Renal failure	Perianal fistulas
	Anal strictures

5. How serious are constipation and obstipation?
Extreme cases may lead to bowel/colon perforation, which results in septic peritonitis. Immediate exploratory surgery is required in such patients.

6. What are the typical clinical signs of constipation and obstipation?
Tenesmus and dyschezia are the more common clinical signs of constipation and obstipation. Anorexia and vomiting are often seen in chronic cases, especially in cats. In animals with urinary obstructions, clinical signs may be similar.

7. What is the typical work-up for constipation and obstipation?
A minimal database, which includes complete blood count, serum biochemical analysis, urinalysis, and abdominal radiographs, points in the right direction and helps to rule out major medical causes of constipation, including renal disease. At times, further diagnostic tests may include an abdominal ultrasound, pneumocolongram, or barium contrast studies.

8. What may result from repeated episodes of constipation or obstipation?
Chronic megacolon is a serious complication, most often seen in cats. Chronic megacolon also may result in cases that are refractory to pharmacologic manipulation.

9. How do you treat constipation and obstipation?
Simple constipation is often treated with mild soapy or mineral oil enemas. Avoid phosphate enemas, especially in cats. Hexachlorophene products also should be avoided. Obstipated animals often need to be sedated and the fecal material digitally removed, along with with administration of enemas. Small sponge forceps are useful for removal of fecal matter and do not create major trauma to the colon. Obstipation rarely needs to be surgically addressed.

10. How are chronic cases of obstipation and constipation medically managed?
Drugs most often used are Lactulose, Propulcid, and bethanechol hydrochloride. Fiber agents such as bran, Metamucil, or canned pumpkin are also helpful in managing chronic cases. Since the advent of Propulcid, bethanechol is rarely used.

Drugs Used for Chronic Constipation or Obstipation

DRUG		DOSE	COMMON SIDE EFFECTS
Lactulose	Dog	5–30 ml 3 times/day orally	Diarrhea, vomiting, cramping
	Cat	1–10 ml 3 times/day orally	
Propulcid	Dog	0.5 mg/kg 3 times/day orally	Diarrhea, abdominal pain
	Cat	2.5–5 mg 2 or 3 times/day orally	
Bethanechol	Dog	5–20 mg 3 times/day orally	GI cramping, vomiting, anorexia,
	Cat	1.25–5 mg 3 times/day orally	diarrhea
Fiber products			
Canned pumpkin		1–5 tbsp daily with food	Flatulence
Psyllium		1–5 tsp daily with food	Flatulence

11. How does Lactulose work?
Lactulose is an osmotic laxative that helps to retain water in the colon. The end result is softer feces.

12. What is mechanism of action of Propulcid?
Propulcid increases physiologic release of acetylcholine from postganglionic nerve endings. This is believed to increase motor activity in the esophagus, stomach, and small and large intestines.

13. Fiber is used for patients with diarrhea. Why is it recommended for patients with obstipation or constipation?
Fiber may be used for patients with either diarrhea or constipation, depending on the type of fiber. Insoluble high fiber leads to softer fecal consistency, decreased transit time, increased fecal weight, and increased frequency of defecation.

14. Can properly managed cases still be refractory?
Yes. In the author's experience, 10–20% of cases are refractory to proper medical management. Subtotal colectomy, which must be performed by a skilled surgeon, is recommended as a last resort. Even then, postoperative dehiscence and peritoneal sepsis are possible complications. Clients also must be informed that some patients still need some medical management.

BIBLIOGRAPHY

1. Holt D, Johnston D: Idiopathic megacolon in cats. Comp Cont Educ 13:1411–1416, 1991.
2. Hoskins J: Management of fecal impaction. Comp Cont Educ 12:1579–1584, 1990.
3. Sherding RG: Diseases of colon, rectum, and anus. In Tams T (ed): Handbook of Small Animal Gastroenterology. Philadelphia, W.B. Saunders, 1996, pp 353–369.

30. FRACTURED TOOTH

Tim Hackett, D.V.M., M.S.

1. How are dental lesions classified?

Type A   Confined to the crown of the tooth with no involvement of the cemantoenamel junction (CEJ) and no exposed pulp.

Type B   Confined to the crown with pulp exposure.

Type C   Centered on or involving the CEJ enamel, cementum, and dentin, but with no exposed pulp.

Type D   Centered on or involving the CEJ enamel, cementum, and dentin with exposed pulp.

Type E   Confined to the root below the CEJ.

Type F   Destructive and degenerative lesions involving the whole root.

2. What finding in a fractured tooth makes further treatment mandatory?

Exposure of the pulp cavity requires definitive care—either extraction or endodontic care with or without reconstruction. An open pulp cavity exposes nerves and the core of the tooth to contact and contamination. Without endodontic therapy the tooth remains painful and becomes infected. Exposed pulp may be treated temporarily by placement of calcium hydroxide paste over the fracture.

3. Do the roots of fractured deciduous teeth need to be removed, or do they simply resorb?

Often the retained primary tooth is in the process of resorption; however, the root may remain intact for a long time. The most important reason to extract the complete tooth is to prevent malocclusion. Orthodontic malocclusion occurs below the gumline; thus, it is in the patient's best interest to remove the roots of primary teeth.

4. Which teeth are most commonly fractured?

The canines, upper fourth premolar (upper carnaissal tooth), and incisors are most commonly fractured in small carnivores.

5. Define endodontics.

Endodontics means *within the tooth* and refers to diseases of the pulp. Pulp is the core of the tooth, consisting of nervous, vascular, and connective tissue. Any condition that exposes the pulp cavity is an indication for endodontic therapy.

6. What are the treatment goals of endodontic therapy?

The entire contents of the pulp cavity are removed with specialized endodontic files and irrigation. The files are used to clear and enlarge the pulp cavity, forming a slight funnel shape tapering toward the apex of the tooth. The apex of the tooth is sealed after the canal is packed with a special endodontic filling material.

7. What is pulpotomy? What are the contraindications to its use?

Pulpotomy is a conservative variation of standard endodontic therapy reserved for acute traumatic injuries of young permanent teeth with pulp exposure. Pulpotomy involves removal of pulp from the pulp chamber in the crown of the tooth while leaving vital pulp in the pulp canals (roots) to function in a healthy condition.

Contraindications to pulpotomy include fractures more than 25 hours old, evidence of sensitivity of the tooth to percussion, suppurative pulp, or radiographic evidence of periapical changes consistent with tooth root abscess. Exposed pulp from injuries less than 25 hours old is red and bleeds freely when probed. Frequent radiographic rechecks are indicated to assess the viability of the tooth.

8. What is the approach to a displaced or avulsed tooth?

If client reports an avulsed tooth, instruct the client to place the tooth in a glass of milk or, if available, a commercial conditioning solution for transport to the veterinary hospital. The periodontal ligament on the root of the tooth must be preserved for reattachment without root resorption. Handle the tooth by the crown, not the root. A human tooth kept in dry storage for 30 minutes undergoes root resorption when replanted. The same tooth is viable for 6 hours in milk and up to 96 hours in Hank's Balanced Salt Solution. Once the patient is anesthetized, radiographs should be taken to assess the extent of injury to the surrounding alveolar bone. Tooth displacement may be accompanied by fracture of surrounding alveolar bone; this is almost always the case with tooth avulsion. The area should then be lavaged with sterile saline or 0.12% chlorhexidine. Lavage the socket, and remove any blood clots. Remove any bone fragments from the wound edges, and replace and reposition the tooth. The fractured alveolar bone can be pressed back into place. Hold the tooth firmly in place for a few minutes before suturing the soft tissue. The tooth should be splinted with either a self-cure composite or an acrylic. Acrylics are not as strong as composites and may cause thermal damage to the oral tissues when they cure. A figure-8 wire should be placed between the canines to act as a framework for the splint.

BIBLIOGRAPHY

1. Bellows J: Radiographic signs and diagnosis of dental disease. Semin Vet Med Surg 8(3):138–145, 1993.
2. Harvey CE, Emily PP: Small Animal Dentistry. St. Louis, Mosby, 1993, pp 213–265.

31. ABSCESSES AND CELLULITIS

Tim Hackett, D.V.M., M.S.

1. Differentiate abscess and cellulitis.

An abscess is a localized collection of pus and debris in a distinct cavity surrounded by firm granulation tissue. Cellulitis is a diffuse inflammation of soft tissues characterized by infection spreading through the fascial planes of the skin and subcutaneous tissues.

2. Why do cats get more percutaneous abscesses than dogs?

The thin sharp teeth and fighting behavior of cats provide a means of entry for resident oral microflora. Cat skin is tough and elastic, sealing over contaminated puncture wounds. Subcutaneous exudates quickly form pus-filled cavities, usually around the cat's legs, face, back, and base of the tail.

3. What are the common systemic consequences of localized infections?

Animals with systemic signs of infection are often febrile and lethargic and may develop septicemia and shock. Large inflammatory reactions recruit white blood cells, causing relative neutropenia. Mature neutrophilia is a common finding with mature, walled-off abscesses. Diffuse cellulitis is more likely to cause neutropenia and fever. Through hematogenous spread of bacteria, animals with local infections may develop pneumonia and other deep infections. Septic shock results from the systemic activation of a cascade of mediators that lead to vasodilation, hypotension, and circulatory failure.

4. What diseases should be ruled out in patients with recurrent bacterial infections?

Outdoor cats, especially adult males, that fight with other cats are at risk for infection with feline leukemia virus (FeLV) or feline immunodeficiency virus (FIV). Such cats often have severe leukopenia with or without anemia. Osteomyelitis, foreign body, neoplasia, infections with L-form bacteria, *Nocardia* and *Mycobacterium* spp., and fungi should also be considered when lesions fail to heal.

5. How does management of cellulitis differ from management of an abscess?

Surgical drainage is the treatment of choice for an abscess. With good drainage, antibiotics may not be necessary in healthy animals. Because of the diffuse nature of cellulitis, immobilization, warm compresses, and antibiotics are the recommended treatment. Animals with cellulitis are often systemically ill and may benefit from intravenous fluids, antibiotics, and analgesics.

6. What direct complications of abscesses and cellulitis may require emergency care?

The location of the abscess may cause a mass effect that impinges on vital structures. Pharyngeal swelling may obstruct airflow. Abscess in the gastrointestinal tract or abdomen may obstruct the bowel. Localized infection may lead to systemic complications, including septicemia and fever. Septic shock may result directly from the effect of endotoxin or from systemic activation of inflammatory mediators. The result is maldistribution of blood flow and multiple organ failure.

7. What is the most important point in treating a localized infection?

Antibiotics do not penetrate well into enclosed infectious foci. Surgical drainage and debridement are necessary to resolve local infections. Antibiotic therapy guided by culture and susceptibility testing is important to prevent systemic complications, but drainage is necessary for resolution.

8. What zoonotic diseases cause abscesses in dogs and cats?

Yersinia pestis (plague) is a potentially lethal bacterial infection in small animals, especially cats. Although infection with *Y. pestis* may take bubonic, pneumonic, or septicemic forms, most cats with *Yersinia* infection have submandibular, cervical, and retropharyngeal lymphadenopathy. *Yersinia* infections may present like any other facial abscess—with lethargy, fever, and a draining wound from enlarged lymph nodes. Cats may develop septicemic plague or pneumonic plague if the lymph nodes do not drain. People may become infected by inhalation of respiratory droplets from animals with pneumonic plague, by handling infected tissues or fluids via broken skin, or through bites of plague-infected fleas. Giemsa-stained tissue aspirates are used to detect bipolar-staining coccobacilli. The diagnosis is confirmed by fluorescent antibody staining of lymph node aspirates or abscess fluid.

Sporothrix schenckii is a dimorphic fungus that favors soils rich in organic matter. Animals become infected via inoculation of the organism into the tissues. People may become infected by contact exposure with infected cats. The cutaneous and cutaneolymphatic forms of sportichosis present with multiple nodules. Nodules may be firm, ulcerated, or draining. In cats, the lesions usually occur on the distal limbs, head, or base of the tail. Animals are often lethargic and febrile. The lesions may appear similar to other draining fight wounds. The organism can be identified in exudates or biopsy specimens, using either periodic acid-Schiff (PAS) or Gomori's methenamine silver (GMS) stain. Organisms are usually easy to find in cats but more difficult in dogs.

9. What common pathogens are found in abscesses? What first-line antibiotics should be considered?

If the abscess is from a cat bite, common pathogens may include *Pasteurella* spp., *Streptococcus* spp., *Escherichia coli, Actinomyces* spp, and *Nocardia* spp. Anaerobes such as *Bacteroides, Fusobacterium, Peptostreptococcus,* and *Clostridium* spp. are also potential pathogens. Actinomyces and Nocardia infections are common causes of abscesses in dogs, especially intact, large-breed, male hunting dogs. Effective antibiotics include penicillin products because of their anaerobic spectrum and chloramphenicol because of its broad spectrum and ability to penetrate tissues. Most antibiotics do not penetrate to the center of a walled-off abscess. Surgical drainage and debridement reduce the infectious burden and allow antibiotic penetration into surrounding tissues.

BIBLIOGRAPHY

1. Eidson M, Thilsted JP, Rollag OJ: Clinical, clinicopathologic, and pathologic features of plague in cats: 119 cases. J Am Vet Med Assoc 199:1191–1197, 1989.
2. Kirpensteijn J, Fingland RB: Cutaneous actinomycosis and nocardiosis in dogs: 48 cases (1980–1990). A Am Vet Med Assoc 201:917–920, 1991.
3. Rosser EJ, Dunstan RW: Sporotichosis. In Greene CE (ed): Infectious Diseases of the Dog and Cat. Philadelphia, W.B. Saunders, 1990, pp 707–710.

32. RATTLESNAKE ENVENOMATION

Tim Hackett, D.V.M., M.S., and Wayne E. Wingfield, D.V.M., M.S.

1. What groups of poisonous snakes cause the most problems for domestic animals in the United States?

There are three groups of poisonous snakes in the United States:

Pit vipers. Pit vipers are the largest group and include rattlesnakes, copperheads, and water moccasins. Pit vipers have thermoreceptor organs ("pits") between the eye and nostril, triangular-shaped heads, and retractable fangs.

Elapids. Elapids include coral snakes. They are brightly colored and have fixed fangs. The coloring of coral snakes differentiates them from the similar but harmless king snake:

• *Red on yellow, kill a fellow* (coral snake)
• *Red on black, venom lack* (king snake)

Colubrids. Colubrids include the Sonoran lyre snake, vine snake, and night snake. They have fixed fangs and are of minor importance.

2. What first aid should be rendered in the field after a rattlesnake bite?

Rescuers should be careful not to get bitten. The best treatment for rattlesnake envenomation is to take the animal to a veterinary hospital as soon as possible. Tourniquets, suction devices, and local application of electrical current have been reported for early management of rattlesnake envenomation. These interventions may delay transport, and none has proved efficacious.

3. What are the common clinical signs associated with pit viper attack?

"Snakebite" can be difficult to diagnose. In general, pit viper envenomation produces a local reaction. Look for fang marks, rapid swelling, edema, and pain at the site. Other symptoms may include erythema, petechia, ecchymosis, and tissue necrosis. Clinical signs of systemic illness include vomiting, respiratory distress, tachycardia or arrhythmia, hypotension, bleeding disorders, nystagmus, and fever.

4. Once the animal arrives at the hospital, how can you determine whether the animal was envenomated by a rattlesnake?

Owners may present their animals after coming in close contact with a rattlesnake, unsure whether the animal was bitten. If envenomation has occurred, the affected areas usually develop marked edema and erythema within 1 hour of the strike. The face, neck, and forelimbs should be examined carefully for fang marks, swelling, and bleeding; the animal may be in extreme pain.

Measurement of swollen areas should be repeated, because rapid swelling indicates probable snakebite. One useful test for envenomation is to examine a peripheral blood smear for echinocytes.

5. How do you examine for echinocytes? What do they look like?

A drop of the patient's blood is placed on a slide with a drop of saline and examined under the microscope for echinocytosis. Small, finely crenated echinocytes are present and affect most of the red blood cells (see figure below). Often this change is seen before swelling and systemic illness become apparent. As you monitor the peripheral blood smear, the number of echinocytes decreases each day; by day 3–5, it is nearly impossible to find these abnormal cells. The mechanism of echinocytosis is unknown in envenomation but probably involves uncoupling of oxidative metabolism. In addition, dogs bitten by rattlesnakes do not have increased levels of bilirubin, as one may expect if the echinocytes were destroyed by the spleen. For some reason, perhaps because of massive tissue injury by envenomation, dogs often show increased fractional excretion of potassium in the urine.

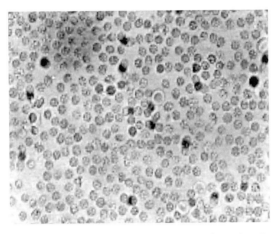

Echinocytosis affecting 100% of the red blood cells in a dog after rattlesnake envenomation.

6. What determines the severity of a snakebite?

Many factors influence the amount and type of venom received and the host's reaction. Host size and health are important, as are regional and species differences among snakes. Bites from copperheads and prairie rattlesnakes are usually minimally symptomatic. Conversely, in some southwestern desert areas the Mojave rattlesnake may cause respiratory paralysis and rapid death. The age and size of the snake, time of day, time since the snake's last meal, and season affect the amount of venom administered in a bite. Many bites are dry and nonpoisonous. They may be painful but usually show no signs of swelling. Wounds still should be considered contaminated, and appropriate cleaning and antibiotic therapy are indicated.

7. What is a dry snakebite?

A dry snakebite is present if no venom is released at the time of the bite. Clinically a dry snakebite is assumed if no pain or swelling occurs within 1 hour of envenomation.

8. What toxic components are found in pit viper venoms?

Rattlesnake venom contains various proteolytic enzymes. An early, direct effect of an enzyme called kininogenase is bradykinin activation. Bradykinin is a potent vasodilator on its own, but it also stimulates endogenous phospholipase A, which stimulates the arachidonic cascade to produce various inflammatory eicosanoids, including prostaglandins I_2, E_2, and $F_{2\alpha}$ and thromboxane A_2. The results are systemic inflammation, vasodilation, and severe hypotension. Rattlesnake venom also disrupts the basal lamina and collagen of the capillaries, allowing leakage of blood cells and plasma into the surrounding tissues. Signs include edema and petechia. Venom may cause platelet aggregation and margination through damage to the endothelium. Activated platelets then produce thromboxane and prostaglandins, which attract more platelets and white blood cells. Activation of platelets and the coagulation cascade may lead to consumption of clotting factors. The snake's venom also has a thrombinlike enzyme that cleaves fibrin and adds to the mechanisms of disseminated intravascular coagulation (DIC).

9. What are the first steps to treat snake envenomation?
When an animal presents in distress after rattlesnake envenomation, the clinician should first assess the ABCs of resuscitation:

A Airway patency should be assessed. The airway may become obstructed if swelling and edema affect the face or throat. If necessary, the patient should be intubated or a tracheostomy performed.

B Breathing should be assessed by auscultation and examination of mucous membranes.

C Circulation is assessed by palpating pulses, auscultating the heart, and again assessing mucous membrane color and capillary refill. If possible, blood pressure also should be checked.

Because the most serious early complication of rattlesnake bite is hypotension, a large-bore intravenous catheter should be placed and a balanced crystalloid solution started. Volumes and fluid rate should be based on clinical signs. In general, be prepared to give a whole blood volume (90 ml/kg in dogs) in the first hour. The patient's response to fluids should guide further therapy. Be aware of the potential fluid loss associated with increased capillary permeability. Patients presented within a few hours of a bite usually swell much more in the hospital. Continuous reassessment of vital functions is mandatory. Blood and urine should be collected for baseline data, coagulation testing, and identification of early myoglobinuria.

10. When should antivenin be given?
Rattlesnake antivenin is a polyvalent compound containing serum globulins from horses immunized with venoms of the major pit vipers (family: Crotalidae). Antivenin is contraindicated only in patients with known hypersensitivity. Unfortunately, there is no correlation between positive intradermal skin reactions and identification of early antivenin reactions. Normally, the antibodies in horse serum combine with the snake's venom to neutralize it. It may be life-saving in severely affected animals and limits the morbidity of relatively minor envenomation. Use of antivenin is controversial because many animals recover without it, it is expensive, and it is not without some risk of anaphylaxis. The dose may be quite variable. In people 2–4 vials are recommended for moderate envenomation (large swelling and abnormal laboratory tests) and up to 15 vials for severe envenomation (systemic manifestations). In animals, the number of vials depends on the severity of clinical signs, size of the patient, and location of the bite (smaller patients and snakebites on the digits generally require 50% more antivenin than larger patients and nondigital bites). Routine antivenin therapy may be cost-prohibitive. Mild envenomation may be treated successfully with supportive therapy alone. Clients should be informed of the potential benefit of antivenin and the possible need to give multiple doses. Antivenin administration should be monitored closely. If a patient shows signs of anaphylaxis, discontinue the antivenin and administer corticosteroids and epinephrine.

11. Is serum sickness a common complication of antivenin therapy?
About 50–75% of humans who are given antivenin develop serum sickness, a type II hypersensitivity reaction that may occur up to 30 days after administration. Clinical signs in humans include lymphadenopathy, skin rashes, fever, and arthralgia. Evidence indicates that patients given systemic glucocorticoids have a significantly decreased risk for development of serum sickness. Serum sickness may not be a common complication in animals because of the expense of using several vials of antivenin.

12. Are any treatments contraindicated in patients with snakebite?

Tourniquets are useful only if applied immediately and should not be used for head or neck wounds. Cold packs may delay the spread of venom but also can increase the amount of tissue damage. Electroshock therapy has been advocated to denature the protein constituents of venom. It is now believed that this treatment merely contributes to local tissue damage and should not be used. Patients with rhabdomyolysis and metabolic acidosis should not receive lactated Ringer's solution. A non–lactate-containing buffered crystalloid solution should be used. Although het-astarch is a useful colloid to manage increased vascular permeability, it should not be used in patients with coagulopathies.

13. What complications should you anticipate?

The proteolytic enzymes associated with rattlesnake venom may induce rhabdomyolysis and myoglobinuria. Myoglobin is nephrotoxic, and renal failure is a potential complication. Intravenous fluid therapy and close attention to urine character and output should identify problems early. DIC is a common complication. Patients should be screened once or twice daily with activated clotting times. Blood smears identify schistocytes, and laboratory evaluation of fibrin degradation products and antithrombin III identifies DIC.

14. How should you treat DIC associated with snakebite?

DIC should be anticipated. Aggressive supportive care, including intravenous fluid therapy, helps to treat the primary problem, dilutes the toxin, and enhances renal clearance. Antivenin may decrease the incidence of DIC but is most effective before serious complications develop. The use of fresh and fresh frozen plasma to provide clotting factors and antithrombin III can be augmented by incubating the plasma with heparin before administration. If severe anemia also develops, fresh whole blood also provides needed factors and can be incubated with heparin.

CONTROVERSIES

15. Are corticosteroids indicated for treatment of rattlesnake envenomation?

Corticosteroids are advocated by many for treatment of shock related to rattlesnake envenomation. Corticosteroids inhibit phospholipase A, the arachidonic acid cascade, complement activation, and leukocyte accumulation and activation. They may increase the response to catecholamines, resulting in bronchodilation. Steroids also may help to reduce increased capillary permeability by decreasing leukocyte aggregation. Controversy about steroid use stems from work in other forms in septic shock, which has shown increased morbidity and mortality. A major concern with corticosteroids is that decreasing the immune response leaves the host open to bacterial pathogens. Experimental and retrospective studies in patients with snakebite have demonstrated the potential benefit of steroids and to date have revealed no problems with their use.

16. What is the role of antihistamines and fasciotomy?

Although antihistamines may be used for their sedative effects, no evidence shows that they have any effect on snake venom or patient response. Fasciotomies to relieve pressure on extremities in dogs are rarely helpful.

BIBLIOGRAPHY

1. Brown DE, Meyer DJ, Wingfield WE, et al: Echinocytosis associated with rattlesnake envenomation in dogs. Vet Pathol 31:654–657, 1996.
2. Hudelson S, Hudelson P: Pathophysiology of snake envenomation and evaluation of treatment. Part I. Comp Cont Educ Pract Vet 17:889–896, 1995.
3. Hudelson S, Hudelson P: Pathophysiology of snake envenomation and evaluation of treatment. Part II. Comp Cont Educ Pract Vet 17:1035–1040, 1995.
4. Hudelson S, Hudelson P: Pathophysiology of snake envenomation and evaluation of treatment. Part III. Comp Cont Educ Pract Vet 17:1385–1394, 1995.

33. LAMENESS

Maura G. O'Brien, D.V.M.

1. What four principles are used to determine the location and cause of lameness?

1. **Historical information** important in determining the cause of lameness includes known traumas, duration of lameness, and response to medical management.

2. **Observation** of the dog standing, walking, and trotting demonstrates which limb(s) is affected.

3. **Physical examination,** including palpation of the muscles and joints, detects asymmetry of muscle groups as well as fractures, joint effusions, joint instabilities, or swelling.

4. **Diagnostic imaging,** such as radiography, nuclear scintigraphy, magnetic resonance imaging, and computed tomography, best define the cause of the lameness once it is localized to a specific region of the body.

2. What initial evaluations should be performed in animals presenting with lameness or fracture?

Some form of trauma is behind most lameness. Owners may notice only an obvious fracture or lameness; subtle signs of internal injury may be missed. All animals with suspected trauma should be carefully evaluated for cardiopulmonary complications and evidence of abdominal and neurologic injury. Pulmonary and myocardial contusions, head trauma, diaphragmatic hernia, uroabdomen, and internal hemorrhage are among the common sequelae of blunt force trauma. Careful physical examination, neurologic examination, thoracic and abdominal radiographs, and eletrocardiogram should be considered before attempting to correct the cause of lameness.

3. What questions provide the most information about a patient presenting with lameness?

Signalment often provides important clues to the cause of the condition. Young, rapidly growing animals may have a congenital or developmental cause of lameness, such as osteochondrosis or hip dysplasia. Older animals are more likely to develop lameness due to degenerative conditions such as arthritis or neoplasia. The onset of lameness may be associated with a known traumatic event. The clinician should ask which limb is affected, whether more than one limb is affected, how severe the lameness is, and whether the onset was acute or gradual. Additional helpful information includes duration of lameness, whether the animal will place weight on the affected limb, response to rest or exercise, and response to previously administered antiinflammatory medication.

4. What points are important in the physical examination of patients with lameness?

- Can the animal stand or support its own weight? If the animal is non–weight-bearing, is the reason due to a muscloskeletal problem, neurologic problem, or generalized weakness suggestive of metabolic or cardiovascular disease?
- Does the patient exhibit conscious proprioceptive deficits, which suggest a neurologic cause?
- Does examination reveal asymmetry of major muscle groups or alignment of limbs?
- Is joint effusion present?
- Neck or back pain elicited on palpation suggests nerve root injury as the cause of lameness.
- Evaluate the animal at a walk or trot. Does the animal's head rise abruptly when weight is placed on the affected forelimb? Do the hips move synchronously, or is an imbalance apparent, suggesting pain in a hind leg? Is the stride shortened?

• Examine the patient from the side. Are all joints moving through full range of motion?
• If lameness is not evident with gait analysis, the patient should undergo palpation of limbs and joints to see whether pain can be elicited or lameness exaggerated.

5. What is the Ortolani sign?

The Ortolani sign is significant in examining a patient for hip dysplasia. With the patient positioned in dorsal recumbency, the hindlimbs are held parallel to each other and perpendicular to the long axis of the body with the stifles flexed. Pressure is applied to the shaft of the femur proximally toward the hip. Each limb is slowly abducted. The hip is initially subluxated in dysplastic patients. As the limb is abducted, the femoral head drops into the acetabulum. This sudden reduction, which can be felt by the thumb on the trochanter, is a positive Ortolani sign. The maneuver also can be performed with the patient in lateral recumbency, but laxity of the hip joint may not be as evident.

6. What should be suspected in a dog with acute non–weight-bearing lameness of the rear limb and stifle pain?

• Rupture of the anterior cruciate ligament
• Injury to the menisci or collateral ligament
• Luxation of the medial patellar tendon
• Fracture

7. What additional tests should be performed?

The stifle is gently palpated, compared with the opposite stifle joint, and evaluated for joint effusion. Radiographic evaluation of the joint identifies fractures or joint effusion. Palpation of the joint to assess integrity of the collateral ligament and patellar luxation includes checking for the cranial drawer sign.

8. What is the cranial drawer sign?

The cranial drawer is a test of the integrity of the cranial cruciate ligament (CCL). With the stifle in flexion and extension, the tibia is pushed in an anterior direction while the femur is held in place. In a normal joint the tibia is fixed and cannot be displaced cranially to the femur. With complete rupture of the CCL, the tibia moves cranially to the femur in flexion and extension. Partial tears of the CCL may have only cranial movement when the stifle is in flexion because the craniomedial band of the CCL is more commonly torn than the thicker caudolateral band. The caudolateral band is taut in extension but relaxed in flexion, whereas the craniomedial band is taut throughout the range of motion.

9. How does an animal with luxation of the coxofemoral joint present?

Most coxofemoral luxations are craniodorsal. The dog presents with non–weight-bearing lameness, and the distal limb is rotated outward. Palpation reveals asymmetry in the location of the greater trochanter and ischium. Radiographs in both lateral and ventrodorsal positions confirm the diagnosis, evaluate for fractures, and assess the coxofemoral joint for hip dysplasia and arthritis to ensure that closed reduction is practical.

10. Describe methods to reduce and treat coxofemoral luxation.

With the patient under general anesthesia, the muscles are allowed to relax. The patient is placed in lateral recumbency, the limb is grasped by the distal femur, and pressure is applied proximally. The limb is externally rotated to free the femoral head from the shaft of the ilium. It is then abducted while pressure is applied to the greater trochanter until the femoral head pops into place. Once the femoral head is in place, the limb is placed in an Ehmer sling to prevent weight-bearing and to force the femur into the acetabulum.

If the closed procedure fails, open surgical reduction of the joint should be performed. The joint can be stabilized by capsulorrhaphy, prosthetic, toggle pin fixation, or Devita pin stabilization. As a last resort, ostectomy of the femoral head and neck provides relatively normal function.

10. What potential causes of fractures should be considered in animals with minor trauma or no history of trauma?

Pathologic fracture is more common in older animals but may affect animals of all ages. There may or may not have been a subtle lameness before fracture of the bone. Pathologic fractures may be due to neoplasia or nutritional disorders. Nutritional disorders causing lameness are seen in young animals with congenital disease or as the result of an all-meat diet. Primary bone tumors, such as osteosarcoma and multiple myeloma, and metastatic cancers, including mammary gland adenocarcinoma and prostatic carcinoma, may present with lameness or fractures. Owners should be questioned about previous diagnosis of cancer. Possible masses should be noted by careful physical examination. Radiographs should be taken of the thorax and abdomen to look for primary or metastatic disease. Careful evaluation of bone quality at the fracture site should focus on destruction of cortical bone, mottling of the medullary canal, and any periosteal component to a recent fracture. If the cause of the fracture is in doubt, the bone should be submitted for histopathologic evaluation.

11. What is the most common type of fracture in young animals?

Physeal fractures occur in young, skeletally immature animals. The physis is the weakest region of developing bone. Physeal fractures are classified according to the Salter-Harris system:

Type 1 Separation of the epiphysis from the rest of the bone at the physis
Type 2 Fracture across the physis and into the metaphysis
Type 3 Fracture through the physis and epiphysis, entering the joint
Type 4 Fracture across the physis, involving both the epiphysis and metaphysis
Type 5 Crushing type of fracture to the physis, which usually results in permanent damage to the growing cells, shortened limb, and potentially an angular limb deformity

12. What is an open fracture? How is an open fracture classified?

In an open fracture, bone is exposed through a wound. In a grade I open fracture, a small puncture wound is created by the bone fragment. A grade II open fracture is characterized by exposed bone and a larger wound than a grade I fracture. Grade III open fractures have extensive loss of skin and connective tissue around the fracture and are often referred to as shear wounds. Grade III wounds also may be caused by gunshot injuries.

13. Describe the initial management of an open fracture.

During assessment and treatment of any life-threatening traumatic complication, the wound is covered with a sterile dressing or clean cloth. When the patient is stable, the dressing is removed, and the fracture and wound are assessed for vascular and neurologic integrity. If possible, the patient should be sedated or a local anesthetic block should be applied to allow clipping of hair from the wound edges and irrigation with sterile saline. Another sterile dressing can be applied while waiting for primary debridement and fracture stabilization. Broad-spectrum antibiotics are administered parenterally, and the patient is prepared for surgery. It is preferable to repair open fractures as soon as possible, but the patient's respiratory and cardiovascular status takes precedence over repair. When the fracture is repaired, the wound is debrided of devitalized or contaminated tissue and closed. If the degree of contamination and tissue loss is too great, the wound can be left open and the dressing changed daily. Debridement is done intermittently until it is appropriate to close the wound (delayed closure) or until the wound heals by second intention.

14. What causes swelling and pain of the metaphyseal region of the long bones in immature large or giant-breed dogs?

The underlying condition is hypertrophic osteodystrophy, which usually affects the distal radius but may involve other bones. Vascular supply to the metaphyseal area is disrupted, and ossification of the hypertrophic zone is delayed. The results are inflammation, hemorrhage, necrosis, fracture, and remodeling in the metaphysis. Radiographs may reveal a periosteal reaction adjacent to the metaphysis, but this finding is not consistent. Affected puppies usually present between the ages of 2 and 8 months; they may exhibit only lameness or be systemically ill with pyrexia and weight loss. Pain, heat, and swelling on palpation of the metaphysis of affected bones are variable. The cause is not known, but potential factors include vitamin C deficiency, respiratory viral infection, and congenital factors. Treatment is supportive, with analgesics such as buffered aspirin for mildly affected patients. Systemically ill patients may require intravenous fluid therapy and nutritional support in addition to analgesics. Nursing care with attention to hygiene is important to prevent urine scald and decubital ulcers.

15. After trauma, a dog is presented with non–weight-bearing lameness of the foreleg and no palpable fractures. The limb hangs limp with no pain or sensation elicited on palpation. During physical examination the dog is found to have Horner's syndrome. What is the most likely diagnosis? What causes the Horner's syndrome?

The patient most likely has a brachial plexus avulsion. The nerves of the brachial plexus are stretched or torn from either the spinal cord or the plexus when the forelimb is forcefully abducted from the body wall. The presence of Horner's syndrome indicates that the injury is at the level of the nerve roots instead of the plexus. Damage to the nerve roots in the spinal cord segment from C6 to T1 results in loss of sympathetic innervation to the ipsilateral eye, with a miotic pupil, enophthalmos, ptosis, and protrusion of the third eyelid. Prognosis for return of innervation to the limb after brachial plexus avulsion is extremely poor, and often the limb is amputated to prevent or treat self-trauma to the denervated limb.

16. Hypertrophic osteopathy is reported to cause lameness most commonly in humans and dogs. What is this condition? What tests should be performed to confirm the diagnosis?

Hypertrophic osteopathy (HO) is a condition in mature animals characterized by symmetrical swelling of the distal extremities. Pain is elicited when these areas are palpated, and radiographs of the bones reveal a diffuse periosteal reaction. HO is associated with a primary pulmonary condition. The pathogenesis is not understood, but it is theorized that the pulmonary condition results in an increase of blood flow. The increase in blood flow is believed to be due to a neurologic process and results in congestion of connective tissues, such as periosteum. The periosteum responds by laying down new bone. HO is most commonly seen with pulmonary metastasis but also may be seen with a primary lung tumor, abscess, and bronchopneumonia. Patients with abdominal conditions such as rhabdomyosarcoma of the bladder and adenocarcinoma of the liver also have developed this secondary condition. If a primary pulmonary condition is not found, abdominal radiographs or ultrasound should be pursued. If the primary condition can be treated (e.g., lung lobectomy for a primary tumor), HO usually resolves.

BIBLIOGRAPHY

1. Brinker WO, Piermattei DL, Flo GL: Handbook of Small Animal Orthopedics and Fracture Management, 2nd ed. Philadelphia, W.B. Saunders, 1990.
2. Slatter D, Vasseur PB: The musculoskeletal system. In Slatter D (ed): Textbook of Small Animal Surgery, 2nd ed. Philadelphia, W.B. Saunders, 1993, pp 1577–2026.
3. Wingfield WE, Henik RA: Treatment priorities in multiple trauma. Semin Vet Med Surg 3(3):193–210, 1988.

34. INFECTIOUS DISEASE

Derek P. Burney, D.V.M.

1. Why is recognition of infectious disease important in the critical care setting?

Infectious diseases must be recognized so that effective methods of preventing spread of contagious organisms to animals or humans can be implemented. In a critical care setting, a large number of critically ill patients with varying degrees of immuncompromise may be in close proximity; therefore, it is important to minimize infectious disease transmission.

2. How can transmission of zoonotic agents to hospital staff be avoided?

Some infectious agents are zoonotic; thus, the risk to hospital personnel must be carefully evaluated. Proper measures to dispose of contaminated materials and proper disinfection procedures for the suspected organism should be followed. Personnel should wear protective clothing, such as surgical caps, masks, disposable gowns, and shoe covers, to protect the most likely routes of infection by the suspected organism.

3. How are most infectious agents of dogs and cats transmitted?

Most infectious agents are transmitted by contact with fecal material, respiratory secretions, reproductive tract secretions, or urine or by bites, scratches, reservoirs, or vectors. Some animals may be contagious but not clinically affected.

4. What are the most common means of transmission and prevention of nosocomial infection?

Hospital employees are the most common mode of transfer of nosocomial infections. To prevent transmission of disease, hospital employees should wash hands thoroughly with a disinfectant soap between patients. Employees should be encouraged to wear disposable gloves and to obtain a clean pair for each patient. Soiled gloves should be thrown away, and soiled hands should be washed immediately. All personnel should wear a smock or scrub suit, and clothes should be changed after contact with feces, secretions, and exudates. Equipment such as stethoscopes, pen lights, scissors, clipper blades, and percussion hammer serve as excellent fomites and should be cleaned and disinfected in 0.5% chlorhexidine solution between patients. Disposable thermometer covers should be used.

5. What clinical signs should alert hospital employees to potentially contagious diseases?

Animals with gastrointestinal or respiratory disease are likely to be the most contagious. All diarrhea, acute or chronic, should be considered infectious until proved otherwise. Infectious respiratory disease should be suspected in all sneezing or coughing animals, especially if purulent nasal discharge or productive cough is present. Cats with acute high fever, particularly if from a breeding facility, humane society, or boarding facility, carry a high index of suspicion for infectious disease.

6. How can reception personnel help to decrease contagious disease spread within the hospital?

Often clients indicate by telephone what clinical signs the pet is showing. Animals with suspected gastrointestinal or respiratory disease should be sent straight to an examination room or isolation. They should be transported by gurney to minimize contamination of the hospital facility. The gurney should be disinfected immediately after use. If possible, the clinician should examine animals with suspected infectious disease immediately to decrease hospital contamination by minimizing the time an infected patient is in the hospital.

7. What patients should be kept in isolation facilities?

Patients with suspected salmonellosis, campylobacteriosis, parvovirus, coronavirus, kennel cough syndrome, feline upper respiratory disease syndrome, rabies, and plague have contagious diseases and should be kept in isolation.

8. Where should cats with feline leukemia virus (FeLV) and/or feline immunodeficiency virus (FIV) be housed?

Cats with FeLV and/or FIV should not be kept in infectious disease isolation facilities because their immunodeficient state places them at high risk of contracting further infectious disease. Seropositive cats should not be caged next to or above seronegative cats.

9. What biosecurity measures should be used in an isolation facility?

Disposable foot covers or a foot bath with 1:64 dilution of disinfectant should be used on entering and exiting the isolation facility. Employees should remove outerwear and put on disposable gowns and Latex gloves. If working with plague-infected cats, personnel should wear masks. All sharps should be placed in dedicated containers with biohazard warnings. The isolation facility should have separate equipment and supplies, and supplies or equipment should not be moved into and out of isolation. All biologic materials submitted for laboratory analysis should be clearly labeled with the suspected infectious disease. Feces for analysis should be collected by tongue depressor or wooden applicator stick, placed in a screw-top plastic vial, and bagged in a plastic bag. The fecal sample bag should be clearly labeled with the suspected infectious disease. All disposables should be placed in heavy-duty plastic bags and sealed. The bags should be sprayed with disinfectant before removal from the isolation facility. All equipment should be cleaned and disinfected, and staff should wash their hands on conclusion of procedures in isolation.

10. How should cages be cleaned and maintained to minimize transmission of infectious disease?

Animals should stay in the same cage during their hospital stay and should not be moved from cage to cage. Soiled items should be removed from cages as soon as possible. Contaminated surfaces should be cleaned and disinfected. All surfaces should be in contact with the disinfectant for 10–15 minutes, if possible. Do not forget to clean the tops of the cages, which are often overlooked.

11. How can transmission of parasites be minimized in the hospital environment?

Cleanliness is crucial to inhibit parasite problems. Detergent and steam cleaning inactivate most parasite ova. Prompt removal of fecal material from outdoor exercise areas is extremely important.

12. What patients are at highest risk for contracting diseases in the hospital?

Immunocompromised patients, such as puppies, kittens, old animals, debilitated animals, animals with immunosuppressive diseases (e.g., hyperadrenocorticism, diabetes mellitus), animals with concurrent infections, and animals treated with glucocorticoids or cytotoxic agents, are at risk for contracting infectious diseases.

13. What environments are at most risk for transmission of infectious disease?

Veterinary hospitals, pet shows, kennels, humane societies, and parks are great reservoirs of infectious disease, especially parasites and parvovirus. Any area in which large numbers of animals from many different environments congregate is a potential infectious disease clearinghouse.

14. How can hospitals decrease transmission of disease when treating patients with infectious diseases?

Animals with infectious diseases should be treated as outpatients if at all possible. If hospitalization is required, all procedures, such as radiographs or surgery, should be delayed until the end of the day if possible. Cage identification should be used for all hospitalized animals, and the cage identification of animals suspected of contagious disease should be clearly marked with the suspected infectious agent. As the diagnosis becomes updated, the cage information should be updated. A hospitalwide biosecurity system committee may be formed to design guidelines for infectious diseases and to ensure that all personnel are familiar with the guidelines. The biosecurity committee also can periodically review procedures to ensure that the infectious disease protocol is followed and to make changes as necessary.

BIBLIOGRAPHY

1. Greene CE: Environmental survival of certain microorganisms and some effective biocidal agents. In Infectious Diseases of the Dog and Cat, 2nd ed. Philadelphia, W.B. Saunders, 1990, pp 905–907.
2. Hartmann FA, Callan RJ, McGuirk SM, West SE: Control of an outbreak of salmonellosis caused by drug-resistant *Salmonella anatum* in horses at a veterinary hospital and measures to prevent future infections. J Am Vet Med Assoc 209:629–631, 1996.
3. Lappin MR: Prevention of infectious diseases. In Essentials of Small Animal Internal Medicine, 2nd ed. St. Louis, Mosby, 1997 [in press].

IV. Ophthalmic Emergencies

Section Editors: Cynthia C. Powell, D.V.M., M.S.,
and Steven M. Roberts, D.V.M., M.S.

35. ACUTE OCULAR TRAUMA

Cynthia C. Powell, D.V.M., M.S., and Steven M. Roberts, D.V.M., M.S.

1. What are the major considerations in evaluating acute ocular injury?

Overall patient condition is the first consideration with acute trauma. Once the patient is stable, attention then should be focused on the eye. Prognosis and therapeutic options vary depending on cause and duration of injury and ocular structures involved. If other injuries preclude immediate evaluation and attention to the injured eye, it should be protected from further damage with lubricants and a protective collar if necessary. In cases of chemical injury, the globe should be examined to determine its integrity, and lavage should be instituted immediately.

2. Are certain injuries more threatening to vision or the integrity of the globe?

Ocular proptosis and injuries that rupture or perforate the globe often result in vision loss or require enucleation and carry a guarded prognosis. In general, blunt traumatic injury carries a worse prognosis than sharp penetrating injury because of the increased incidence of retinal detachment and broader scope of uveal damage. Alkali chemical burns, such as those due to ammonia, lye, lime, and magnesium hydroxide, are more likely to cause globe or sight-threatening injury.

3. Why are alkali injuries worse than acid injuries?

Most acids coagulate corneal epithelial and stromal proteins, thus forming a barrier and limiting corneal penetration. Alkalis, however, saponify plasma membrane lipids, denature collagen, and readily penetrate the cornea, increasing possibility of anterior segment damage.

4. How do you treat chemical burns of the eye?

Copious irrigation to decrease contact time and concentration should be instituted immediately if a chemical burn is suspected or confirmed. Continuous lavage with a sterile solution of lactated Ringer's and 5% dextrose in water or saline can be delivered through a standard IV set. During irrigation the conjunctival and corneal surfaces should be inspected and cleaned of chemical residue. Lavage should be continued for 30 minutes or until the pH of the ocular surface returns to normal range (7.3–7.7). After irrigation the eye should be treated for corneal ulceration, uveitis, and glaucoma when present.

5. Do any specific therapies for alkali burns help treatment and improve prognosis?

Alkali corneal burns decrease aqueous and corneal ascorbic acid levels and may result in impaired collagen synthesis in the injured cornea. Evidence suggests that topical 10% sodium ascorbate applied hourly and high dosages of oral ascorbate 4 times/day may decrease the incidence (but not progression) of sterile stromal ulceration after alkali chemical injury. Treatment is continued at this level for 1 week when the topical medication is decreased to 4 times/day. Both medications are continued until the cornea is reepithelialized.

6. What are some of the long-term sequelae of chemical burn?

Long-term complications of chemical burns include corneal scarring, glaucoma, keratoconjunctivitis sicca, symblepharon and entropion. If uveitis is severe, synechia and cataract formation are also possible.

7. What causes proptosis of the eye?

Trauma to the head either by a car or dog fight is the most common injury associated with prolapse of the globe from the orbit. However, in extremely exophthalmic breeds, proptosis may result from grasping the scruff of the neck or tension on the skin of the face from excessive restraint. Ocular damage is related to the amount of force needed to cause proptosis. Cats and dolicocephalic breeds of dogs are more likely than brachycephalic animals to sustain severe ocular injuries during proptosis.

8. How can you assess prognosis for vision or retention of the globe?

The amount of damage to the optic nerve, blood supply and musculature may be difficult to establish, but they determine the prognosis. Unless the eye, optic nerve, or extraocular muscles are obviously ruptured, the prognosis for vision is difficult to judge and in general should be considered guarded. Optic nerve damage results in blindness in most cases of proptosis. Indicators of prognosis are summarized below:

Favorable	*Unfavorable*
Positive menace	Negative consensual pupillary light response
Miotic pupil	Midpoint or dilated and unresponsive pupil
Positive direct or consensual pupillary light response	Severe hyphema
Normal-appearing fundus	Extraocular muscle avulsion
Normal intraocular pressure	Hypotony
Good extraocular muscle tension	Retinal detachment
Short time ($< \frac{1}{2}$ hr) from injury to treatment	Long time from injury to treatment

9. What emergency treatment is appropriate for the proptosed globe?

The owner should be told to keep the cornea protected and lubricated until the patient arrives at the clinic. Sterile ocular lubricants, artificial tears, or collyrium are ideal but petroleum jelly may also be used. In most cases of acute proptosis, the eye should be surgically replaced as soon as possible. Enucleation should be done if the eye is ruptured or the extraocular muscles are severely avulsed. If there is any question about the status of the eye, it should be replaced; enucleation may be done later, if needed. After the globe is replaced, temporary tarsorrhaphy prevents reprolapse and protects the cornea. Often, medical therapy for the treatment or prevention of uveitis, optic neuritis, or corneal ulceration is also needed.

10. How do you replace the globe?

When the eye prolapses, the eyelid margins become entrapped behind the globe. Relief of entrapment is necessary for globe replacement and usually requires general anesthesia. The lid margins must be pulled forward while simultaneously placing gentle pressure on the globe to replace it in the orbit. To expose the eyelid margins, grasp the rolled skin adjacent and parallel to the lid margin with a hemostat and roll the instrument outward. Alice tissue clamps are used to hold and pull the margins gently forward while the globe is pushed back into the orbit with firm, even pressure applied over several minutes. A lateral canthotomy may be required to facilitate globe replacement in some cases.

11. How is temporary tarsorrhaphy done? How long should it be left in place?

Four to six horizontal mattress sutures of split thickness should be placed through the eyelid margins with 2-0 to 4-0 nonabsorbable suture. Because of the considerable swelling that accompanies proptosis, tents (rubber band or IV tubing) should be used and the sutures tied tightly. Leaving a small space at the medial canthus allows application of topical medications. Tarsorrhaphy sutures should be left in place until retrobulbar swelling has decreased sufficiently for complete eyelid closure. This may take up to 3 weeks. Frequent rechecks are recommended because sutures loosen as swelling subsides and may contact the cornea. Sutures tied too tightly result in necrosis of the lid margin.

12. What follow-up therapy is recommended?

Corneal ulceration, traumatic uveitis, and traumatic optic neuritis may accompany globe proptosis. Corneal ulcers should be treated with a topical broad-spectrum antibiotic 3 times/day and with topical 1% atropine sulfate if the pupil is miotic. Conservative use of atropine is recommended because it decreases tear production; often a single application or once daily application for a few days is sufficient. Uveitis and optic neuritis are treated with systemic corticosteroids (e.g., 0.125–0.5 mg/kg dexamethasone once daily) for 7 days, then tapered over the next 2 weeks. The higher dosages are used to treat optic neuritis and more severe cases of uveitis. Topical corticosteroids are not recommended because of the high incidence of corneal ulceration. Cold compresses may help to relieve swelling.

13. What are the long-term sequelae of proptosis?

In most cases, the eye is blind as a result of optic nerve damage; however, the eye often has a cosmetic appearance. The pupil is dilated with parasympathetic denervation or mid-point with both parasympathetic and sympathetic denervation. Most eyes have permanent lateral or dorsolateral strabismus, although it sometimes improves over several weeks. Lagophthalmos and exposure keratitis are common, especially in brachycephalic breeds of dogs, and may require permanent blepharoplastic procedures to reduce palpebral fissure size. Other sequelae include keratoconjunctivitis sicca, neurotropic keratitis, and phthisis bulbi.

14. What clinical signs indicate the extent of ocular injury?

Physical ocular trauma may be blunt or sharp, perforating or nonperforating. The degree of injury depends on the force of the injury, depth of penetration, and involvement of intraocular structures. Blunt injury causing globe rupture almost always carries a poor prognosis because it often is accompanied by severe uveal herniation, hemorrhage, and retinal detachment. Penetrating wounds by sharp objects and nonperforating blunt trauma vary greatly in the amount of damage. Clinical signs indicating a guarded or poor prognosis include large or deep corneal laceration, collapsed anterior chamber, severe hyphema (anterior chamber > $1/3$ full of blood), inability to visualize the iris due to corneal edema or anterior chamber opacity, uveal prolapse, lens luxation, vitreous hemorrhage, and retinal detachment.

15. How can you tell if the eye has been perforated?

Large perforating scleral wounds result in severe hypotony and often marked subconjunctival and intraocular hemorrhage. Small perforating scleral wounds are harder to detect because chemotic conjunctiva obscures the point of entry and intraocular pressure may be affected only mildly. Large, full-thickness corneal lacerations result in anterior chamber collapse and iris incarceration in the wound. Small, full-thickness lacerations may self-seal as a result of swelling of the stroma when aqueous and tears enter the cornea. The Seidel test helps to detect small perforating corneal injuries.

16. What is the procedure for the Seidel test?

A sterile fluorescein strip is moistened with sterile saline or eye wash, and a drop is administered to the wound area. As aqueous fluid mixes with fluoresceine, a bright green stream of fluid will form. If the animal is under general anesthesia, gentle digital pressure can be applied to the cornea to check for wound leakage.

17. What is the significance of a perforating wound if it has already sealed?

Eyes with full-thickness lacerations or perforations are at risk for endophthalmitis and should be treated aggressively with broad-spectrum, systemic antibiotics. In addition, perforating injuries may involve intraocular damage not easily detected, such as lens rupture or retinal tear. If the cause of the injury is not known, radiography or ultrasonography to look for a metallic foreign body (BB or pellet) is warranted.

18. What treatment should be provided by the emergency care clinician?

The primary goal of emergency therapy is to prevent or treat infection, to protect and support the wound, and to prevent sequelae by controlling intraocular inflammation. If perforation of the eye is suspected, a broad-spectrum systemic antibiotic, such as a first-generation cephalosporin, should be started as soon as possible. Trauma to the globe almost always results in some degree of anterior uveitis and should be treated with topical and/or systemic nonsteroidal antiinflammatory drugs (NSAIDs) and topical cycloplegics (see chapter on uveitis). Topical corticosteroids should be avoided in the presence of ulcerative keratitis, and ophthalmic ointments should not be used if the globe is perforated.

1. To control or prevent infection
   - If not perforated—topical antibiotic ointment or solution
   - If perforated—systemic antibiotic (e.g., cefazolin) with or without topical antibiotic solution
2. To protect and support wound
   - Suture—if > half thickness laceration
   - With or without conjunctival graft
3. To control intraocular inflammation
   - Corticosteroids—systemic (e.g., prednisolone, dexamethasone)
   - NSAIDs—topical (e.g., Voltaren, Profenal, Ocufen)
   - Cycloplegic—topical (e.g., atropine, tropicamide)

19. What kinds of protection and support should be used?

Partial tarsorrhaphy decreases the palpebral fissure size and thus helps to protect the cornea and maintain an adequate tear film. This is especially important in exophthalmic or lagophthalmic animals. A nictitans flap should be used with caution because it interferes with topical medication of the cornea and prevents observation of the wound. If self-trauma is a consideration, a protective collar should be used. Other methods of support include a conjunctival graft or flap, tissue adhesive, and collagen shields.

20. When should a corneal laceration be sutured?

Corneal lacerations of less than half thickness may be treated as a corneal ulcer with topical antibiotics and mechanical support (see chapter on corneal ulceration). Deeper lacerations should be closed with 7-0 to 9-0 suture. If the iris is incarcerated in the wound, it should be amputated or replaced into the anterior chamber before closure. A conjunctival graft placed over the sutured wound may be used for added support if necessary.

21. When should a conjunctival graft or flap be used?

Conjunctival flaps not only provide mechanical support and surface protection to the cornea but also furnish blood supply. Leukocytes, antibodies, anticollagenases, antiproteases, and nutrients for healing and wound repair are thus brought directly to the injury. Lacerations with loss of deep stromal tissue that prevents adequate primary closure and lacerations in which the viability of the sutured tissue is in question should be supported with a conjunctival flap.

22. How can the collapsed anterior chamber be reformed?

In a healthy eye, the aqueous humor reforms at a rate of 2.5 μl/min and 15 μl/min in dogs and cats, respectively. If the eye is not severely damaged, the aqueous production rate may be sufficient to reform the anterior chamber within several minutes after the eye has been sealed.

Usually, however, the anterior chamber is reformed with lactated Ringer's or balanced salt solution. A 25- or 27-gauge needle is inserted at the limbus, parallel to the iris plane, and enough fluid is injected to restore the anterior chamber to its normal depth without creating high intraocular pressure (IOP). The IOP should be in the low-normal range (10–15 mmHg).

23. How and when should the entrapped iris be amputated or replaced?

When a prolapsed iris should be excised rather than repositioned is controversial. Recommendations are based on the time it takes for the exposed iris to become sufficiently contaminated to cause infection if replaced. Recommended times range from 1–24 hours. It is safe to assume that smaller prolapses take longer to pose a threat of infection. Tissue to be excised should be gently grasped with fine forceps and cut flush with the cornea. A dilute solution of epinephrine (1:10,000 in lactated Ringer's or balanced salt solution) aids hemostasis. To replace the iris, it is carefully freed from corneal attachments with an iris spatula or irrigating cannula. Care must be taken to avoid trauma to the corneal endothelium, iris, and lens.

24. What type of suture pattern should you use in the cornea?

Simple interrupted sutures are the easiest to place correctly. If you experience a lot of tension, horizontal mattress sutures may be placed first, followed by interrupted sutures. Correct suture placement is important to avoid internal wound gape (too shallow), wound override (sutures of unequal depth and length on each side of the wound), and intraocular contamination (too deep). Sutures should be approximately 90% of corneal depth, 1.5–2 mm in length, equal depth on each side of the wound, and 1–1.5 mm apart.

25. What are the common types of foreign body-related injuries?

Corneal and conjunctival foreign bodies from plant material and sand are frequently encountered in dogs, especially those used for hunting or field trials. Patients often present with an acutely red and painful eye. Linear abrasions of the cornea are an indication for eversion of the lid to examine for foreign material lodged in the upper palpebral conjunctiva. Superficial corneal foreign bodies may present with variable amounts of discomfort and usually can be detected with simple magnification (e.g., loupe or diagnostic otoscope head). Deeper corneal foreign bodies may have the appearance of a puncture wound and are harder to detect without the use of a slit lamp. Foreign body penetration into deeper ocular structures is often associated with BB-pellet, bird shot, and glass. Involvement of orbital structures, iris, lens, retina, and/or vitreous humor is possible, and the prognosis is affected accordingly.

26. How should foreign bodies involving the ocular surface be treated?

Superficial foreign bodies can be removed with topical anesthesia in many cases, but some animals may require sedation or general anesthesia. A spatula, corneal forcep, or hypodermic needle (25- or 27-gauge) is used to elevate the foreign body from the ocular surface. If loosened foreign material remains on the eye, it can be picked up with a moistened cotton tipped swab. Hypodermic needles should be held at a shallow angle to the cornea to avoid perforation. After removal, treat topically with a broad-spectrum antibiotic drop or ointment 3 times/day for 5–7 days. A single application of 1% atropine sulfate is given if the eye is miotic.

27. What should be done to manage an intraocular foreign body?

Management of intraocular foreign bodies depends on how long the foreign body has been in the eye, its location, and what it is made of. The potential for damage during removal should be compared with the potential for damage if it is left in the eye. Organic material leads to sepsis if not removed soon after penetration. Some metals and glass, however, may cause little reaction if left alone and eventually become anchored by fibrin or scar tissue. If the foreign body is recent and located in the anterior chamber, it should be removed through a limbal incision. Surgery to remove a foreign body from the posterior segment often results in complications leading to a blind eye and carries a poor prognosis. Broad-spectrum topical and systemic antibiotics should be used to control infection. Topical corticosteroids, cycloplegics, and oral corticosteroids (anti-inflammatory dosages) or NSAIDs may be used to treat uveitis. Corticosteroids should be used with caution because of the potential for sepsis.

Organic Foreign Body	Nonferrous Metal, Glass, or Plastic Foreign Body	Ferrous Metal Foreign Body
• Reactive	• Minimal reaction	• Highly reactive
• Sepsis possible	• Becomes walled off by fibrin and fibrous tissue	• Toxic to intraocular tissues
• Early removal recommended		• Early removal essential

BIBLIOGRAPHY

1. McCalla TL, Moore CP: Exophthalmos in dogs and cats. Part II: Causes and treatment. In the Compendium Collection: Ophthalmology in Small Animal Practice. 1996, pp 129–141.
2. Morgan RV: Ocular emergencies. Comp Cont Educ Vet 4(1):37–45, 1982.
3. Roberts SR: Assessment and management of the ophthalmic emergency in cats and dogs. In The Compendium Collection: Ophthalmology in Small Animal Practice. Trenton, NJ, Veterinary Learning Systems, 1996, pp 252–267.

36. OCULAR HEMORRHAGE

Steven M. Roberts, D.V.M., M.S., and Cynthia C. Powell, D.V.M., M.S.

1. What are common causes of ocular hemorrhage?
  • Trauma—hemorrhage of the eyelids, conjunctiva, and uvea
  • Coagulopathies and thrombocytopenia—hemorrhage of the subconjunctival tissues, uvea, and retina
  • Vasculitis due to infectious disease or immune-mediated disorders—hemorrhage of the uvea and retina

2. What forms of ocular hemorrhage have emergency significance?
Depending on the cause, all forms of ocular hemorrhage may be of emergency significance. The high vascularity of ocular tissues results in tissue hemorrhage from minor or severe ocular problems. A simple eyelid or conjunctival laceration may yield what the owner perceives as copious blood loss. Such injuries are not really emergencies from patient status standpoint but should be considered urgent. Emergency ocular hemorrhage situations include:
  • Petechial conjunctival or intraocular hemorrhage, which may represent life-threatening systemic disease or simply the result of blunt or sharp trauma.
  • Diffuse conjunctival petechial hemorrhage or hyphema (blood in the anterior chamber), which may indicate a need to check platelet numbers and coagulation parameters.
  • Hyphema due to trauma, thrombocytopenia, or coagulopathies, which may result in glaucoma; thus immediate medical management is important.
  • Retinal hemorrhage, which may be due to trauma, vasculitis, or hypertension.

3. Why is blunt trauma so potentially damaging to intraocular tissues?
Tremendous tissue distortion results from blunt ocular trauma. The four phases of blunt injury that induce tissue damage are as follows:
  • Compression   • Overshooting
  • Decompression • Oscillations

The initial anteroposterior globe compression at the cornea causes equatorial expansion and shortening of the globe along the anteroposterior axis so that the cornea may touch the iris and lens. As the momentary force of deformation is removed, the anteroposterior globe diameter increases, whereas the equatorial diameter decreases and the tissues overshoot so that the anteroposterior diameter becomes momentarily greater than normal and the equatorial diameter less than normal. The globe subsequently oscillates between these maximums and minimums with decreasing amplitude for a brief time. This extreme stretching of the ocular tissues causes injury to the choroid, lens, optic nerve, retina, and vitreous gel.

4. Describe the implications of hyphema.

Hyphema is the presence of blood within the anterior chamber. Blunt or sharp trauma to the globe is the most common cause. However, hyphema may be due to thrombocytopenia, coagulopathies, iritis, intraocular neoplasia, congenital ocular anomalies, and chronic glaucoma. Initial examination should determine whether the globe has been penetrated. Hyphema often causes little damage to the eye itself but may result in glaucoma, anterior uveitis, iris adhesions secondary to clot contraction, and capsular cataract formation. Anterior chamber bleeding may not clot completely because the iris produces fibrinolysin. Maximal clot integrity requires 4–7 days. Hyphema should be treated as a clinical sign, and its cause should be determined as soon as possible.

5. What clinical parameters should be evaluated in cases of hyphema?

Not only should a complete eye examination be performed, but the entire animal must be evaluated to assess concomitant injury or disease. In particular, globe rupture should be ruled out. Vision should be estimated based on the degree of menace when bright light is suddenly directed into the eye. Assuming the examination light penetrates to the posterior part of the globe, the consensual pupillary light reflex indicates whether the retina and optic nerve are functional. If a globe rupture is not present, intraocular pressure should be measured. Finally, the hyphema should be graded by the anterior chamber volume occupied by the blood. The grading system is helpful prognostically because it indicates the severity of hemorrhage and the degree of intraocular tissue damage in trauma cases. Hyphema of grade 1 severity generally clears in less than 1 week. Grades 2 and 3 take several weeks or longer to resolve. Grade 4 hyphema often is associated with globe atrophy (phthisis bulbi).

- Grade 1: less than $1/3$ of the anterior chamber
- Grade 2: $1/3$–$1/2$ of the anterior chamber
- Grade 3: $1/2$ to nearly total
- Grade 4: total

6. How should hyphema be treated?

If a primary cause other than trauma is determined, specific treatment must address the underlying problem rather than the hyphema. Animals with traumatic hyphema should be kept quiet and subdued, possibly by use of sedation. A wide variety of medical treatments has been proposed, but no studies have evaluated their effectiveness. Interest in some treatments continues, whereas others remain controversial. Basically the treatments can be separated into the following categories:

- Cycloplegics
- Miotics
- Adrenergic agonists
- Corticosteroids
- Antifibrinolytic agents
- Fibrinolytic agents
- Surgical intervention

7. What cycloplegics may be useful and why?

Cycloplegics are parasympatholytic drugs that cause paralysis of ciliary body and iris sphincter smooth muscles. Thus the ocular accommodation by the ciliary body is prevented and the pupil dilates. Prevention of smooth muscle spasm may enhance patients' comfort and facilitates fundus examination. Topical atropine 1% solution once or twice daily is sufficient. Once mydriasis (pupil dilation) occurs, the frequency of treatment may be reduced and the drug used to effect.

8. What miotics are useful and why?

Parasympathomimetic agents are miotics that induce spasm of the ciliary body and iris sphincter smooth muscles. In theory, use of a miotic such as pilocarpine 1% should open the filtration angle. However, miotics tend to increase intraocular inflammation. No scientific evidence suggests that they enhance the clearance of blood from the anterior chamber. Miotics should be avoided in general.

9. What adrenergic agonists have been advocated and why?

Sympathomimetic agents such as topical epinephrine 1% and phenylephrine 2.5% have been advocated as a means of decreasing anterior chamber hemorrhage by way of vasoconstriction. Such treatment may be helpful with evidence of ongoing hemorrhage but usually provides little effect. It is rarely considered an option in the treatment of hyphema in humans.

10. Which corticosteroids are best to use?

Invariably, traumatic hyphema is associated with anterior uveitis ranging from mild to severe. Thus, topical steroids such as prednisolone acetate, prednisolone sodium phosphate, and dexamethasone ophthalmic drops are used 4 times/day. Their efficacy in improving the actual hyphema outcome is unproved. Systemic steroid use is more controversial, yet commonly used as a treatment. Certainly any concurrent anterior uveitis will be lessened, and theoretical evidence suggests that steroids may enhance clot stabilization; however, controlled studies are lacking.

11. When is antifibrinolytic treatment indicated?

Agents such as aminocaproic acid have been proposed as a means of reducing traumatic hyphema rebleeding that results from premature clot lysis mediated by the fibrinolytic system. The theoretical rationale is that the reduced rate of clot lysis allows more time for the damaged blood vessels to heal. In humans, the current recommended dosage is 50 mg/kg orally every 4 hr for 5 days. Antifibrinolytic drugs are contraindicated in cases with intravascular clotting disorders, pregnancy, and cardiac, hepatic, or renal disease.

12. What is the purpose of fibrinolytic treatment?

Hyphema typically progresses from free blood to varying degrees of blood clot formation 1–7 days after traumatic injury. Once fibrin formation has occurred, clot lysis may be induced with fibrinolytic agents such as tissue plasminogen activator (tPA). Clinically, tPA is used by injecting 25 µg in a 100-µl volume into the anterior chamber. Clot lysis typically occurs within 30–60 minutes of injection. As clot lysis occurs, red blood cell clearance is facilitated. Topical application of tPA is also promising.

13. What surgical interventions are used for hyphema?

If hyphema persists beyond 5–10 days or intraocular pressure increases, surgical removal may be necessary. An anterior chamber wash-out is the simplest and safest surgical procedure to clear free blood from the anterior chamber. Removal of the clotted blood is not required, but rather evacuation of loose blood cells and debris. A 30-gauge needle or cannula is used to irrigate a balanced salt solution into the anterior chamber, and a second 2-mm incision is made to allow fluid egress. Removal of the entire clot is possible but may result in lens, iris, and corneal endothelial trauma. Other surgical procedures are available but should be performed by someone experienced and equipped for intraocular surgery.

14. What drugs may be contraindicated in cases of hyphema?

Based on the antiplatelet effect of the cyclooxygenase inhibitors, nonsteroidal antiinflammatory agents such as aspirin, flunixin megulamine, and topical ocular nonsteroidals should be avoided. Although cycloplegics such as atropine are advocated for medical management of hyphema, a small percentage of patients develop glaucoma associated with use of atropine.

15. How can vitreal hemorrhage be recognized?

Disorders of the posterior segment (ocular tissues posterior to the lens) are more difficult to detect and characterize because direct examination must be performed through the pupil, or indirect imaging techniques such as ultrasound must be used. Direct examination is impaired with disease of the anterior ocular tissues. Dilation of the pupil, if possible, greatly facilitates evaluation of the posterior globe. If vitreous hemorrhage is near the lens, it may be visible with a penlight or transilluminator. Otherwise, an indirect ophthalmoscopic examination is the best way to evaluate the vitreous cavity. Vitreous hemorrhage appears as strands, sheets, or diffuse areas of blood accumulation. If the hemorrhage is subvitreal (between the vitreous and retina), it may resemble a "boat keel" because of gravitational settling of the erythrocytes.

16. Does vitreal hemorrhage have special implications?

The most common cause of vitreal hemorrhage is trauma-induced rupture of uveal or retinal blood vessels. The animal should be evaluated closely for rupture of the cornea or sclera. Causes of vitreal hemorrhage may be grouped as follows:

- Tearing of a blood vessel in a congenital or acquired retinal detachment
- Retention of the fetal hyaloid artery system
- Widespread ocular disease (inflammation of the choroid and retina, optic neuritis, chronic glaucoma, and intraocular neoplasia)
- Systemic disease (hypertension, coagulopathies, and thrombocytopenia)

17. How is vitreal hemorrhage treated?

Other than dealing with the underlying ocular or systemic disorder associated with vitreal hemorrhage, no simple treatment is available. If hemorrhage occurs into the solid vitreous gel, clotting is rapidly activated because the gel matrix serves as a collagen framework for platelet adhesion. Infiltration of neutrophils and macrophages hasten clot removal but cause further vitreous gel breakdown and inflammation. Subvitreal hemorrhage clots poorly. Concurrent use of topical and systemic corticosteroids is appropriate and may ameliorate the inflammatory reaction. If anterior uveitis is present, the use of topical atropine as a cycloplegic is appropriate. Depending on the hemorrhage area and density, resolution may take many months.

18. What does retinal hemorrhage look like?

The appearance of retinal hemorrhage depends on the retinal layer involved. Because of the relatively loose attachment between the retina and vitreous gel and the retina and retinal pigment epithelium, hemorrhage of large size may develop in either space. Preretinal hemorrhage (between the retina and vitreous gel) frequently has a "keel boat" shape due to gravitational settling of the erythrocytes. Intraretinal hemorrhages primarily are aligned vertically; their end on appearance is round, and the hemorrhages are small. Nerve fiber layer hemorrhages are typically feathered or striated and flat, because the hemorrhage follows the path of the nerve fibers. The retinal depth of a focal hemorrhage may be estimated based on which structures are positioned beneath and thus obscured or positioned above and thus visible.

19. Explain the significance of retinal hemorrhage.

Retinal hemorrhage indicates disruption or inflammation of the vasculature. If there is no clear history or physical evidence of trauma, systemic disorders must be considered. Infectious diseases capable of causing vasculitis or retinitis must be considered. Disorders that may be immediately life-threatening are coagulopathies, severe anemias, and blood dyscrasias. Chronic disorders such as hypertension, hyperviscosity syndromes, and neoplasia may cause retinal hemorrhage. Although not immediately life-threatening, such conditions may cause ocular signs that can be confused with a more acute process. The clinician should consider performing a complete blood count and clotting profile if retinal hemorrhage is noted. Serum should be collected and a portion saved for potential serologic testing before corticosteroids are administered and dispensed.

20. Is there any specific treatment for retinal hemorrhage?

There is no specific treatment in an emergency setting. If an underlying systemic disorder is identified or suspected, appropriate treatment is indicated. Severe subretinal or preretinal hemorrhage can be surgically removed or lysed with intracameral injection of tissue plasminogen activator, but these procedures must be performed by someone well-versed in intraocular and posterior segment surgery.

BIBLIOGRAPHY

1. Aguirre GL, Gross SL: Ocular manifestations of selected systemic diseases. In The Compendium Collection: Ophthalmology in Small Animal Practice. Trenton, NJ, Veterinary Learning Systems, 1996, pp 89–98.
2. Lane IF, Roberts SM, Lappin MR: Ocular manifestations of vascular disease: Hypertension, hyperviscosity, and hyperlipidemia. J Am Animal Hosp Assoc 29:28–36, 1993.
3. Roberts SM: Assessment and management of the ophthalmic emergency in cats and dogs. In The Compendium Collection: Ophthalmology in Small Animal Practice. Trenton, NJ, Veterinary Learning Systems, 1996, pp 252–267.

37. SUDDEN BLINDNESS

Cynthia C. Powell, D.V.M., M.S., and Steven M. Roberts, D.V.M., M.S.

1. What are the common causes of sudden blindness as a presenting complaint?

Opacification of normally clear ocular structures or neurologic abnormalities related to the visual system result in vision loss. In animals, gradual or incomplete loss of vision often goes undetected, and the veterinarian is presented with what the owner interprets as an acutely blind animal. A good history including questions about changes in environment, night vision, and behavioral changes, helps to establish the true onset. Common causes of acute blindness as the presenting complaint include bilateral retinal detachment, sudden acquired retinal degeneration, and bilateral optic neuritis. Although there are many other causes of blindness, they are often slower in onset (e.g., progressive retinal atrophy, cataracts) or have other primary presenting complaints (e.g., toxic causes, central nervous system [CNS] disorders, trauma).

2. Describe appropriate diagnostic tests for patients with sudden blindness.

Bilateral ophthalmic disease should raise the suspicion of a systemic cause. Because optic neuritis and retinal detachment are often treated with high dosages of corticosteroids, a complete blood count, platelet count, urinalysis, and serum chemistry profile are indicated to screen for infectious disease or other contraindications of corticosteroid use. In addition, retinal detachment is associated with hypertension, especially in older cats, and evaluation of renal function, thyroid hormone level, and blood pressure is warranted.

3. What disorders causing acute blindness result in abnormal pupillary light reflexes (PLR)?

Bilateral optic neuritis and sudden acquired retinal degeneration always present with PLR abnormalities. The pupils are usually widely dilated in room light and are not responsive or poorly responsive to light stimulation. If optic neuritis is not symmetrical, there may be variations in the amount of response to light in each eye. Pupil abnormalities related to bilateral retinal detachment are more subtle, with the resting pupil size usually larger and the PLRs less brisk than normal. CNS lesions of the optic radiation or visual cortex have normal pupil size and PLRs; however, complete blindness is rare without other signs of nervous system dysfunction.

4. What is SARDS?

Sudden acquired retinal degeneration syndrome (SARDS) is a degenerative retinal disease of dogs. Older animals are predisposed, and females are more likely to be affected than males. Dogs with SARDS are often obese and may have a history of polyuria/polydypsia or polyphagia. Laboratory changes frequently resemble those of hyperadrenocorticism, but specific tests for hyperadrenocorticism (low-dose dexamethasone suppression, adrenocorticotropic hormone [ACTH] stimulation) are usually normal. The cause of SARDS is unknown; toxic and autoimmune etiologies and apoptosis have been suggested.

5. How is SARDS recognized and confirmed?

The hallmark of SARDS is acute or subacute onset of blindness coupled with an ophthalmoscopically normal fundus. A nonrecordable electroretinogram (ERG) confirms the diagnosis. Bilateral retrobulbar optic neuritis has the same clinical presentation as SARDS, but the ERG is normal.

6. Can SARDS be treated or managed?

Unfortunately, there is no treatment for SARDS. Blindness is permanent. The best way to manage an acutely blind animal is to give time for adjustment and maintain a familiar environment.

7. What are the clinical signs of optic neuritis compared with retinal detachment?

Retinal detachments severe enough to cause blindness are usually complete or almost complete and easy to diagnose with an indirect ophthalmoscope or focal light source. If not disinserted (detached at the ora ciliaris), the retina floats in the vitreous gel and often can be seen directly behind the lens. It has the appearance of a gray to white veil with blood vessels. Retinal hemorrhages also may be present, and the optic nerve may be partially covered by the floating retina, making it difficult to see. A disinserted retinal detachment hangs from and completely obscures the optic disk. As mentioned before, with acute detachment, the pupillary light responses may have only subtle abnormalities and on cursory examination may appear normal.

Optic neuritis causes dilated pupils poorly responsive to light. Funduscopic changes are found only if the inflammation involves the optic papilla (disk). Hyperemia, swelling, and hemorrhage of the optic nerve head and edema and hemorrhage of the adjacent (peripapillary) retina are evident ophthalmoscopically. Retrobulbar optic neuritis (inflammation of the optic nerve that does not extend to the nerve head) has a normal-appearing fundus and clinically resembles SARDS. Optic neuritis and retinal detachment affecting one eye often go undetected because behavioral changes and PLR abnormalities are usually subtle.

8. What are the common causes of optic neuritis?

The cause of optic neuritis is often elusive and classified as idiopathic. Causes that have been identified most frequently include systemic infection (canine distemper, cryptococcosis, toxoplasmosis), retrobulbar abscess or cellulitis, granulomatous meningoencephalitis (GME), neoplasia, and trauma. Cerebrospinal fluid analysis and cytology or CT scan may be helpful in the diagnosis.

9. How rapidly should optic neuritis be treated and by what means?

Treatment of optic neuritis should be instituted as soon as possible to minimize permanent structural damage to the optic nerve. When a primary cause is identified, specific therapy is required. The goal of treating idiopathic optic neuritis and GME is rapid reduction of inflammation, which is achieved with high dosages of systemic corticosteroids. Standard protocol is oral prednisolone given at an initial dose of 2–4 mg/kg/day and tapered over 3–4 weeks. In severe cases of inflammation, pulsed corticosteroid therapy should be considered. Pulsed therapy uses suprapharmacologic doses of methylprednisolone sodium succinate (15–30 mg/kg IV), followed by maintenance prednisolone (1–2 mg/kg/day) tapered over 3–4 weeks. Cases suspected of GME should be tapered from steroids at a slower rate.

10. When should response to treatment be expected? What is the prognosis?

Irreversible damage has often occurred by the time optic neuritis is diagnosed; thus, the prognosis for return of vision is guarded. Response to treatment usually occurs within 1–10 days if at all.

11. What are the common causes of retinal detachment?

Causes of retinal detachment are either congenital or acquired. Retinal dysplasia and optic nerve coloboma are common congenital defects associated with detachment and may affect one or both eyes. Acquired conditions include infectious and immune-mediated chorioretinitis, vascular disorders leading to edema or hemorrhage, neoplasia, hypertension, postinflammatory traction bands, and trauma. Hypertension is a common cause of retinal detachment in older cats.

12. How should retinal detachment be treated initially?

Cases of retinal detachment presented as an emergency are generally severe and require aggressive therapy if any vision is to be saved. In cases of systemic disease, treat the underlying cause. Idiopathic cases with active inflammation and serous detachments may be immune-mediated and often respond dramatically to combined corticosteroid and diuretic therapy. Conventional therapy with oral prednisolone (1–2 mg/kg/day) or pulsed therapy with methylprednisolone sodium succinate (15 mg/kg IV) followed by maintenance prednisolone (0.5–1 mg/kg/day) is recommended in combination with standard dosages of furosemide or a carbonic anhydrase inhibitor, such as methazolamide (1 mg/kg 2 times/day) or dichlorphenamide (0.5 mg/kg 2 times/day). Treatment should continue until reattachment and then be tapered and discontinued as response dictates.

13. Does vision return after reattachment?

Cell degeneration and death begin within hours to several days after detachment. The amount of cell death increases with duration of detachment and may continue after reattachment. The prognosis for return of vision is always guarded. Although some vision may return, normal vision is not expected.

Optic Neuritis	*Retinal Detachment*
• Mydriasis or afferent PLR defect	• If blind, usually large or total detachment

• Optic disk changes
   Hyperemia
   Swelling
   Hemorrhage
	• Veil with blood vessels floating in vitreous

	• Retinal hemorrhages
	• Optic disk possibly obscured

• Retinal peripapillary changes
   Edema
   Hemorrhage
	• Normal to slightly reduced PLR

	• Unilateral cases often unrecognized
• Normal ocular fundus if retrobulbar neuritis	
• Unilateral cases often unrecognized	

BIBLIOGRAPHY

1. Hendrix DV, Nasisse MP, Cowen P, Davidson MG: Clinical signs, concurrent disease and risk factors associated with retinal detachment in dogs. Prog Vet Comp Ophthal 3(3):87–89, 1993.
2. Krohne SD, Vestre WA: Ocular use of antiinflammatory drugs in companion animals. In The Compendium Collection: Ophthalmology of Small Animal Practice. Trenton, NJ, Veterinary Learning Systems, 1996, pp 239–251.
3. Mattson A, Roberts SM, Isherwood JME: Clinical features suggesting hyperadrenocorticism associated with sudden acquired retinal degeneration syndrome in a dog. J Am Animal Hosp Assoc 28(3):199–202, 1992.
4. Roberts SM: Assessment and management of the ophthalmic emergency in cats and dogs. In the Compendium Collection: Ophthalmology in Small Animal Practice. Trenton, NJ, Veterinary Learning Systems, 1996, pp 252–278.

38. UVEITIS

Steven M. Roberts, D.V.M., M.S., and Cynthia C. Powell, D.V.M., M.S.

1. What is the uvea or uveal tract?
The eyeball structure consists of an outer wall (cornea and sclera), inner retinal layer, and highly vascular and pigmented tissue layer sandwiched between the sclera and retina. This vascular and pigmented intraocular tissue is called the uvea. It consists of the iris, ciliary body, and choroid. The iris and ciliary body are collectively referred to as the anterior uvea. The posterior uvea is the choroid. Although the anatomic regions have different names, the tissues are basically continuous with each other.

2. How is the uvea different from the uvula?
In contrast to the ocular uvea, the term *uvula* stems from a Latin word that means "little grape." The palatine uvula is a small, pendulous, fleshy mass hanging from the posterior soft palate edge above the root of the tongue in humans. Other structures associated with the term *uvula* include the bladder (uvula vesicae = a rounded elevation at the bladder neck) and cerebellum (uvula vermis = part of the cerebellum vermis between the pyramis and nodulus).

3. What is uveitis?
Uveitis is inflammation of one or more of the uveal tissues. Inflammation that involves a single tissue is termed iritis, cyclitis, or choriditis if the iris, ciliary body, or choroid is inflamed, respectively.

4. What is anterior uveitis?
Anterior uveitis denotes inflammation of both the iris and ciliary body.

5. What is posterior uveitis?
Posterior uveitis refers to choridal inflammation.

6. Can inflammation involve the anterior and posterior uvea simultaneously?
The division of the uvea into anterior and posterior region tissues does not imply a physical barrier between the regions. Inflammation often involves both anterior and posterior portions. The terms uveitis, endophthalmitis, and panophthalmitis are used to describe diffuse uveal inflammation.

7. What is endophthalmitis?
If the entire uveal tract is involved, the term *endophthalmitis* is used to indicate inflammation of the vascular intraocular tissues. Such inflammation affects not only the uveal tissues but also the retina. The prognosis for vision preservation if endophthalmitis develops is poor.

8. What is panophthalmitis?
Uveal tract inflammation coupled with scleral and corneal inflammatory changes is termed *panophthalmitis*. Such inflammation involves the entire globe (inner contents and outer wall). It is difficult to maintain a normal-appearing globe with inflammation of this severity and distribution. Preserving vision is hopeless.

9. What are the major clinical signs of uveitis?
Anterior uveitis typically causes a painful globe with conjunctival and episcleral vascular hyperemia, miosis, aqueous humor flare and cell accumulation, perilimbal to generalized corneal

edema, iris swelling and hyperemia, and reduced intraocular pressure (hypotony). Vision is impaired but rarely lost with simple anterior uveitis. Vision loss indicates more extensive ocular tissue damage. Clinical signs of posterior uveitis are not easily observable without anterior uveal involvement. An ophthalmoscope is required for assessment of posterior uveitis. Ophthalmoscopic signs include loss of the normal tapetal color, retinal detachment, subretinal transudation or exudation, and loss of retinal pigment epithelial cell and choroidal pigmentation. Posterior uveitis may cause blindness.

10. Can the clinical signs be used as an indication of chronicity, severity, or prognosis?

The spectrum and magnitude of signs depend on the severity of insult. The list below differentiates acute vs. chronic anterior uveitis based on clinical signs. If trauma, vasculitis, or bleeding disorders are underlying causes of uveitis, hyphema and anterior chamber fibrin clots are common. Septic or neoplastic disorders induce the above changes and are often bilateral with varying degrees of hypopyon (white blood cells within the aqueous humor) or keratic precipitates (white blood cells and fibrin adherent to the corneal endothelial surface). Posterior uveitis warrants a guarded prognosis for vision. Acute signs include retinal edema, retinal hemorrhage, loss of normal tapetal color, subretinal fluid accumulation, and decreased vision. Chronic signs consist of hyperreflective areas in the tapetal fundus (caused by retinal atrophy and thinning), abrupt color changes of the tapetum, and pigment proliferation or loss.

Clinical Signs

ACUTE ANTERIOR UVEITIS	CHRONIC ANTERIOR UVEITIS
Mild conjunctival hyperemia	Deep corneal vascularization
Iris swelling	Iris hyperpigmentation
Aqueous humor flare reaction	Iris neovascularization
Mild episcleral hyperemia	Synechia formation
Miosis	Cataract
Photophobia	Secondary glaucoma

11. What is the significance of aqueous humor flare and cell accumulation?

The blood-ocular barrier maintains the low total protein content (20–30 mg/dl) and cell-free state of the aqueous humor. Uveal inflammation disrupts this barrier, resulting in an increased amount of protein and influx of cells within the aqueous humor. The increased protein causes light directed into the eye to back-scatter, thus imparting a turbid characteristic to the aqueous humor. This phenomenon is termed *flare* and is subjectively graded using a scale ranging from 0–4+ (0 = normal, and 4+ = fibrin clot formation). The accumulation of cellular material is termed *cell* and may consist of white blood, red blood, pigment, or tumor cells as well as pigment granules. The presence of increased amounts of aqueous protein indicates inflammation (with the severity approximating the magnitude of the flare reaction). Likewise, cell accumulation indicates inflammation but suggests a more severe inflammatory response and poorer prognosis than simple flare. Flare and cell may be sterile inflammatory responses or result from sepsis.

12. Which is more common—anterior uveitis or posterior uveitis?

Anterior uveitis is more common, especially considering the propensity for the globe to suffer traumatic injury. The anterior segment (cornea, iris, ciliary body, and lens) is more frequently damaged than the posterior segment (vitreous, retina, optic nerve, and choroid) in ocular trauma. The orbital protection and posterior location of the choroid affords considerable protection, but contrecoup forces may result in choridal contusion. Inflammation of both anterior and posterior uveal tissues often results when septic, toxic, or neoplastic processes are present.

13. What are the common causes of uveitis?

Uveitis is a component of most intraocular disease processes and a frequent result of blunt trauma to the globe. In an emergency setting, trauma or fulminating sepsis or toxemia commonly is associated with uveitis. Despite the ease with which uveitis can be recognized clinically, most cases are classified as idiopathic. Many endogenous causes of uveitis have been recognized (see table below). Common causes of uveitis in companion animals presented for emergency care include blunt trauma, corneal ulceration, and perforation of the cornea or globe.

Causes of Endogenous Uveitis in Dogs and Cats

CANINE UVEITIDES	FELINE UVEITIDES
Infectious disease	**Infectious disease**
Algae	**Fungal**
Prototheca spp.,	*Blastomyces dermatitidis* (rare)
Bacterial	*Candida albicans* (rare)
Brucella canis	*Coccidioides immitis* (very rare)
Borrelia burgdorferi	*Cryptococcus neoformans*
Fungal	*Histoplasma capsulatum* (most
Blastomyces dermatitidis	common)
Coccidioides immitis	**Parasitic**
Cryptococcus neoformans	*Cuterebra* larva
Histoplasma capsulatum	*Dirofilaria immitis*
Parasitic	Metastrongylidae nematodes
Dirofilaria immitis	**Protozoan**
Diptera spp. (fly larvae)	*Toxoplasma gondii*
Ocular larval migrans (*Toxocara* and *Balisascaris*	**Viral**
spp.)	Feline immunodeficiency virus
Protozoan	Feline infectious peritonitis
Leshmania donovani	Feline leukemia virus (tumor
Toxoplasma gondii	formation)
Rickettsial	**Miscellaneous causes**
Ehrlichia canis or *platys*	Idiopathic
Rickettsia rickettsii	Trauma
Viral	
Adenovirus	**Neoplastic disorders**
Distemper virus	Fibrosarcoma
Herpesvirus	Primary tumor (melanoma)
Idiopathic	Secondary tumor (lymphosarcoma)
Trauma	
Toxemia (e.g., pyometra, pancreatitis	
Ulcerative keratitis	
Neoplastic and paraneoplastic disorders	
Hyperviscosity syndrome	
Granulomatous meningoencephalitis	
Primary neoplasia (ocular melanoma, adenocarcinoma)	
Secondary neoplasia (lymphosarcoma most common	
Uveodermatologic syndrome	
Metabolic disorders	
Diabetic cataract (lens-induced uveitis)	
Miscellaneous causes	
Coagulopathy	
Immune mediated vasculitis	
Lens trauma (phacoclastic uveitis)	
Cataract (lens-induced uveitis)	
Immune-mediated disorders	

14. What significance can be attributed to anterior uveitis?

Depending on the cause, uveitis may indicate uveal tissue trauma and necrosis due to traumatic injury or serve as an index of the type of systemic disease. Bilateral uveitis is more likely to result from systemic disease. The mere presence of uveitis is not necessarily an indicator of sepsis. Any pathophysiologic mechanism that results in uveal tissue damage will trigger an inflammatory response. Because many intraocular tissue antigens are not recognized by the host as self, nonspecific immunologic responses to antigenic material released as a result of the inflammation serves to propagate the inflammatory processes.

15. Can a prognosis be determined in emergency cases with uveitis?

Obviously the prognosis depends on the actual condition or injury. However, the prognosis for vision in cases with mild-to-moderate degrees of uveitis is favorable. Severe cases have a guarded prognosis. Within 24–48 hours of treatment initiation, the prognosis needs to be reevaluated and possibly upgraded or downgraded. In cases of endophthalmitis or panophthalmitis, the prognosis for vision is poor, and the prognosis for globe salvage is guarded to poor. If secondary conditions develop as a result of uveitis (e.g., hyphema, glaucoma, intensified pain), a guarded-to-poor prognosis is warranted.

16. How should anterior uveitis be treated in an emergency setting?

If the patient's overall condition does not suggest contraindications for ocular treatment, nonspecific antiinflammatory therapy with systemic corticosteroids or cyclooxygenase inhibitors is optimal. Cyclooxygenase inhibitors should be avoided in cases associated with coagulopathies or intraocular hemorrhage. Topical preparations should be used with caution in cases of globe perforation, because the drug, vehicle, or preservatives may damage the intraocular tissues. If an infectious cause is suspected, topical and/or systemic antimicrobial agents can be used. If antibiotics are indicated, use of a triple antibiotic ophthalmic solution topically and first-generation cephalosporine systemically is appropriate. The following treatment goals and grades of inflammation severity provide guidelines for initial therapy:

Mild inflammation (miosis, subtle flare, photophobia)
  • Topical corticosteroids, 3 times/day
  • Topical cyclooxygenase inhibitors, 3 times/day
  • Topical cycloplegics (e.g., atropine), every 24 hr

Moderate inflammation (aqueous flare and cell, iris swelling, blepharospasm, corneal edema)
  • Systemic corticosteroids (e.g., prednisone, 1 mg/kg/day)
  • Topical corticosteroids (e.g., 1% prednisolone or 0.1% dexamethasone, 4 times/day to every 24 hr)
  • Topical cyclooxygenase inhibitors, 4 times/day
  • Topical cyclosporin A, twice daily
  • Cycloplegics, twice daily until mydriasis occurs

Severe inflammation (hyphema, hypopyon, aqueous fibrin, irregular pupil shape and iris roughening)
  • Systemic corticosteroid pulse-therapy initially (e.g., methylprednisolone sodium succinate, 30 mg/kg IV over 20–30 min)
  • Systemic corticosteroids (e.g., prednisone 2 mg/kg/day 6–12 hours after pulse-therapy)
  • Topical corticosteroids (e.g., 1% prednisolone or 0.1% dexamethasone, every 1–2 hr until improved, then 4 times/day)
  • Topical cyclooxygenase inhibitors, 4 times/day
  • Topical cyclosporin A, 4 times/day

BIBLIOGRAPHY

1. Aguirre GL, Gross SL: Ocular manifestations of selected systemic diseases. In The Compendium Collection: Ophthalmology in Small Animal Practice. Trenton, NJ, Veterinary Learning Systems, 1996, pp 89–98.

2. Bistner S, Shaw D, Riis RC: Diseases of the uveal tract (Part I, Part II, and Part III). In The Compendium Collection: Ophthalmology in Small Animal Practice. 1996, pp 161–185.
3. Bistner SI: Recent developments in comparative ophthalmology. Comp Cont Educ 14:1304–1323, 1992.
4. Davidson MG, Nassisse MD, Jamieson VE, et al: Traumatic anterior lens capsule disruption. J Am Animal Hosp Assoc 27:410–414, 1991.
5. Hakanson N, Forrester SD: Uveitis in the dog and cat. Vet Clin North Am Small Animal Pract 20:715–735, 1990.
6. Kural E, Lindley D, Krohne S: Canine glaucoma: Medical and surgical therapy. In The Compendium Collection: Ophthalmology in Small Animal Practice. Trenton, NJ, Veterinary Learning Systems, 1996, pp 226–233.
7. Rathbone-Gionfriddo J: The causes, diagnosis, and treatment of uveitis. Vet Med 90:278–284, 1995.
8. Roberts SM: Assessment and management of the ophthalmic emergency in cats and dogs. In The Compendium Collection: Ophthalmology in Small Animal Practice. Trenton, NJ, Veterinary Learning Systems, 1996, pp 252–267.
9. Schmeitzel LP: Recognizing the cutaneous signs of immune-mediated diseases. Vet Med 86:138–163, 1991.

39. GLAUCOMA

Steven M. Roberts, D.V.M., M.S., and Cynthia C. Powell, D.V.M., M.S.

1. What is acute glaucoma?

Glaucoma occurs when the intraocular pressure (IOP) is increased above normal and results in optic nerve degeneration. Normal intraocular pressure for companion animals is 15–20 mmHg. Acute glaucoma results from a rapid increase in IOP over a course of several hours. Once glaucoma has been present for more than several days, the problem should be considered subacute; after several weeks, chronic glaucoma is present. Because most cases of canine glaucoma do not resolve, chronic glaucoma is inevitable. Many canine glaucoma cases are chronic by the time veterinary care is sought.

2. What is the difference between primary and secondary glaucoma?

In primary glaucoma, no discernible ocular abnormalities on routine examination account for the increased IOP, which is due to impairment of aqueous humor outflow through the filtration angle by poorly understood mechanisms. Secondary glaucoma results from filtration angle dysfunction due to or associated with other intraocular problems such as lens subluxation, neoplasia of the iris or ciliary body, intraocular hemorrhage, or intraocular inflammation (e.g., anterior uveitis, endophthalmitis, panophthalmitis).

3. Are the glaucoma classifications of open-angle and closed-angle appropriate for veterinary medicine?

This controversial area is confused by the fact that veterinary medicine has adopted the human classification system for animal species whose filtration angle has anatomic and physiologic features quite different from humans. The real issue in companion animals is whether the ciliary cleft is open, narrowed, or closed. The ciliary cleft is located posterior to the iris and is examined either in vivo by high-frequency ultrasound techniques (50 MHz) or in vitro by histology.

4. What are the common causes of glaucoma in companion animals?

Glaucoma is due to impairment or obstruction of aqueous humor outflow from the globe. Primary glaucoma results from structural and functional abnormalities of the filtration angle and is most common in dogs. More than 40 breeds of dogs are predisposed to primary glaucoma. Secondary glaucoma is due to problems such as anterior uveitis, lens subluxation or luxation, and intraocular neoplasia. Secondary glaucoma is most common in cats (secondary to chronic uveitis). If glaucoma is truly acute, the cause is most likely a primary filtration angle abnormality. Secondary glaucoma frequently results from chronic ocular disorders and is usually subacute or chronic by the time the animal is brought to a veterinarian.

Primary Glaucoma	Secondary Glaucoma
• Breed-associated filtration angle abnormality (common in dogs) • Open ciliary cleft progressing to narrowed and closed cleft • Final stages have closed filtration angle	• Associated chronic intraocular disease causing ciliary cleft collapse and closure (common in cats) • Filtration angle closure occurs with disease progression

5. What is the cause of primary glaucoma?

The initiating cause is not known but involves poorly understood changes in the pathways of aqueous humor outflow that restrict and eventually obstruct aqueous outflow from the eye. Once the IOP increases, the ciliary body and peripheral iris are forced toward the sclera, thus narrowing or collapsing the ciliary cleft and filtration angle. When the peripheral iris and ciliary body come into appositional contact with the sclera, aqueous humor outflow through the angle is further impaired. Eventually the iris and ciliary body become adherent to the sclera (synechia), and the filtration angle is closed. As the IOP increases, pathologic degenerative changes occur throughout the globe.

6. Which breeds of dog are at greatest risk for developing glaucoma?

Breeds that have a high risk of developing primary glaucoma include the American cocker spaniel, Basset hound, chow chow, samoyed, Shar Pei, and Siberian husky.

7. How is acute glaucoma diagnosed?

Glaucoma is confirmed by measurement of the IOP, but ample clinical signs provide clinicians with a strong presumptive diagnosis. Acute cases often present with a history of rapid onset of diffuse corneal clouding, conjunctival and episcleral hyperemia, ocular pain, and loss of vision (if the case is unilateral, owners often do not notice vision impairment). Examination reveals an abnormal pupillary light reflex (PLR). Miosis appears in acute cases that are afferent-deficit with loss of the direct and consensual PLR, and mydriasis is seen in most cases. The affected eye is usually blind. The magnitude of increased IOP is proportional to the severity of clinical signs.

8. What is a good method of measuring intraocular pressure?

There are two basic methods of indirectly estimating the IOP:

1. Indentation tonometry uses the inexpensive Schiotz tonometer, which correlates corneal indentation caused by the instrument plunger with IOP.

2. Applantation tonometry estimates IOP by the force required to flatten the corneal epithelial surface by use of various electronic or pneumatic devices.

Both are good estimators of IOP in the normal range and give a reasonable approximation of abnormal pressure values. Topical anesthesia is required, and the animal must be gently restrained so that external forces are not directly or indirectly applied to the globe.

9. How is the actual IOP determined by a Schiotz tonometer?

A Schiotz tonometer provides indirect determination of the IOP. The instrument measures the amount of corneal indentation, with each unit on the scale representing 0.05 mm of indentation. The scale is therefore an inverse scale; that is, high IOP yields a low-scale reading. As a general rule, the Schiotz tonometer scale reading of a normal eye should approximate the plunger mass load. Thus, with a 5.5-gm plunger load, the scale reading should be between 4 and 7. If the scale reading is less than 4, the IOP is increased. Conversely, if the scale reading is greater than 7, the IOP is below normal. This same rule holds true for plunger loads of 7.5 and 10 gm. The table below allows conversion of scale reading to mmHg for dogs and cats using the accepted human conversion table.

Calibration Table for Schiotz Tonometry

SCHIOTZ SCALE READING	IOP (mmHg) 5.5 GM WT	IOP (mmHg) 7.5 GM WT	IOP (mmHg) 10.0 GM WT
0	42	59	82
1	34	50	69
2	29	43	59
3	24	36	51
4	21	30	43
5	17	26	37
6	15	22	32
7	12	18	27
8	10	16	23
9	8	13	20
10	7	11	16
11	6	9	14
12	5	8	12
13	4	6	10
14		5	8
15		4	6
16			5
17			4

Modified from Friendenwald JS: Tonometer calibration: An attempt to remove discrepancies found in the 1954 calibration scale for Schiotz tonometers. Trans Am Acad Ophthalmol Otol 61:108–123, 1957.

10. What signs indicate that the problem is due to chronic glaucoma?

Chronic glaucoma should be suspected if the history indicates that the problem has been present for several weeks or that several repetitive episodes have occurred. Clinical signs associated with chronicity include an enlarged globe, Haab's striae (breaks in Descemet's membrane), keratitis (vascular and pigmentary), lens subluxation, optic nerve atrophy and cupping, and peripapillary retinal atrophy (hyperreflectivity).

11. What are Haab's striae?

Persistent increased IOP causes stretching of the cornea and sclera, resulting in overall globe enlargement. Descemet's membrane is the corneal endothelial cell basement membrane along the posterior cornea. Pressure-induced stretching of Descemet's membrane causes single or branching curvilinear ruptures. As the basement membrane wound heals, permanent ridges remain and appear as white-to-gray, deep corneal opacities. Thus Haab's striae are specific for glaucoma, although the process may not be active at the time of examination.

12. How should emergency treatment of glaucoma be approached?

Emergency treatment must first focus on underlying problems that may contribute to increased IOP. If primary glaucoma is suspected or underlying problems are being addressed, focus shifts to dealing with the acute increase in IOP. Permanent retinal nerve fiber and optic nerve damage occurs within hours to days of the IOP increase; thus, rapid intervention is essential. Emergency medical treatment should consist of administration of a hyperosmotic agent (mannitol, 2 gm/kg IV over 30 minutes, or glycerin, 2 ml/kg orally) and a carbonic anhydrase inhibitor (dichlorphenamide, 2 mg/kg orally 2 or 3 times/day, or methazolamide, 4 mg/kg orally 2 or 3 times/day.

13. What topical drugs should be used in acute glaucoma?

A wide variety of topical drugs is available. If a veterinary ophthalmologist will eventually manage the case, he or she should be consulted early to determine appropriate topical treatment. Topical agents are expensive and must be used only if likely to be effective. Pilocarpine, a cholinergic drug, is commonly administered, but because of inherent problems with the filtration angle in dogs, it is often not effective or effective only for a brief time. Adrenergic agonists and antagonists are the most useful topical agents. Latanoprost is a prostaglandin $F_{2\alpha}$ analog that shows tremendous potential because the mechanism of action is to increase aqueous humor outflow by an alternative route (the uveoslceral pathway).

Adrenergic Agonists	*Adrenergic Antagonists*	*Prostaglandin Analog*

• Beta agonist
  Epinephrine 1%
  Dipivefrin 0.1%
 	
• Alpha agonist
  Apraclonidine 0.5%
	• Beta 1 and 2 blockers
	  Carteolol 1%
	  Levobutanol 0.5%
	  Metipranolol 0.3%
	  Timolol 0.5%
	
	• Beta 1 blocker
	  Betaxolol 0.5%
		• Latanoprost 0.005%

14. If immediate referral to an ophthalmologist is not feasible, what agents are best?

An optimal medical protocol consists of a carbonic anhydrase inhibitor (dichlorphenamide or methazolamide) twice daily, dipivefrin drops twice daily, a beta-blocker twice daily, and latanoprost every 24 hr. If the IOP remains controlled for several weeks, the drug dosages can be gradually decreased by changing the frequency of administration, sequential (not simultaneous). Long-term medical management is difficult and requires careful monitoring, dosage adjustments, and drug changes.

15. What is the prognosis for acute glaucoma?

The prognosis for preserving vision is guarded to poor. Early during the course of treatment, the owner should be asked to determine one of the following primary goals: to provide the maximal chance of vision preservation, to maintain a blind but comfortable and cosmetic globe, or to achieve a comfortable or disease-free state. The degree of vision present on initial evaluation or vision returning after 24–48 hours of treatment is the best that can be hoped for.

16. What causes the loss of vision associated with glaucoma?

Vision loss occurs rapidly as increased IOP damages the innermost retinal layers, retinal nerve fiber layer, and ganglion cells. The retinal nerve fiber layer is comprised of ganglion cell axons that exit the globe as the optic nerve. These central nervous system neurons do not repair cellular damage well. A few hours of increased IOP result in permanent loss of some ganglion cells and axons. As the duration and magnitude of IOP elevation continues, more neuronal damage occurs; within hours to days, the neurons have minimal-to-no remaining function. Thus, blindness is inevitable unless the IOP is quickly reduced and maintained in a normal range.

17. When is surgery indicated for glaucoma?

Long-term management of glaucoma usually requires surgical intervention, often coupled with continued medical treatment. If the animal owner is interested in surgery, procedures are best performed soon after other serious medical conditions have been stabilized. Procedures suitable for visual eyes include placement of an anterior chamber shunt, transscleral laser ciliary body coagulation, and transscleral ciliary body cryosurgery. Blind eyes can be treated surgically by transscleral laser or cryosurgery of the ciliary body, pharmacologic ciliary ablation with intravitreal gentamicin, evisceration, or enucleation.

BIBLIOGRAPHY

1. Brooks DE: Glaucoma in the dog and cat. Vet Clin North Am Small Animal Pract 20:775–797, 1990.
2. Kural E, Lindley D, Krohne S: Canine glaucoma: Clinical signs and diagnosis. In The Compendium Collection: Ophthalmology in Small Animal Practice. Trenton, NJ, Veterinary Learning Systems, 1996, pp 38–44.
3. Kural E, Lindley D, Krohne S: Canine glaucoma: Medical and surgical therapy. In The Compendium Collection: Ophthalmology in Small Animal Practice. Trenton, NJ, Veterinary Learning Systems, 1996, pp 226–233.
4. Miller PE, Pickett JP: Comparison of the human and canine Schiotz tonometry conversion tables in clinically normal cats. J Am Vet Med Assoc 201:1017–1020, 1992.
5. Miller PE, Pickett JP: Comparison of the human and canine Schiotz tonometry conversion tables in clinically normal dogs. J Am Vet Med Assoc 201:1021–1025, 1992.
6. Renwick P: Diagnosis and management of glaucoma. Practice 17:10–20, 1995.
7. Roberts SM: Glaucoma in companion animals: Current management and new trends. Calif Vet 48:9–16, 1994.
8. Roberts SM: Assessment and management of the ophthalmic emergency in cats and dogs. In The Compendium Collection: Ophthalmology in Small Animal Practice. Trenton, NJ, Veterinary Learning Systems, 1996, pp 252–267.
9. Wilcock BP, Peiffer RL Jr, Davidson MG: The causes of glaucoma in cats. Vet Pathol 27:35–40, 1990.

40. VISION-THREATENING CORNEAL ULCERS

Steven M. Roberts, D.V.M., M.S., and
Cynthia C. Powell, D.V.M., M.S.

1. When does a corneal ulcer threaten vision?

By definition, a corneal ulcer represents a break or disruption in the corneal epithelium. If an ulcer involves only the epithelium, healing is usually rapid with no significant loss of corneal transparency. If the epithelial defect becomes infected or involved with a purulent inflammatory response, the deeper corneal stroma are affected. Of course, the initial insult causing ulceration may directly result in stromal damage. Once the stroma is damaged, healing occurs with some degree of fibrosis and collagen disorganization, which result in loss of corneal transparency and potentially significant loss of vision. Because the cornea is less than 1 mm thick, ulceration may pose a threat to overall globe integrity. Optimal treatment of a corneal ulcer needs to be rapid and effective to minimize the chance of vision impairment.

2. What initial diagnostics should be done when evaluating a corneal ulcer?

The first objective is to determine the area of corneal involvement and lesion depth. If the ulcer margins are not readily apparent, fluorescein stain may be applied, using a sterile strip moistened with a drop of sterile saline or artificial tears. The moistened strip is momentarily touched to the superior bulbar conjunctiva, anterior nictitans surface, or the inferior conjunctival area. The animal is allowed to blink, and the excessive stain is irrigated with sterile saline. The region of denuded corneal epithelium stains a green color. Depth can be estimated by viewing the ulcer from an oblique angle across the cornea. Normal corneal thickness is about 0.75 mm. Most ulcers are associated with corneal edema that increased the corneal thickness to 1.5–2.5 mm. Ulcer depth should be classified into one of the following categories.

- Epithelial erosion
- Superficial stromal (< $\frac{1}{4}$ thickness)
- Anterior stromal ($\frac{1}{4}$ thickness)
- Midstromal ($\frac{1}{2}$ thickness)

- Deep stromal ($\frac{3}{4}$ thickness)
- Impending perforation (descemetocele)
- Perforation without iris prolapse
- Perforation with iris prolapse

3. What is the second diagnostic step that an emergency clinician should perform in evaluating a serious corneal ulcer?

The second objective is to determine the cause of the ulcer. If the cause is not apparent from the history or initial physical examination, further diagnostic tests are indicated. Culture and cytology specimens should be collected from the ulcer margins and center. If epiphora is not present, a Schirmer tear test should be performed. Inspection of the cornea with a magnifying aid (head loupe or diagnostic otoscope head) allows detection of vascularization and pigmentation, both of which are indicators of chronic disease. Immediate cytologic evaluation with a Wright-Giemsa stain allows characterization of the ulcer process into suppurative inflammation, septic, and noninflammatory categories. Other cytology staining methods can be used if indicated. If the ulcer is deep, minimal pressure should be applied to the ocular tissues because rupture and uveal prolapse may result.

4. Discuss the common causes of deep corneal ulcers.

Ulcerations involving at least 30% of the corneal thickness are often due to traumatic injuries, chronic underlying disease, or direct corneal infection with bacteria, fungi, or viruses. Septic ulcers are particularly dangerous because progression may be rapid because of stromal inflammation, necrosis, and melting. Specific causes of deep corneal ulcers include trauma (blunt, foreign body, sharp), eyelid disorders (distichiasis, ectopic cilia, entropion), keratoconjunctivitis sicca, lagophthalmos (buphthalmos, exophthalmos, facial nerve paralysis), thermal injuries, chemical burns (acids, alkaline agents, detergents), and infection. Common infectious agents in companion animals are *Staphylococcus intermedius* or *aureus*, *Pseudomonas aeruginosa*, *Aspergillus* spp., *Fusarium* spp., and feline herpesvirus. Bacterial agents are often associated with rapid progress to deep ulceration.

5. What first-aid steps should be taken at home before bringing the pet with a corneal ulcer to the veterinarian?

Because the lesion depth is unknown, owners must be careful when manipulating the periocular region. At the least, the animal should be restrained to prevent self-mutilation from rubbing with the paws or against objects. Other pets should not be allowed to lick the facial area of the affected animal. If it is known that the eye is not perforated, the owner may attempt to clean the eye with sterile saline eye rinse (however, this is usually not readily available). In certain situations, the owner may be instructed to instill an antibiotic eyedrop. Potential problems include the following: (1) the medication may have been used for another problem, (2) culture results may be influenced by antibiotic use, (3) treatment may induce more trauma, and (4) the owner may be injured by the animal. Generally, the owner should be encouraged to take the animal to a veterinarian immediately.

6. When is medical treatment the only appropriate approach to corneal ulcer management?

Superficial ulcers respond well to medical treatment because of the tremendous corneal healing response. The primary concern is that the ocular surface is not sterile; if the ulcer is not contaminated or infected, it may soon become so. Thus, topical antibiotics should be instilled frequently (4 times/day). If stromal involvement is present, the frequency should be increased to every 1–2 hr. Anterior uveitis is often present to some degree; thus, topical atropine should be instilled several times to induce cytoplegia and mydriasis, then maintained to effect so that mydriasis is perpetuated during healing. Systemic nonsteroidal agents are also useful for combating ulcer-induced anterior uveitis. If feline herpesvirus is suspected, topical trifluorthymidine solution or idoxuridine ointment and oral acyclovir should be administered. All corneal ulcers should be reevaluated several days to a week or so after starting the initial topical treatment.

7. What antibiotics are best for treating a corneal ulcer?

Ideally a broad-spectrum, bactericidal drug or drug combination should be used. Gram-positive bacteria are the most frequently isolated organisms from pet companion animals. A good combination preparation to keep in a hospital setting is Polymyxin B/Neomycin/Bacitracin or Polymyxin B/Neomycin/Gramicidin ophthalmic solutions. Gentamicin is a good single agent ophthalmic solution, but because of widespread clinical use, some gram-negative organisms are resistant and most streptococcal organisms are resistant. If necessary, prescriptions can be written for ophthalmic ciprofloxacin, ofloxacin, and tobramycin ophthalmic drops. Various injectable antibiotics can be added to artificial tear solutions as single or combination agents. However, most penicillins and cephalosporins are physically incompatible with aminoglycosides. A pharmacist should be consulted before using custom-prepared antibiotics or mixtures.

8. If surgery is anticipated, how should the patient be managed preoperatively?

Because ocular tissue is not essential for life, the animal must be stabilized and restored to a state of physiologic homeostasis that permits general anesthesia and ocular surgery. If the ocular tissues are contaminated or infected with bacteria, topical and, if indicated, systemic antibiotics should be used in preparation for surgery. Unless otherwise indicated, perioperative systemic antibiotics are usually sufficient for ocular surgery. If anterior uveitis is present, parenteral nonsteroidal or corticosteroid drugs are administered (unless contraindicated by the animal's condition). Analgesics such as oxymorphone or butorphanol improve patient comfort and decrease the chance of self-trauma.

9. What surgical repairs should the emergency clinician consider?

Simple protective eyelid flaps, such as a nictitans flaps or temporary tarsorrhaphy, provide good protection and facilitate wound healing. Tarsorrhaphy prevents clinical evaluation of the healing process and is not an ideal protective method. Conjunctival grafts are more difficult to perform but require limited instrumentation. Emergency clinicians should be able to perform a primary suture closure of a ruptured ulcer, if immediate case referral is not possible. Eyelid flaps should be placed using 4-0 to 5-0 sutures; corneal sutures should be 7-0 or 8-0 in size.

BIBLIOGRAPHY

1. Hakenson N, Lorimer D, Merideth RE: Further comments on conjunctival pedicle grafting in the treatment of corneal ulcers in the dog and cat. J Am Animal Hosp Assoc 24:602–605, 1988.
2. Nasisse MP: Canine ulcerative keratitis. In The Compendium Collection: Ophthalmology in Small Animal Practice. Trenton, NJ, Veterinary Learning Systems, 1996, pp 45–59.
3. Nasisse MP: Manifestations, diagnosis, and treatment of ocular herpesvirus infection in cats. In The Compendium Collection: Ophthalmology in Small Animal Practice. Trenton, NJ, Veterinary Learning Systems, 1996, pp 210–218.
4. Roberts SM: Assessment and management of the ophthalmic emergency in cats and dogs. In The Compendium Collection: Ophthalmology in Small Animal Practice. Trenton, NJ, Veterinary Learning Systems, 1996, pp 252–267.
5. Williams D: The treatment of corneal ulcers. Vet Pract 27(13):3–4, 1994.

V. Respiratory Emergencies

Section Editor: Deborah R. Van Pelt, D.V.M., M.S.

41. ASTHMA IN CATS

Kelly J. Diehl, D.V.M., M.S.

1. What is asthma? What criteria are used to make the diagnosis?

Asthma is reversible bronchospasm resulting in airway obstruction. Criteria to diagnose asthma in cats (feline bronchial disease) include the following:
- Historic and clinical findings, coupled with response to treatment for airway obstruction
- Radiographic changes consistent with asthma (bronchial thickening with evidence of hyperinflation)
- Clinicopathologic evidence of airway inflammation

2. Give the signalment, clinical signs, history, and physical findings in cats with asthma.

Asthma is a disease of all breeds of cats, with a possible predilection for Siamese and Himalayans. There is no gender predilection, and all ages of cats may be affected. The most common historical finding is cough, although some cats present with acute respiratory distress as the first sign of asthma. Physical examination between attacks may be unremarkable. Expiratory dyspnea, wheezing, and increased bronchovesicular sounds may be auscultated in some cases.

3. What other disorders should be considered in the differential diagnosis?
- Primary cardiac disease
- Neoplasia
- Infectious pulmonary diseases
- Pulmonary foreign body
- Pulmonary thromboembolism
- Heartworm disease
- Upper airway disease
- Pleural diseases

4. What tests are most helpful in establishing a diagnosis of asthma?

Although they are often normal in cats with asthma, thoracic radiographs are helpful in ruling in or out other diagnoses and may be useful in establishing a diagnosis of asthma.

5. What radiographic changes are associated with asthma?

Radiographic abnormalities may include thickening of bronchial walls, flattening of the diaphragm (overinflated lungs), increased lucency of lung fields (suggestive of air trapping), and, occasionally, atelectasis of the right middle lung lobe (11% of cats).

6. What ancillary tests are recommended in cases of asthma? What are the most common findings?

Complete blood counts may reveal peripheral eosinophilia, but the presence or absence of eosinophilia should not be the only guideline to rule in or out asthma. Biochemical profiles and urinalysis are not helpful in establishing a definitive diagnosis but may help to eliminate other disorders. Fecal examination for parasites is indicated in all cases. Sampling of cells from airways (via transtracheal wash, bronchoalveolar lavage, or bronchial brushing) may demonstrate eosinophils, but they are not pathognomonic for asthma. Bacterial and mycoplasmal cultures of tracheal or bronchial secretions are controversial; some authors believe that microorganisms contribute directly to airway reactivity, some believe that they may be secondary invaders, and others consider them irrelevant. Studies show that 24% of cats with bronchial disease have positive bacterial cultures, and *Mycoplasma* sp. has been cultured from cats with airway disease. Therefore, submission of fluid for culture may be indicated in cats with asthma.

7. What are proposed mediators of asthma in cats?

Research suggests that serotonin is the primary mediator in feline mast cells. Interleukin 5, which is a chemoattractant for eosinophils, also may play a role. Eosinophils are the primary effector cells responsible for pathologic lung changes in cats. They release substances from granules that result in airway inflammation and cellular damage. These substances also sensitize airway smooth muscle cells, making them hyperresponsive.

8. What are the histopathologic findings in cats with asthma?

Inflammatory cellular infiltrates (predominantly eosinophils) are found in the submucosa, sometimes extending into the lamina propria. Evidence of chronic inflammation (epithelial, glandular, and muscular hypertrophy; fibrosis; and emphysema) may be noted on histopathologic evaluation.

9. What is the treatment for cats with acute respiratory distress secondary to asthma?

Cats with severe respiratory distress should be treated with a rapidly acting corticosteroid administered intravenously, if possible. Oxygen therapy is beneficial, along with cage rest. Even severely distressed cats respond positively to this approach. Aminophylline or terbutaline may be used for bronchodilation in cats with acute respiratory distress. Occasionally, epinephrine may be administered in life-threatening situations. Epinephrine may cause arrhythmias (sometimes fatal) and should be used judiciously.

Drugs Used in the Treatment of Asthma in Cats

DRUG	DOSE	USE
Corticosteroids		
Prednisone sodium succinate	50–100 mg/cat	Emergency treatment
Dexamethasone	1 mg/kg IV or IM	Emergency treatment
Prednisone	1–2 mg/kg orally 2–4 times/day	Maintenance therapy
Methylprednisone acetate	10–20 mg/cat IM every 2–4 wk, then every 2–8 wk	Maintenance therapy
Bronchodilators		
Methylxanthines—sustained-release tablets (Theo-Dur or Slo-Bid)	50–100 mg/cat every 24 hr at night	Maintenance therapy
Beta agonists		
Epinephrine	20 µg/kg IV, IM, IT, SC	Emergency treatment
Terbutaline	0.01 mg/kg SC	Emergency treatment
	0.1 mg/kg or 0.625 mg/cat orally every 12 hr	Maintenance therapy
Miscellaneous		
Cyproheptadine	1–2 mg/cat orally every 12 hr	Maintenance therapy
Cyclosporin A	10 mg/kg orally every 12 hr (measure blood levels)	Maintenance therapy

10. What environmental considerations are relevant to long-term management of asthma?

Clients need to be counseled that, although asthma can be controlled, it is seldom cured and some degree of coughing may always be present. Although most environmental triggers are never identified, in people with asthma tobacco smoke, air pollution, and dusty central heating systems aggravate the condition (but are exceedingly hard to eliminate). Changing kitty litter to newspaper or low dust forms is helpful. The vast majority of cases do not have an obvious trigger, necessitating the use of medications.

11. Describe the long-term pharmacologic treatment of asthma.

Corticosteroids remain the mainstay of long-term therapy in cats (see table in question 9). High doses are used initially, gradually tapering the amount, as clinical response is seen, to the lowest dose needed to reduce acute asthma attacks and to minimize coughing episodes. If oral corticosteroids cannot be administered, injectable repositol steroids also have been used. Bronchodilators are often used to ameliorate the signs of asthma, potentially lowering the doses of corticosteroids needed for long-term management. Theophylline (a methylxanthine), given once daily at night, or terbutaline (beta$_2$ agonist) are commonly used bronchodilators. In addition, owners can be instructed how to give injectable terbutaline at home if an acute attack begins. Chronic use of beta$_2$ agonists has been associated with increased morbidity and mortality in humans. In addition, beta agonists should not be used in cats with cardiac disease. Because serotonin is an important mediator of bronchoconstriction in cats, cyproheptadine also may be used in cats with refractory asthma. Cyclosporin A, which blocks T-cell activation (and therefore interleukin production), has been used successfully in humans and experimentally in cats to treat asthma; it is suggested for cases of severe, refractory asthma. If an infectious etiology is identified, appropriate therapy based on culture and sensitivity testing is started (although a purely infectious cause of asthma is rare).

12. How should patients be monitored over the long term?

Recommendations vary, depending on the severity of disease. Severely affected patients may need to be evaluated frequently until signs are controlled, then every 3–6 months, as needed. Owners should contact the veterinarian if signs of worsening airway disease or acute respiratory distress occur.

CONTROVERSIES

12. How should asthma in cats be classified?

Several authors have proposed a more precise description of feline lower airway disease, dividing lower airway disease into categories based on human classification schemes: bronchial asthma, acute bronchitis, chronic bronchitis, chronic asthmatic bronchitis, and chronic bronchitis with emphysema. Other authors make no such distinctions.

13. What is the role of histamine in feline asthma?

Although histamine is unquestionably an important mediator of asthma in people, research has raised questions about its role in the pathogenesis of feline asthma. In fact, some antihistamines may exacerbate the signs of feline asthma.

BIBLIOGRAPHY

1. Johnson L: Bronchial disease. In Consultations in Feline Internal Medicine, vol. 3. Philadelphia, W.B. Saunders, 1997, pp 303–309.
2. Moise SN, Wiedenkeller D, Yeager AE, et al: Clinical, radiographic and bronchial cytologic features of cats with bronchial disease: 65 cases (1980–1986). J Am Vet Med Assoc 194:1467–1473, 1989.
3. Padrid PA: Asthma, bronchitis—Cats. In Five Minute Veterinary Consult. Baltimore, Williams & Wilkins, 1997, pp 370–371.
4. Padrid PA: Chronic lower airway disease in the dog and cat. In Problems in Veterinary Medicine. Philadelphia, J.B. Lippincott, 1992, pp 320–345.
5. Padrid PA: New strategies to treat feline asthma. Vet Forum 46–50, 1996.

42. ASPIRATION PNEUMONITIS

Deborah R. Van Pelt, D.V.M., M.S.

1. What underlying conditions predispose to the development of aspiration pneumonitis?
- Altered consciousness (sedation, central nervous system disorders, anesthesia)
- Oropharyngeal conditions (cleft palate, force feeding)
- Esophageal disorders (vascular ring anomaly, motility disorders, megaesophagus)
- Mechanical disruption of the normal defense barriers (pharyngostomy tube, endotracheal tube, tracheostomy tube)
- Gastroesophageal reflux
- Any cause of persistent vomiting

2. Which bacteria are commonly isolated in patients with aspiration pneumonitis?
Typically, bacteria involved in aspiration pneumonia originate from the oropharynx and include a wide variety of both aerobic and facultative bacteria, such as *Escherichia coli, Klebsiella* sp., *Pasteurella* sp., *Pseudomonas* sp., *Bordetella* sp., and *Streptococcus* sp.

3. List the four different types of aspiration pneumonitis.
1. Chemical pneumonitis (pulmonary inflammatory reaction to any fluid toxic to the lower respiratory tract)
2. Reflex airway closure with aspiration of inert fluids
3. Mechanical obstruction with aspiration of inert fluids or particulate matter
4. Infection by inoculation of oropharyngeal flora

4. What determines the severity of pulmonary reaction in chemical aspiration pneumonitis?
- pH
- Volume of gastric acid
- Presence of particulate matter

With aspiration of material with pH < 2.5, pathologic changes occur within minutes. Material with pH > 2.5 was once thought to be benign. However, it has been demonstrated that aspiration of gastric contents with pH of 5.9 causes severe hypoxia and intrapulmonary shunting. If particulate matter is present, a significant pulmonary reaction occurs whether the pH is < 2.5 or more neutral, although a more severe reaction occurs with lower pH aspirate.

5. Describe the thoracic radiographic changes in patients with chemical pneumonitis.
Radiographic changes are minimal immediately after aspiration unless a large volume of acid is aspirated. Over the following 12–36 hours, diffuse or localized alveolar infiltrates may appear and progress as a result of pulmonary inflammation.

6. What pathologic and clinical signs result from aspiration of inert substances such as saline, water, or barium?
Aspiration of inert substances typically causes only transient damage to the lung, which usually results in transient respiratory distress and self-limiting hypoxia. However, if large volumes are aspirated, mechanical obstruction of the airways may result, causing respiratory distress and asphyxiation.

7. In cases of chemical pneumonitis resulting from aspiration of acid, should neutralization of the aspirated material be attempted?
With aspiration of acidic material, the full extent of pulmonary injury typically occurs within seconds to several minutes after the insult. Aspirated acid is usually neutralized within minutes

by tracheobronchial secretions. Adding diluents may further compromise the airways by causing mechanical obstruction. If lavage is attempted, it should be done immediately after aspiration, and only saline should be used.

8. What is the pathophysiologic reason behind the limited response to supplemental oxygen in some patients with aspiration pneumonitis?

In patients with severe cases of aspiration pneumonia, ventilation/perfusion (V/Q) imbalance results from perfusion of partially collapsed alveoli. Intrapulmonary shunting occurs with perfusion of completely collapsed alveoli as a result of small airway obstruction. Hypoxemia due to intrapulmonary shunting typically responds poorly to oxygen supplementation because nonventilated alveoli do not contribute to increasing the PaO_2 of the pulmonary arterial blood. In patients with hypoxemia poorly responsive to oxygen, positive pressure ventilation may be necessary to correct hypoxemia.

9. Are antibiotics necessary in the treatment of aspiration pneumonitis?

Antibiotics are not indicated in most cases of isolated chemical pneumonitis and inert substance aspiration, because such episodes are rarely associated with infection. In cases of pneumonia secondary to aspiration of normal upper airway flora, antimicrobial agents should be used.

10. List the clinical signs that should lead the clinician to suspect pulmonary infection in patients with a history of aspiration.
- Fever
- Leukocytosis
- Mucopurulent nasal or oropharyngeal discharge
- Radiographic evidence of consolidating lung lobes with air bronchograms

11. Pending results of sputum or transtracheal wash culture, which antibiotics should be used in the treatment of aspiration pneumonia?

Broad-spectrum aggressive antimicrobial therapy with activity against all potentially pathogenic organisms should be initiated. Examples include a combination of cephalosporins with aminoglycosides or enrofloxacin. In less severe cases, trimethoprim-sulfa or chloramphenicol also may be used.

12. Describe the classic distribution of affected lung lobes in patients with aspiration pneumonia.

Most frequently the right middle lung lobe is involved, although any dependent lung lobe (including the left and right cranial) may be affected.

13. Are bronchodilators useful in the treatment of aspiration pneumonitis?

Because bronchoconstriction is a frequent sequela of aspiration, emergency bronchodilation may be beneficial in cases with significant respiratory distress. Aminophylline or isoproterenol may be used.

CONTROVERSY

14. Discuss the pros and cons of corticosteroid administration in the treatment of aspiration pneumonitis.

Pros: Corticosteroids decrease platelet and polymorphonuclear aggregation, stabilize lysosomal membranes, and have an antiinflammatory effect.

Cons: Corticosteroids interfere with normal defense mechanisms that act to localize and wall off foreign materials (it has been reported that the inflammatory response persists longer in patients treated with corticosteroids than in patients without corticosteroids). No improvement in arterial oxygenation, cardiac output, pulmonary arterial pressure, or survival has been reported in patients treated with corticosteroids.

BIBLIOGRAPHY

1. Boothe DM, McKiernan BC: Respiratory therapeutics. Vet Clin North Am (Small Animal Pract) 22:1231–1258, 1992.
2. Hawkins EC: Aspiration pneumonia. In Bonagura JD (ed): Current Veterinary Therapy XII. Philadelphia, W.B. Saunders, 1995, pp 915–919.
3. Khawaja IT, Buffra SD, Brandstetter RD: Aspiration pneumonia. Postgrad Med 92:165, 1992.
4. Orton EC, Wheeler SL: Continuous positive airway pressure therapy for aspiration pneumonia in a dog. J Am Vet Med Assoc 188:1437, 1986.
5. Schwartz DJ, Wynne JW, Gibbs CP, et al: The pulmonary consequence of aspiration of gastric contents at pH values of greater than 2.5. Am Rev Respir Dis 121:119–126, 1980.
6. Tams TR: Aspiration pneumonia and complications of inhalation of smoke and toxic gases. Vet Clin North Am (Small Animal Pract) 15:971–989, 1985.
7. Tams TR: Pneumonia. In Kirk RW (ed): Current Veterinary Therapy X. Philadelphia, W.B. Saunders, 1989, pp 376–384.

43. DIROFILARIASIS

Kelly J. Diehl, D.V.M., M.S.

1. What is the causative agent of heartworm disease?

Heartworm disease is caused by the filaroid *Diroflaria immitis*.

2. Describe the life cycle of *D. immitis*.

Heartworm disease is spread by infected mosquitoes, which acquire microfilaria when they ingest blood from infected hosts. The microfilaria undergo two molts within the mosquito and are then capable of infecting a dog when the mosquito next feeds. The larvae (L3) enter the skin and migrate through the host for approximately $3\frac{1}{2}$ months. During migration they mature into young adult heartworms (L5), which enter the vascular system and travel to the pulmonary arteries. Adults produce microfilaria (L1), which enter the bloodstream and are available for ingestion by another mosquito.

3. What is the pathogenesis of disease caused by *D. immitis*?

The particular host's immune response to adult heartworms is responsible for the pathologic lesions noted in heartworm infection. Adult heartworms cause endothelial damage; the damaged endothelium attracts leukocytes, stimulates release of various trophic factors, and loses its properties of selective permeability. The pathognomonic histopathologic change is myointimal proliferation on the endothelial surface of pulmonary arteries. These changes result in pulmonary hypertension and local inflammation with interstitial fluid accumulation. Hypertension within the pulmonary vasculature increases the work of the right ventricle; consequently, the right ventricle hypertrophies and dilates in response to increased demand and eventually may fail.

4. What laboratory tests should be performed before initiation of adulticide therapy? Are any tests predictive of future complications?

Complete blood count, biochemical profile, urinalysis, radiography, and echocardiography are recommended before initiation of adulticide treatment. Although blood work is helpful to rule out concurrent disease (particularly liver and renal disease), only radiography may be helpful in determining the extent of pulmonary disease and in predicting which patients may be at increased risk for pulmonary thromboembolism. Echocardiography is helpful in the diagnosis of postcaval heartworm syndrome.

5. What specific screening tests are used to diagnose heartworm disease?

Microfilaria concentration tests and direct smears of whole blood are still occasionally used to screen dogs for heartworm disease. However, newer immunodiagnostic tests are more sensitive and specific, detect microfilaria-negative but infected dogs, and are readily available to most practices, making other techniques obsolete. Tests geared to detect circulating microfilaria are important only in dogs receiving daily diethylcarbamazine (DEC) therapy; life-threatening side effects may develop if DEC is administered to microfilaremic dogs.

6. What are the recommended adulticide treatments? What is the appropriate timing of treatment?

There are two recommended treatments: the organoarsenical thiacetarsamide and the newer melarsomine dihydrochloride. Thiacetarsamide is given over 48 hours, with two treatments on each day. Although originally given at 12-hour intervals, new data support the pairing of doses 8 hours apart, starting in the morning of each day, with no longer than 16 hours between the second dose on day 1 and the first dose on day 2. Melarsomine is administered in 2 doses 24 hours apart, with retreatment in 4 months.

Drugs and Dosages for Heartworm Disease in Dogs and Cats

DRUG	DOSE
Adulticides	
Thiacetarsamide	2.2 mg/kg IV twice daily for 4 doses (dogs and cats; in cats, pretreatment with ketamine is recommended)
Melarsomine	2.5 mg/kg IM every 24 hr for 2 doses (dogs)
Microfilaricides	
Ivermectin	
Adulticide	6–12 µg/kg orally once before (before microfilaricide) (dogs and cats)
Microfilaricide	50 µg/kg orally once (after adulticide) (dogs and cats)
Preventatives	
Milbemycin	500 µg/kg every 30 days (dogs and cats)
Ivermectin	24 µg/kg every 30 days (dogs and cats)
Diethylcarbamazine citrate	2.5–3.0 mg/kg every 24 hr (dogs)
Miscellaneous	
Prednisone	1 mg/kg orally every 24 hr
Aspirin	5–10 mg/kg orally every 24 hr
Heparin	75 U/kg SC every 8 hr
Oxygen therapy	As needed

7. What are the potential complications of adulticide therapy?

Thiacetarsamide is hepatotoxic and extremely caustic if given perivascularly. Melarsomine has the advantage of intramuscular administration, although pain and swelling at the injection site are common. Melarsomine does not cause hepatotoxicity. Pulmonary thromboembolism secondary to worm kill is an important complication of adulticide therapy, occurring 10–21 days after therapy. Strict rest is the single most important treatment of thromboembolism; it is a much more difficult problem to treat than to prevent. Treatment for pulmonary thromboembolism includes oxygen, cage rest, corticosteroid therapy, and antithrombotics.

8. What tests are used to confirm adulticide therapy?

First, clinical improvement in treated dogs is suggestive of at least partial kill of heartworms. Antigenemia disappears in 3 months after treatment if all or most of the adults are eliminated. Periodic monitoring of antigen tests at approximately 3-month intervals is recommended. Affirmative (even weak positive) results indicate the persistence of adults, usually females.

9. What microfilaricides are available? Discuss timing of treatment and complications.

No microfilaricides are approved by the Food and Drug Administration. Extra-label use of ivermectin or milbemycin oxime is accepted as a safe microfilaricide treatment; both drugs are generally given 3–4 weeks after completion of adulticide therapy. Milbemycin oxime is an excellent microfilaricide at prophylactic doses, and one dose is usually sufficient to eliminate microfilaria in adulticide-pretreated dogs. Ivermectin at a dose of 50 µg/kg orally once is also an effective microfilaricide. Side effects of both drugs are related to rapid die-off of microfilaria and include weakness, pale mucous membranes, and tachypnea. The signs are mild and generally subside with supportive care. Most authors recommend that dogs be hospitalized for several hours after therapy.

10. What heartworm preventatives are currently available for dogs? What are their side effects?

Both ivermectin and milbemycin oxime are effective preventatives. They are given on a monthly basis and are quite safe, with no reported side effects. Diethylcarbamazine (DEC) is rarely given as a daily heartworm preventative; microfilaremic dogs may have severe reactions to DEC.

11. Are ivermectin and milbemycin microfilaricidal at preventative doses? If so, how does this change the diagnostic tests used to detect heartworm infections?

After 6–8 months of administration, both are microfilaricidal. Therefore, antigen tests should be used to screen for heartworm infection.

12. How frequently should dogs be tested for heartworm infection?

Frequency of testing is controversial, although most clinicians recommend yearly testing for dogs in endemic areas, with testing every 1–2 years in areas of low prevalence.

13. What other treatments are occasionally used as adjunctive therapy for heartworm disease? What are the criteria for using adjunctive treatments?

The need for other medications and the criteria for their use remain controversial. Corticosteroids are at the center of the controversy. Many recommend their use in both cats and dogs with radiographic evidence of allergic lung disease (eosinophilic pneumonitis). Corticosteroids must be withdrawn 1 week before initiation of adulticide therapy, or kill rates of adult heartworms will be reduced. Aspirin therapy is often initiated before adulticide therapy if signs of pulmonary vascular changes (without pneumonitis) are present. In addition, aspirin therapy may reduce the incidence of pulmonary thromboembolism.

14. What controversies surround pretreatment with ivermectin before adulticide therapy in dogs?

Some clinicians advocate the use of ivermectin before adulticide therapy is started. Ivermectin kills the L4 larvae, which may develop into adults while adulticide therapy and subsequent microfilaricides are administered.

15. What larval stages are destroyed by ivermectin? When?

Evidence suggests that L5 larval stages are killed by ivermectin after 5–6 months of treatment. In addition, some research suggests that ivermectin may destroy even adult heartworms after 18–20 months of continuous use.

16. What is postcaval heartworm syndrome? How is it treated?

Postcaval heartworm syndrome occurs in patients with high worm burdens. It is characterized by circulatory collapse and shock, accompanied by icterus and hemoglobinuria or hemoglobinemia secondary to red blood cell fragmentation. Large numbers of adult worms obstruct the tricuspid valve and right atrium, sometimes extending into the caudal vena cava. Echocardiography is used to confirm the diagnosis. Such patients must be distinguished from dogs with severe heartworm disease without obstruction. The treatment of choice (and necessity) is surgical removal of the worms via the jugular vein.

17. What is the reported prevalence of heartworm disease in cats?

Studies from the Southeast report a prevalence of 2.5–14%. Atkins reported a prevalence of 25% at North Carolina State University. The incidence in cats is approximately 10% of the incidence in dogs in a given area.

18. What are the most common signs of heartworm disease in cats? What is the best diagnostic test in cats?

Vomiting and respiratory signs (coughing) are the most common signs in cats with chronic disease. The heartworm antigen test, if positive, is a strong indicator of heartworm disease in cats.

19. What are the controversies about treatment of heartworm disease in cats?

Atkins recommends treating cats with heartworm prophylaxis in areas with increased incidence of infection, because treatment regimens in cats are not benign and carry a high risk of death. Adulticide therapy with thiacetarsemide is dangerous; normal cats often develop fatal pulmonary reactions. Many cats develop pulmonary thromboembolism after receiving adulticide therapy. Many authors do not recommend adulticide therapy in cats unless clinical signs are of sufficient severity to warrant the risk. Others recommend pretreatment with ketamine because of its antiserotonin activity (serotonin is implicated as a potent bronchoconstrictor in cats). The new adulticide melarsomine has not been used in cats. Microfilaricides are unnecessary because most cats do not exhibit microfilaremia.

BIBLIOGRAPHY

1. Atkins CE: Feline cardiovascular disease: Therapeutic considerations. Proceedings of the 14th ACVIM Forum, San Antonio, TX, 1996, pp 175–177.
2. Blagburn BL: Microfilaricidal therapy: Review and update. Vet Med July:630–638, 1994.
3. Calvert CA, Rawlings CA: Canine heartworm disease. In Canine and Feline Cardiology. New York, Churchill Livingstone, 1988, pp 519–549.
4. Calvert CA: Heartworm disease. In Manual of Canine and Feline Cardiology. Philadelphia, W.B. Saunders, 1995, pp 225–229.
5. Coleman MW: Legal and medical considerations in dispensing heartworm preventives. Vet Med June:552–558, 1994.
6. Dillon R: Feline heartworms: More than just a curiosity. Vet Forum Dec:18–26, 1995.
7. Dzimianski MT: Developing a heartworm prevention program. Vet Med June:545–550, 1994.
8. Knauer KW: State of the art heartworm therapy. Proceedings of the 14th ACVIM Forum, San Antonio, TX, 1996, pp 189–191.
9. Knight DH (ed): Proceedings of the Heartworm Symposium 95. Batavia, IL, American Heartworm Society, 1996.
10. Knight DH: Should every heartworm-infected dog be treated with an adulticide? Vet Med July:620–628, 1994.
11. Knight DH: Guidelines for diagnosis and management of heartworm (*Dirofilaria immitis*) infection. In Current Veterinary Therapy XII. Philadelphia, W.B. Saunders, 1995, pp 879–887.
12. McCall JW, Calvert CA, Rawlings CA: Heartworm infection in cats: A life-threatening disease. Vet Med July:639–647, 1994.
13. McTier TL: A guide to selecting adult heartworm antigen test kits. Vet Med June:528–544, 1994.
14. Miller MW: Therapeutic strategies for dogs with severe heartworm disease. Vet Prev 1:5–7, 15, 1994.
15. Rawlings CA, Calvert CA: Heartworm disease. In Textbook of Veterinary Internal Medicine. Philadelphia, W.B. Saunders, 1995, pp 1046–1068.
16. Rawlings CA, Calvert CA: Heartworm disease—Dogs. In Five Minute Veterinary Consult. Baltimore, Williams & Wilkins, 1997, pp 638–639.

44. PULMONARY THROMBOEMBOLISM

Deborah R. Van Pelt, D.V.M., M.S.

1. What underlying diseases have been associated with the development of pulmonary thromboembolism?

- Autoimmune hemolytic anemia
- Hyperadrenocorticism
- Disseminated intravascular coagulation
- Heart worm disease
- Hypothyroidism
- Pancreatitis
- Protein-losing glomerulopathy
- Cardiac disease
- Neoplasia
- Sepsis

2. Describe the typical radiographic findings in dogs with pulmonary thromboembolism.

Two common radiographic findings in dogs with pulmonary thromboembolism (PTE) are focal atelectasis with regional pulmonary infiltrates and regional oligemia. However, in a significant percentage of patients with PTE, thoracic radiographs are normal. The primary reason to obtain thoracic radiographs in patients with suspected PTE is to rule out other diseases, such as pneumothorax, that may mimic signs of PTE.

3. Describe the typical arterial blood gas in a patient with PTE.

The most common findings of arterial blood gas analysis in patients with PTE are hypoxemia (decreased PaO_2), mild respiratory alkalosis (decreased $PaCO_2$), and increased alveolar–arterial (A–a) gradient (PAO_2–PaO_2).

4. What is the best technique for diagnosis of PTE?

The gold standard for diagnosis of PTE is pulmonary angiography. However, ventilation/perfusion (V/Q) scanning is becoming more readily available and aids in the diagnosis of PTE. A normal V/Q scan rules out the diagnosis of PTE, whereas an abnormal scan (demonstrating areas of decreased perfusion), along with hypoxemia and clinical signs, supports the diagnosis of PTE.

5. Why does a patient with PTE have such a dramatic response to the administration of supplemental oxygen?

Patients with PTE are hypoxemic because they have significant ventilation/perfusion (V/Q) mismatch; ventilation is normal, but perfusion is significantly decreased. Pulmonary arterial blood is diverted to other areas of the lung because of the thrombus. When supplemental oxygen is administered, the entire blood volume is now exposed to increased alveolar oxygen levels and results in increased PaO_2.

6. Should thrombolytic agents be used for treatment of PTE?

Because one of the goals of treatment in patients with PTE is to promote dissolution of the thrombi, in theory administration of thrombolytic agents helps. However, large clinical trials in humans with PTE found no differences in morbidity or mortality rates when heparin alone was compared with thrombolytic therapy. Because thrombolytic therapy may be associated with a higher complication rate, heparin alone may be preferred. In the author's experience, use of thrombolytic agents has not been helpful in decreasing mortality in veterinary patients with PTE.

7. List three modalities for medical treatment of PTE other than treating the underlying disease.

- Oxygen supplementation
- Hemodynamic support of the microvascular circulation with crystalloids
- Anticoagulation

8. What role does anticoagulation play in the treatment of PTE?

Anticoagulation, most commonly with heparin, decreases the formation of additional thrombi as well as prevents the thrombus already present from increasing in size. Anticoagulation also may be accomplished with warfarin. The goal of anticoagulation is to increase the prothrombin time (PT) to 1.5–2 times normal levels.

9. In conjunction with treatment of underlying disease and anticoagulation, what other therapy may be effective in preventing recurrent or ongoing thrombosis?

Low-molecular-weight dextrans, through their effect on platelet function, may be beneficial in preventing continuing thrombosis. By coating platelets in the peripheral circulation, dextrans decrease their adhesion and aggregation, thereby decreasing thrombus formation.

10. Which diagnostic tests should be performed in the initial work-up of patients suspected of having PTE?

- Arterial blood gas analysis
- Complete blood count
- Activated clotting time, PT, partial thromboplastin time
- Electrocardiogram
- Thoracic radiographs

Although these tests do not specifically diagnose PTE, they may uncover another reason for the patient's clinical signs.

11. What is Virchow's triad?

Virchow's triad describes the three pathophysiologic states that contribute to development of thrombi: hypercoagulable state, venous stasis, and endothelial injury.

12. Why do patients with PTE have an increased alveolar–arterial (A–a) gradient?

A–a gradient is the alveolar partial pressure of oxygen (PAO_2) minus the arterial partial pressure of oxygen (PaO_2) and in normal patients should be less then 10 mmHg. However, in patients with PTE, the PaO_2 is typically significantly decreased, whereas PAO_2 is normal. The result is an increased A–a gradient.

13. How do you calculate the A–a gradient?

PaO_2 is obtained from the arterial blood gas sample. PAO_2 is calculated as follows:

$$PAO_2 = (\text{barometric pressure} - \text{water vapor pressure}) \times FIO_2 - 1.2 \times PaCO_2$$

Water vapor pressure is typically 47 mmHg. FIO_2 is the fraction of inspired oxygen, which is 0.21 in room air. $PaCO_2$ is obtained from the arterial blood sample. A–a gradient = $PAO_2 - PaO_2$.

14. What are the most common clinical signs of PTE in dogs?

- Dyspnea
- Tachypnea
- Depression
- Tachycardia

BIBLIOGRAPHY

1. Cuitanic O, Marino PL: Improved use of arterial blood gas analysis in suspected pulmonary embolism. Chest 95:48–51, 1989.
2. D'Alonzo GE, Dantzker DR: Gas exchange alterations following pulmonary thromboembolism. Clin Chest Med 5:411–419, 1984.
3. Dennis JS: Clinical features of canine pulmonary thromboembolism. Comp Cont Educ Pract Vet 15:1595–1603, 1993.
4. Fisher WT, Reilly K, Salluzzo RF, et al: Atypical presentation of pulmonary embolism. Ann Emerg Med 19:1429–1435, 1990.
5. Kelley MA, Carson JL, Palevsky HI, Schwartz JS: Diagnosing pulmonary embolism: New facts and strategies. Ann Intern Med 114:300–306, 1991.
6. Klein JK, Dow SW, Rosychuk RAW: Pulmonary thromboembolism associated with immune-mediated hemolytic anemia in dogs: Ten cases (1982–1987). J Am Vet Med Assoc 195:246–250, 1989.

7. LaRue MJ, Murtaugh RJ: Pulmonary thromboembolism in dogs: 47 cases (1986–1987). J Am Vet Med Assoc 197:1368–1372, 1990.
8. Marder WJ, Sherry S: Thrombolytic therapy: Current status. N Engl J Med 318:1585–1595, 1988.
9. Parsons PE: Deep venous thrombosis and pulmonary embolism. In Markovchick VJ, Pons PT, Wolfe RE (eds): Emergency Medicine Secrets. Philadelphia, Hanley & Belfus, 1993, pp 89–92.
10. Rosenow ED, Osmundson PJ, Brown JL: Pulmonary embolism. Mayo Clin Proc 56:161–178, 1981.
11. Van Pelt DR, Wingfield WE, Wheeler SL, et al: Oxygen-tension based indices as predictors of survival in critically ill dogs. J Vet Crit Care Emerg Med 1:19, 1991.
12. White RA: Pulmonary embolism. In Shoemaker WC, Ayres S, Grenvik A, et al: Textbook of Critical Care. Philadelphia, W.B. Saunders, 1989, pp 666–668.

45. LARYNGEAL PARALYSIS

Deborah R. Van Pelt, D.V.M., M.S.

1. What underlying conditions have been associated with development of laryngeal paralysis?

Congenital laryngeal paralysis has been reported in Siberian huskies, Bouvier des Flandres, English bulldogs, and bull terriers. Other conditions include systemic neuromuscular or metabolic diseases (such as myasthenia gravis and hypothyroidism), trauma (bite wounds or blunt trauma to the neck), and, less often, inflammation or neoplasia.

2. In dogs with acute respiratory distress secondary to laryngeal paralysis, what emergency measures should be undertaken to alleviate the respiratory distress?

• Evaluate for the presence of pharyngeal foreign body.
• Administer supplemental oxygen.
• Administer antiinflammatory doses of dexamethasone sodium phosphate.
• Sedate the patient to decrease anxiety.
• If necessary, provide an airway via placement of an endotracheal tube or tracheostomy.

3. Describe the typical respiratory pattern of a patient with laryngeal paralysis.

Laryngeal stridor with inspiratory distress.

4. List the presenting complaints common in patients with laryngeal paralysis.

• Exercise intolerance
• Increased effort and noise associated with inspiration
• Change in voice
• Gagging, retching, or coughing associated with swallowing food or water

5. Why is laryngeal paralysis one of the first signs in dogs with polyneuropathies?

Laryngeal paralysis results from loss of innervation of the intrinsic muscles of the larynx, which receive motor innervation through the recurrent laryngeal nerves. The recurrent laryngeal nerves are among the longest nerves in the body, originating in the brainstem, accompanying the vagi to the thoracic inlet, and then passing around the aortic arch and right subclavian artery before innervating the larynx. Because of their length, the recurrent laryngeal nerves are often the first to be affected by peripheral neuropathies.

6. Describe the protocol for laryngoscopic evaluation in patients suspected of having laryngeal paralysis.

Laryngoscopic examination should be performed while the patient is lightly sedated. A short-acting thiobarbiturate or propofol may be given intravenously. The dose should be titrated to provide adequate restraint for laryngeal examination but not suppress spontaneous ventilation. The patient must be spontaneously ventilating to allow proper evaluation of laryngeal function. The arytenoid cartilages should be observed with a laryngoscope for abduction during inspiration.

7. List three surgical procedures for treatment of laryngeal paralysis.
- Partial laryngectomy
- Castellated laryngofissure
- Arytenoid lateralization

8. Is unilateral arytenoid lateralization successful in the treatment of laryngeal paralysis?
Yes. Unilateral arytenoid lateralization appears to provide satisfactory functional improvement in as many as 90% of patients treated for laryngeal paralysis. It provides improvement similar to bilateral lateralization with a lower incidence of aspiration pneumonia.

BIBLIOGRAPHY

1. Bjorling DE: Laryngeal paralysis. In Bonagura JD (ed): Current Veterinary Therapy XII. Philadelphia, W.B. Saunders, 1995, pp 901–905.
2. Braund KG, Steinberg S, Shores A, et al: Laryngeal paralysis in immature and mature dogs as one sign of a more diffuse polyneuropathy. J Am Vet Med Assoc 194:1753, 1989.
3. Gaber CE, Amis TC, LeCouteur RA: Laryngeal paralysis in dogs: A review of 23 cases. J Am Vet Med Assoc 186:377–380, 1985.
4. Greenfield CL: Canine laryngeal paralysis. Comp Cont Educ Pract Vet 9:1011–1017, 1987.
5. LaHue TR: Treatment of laryngeal paralysis in dogs by unilateral cricoarytenoid laryngoplasty. J Am Animal Hosp Assoc 25:317, 1989.
6. Venker-van Haagen AJ: Diseases of the larynx. Vet Clin North Am (Small Animal Pract) 22:1155–1172, 1992.

46. NEAR DROWNING

Linda G. Martin, D.V.M., M.S.

1. What is the definition of near drowning?
Drowning refers to dying as a result of underwater immersion. **Near drowning** is survival for at least 24 hours after submersion.

2. What results in the vast majority of deaths after a near-drowning episode?
Almost all patients who ultimately die do so not because of the pulmonary insult and resulting hypoxemia but rather because of anoxic brain injury. The degree of central nervous system insult seems to be the limiting factor for survival. Diffuse anoxic injury to the brain results in intracellular swelling and increased intracranial pressure.

3. What is the mechanism for fresh water drowning?
Aspiration of fresh water causes inactivation of surfactant, which leads to atelectasis and ventilation–perfusion mismatch. In addition, water in the alveoli interferes with gas exchange by diffusion impairment. Once in the alveoli, fresh water tends to move rapidly into the intravascular space. Depending on the initial volume of aspirated water, intravascular volume may significantly increase as the fluid shift takes place. In the vast majority of cases, despite the increase in free water, significant electrolyte disturbances do not occur.

4. What is the mechanism for salt water drowning?

The major pathophysiologic change that accompanies salt water drowning is alveolar flooding. Hypoxemia develops primarily from inability to oxygenate because of fluid-filled alveoli. The fluid probably remains in the alveoli longer than fresh water. The increased osmolarity of salt water predisposes fluid movement from the intravascular space into the alveoli, which results in decreased blood volume and hypotension. Unlike fresh water, salt water does not interfere with surfactant production by type II alveolar cells or inactivate surfactant. Therefore, alveolar collapse is not a predominant feature of salt water drowning.

5. Is it possible for drowning victims not to aspirate significant volumes of water?

Yes. Minute amounts of water drawn into the mouth may cause significant and severe laryngospasm. Hypoxemia may result from persistent laryngospasm. Further attempts to breathe may result in negative pressure pulmonary edema secondary to laryngospasm and glottis closure.

6. What other secondary problems may occur in near-drowning victims?

Hypoxemia may lead to cardiac arrhythmias, myocardial ischemia, cardiac arrest, acute renal failure, acute hepatic failure, and anoxic central nervous system injury.

7. What is the initial therapy for near-drowning victims?

Resuscitation should begin by establishing an airway, breathing for the patient (preferably with 100% oxygen), starting chest compressions if the patient is pulseless, and establishing intravenous access.

8. When is the use of continuous positive airway pressure (CPAP) or positive end-expiratory pressure (PEEP) indicated?

Because of the inactivation of surfactant and atelectasis associated with fresh water near drowning, the use of CPAP or PEEP helps to maintain lung expansion and to improve gas exchange. Salt water near drowning generally does not require the same degree or duration of mechanical ventilation as fresh water near drowning.

9. Is there an indication for glucocorticoid therapy in the treatment of near drowning?

No. No evidence clearly indicates that steroid therapy provides any benefit, nor does it improve the recovery of the lung after near drowning.

10. Do antibiotics have a role in the treatment of near drowning?

Prophylactic antibiotics are of no proven benefit. But antibiotic therapy may be appropriate if immersion has occurred in a body of water known to be contaminated. In addition, loss of consciousness may result in aspiration of stomach contents and require antibiotic therapy.

11. What is the approach to patients exhibiting central nervous system deficits?

Hypoxemia leads to cerebral edema and a subsequent increase in intracranial pressure. Cerebral resuscitation is directed toward reducing intracranial pressure and ensuring efficient oxygen delivery. Emergency treatment of patients who appear to have suffered a severe CNS event includes osmotic diuretics, treatment of seizures if they occur, sedation to reduce agitation, judicious fluid therapy, and controlled ventilation via endotracheal tube and mechanical ventilation, if necessary.

12. Is there an indication for use of sodium bicarbonate during resuscitation?

No. Respiratory and metabolic acidosis should be treated by proper ventilation and fluid therapy.

13. Can hypothermia at the time of immersion provide protective effects?

Yes. Cold water has potentially beneficial effects. Submersion in cold water theoretically induces the mammalian diving reflex in which blood is shunted from the periphery to the central core. Hypothermia also causes a decrease in metabolic demand, thus reducing potential hypoxic injury in prolonged asphyxia.

BIBLIOGRAPHY

1. Bohn DJ, Biggart WD, Smith CR, et al: Influence of hypothermia, barbiturate therapy, and intracranial pressure monitoring on morbidity and mortality after near-drowning. Crit Care Med 14:529–534, 1986.
2. Edwards ND, Timmins AC, Randalls B, et al: Survival in adults after cardiac arrest due to drowning. Intens Care Med 16:336–337, 1990.
3. Gallagher TJ: Drowning. In Parrillo JE, Bone RC (eds): Critical Care Medicine: Principles of Diagnosis and Management. St. Louis, Mosby, 1995, pp 1415–1418.
4. Goodwin SR, Boysen PG, Modell JH: Near-drowning: Adults and children. In Shoemaker WC, Ayres SM, Grenvik A, Holbrook PR (eds): Textbook of Critical Care. Philadelphia, W.B. Saunders, 1995, pp 65–74.
5. Lavelle JM, Shaw KN: Near drowning: Is emergency department cardiopulmonary resuscitation or intensive care unit cerebral resuscitation indicated? Crit Care Med 21:368–373, 1993.
6. Modell JH: Drowning. N Engl J Med 328:254–256, 1993.
7. Orlwoski JP: The hemodynamic and cardiovascular effects of near-drowning in hypotonic, isotonic, and hypertonic solutions. Ann Emerg Med 18:1044–1049, 1989.

47. PULMONARY EDEMA

Deborah R. Van Pelt, D.V.M., M.S.

1. List the six physiologic variables that affect the rate of transvascular fluid transport.
• Intravascular hydrostatic pressure
• Interstitial hydrostatic pressure
• Intravascular colloid oncotic pressure
• Interstitial fluid colloid oncotic pressure
• Vascular surface area capable of fluid transport
• Degree of vascular permeability to solutes, especially proteins

2. What are the four broad categories used to describe the mechanisms of development of pulmonary edema?
1. Increased intravascular hydrostatic pressure (pressure or cardiogenic edema)
2. Increased vascular permeability to fluids and proteins (permeability or low-pressure edema)
3. Combination of pressure and permeability edema
4. Other causes (decreased capillary oncotic pressure, decreased interstitial hydrostatic pressure, altered alveolar surface tension, decreased lymphatic drainage)

3. How can the variables responsible for development of pulmonary edema be quantitatively measured?
Intravascular hydrostatic pressure can be estimated by measuring the pulmonary capillary wedge pressure (which approximates left atrial pressure in the absence of obstructive disease of the pulmonary veins).

Changes in intravascular oncotic pressure can be estimated by determining serum albumin concentrations.

Vascular permeability can be assessed by noninvasive dual radioisotopic marker techniques or by calculating the ratio of alveolar edema/serum protein concentrations.

4. What is the most common cause of pulmonary edema in veterinary patients?

Increased pulmonary vascular pressure is the most common cause. Left heart failure is the most commonly associated primary disease.

5. What is the critical pressure for development of pulmonary edema secondary to left heart failure?

Critical pressure is the pulmonary venous and capillary pressure at which pulmonary edema forms. Although this value is somewhat variable, it is approximately 20–25 mmHg for dogs. Smaller increases in pulmonary vascular pressure are well tolerated with little or no edema formation, probably because of increased pulmonary lymphatic drainage.

6. Other than heart disease, which diseases may cause high-pressure edema?
- **Intravascular volume loading with crystalloids** (crystalloids increase hydrostastic pressure and decrease intravascular colloid oncotic pressure).
- **Kidney disease** may predispose patients to development of pulmonary edema as a result of increased sensitivity to exogenous volume expansion.
- **Neurologic pulmonary edema**, secondary to head trauma, increased intracranial pressure, electrocution, or seizures, initially causes pulmonary venous hypertension but then causes loosening of interendothelial junctions and disruption of alveolar epithelium.

7. What is permeability edema?

Permeability edema is pulmonary edema characterized predominantly by increased leakiness of pulmonary vascular endothelium and alveolar epithelium to water and proteins. Increased leakiness may be due to increased pore size, increased number of pores, or damage to endothelial or epithelial cells with disruption of the normal selective barrier.

8. Describe the cellular mechanisms involved in the pathogenesis of permeability edema.

Underlying diseases such as pancreatitis, sepsis, or trauma activate the complement system. Complement then causes neutrophil sequestration and aggregation within the pulmonary microvasculature. Activated white blood cells liberate a variety of potentially cytotoxic agents, including oxygen radicals, leukotrienes, hydrogen peroxide, platelet-activating factor, and lysosomal enzymes, all of which can cause endothelial and epithelial damage.

9. What are the physiologic consequences of pulmonary edema?
- Decreased pulmonary compliance
- Decreased lung volume
- Decreased regional ventilation in affected areas
- Decreased regional perfusion in areas with alveolar edema
- Ventilation/perfusion mismatch
- Shunting

10. Is analysis of arterial blood gases necessary for diagnosis and treatment of pulmonary edema?

No. The presence and magnitude of arterial hypoxemia correlate poorly with the severity of pulmonary edema in dogs. However, arterial and venous blood gases may be useful in gauging the need and effectiveness of oxygen and ventilatory therapy.

11. What simple diagnostic test can be done to determine whether permeability changes contribute to edema formation?

Protein levels of edema fluid act as an estimator of interstitial protein levels and provide some idea about the integrity of the pulmonary endothelial barrier. Calculating the ratio of edema fluid to serum protein levels may be useful. Typically, pure high-pressure edema fluid has lower than normal protein levels because of dilution, whereas permeability edema fluid has normal or increased protein levels. Edema with serum protein levels < 0.5 are suggestive of high-pressure edema, whereas values > 0.5 are suggestive of increased permeability.

12. What are the goals of treatment in patients with pulmonary edema?
- Decrease excessive extravascular lung water.
- Normalize the physiologic consequences of pulmonary edema.
- Meet minimal whole body oxygen requirements.
- Normalize systemic arterial oxygen content and tissue oxygen delivery.
- Eliminate the cause.

13. How can morphine be useful in the treatment of patients with pulmonary edema?
Morphine may relax and sedate the patient, thereby decreasing whole body oxygen requirements. It also increases venous capacitance, resulting in decreased venous return. Morphine also acts centrally to slow the respiratory rate and to increase tidal volume, both of which improve lymphatic drainage and aid in removing pulmonary edema fluid.

14. When is ventilatory therapy indicated in the treatment of pulmonary edema?
If spontaneous ventilation and tidal volume are insufficient to maintain adequate PaO_2 despite supplemental oxygenation, ventilatory therapy is indicated (i.e., if PaO_2 remains < 70 mmHg on 40% oxygen).

15. How does ventilatory therapy help to relieve hypoxemia in patients with pulmonary edema unresponsive to oxygen supplementation?
Ventilatory therapy, such as positive end-expiratory pressure (PEEP) or continuous positive airway pressure (CPAP), increases pulmonary compliance and improves regional ventilation changes associated with pulmonary edema. PEEP increases the functional residual capacity and prevents alveolar collapse at end expiration, decreasing the work of breathing and ventilating areas of the lung that otherwise may be atelectic.

16. List four pharmacologic agents that may be used to decrease venous return in the treatment of high-pressure edema. Give their mechanisms of action.
1. **Furosemide:** loop diuretic that also acts as a systemic venodilator when given in large doses.
2. **Nitroglycerin**: venodilator that increases systemic venous capacitance and decreases venous return.
3. **Captopril:** angiotensin-converting enzyme (ACE) inhibitor.
4. **Nitroprusside:** balanced vasodilator that causes both systemic venous and arterial dilation, decreases cardiac preload by decreasing venous return, and decreases afterload.

17. Discuss the treatment of patients with permeability edema.
1. Controlling the primary disease is the major objective.
2. Oxygen and ventilatory therapy may be helpful, nonspecific therapeutic measures.
3. The goal should be to maintain the minimal pulmonary intravascular pressure compatible with adequate cardiac output. Because pulmonary transvascular fluid movements are highly sensitive to changes in pulmonary intravascular pressure when vascular permeability is increased, maintaining a relatively low pulmonary intravascular pressure helps to decrease edema formation.

18. What is reexpansion pulmonary edema?
Reexpansion pulmonary edema results when protein-rich fluid leaks into the alveoli or re-expanded lungs and has been reported in association with pneumothorax, pleural effusion, and bronchial obstruction in humans and after surgical repair of diaphragmatic hernias in cats. Increased capillary permeability in reexpansion pulmonary edema may be due to decreased

surfactant concentrations, negative interstitial pressures, or formation of oxygen-derived free radicals in association with chronic hypoxia.

19. How can upper airway obstruction lead to development of pulmonary edema?
Pulmonary edema secondary to upper airway obstruction is thought to be neurogenic in origin. Severe inspiratory efforts during an acute episode of airway obstruction produce marked negative intrathoracic pressure, which results in decreased interstitial hydrostatic pressure. Net flow of fluid into the interstitium exceeds the capacity of lymphatic removal.

20. Which respiratory diseases have been associated with development of pulmonary edema secondary to upper airway obstruction?
- Laryngeal paralysis
- Laryngeal edema
- Laryngeal polyp
- Pharyngeal fibrosarcoma
- Choking (due to choke-chain injuries or pharyngeal foreign bodies)

21. Describe the radiographic changes associated with pulmonary edema due to left heart failure, altered permeability, and overhydration.
In **cardiogenic edema due to left heart failure**, interstitial edema progresses to alveolar edema as evidenced by airbronchograms. The distribution is primarily perihilar; the lung periphery is normal. Distribution of edema is usually symmetrical. Pulmonary venous distention is evident. Changes consistent with left heart failure, such as enlargement of the heart, particularly the left atrium, and elevation of the trachea, also may be seen.

Permeability edema also may be interstitial or alveolar, but the distribution is highly irregular and patchy.

Pulmonary edema due to overhydration is usually associated with perihilar interstitial changes, which may progress to alveolar patterns with severe overhydration. The pulmonary vasculature is typically prominent.

BIBLIOGRAPHY

1. Boysen PG, Modell JH: Pulmonary edema. In Shoemaker WC, Ayres S, Grenvik A, et al (eds): Textbook of Critical Care. Philadelphia, W.B. Saunders, 1989, pp 515–518.
2. Cope D, Grimbert F, Downey J, et al: Pulmonary capillary pressure: A review. Crit Care Med 20:1043–1056, 1992.
3. Demling RH, LaLonde C, Ikegami K: Pulmonary edema: Pathophysiology, methods of measurement and clinical importance in acute respiratory failure. New Horizons 1:371–380, 1993.
4. Ilne E, Pistoleau M, Miniati M, et al: The radiologic distribution of cardiogenic and noncardiogenic edema. AJR 144:1–6, 1985.
5. Jackson RM: Veal CF, Alexander CB, et al: Re-expansion pulmonary edema. Am Rev Resp Dis 137:1165–1171, 1988.
6. Kerr LY: Pulmonary edema secondary to upper airway obstruction in the dog: A review of nine cases. J Am Animal Hosp Assoc 25:207–212, 1989.
7. Milne R, Pistolesi M, Miniati M: The radiologic distinction of cardiogenic and noncardiogenic edema. AJR 144:879–894, 1985.
8. Oliver NB: Primary edema. Vet Clin North Am (Small Animal Pract) 15:1011–1103, 1985.
9. Stampley AR, Waldron DR: Re-expansion pulmonary edema after surgery to repair a diaphragmatic hernia in a cat. J Am Vet Med Assoc 203:1699–1701, 1993.
10. Staub NC: Pulmonary edema. Physiol Rev 54:678–811, 1979.
11. Suter PF: Thoracic Radiography. Davis, CA, Stonegate Press, 1984.
12. Van Pelt DR, Wingfield WE, Martin LG, Hackett TB: Application of airway pressure therapy to veterinary critical care. Part I: Respiratory mechanics and hypoxemia. J Vet Emerg Crit Care 3(2):63–70, 1993.
13. Van Pelt DR, Wingfield WE, Martin LG, Hackett TB: Application of airway pressure therapy to veterinary critical care. Part II: Airway pressure therapy. J Vet Emerg Crit Care 3(2):71–81, 1993.

48. HEMOPTYSIS

Kelly J. Diehl, D.V.M., M.S.

1. What is hemoptysis?

Hemoptysis is the expectoration of blood from the lower airways.

2. What is the significance of hemoptysis in small animals?

Hemoptysis is uncommon in small animals and suggests lower airway hemorrhage or coagulopathy. True hemoptysis should be considered a significant finding in animals and pursued aggressively.

3. What is the differential diagnosis for hemoptysis?

- Rodenticides
- Dirofilariasis
- Pulmonary edema (severe cases)
- Pulmonary thromboembolism
- Pulmonary contusions or trauma
- Coagulopathies
- Lung tumors (usually primary)
- Iatrogenic secondary to diagnostic procedures
- Cavitary pulmonary lesions
- Infectious agents or pneumonia
- Parasites
- Foreign bodies

4. What other pathologic conditions may mimic hemoptysis?

True hemoptysis suggests hemorrhage originating in the lower respiratory tract. It must be distinguished from hematemesis and oral cavity or upper airway bleeding. A thorough history and physical examination are essential to differentiate true hemoptysis from other conditions.

5. What diagnostic procedures should be performed in patients with hemoptysis?

Unless an iatrogenic cause of hemoptysis is suspected, a minimal database of complete blood count and platelet count, biochemical profile, heartworm test, fecal examination for parasites, urinalysis, and chest radiograph should be obtained. If a coagulopathy is highly suspected based on historical and physical findings, platelet count, prothrombin time, partial thromboplastin time, and mucosal bleeding time should be measured. Further diagnostic tests, such as echocardiography, transtracheal washes, transthoracic pulmonary aspiration, and bronchoscopy, may be indicated if other routine tests are not suggestive of a particular problem.

6. How should patients presenting with hemoptysis and respiratory difficulty be treated?

Patients are handled in the same manner as any acutely dyspneic patient. Initial stabilization is achieved with oxygen therapy and cage rest. Intubation, suction, and ventilatory support should be reserved for the most compromised patients. If possible, a thoracic radiograph and assessment of blood clotting ability should be attempted. Drug therapy should be aimed at the underlying problem.

BIBLIOGRAPHY

1. Hanley ME: Hemoptysis. In Critical Care Secrets. Philadelphia, Hanley & Belfus, 1992, pp 107–112.
2. Mahony OM, Cotter SM: Bleeding disorders: Epistaxis and hemoptysis. In Textbook of Veterinary Internal Medicine. Philadelphia, W.B. Saunders, 1995, pp 203–204.

49. SMOKE INHALATION AND BURN INJURIES

Linda G. Martin, D.V.M., M.S.

1. What is the leading cause of death in fires?

Smoke inhalation—not burn injuries.

2. Why is smoke inhalation lethal?

Carbon dioxide and carbon monoxide, the major components of smoke, are responsible for a drop in the concentration of ambient oxygen from 21% to 5–10%. Carbon monoxide also preferentially binds with hemoglobin in place of oxygen, thus decreasing oxygen delivery. Carbon monoxide and, more rarely, hydrogen cyanide block the uptake and utilization of oxygen, leading to severe tissue and cellular hypoxemia.

3. What are the primary mechanisms of direct tissue injury to the respiratory tract caused by smoke inhalation?

Thermal injury and chemical irritation.

4. Which portion of the respiratory tract is primarily injured as a result of inhaling hot gas and smoke?

Thermal injury is usually limited to the upper airway (above the vocal cords) and trachea.

5. What levels of the respiratory tract can be damaged by smoke inhalation?

Upper airway, lower airway, and alveoli.

6. The anatomic level(s) at which smoke inhalation causes damage to the respiratory system depend on what factors?

- Ventilatory pattern
- Smoke constituents (particular concentration, particulate size, chemical components)
- Anatomic distribution of particulate deposition

7. What mechanisms limit thermal injury of the lower airway?

The nasopharynx and oropharynx together provide a highly effective mechanism for cooling inspired air because of their relatively large surface area and associated air turbulence as well as their mucosal water lining, which acts as a heat reservoir. Sudden exposure to hot air also may trigger reflex closure of the vocal cords, reducing the potential for lower airway injury.

8. What are common thermal injuries to the airway?

Common thermal injuries include mucosal and submucosal edema, erythema, hemorrhage, and ulceration of the upper airway structures, generally above the vocal cords, but the trachea also may be affected.

9. How does smoke inhalation cause pulmonary injury by direct chemical irritation?

Smoke particles may interfere with normal physiologic mechanisms, such as inhibition of mucociliary clearance and surfactant inactivation. In addition, activation and recruitment of circulating leukocytes, stimulation of intrapulmonary macrophages, and release of chemotactic factors, oxygen radicals, and tissue proteases cause changes in vascular permeability. The results are pulmonary injury and edema.

10. How common is alveolar injury after smoke inhalation?

Alveolar injury occurs in a small percentage of cases, and clinical signs usually appear hours to days after smoke inhalation. The injury resembles increased permeability pulmonary edema or acute respiratory distress syndrome (ARDS). Alveolar injury is more likely to be seen after inhalation of smoke generated from plastics and poorly water-soluble gases, after combined inhalation and burn injury, and after onset of sepsis or systemic inflammatory response syndrome (SIRS).

11. How is the inhalation of superheated steam different from most other thermal injuries caused by smoke inhalation?

Superheated steam inhalation may cause severe injury to the lower airways and alveoli because energy is released in the respiratory tract as the steam condenses to water.

12. What mechanisms may lead to both small and large airway obstruction secondary to smoke inhalation?

- Airway edema
- Sloughing of necrotic epithelial mucosa
- Impairment of mucociliary clearance of secretions
- Bronchoconstriction due to release of inflammatory mediators such as thromboxane A_2

13. Victims of smoke inhalation are commonly hypoxemic. Name the mechanisms that result in hypoxemia.

- Decreased FiO_2 (decrease in ambient oxygen concentration due to production of carbon dioxide and carbon monoxide)
- Hypoventilation (pain, decreased elastic compliance associated with burns to the thorax, or CNS depression due to carbon monoxide or cyanide poisoning)
- Shunt (atelectasis due to surfactant inactivation, airway obstruction due to edema and sloughing mucosa, or impaired clearance of secretions)
- Ventilation/perfusion mismatch (release of inflammatory mediators and cytokines that alter pulmonary blood flow)
- Diffusion impairment (increased permeability pulmonary edema)

14. How does carbon monoxide affect the oxyhemoglobin dissociation curve?

Carbon monoxide shifts the curve to the left, thereby impairing oxygen unloading at the tissue level.

15. What are common complications after smoke inhalation and burn injuries?

Pneumonia, ARDS, and sepsis or SIRS.

16. What information is important in asking about the fire?

In obtaining a history, emphasis should be placed on data specific to the smoke exposure. Exposure in a closed space, such as a building, indicates that smoke was less diluted by ambient air, resulting in greater pulmonary exposure to carbon monoxide and smoke constituents than open-space exposure. The duration of exposure is also helpful, because it correlates with the severity of lung injury. Information about the probable fuel types burned at the scene may alert the clinician to the possibility of parenchymal lung injury and systemic side effects.

17. Should thoracic radiographs be done for all patients with a history of smoke inhalation?

No. Thoracic radiographs are notoriously insensitive in detecting severely injured lungs early after smoke exposure. False-negative results as high as 92% have been reported in human studies. Radiographic abnormalities are delayed and may be confused with pneumonia, pulmonary edema, or ARDS rather than the inhalation injury. Therefore, thoracic radiographs are generally not indicated in asymptomatic patients and only as a baseline in symptomatic patients.

18. If pulse oximetry is normal, does arterial blood gas analysis yield additional information?

Yes. Pulse oximetry cannot differentiate oxygenated hemoglobin (oxyhemoglobin) from carboxyhemoglobin. Therefore, it consistently overestimates the true oxyhemoglobin saturation. In addition, pulse oximetry gives no information about ventilatory status or acid–base balance.

19. If blood cyanide levels cannot be measured, what is the best alternative diagnostic test?

Plasma lactate concentrations correlate well with cyanide levels because of anaerobic metabolism and lactic acidosis.

20. What are indications for active airway management?

Evidence of progressive airway obstruction demands immediate action. Edema may develop acutely in the upper airway and lead to airway obstruction within 12–24 hours, if not sooner. Early airway management under controlled conditions is preferable to potentially hazardous circumstances that may develop later (unwitnessed airway obstruction and increasingly difficult intubation due to progressive edema).

21. Which routes of intubation are appropriate?

Orotracheal intubation allows direct visualization of the oropharynx and larynx as well as atraumatic placement of the endotracheal tube. Emergency tracheostomy is indicated if edema is severe enough to prevent the passage of the endotracheal tube.

22. How should victims of smoke inhalation be managed?

All victims should be placed on 100% oxygen as soon as possible, even if they are asymptomatic, to accelerate wash-out of carbon monoxide. The concentration of carboxyhemoglobin is reduced by approximately 50% every 30 minutes if 100% oxygen is breathed. Endotracheal intubation should be performed for patients in respiratory distress.

23. How is the need for mechanical ventilation in addition to supplemental oxygen assessed?

By repeated arterial blood gas analysis. Refractory hypoxemia in patients on supplemental oxygen and hypoventilation that results in respiratory acidosis with a pH < 7.25 are evidence of serious parenchymal lung injury and ventilatory failure, which indicate the need for intubation and ventilation with high inspired oxygen fractions or positive-end-expiratory pressure (PEEP).

24. Why is PEEP particularly helpful to patients with smoke inhalation?

Because of the frequent presence of atelectasis after exposure to smoke, PEEP is often necessary to maintain small airway patency.

25. How should fluids be administered to patients with smoke inhalation?

A combination of isotonic crystalloid and colloid solutions may be used during the resuscitation phase at a rate needed to restore and maintain adequate perfusion based on standard monitoring parameters. Biologic or synthetic colloids should be used if hypoproteinemia is present. Patients with smoke inhalation and dermal burns usually have considerable losses of fluid and protein from the skin surface and therefore may have high fluid requirements. Underhydration in an attempt to keep the lungs "dry" is known to increase cardiopulmonary instability and morbidity.

26. Do prophylactic antibiotics have a role in patients with smoke inhalation?

Prophylactic antibiotics are not indicated in the acute treatment of inhalation injury. Their use has not been shown to protect against development of pulmonary infection. However, specific antibiotics are indicated in treating subsequent bacterial pneumonias. Antibiotic choice ideally should be based on culture and sensitivity results.

27. Are corticosteroids indicated in smoke inhalation?

Acute administration of corticosteroids after smoke inhalation is not recommended as a means of protecting against airway obstruction due to edema. Although their antiinflammatory effects may reduce the peak edema response, corticosteroids require hours to take effect and do not guarantee airway patency. After isolated inhalation injury in humans, corticosteroids have been shown to be of no benefit, and in cases of combined inhalation and burn injuries their use is associated with increased mortality and infection rates. Corticosteroids may be of use in patients who depend on exogenous steroids for preexisting medical illness or patients who present with severe bronchospasm unresponsive to bronchodilators.

BIBLIOGRAPHY

1. Baxter CR: Burns. In Parrillo JE, Bone RC (eds): Critical Care Medicine: Principles of Diagnosis and Management. St. Louis, Mosby, 1995, pp 849–865.
2. Baxter C, Waeckerle J: Emergency treatment of burn injury. Ann Emerg Med 17:1305–1315, 1989.
3. Blinn DL, Slater H, Goldfarb W: Inhalation injury with burns: A lethal combination. J Emerg Med 6:471–473, 1988.
4. Brazeal BA, Honeycutt D, Traber LD, et al: Pentafraction for superior resuscitation of the ovine thermal burn. Crit Care Med 23:332–339, 1995.
5. Demling RH: Management of the burn patient. In Shoemaker WC, Ayres SM, Grenvick A, Holbrook PR (eds): Textbook of Critical Care. Philadelphia, W.B. Saunders, 1995, pp 1498–1506.
6. Demling RH: Smoke inhalation injury. In Shoemaker WC, Ayres SM, Grenvick A, Holbrook PR (eds): Textbook of Critical Care. Philadelphia, W.B. Saunders, 1995, pp 1506–1516.
7. Demling R, Picard L, Campbell C, et al: Relationship of burn-induced lung lipid peroxidation and the degree of injury after smoke inhalation and a body burn. Crit Care Med 21:1935–1943, 1993.
8. Gunn ML, Hansbrough JF, Davis JW: Prospective randomized trial of hypertonic sodium lactate versus lactated Ringer's solution for burn shock resuscitation. J Trauma 29:1261–1267, 1989.
9. Lalonde C, Knox J, Youn YK, et al: Burn edema is accentuated by a moderate smoke inhalation injury in sheep. Surgery 112:908–917, 1992.
10. Lalonde C, Knox J, Youn YK, et al: Relationship between hepatic blood flow and tissue lipid peroxidation in the early postburn period. Crit Care Med 20:789–796, 1992.
11. Nieman GF, Clark WR, Paskanik A, et al: Segmental pulmonary vascular resistance following wood smoke inhalation. Crit Care Med 23:1264–1271, 1995.
12. Sharar SR, Hudson LD: Toxic gas, fume and smoke inhalation. In Parrillo JE, Bone RC (eds): Critical Care Medicine: Principles of Diagnosis and Management. St. Louis, Mosby, 1995, pp 849–865.

VI. Cardiovascular Emergencies

Section Editor: Steven L. Marks, B.V.Sc., M.S., M.R.C.V.S.

50. MITRAL VALVULAR INSUFFICIENCY DUE TO ENDOCARDIOSIS

Steven L. Marks, B.V.Sc., M.S., M.R.C.V.S

1. What is the basic pathophysiology of mitral valve disease and left-sided congestive heart failure?

The basic pathophysiology of mitral valve disease is multifactorial and complex. Endocardiosis or myxomatous change in the valve causes inappropriate apposition of the valve leaflets, which leads to a regurgitant volume of blood into the left atrium. The result is a decrease in left ventricular forward cardiac output and an increase in left atrial pressure. In response to reduced cardiac support and organ perfusion, the renin-angiotensin-aldosterone pathway and sympathetic nervous system are activated. Although initially compensatory, these mechanisms eventually lead to decompensation. Structural changes in the heart, such as hypertrophy or dilation, occur. When left atrial pressures peak, pulmonary edema forms, and congestive heart failure is present.

2. Describe the sound and location of the murmur associated with mitral valve disease.

The typical murmur associated with mitral valve disease is a midsystolic regurgitant murmur early in the disease; it may progress to a holosystolic or pansystolic murmur with increased intensity. The location of the murmur on auscultation or point of maximal intensity is at the left apex between intercostal space 3–5 on the left hemithorax. The murmur may radiate to the right hemithorax.

3. How are murmurs graded?

Murmurs are graded from I–VI:

Grade I	Murmur barely audible
Grade II	Murmur softer than S_1 (first heart sound)
Grade III	Murmur equal to S_1
Grade IV	Murmur louder than S_1
Grade V	Murmur with palpable thrill
Grade VI	Murmur with palpable thrill can be heard with stethoscope off chest

4. What is the incidence of mitral valve disease?

Mitral valve insufficiency is the most common cardiovascular disease in dogs. The prevalence increases with age and is reported as high as 75% in dogs 16 years of age. All breeds may be affected, but small and toy breeds are affected more commonly. Males appear to be more commonly affected than females. The King Charles spaniel is predisposed to mitral valve disease.

5. What is the clinical significance of mitral valve disease?

Mitral valve disease may be a common finding in older, small-breed dogs. During physical examination a mitral murmur is often an incidental finding. Because mitral valve disease is a progressive disorder and may lead to congestive heart failure, it should be carefully monitored. The incidence of mitral valve insufficiency in cats without primary myocardial disease is low, and the significance is unknown.

6. What are the clinical signs of mitral valve disease?

The clinical signs of mitral valve disease are related to the severity of lesions. Many animals with early lesions are asymptomatic. Weakness, exercise intolerance, or syncope may be seen with decreased left ventricular forward flow. Coughing may be seen with left atrial enlargement, causing bronchial compression, and dyspnea or tachypnea may be seen with increased left atrial pressures, leading to congestive failure and pulmonary edema. The most common clinical sign in dogs is a nonproductive cough, which is generally worse at night or with exercise. Animals with late-stage disease may present in fulminant congestive heart failure and display all of the above clinical signs as well as cyanosis.

7. What diagnostic tests should be done to evaluate mitral valve disease?

The diagnostic evaluation of mitral valve disease is similar to that of any cardiopulmonary disease. A thorough physical examination and cardiac auscultation should be performed as well as thoracic radiographs and electrocardiography. Echocardiography should be considered if further documentation is required. Because of the therapeutic options available, the minimal database also should include blood urea nitrogen, creatinine, electrolytes, and urinalysis.

8. What electrocardiographic (EKG) changes are commonly seen with mitral valve disease?

The most common EKG abnormality in dogs with mitral valve disease is a widened P-wave or P-mitrale, suggestive of left atrial enlargement. If animals have significant atrial enlargement, premature supraventricular contractions also may be seen as well as supraventricular tachycardia and atrial fibrillation. Sinus tachycardia may be seen in both compensated and decompensated left-sided congestive heart failure. If myocardial hypoxia or myocardial disease is present, ventricular premature contractions may be seen and progress to ventricular tachycardia. Changes in the left ventricle may be seen as tall or wide QRS complexes.

9. What radiographic changes are seen with mitral valve disease?

Thoracic radiographs often provide valuable information for the clinician. The major goal of thoracic radiography is to identify anatomic changes in pulmonary vasculature, left atrium, left ventricle, and mainstem bronchi. It is also valuable to assess for the presence of pulmonary edema. Left atrial enlargement, which is the earliest and most common radiographic finding with mitral regurgitation, leads to loss of the caudal waist of the cardiac silhouette and elevation of the airway on lateral thoracic radiographs. On the dorsoventral projection, the enlarged left atrium can be seen overlying the cardiac silhouette and caudal to the tracheal carina. Pulmonary veins enlarge before pulmonary edema forms. Early pulmonary edema may appear as a peribronchial pattern before progressing to an alveolar pattern. In dogs, pulmonary edema first appears in the perihilar region. In cats, pulmonary edema starts in the periphery and has a patchy distribution.

10. Is coughing due to respiratory disease or heart disease?

This distinction can be one of the most challenging tasks facing the veterinary clinician.

11. A small-breed, coughing dog with a systolic murmur is presented for examination. How can respiratory disease be differentiated from cardiac disease?

Clinical signs discovered on physical examination are often helpful, but some overlap is common. A cough of cardiac origin is most often nonproductive, whereas the cough of respiratory origin may be productive or nonproductive. As a sweeping overgeneralization, dogs with respiratory disease usually do not have higher than normal heart rates. Dogs with heart disease may have normal to higher than normal heart rates. Thoracic radiographs may help to differentiate pulmonary disease and airway disease from heart disease. If the pulmonary pattern is equivocal, a trial of diuretic therapy may help to distinguish early pulmonary edema from airway disease. Electrocardiographic and echocardiographic studies also may be beneficial. Sinus arrhythmia, wandering pacemaker, and bradycardia—all of which are signs of increased vagal tone—suggest respiratory disease. Electrocardiographic findings such as P-mitrale, wide or tall QRS complex morphology, and arrhythmias suggest cardiac disease.

12. What therapy is provided for mitral valve disease?
Therapy for mitral valve disease is based on the stage of disease. For asymptomatic animals in early stages of disease, no therapy may be required. If any signs of heart failure are present, therapy with a diuretic, angiotensin-converting enzyme (ACE) inhibitor, and low sodium diet is suggested. The use of digoxin at this stage is at the discretion of the clinician. If advanced progressive heart failure is present, digoxin is added to the above therapy. If the animal does not improve, other vasodilators, such as hydralazine, should be considered.

13. What therapy is suggested for life-threatening heart failure?
- Oxygen therapy
- Intravenous furosemide
- Topical nitroglycerin
- Hydralazine or nitroprusside
- Dobutamine infusion
- Morphine
- Theophylline
- Antiarrhythmic therapy

CONTROVERSIES

14. Should asymptomatic animals be treated?
Although some evidence in experimental models of heart failure suggests that vasodilator therapy delays progression of disease in animals with acquired mitral valve disease, no consistent evidence indicates that this finding can be extrapolated to asymptomatic cases. Some cardiologists believe that if significant cardiomegaly is present, ACE inhibitors should be used. In considering this therapy in asymptomatic animals, cost may be the limiting factor.

15. Is diuretic monotherapy a viable treatment option?
A diuretic agent has historically been the drug of choice for congestive heart failure for many clinicians. Specifically, furosemide has commonly been used as a single agent. Understanding the pathophysiology of congestive heart failure argues against the use of diuretics as monotherapy. Overzealous use of diuretics may lead to decreased venous return, decreased cardiac output, and initiation of compensatory mechanisms that may lead to decompensation. People with congestive heart failure who are treated with diuretic monotherapy deteriorate more rapidly than people using combination therapy with digoxin and ACE inhibitors.

BIBLIOGRAPHY

1. Braunwald E: Pathophysiology of heart failure. In Braunwald E (ed): Heart Disease: A Textbook of Cardiovascular Medicine, 4th ed. Philadelphia, W.B. Saunders, 1992, pp 1007–1077.
2. Ettinger SJ, Bintz AM, Ericsson GF: Relationships of enalapril with other CHF treatment modalities. Proceedings of the Twelfth ACVIM Forum, San Francisco, 1994.
3. Ettinger SJ, Lusk R, Brayley K, et al: Evaluation of enalapril in dogs with heart failure in a large multi-center Cooperative Veterinary Enalapril (COVE) study group. Proceedings of the Tenth Annual ACVIM Forum, San Diego, 1992.
4. Keene BW: Chronic valvular disease in the dog. In Fox PR (ed): Canine and Feline Cardiology. New York, Churchill Livingstone, 1988, pp 409–418.
5. Keene BW, Bonagura JD: Therapy of heart failure. In Bonagura JD (ed): Kirk's Current Veterinary Therapy XII (Small Animal Practice). Philadelphia, W.B. Saunders, 1995, pp 780–786.
6. Kittleson MD: Left ventricular failure. Part I. Comp Cont Educ Pract Vet 16:287–306, 1994.
7. Kittleson MD: Left ventricular failure. Part II. Comp Cont Educ Pract Vet 16:1001–1017, 1994.
8. Sisson DD: The Invasive Multicenter Prospective Randomized Veterinary Enalapril (IMPROVE) Study Group: Hemodynamic, echocardiographic, radiographic, and clinical effects of enalapril in dogs with chronic heart failure. Proceedings of the Tenth ACVIM Forum, San Diego, 1992.

51. DILATED CARDIOMYOPATHY

Jonathan A. Abbott, D.V.M.

1. What is dilated cardiomyopathy?

Cardiomyopathy is a myocardial disease that is unrelated to coronary vessel disease, pericardial disease, valvular disease, or congenital anomalies of cardiac structure. Specifically, dilated cardiomyopathy (DCM) is a disorder of impaired systolic myocardial function that is unrelated to systemic disease or mechanical overloads imposed on the heart. DCM is a morphopathologic and functional designation; it is characterized by ventricular and atrial dilation as a consequence of systolic myocardial dysfunction. Most often, left ventricular or biventricular dilation is present. In occasional cases, the right ventricle is affected primarily.

2. What is the pathophysiology of DCM?

When stroke volume declines as a result of systolic myocardial dysfunction (decreased contractility), the end-systolic ventricular volume is increased. This residual volume augments pulmonary venous return and results in ventricular dilation and elevated end-diastolic wall stress. In addition, the renin-angiotensin-aldosterone system (RAAS) is activated by diminished cardiac output. One effect of RAAS activation is the retention of salt and water, which serves to expand the intravascular volume. Expansion of intravascular volume further increases preload and contributes to progressive ventricular dilation. Elevated ventricular filling pressures, along with atrioventricular (AV) valve incompetence due to dilation of the valve anulus, causes atrial dilation.

Loss of systolic myocardial function causes ventricular hypokinesis and initiates a series of events that leads to progressive ventricular dilation. Systolic myocardial dysfunction may result from loss of cardiomyocytes due to necrosis or from functional disorders that affect the contractile apparatus. However, the hemodynamic consequences of impaired systolic myocardial function are generally the same, regardless of the cause.

3. Suggest causes of dilated cardiomyopathy.

DCM is a syndrome rather than a specific disease; in a sense, it is an end-stage heart and likely represents the common expression of virtually any pathologic insult to the myocardium. This insult may take the form of a viral infection, toxin, metabolic derangement, or nutritional deficiency. For example, taurine deficiency has been associated with DCM in cats; supplementation of commercial foods with taurine has radically reduced the prevalence of DCM in cats. In some dogs, myocardial carnitine deficiency likely has a role in the pathogenesis of DCM. In addition, antineoplastic agents such as doxorubicin may result in irreversible myocardial dysfunction. Spontaneous DCM in dogs is generally idiopathic.

4. Suggest a typical signalment for a patient with dilated cardiomyopathy.

Large- and giant-breed dogs, including Doberman pinschers, Labrador retrievers, Great Danes, and boxer dogs are most commonly affected. Males are more commonly affected than females, and dogs with DCM are often middle-aged or older. A 4-year-old male Doberman pinscher is a typical signalment for DCM.

5. Are there differences in presentation among the breeds commonly afflicted?

In general, the course of DCM is similar in all dogs. However, two breeds develop myocardial disease that is sufficiently distinctive in its presentation to warrant mention. DCM of boxer dogs is characterized by a high incidence of ventricular tachyarrhythmias and sudden death. Harpster classified the manner of presentation of boxer dogs with DCM as follows:

Category 1: Ventricular arrhythmias with no associated clinical signs
Category 2: Syncope presumably related to ventricular tachyarrhythmia
Category 3: Congestive heart failure (CHF) due to systolic myocardial dysfunction

There are similarities between the DCM of boxer dogs and Doberman pinschers. The incidence of ventricular tachyarrhythmia in affected Dobermans is high, as is the incidence of sudden cardiac death. CHF in Doberman pinschers with DCM is often associated with a short and rapidly progressive course. Giant-breed dogs with DCM are more likely to have signs of biventricular congestive failure, and the disease is often complicated by atrial fibrillation. However, in the author's experience, Doberman pinschers with DCM commonly develop atrial fibrillation in addition to ventricular tachyarrhythmia. Furthermore, all patients with DCM should be considered at risk for sudden cardiac death.

6. What prompts the owner of a dog with DCM to seek veterinary attention?

Patients with DCM are usually presented for evaluation of clinical signs related to CHF. In the emergency setting, the history may reveal respiratory distress, cough, abdominal distention due to ascites, and syncope. In addition, the owner may observe exercise intolerance, weight loss, depression, and inappetance.

7. The physical findings in DCM often suggest the diagnosis. What may be expected on auscultation of the heart?

Because patients with DCM often present with CHF, tachycardia is common, and arrhythmia may be evident on auscultation. Often, but not invariably, a murmur of functional AV valve incompetence results from dilation of the AV valve anulus. This murmur is due to mitral valve regurgitation and is heard best over the left cardiac apex. The murmur is plateau-shaped, occurs during systole, and is usually soft.

In some affected dogs, audibility of the third heart sound results in a gallop rhythm. Rapid deceleration of early diastolic transmitral flow is the hemodynamic association of an S_3 gallop. Thus, the gallop rhythm results from accentuation of a physiologic event. The rapid deceleration of early diastolic flow is probably related to the presence of a large end-systolic volume and reduced ventricular compliance. In the presence of an audible third heart sound, pulmonary crackles suggest the presence of pulmonary edema.

8. What is the most specific abnormality detected on physical examination?

In small animals, audibility of the third heart sound is usually a specific indicator of myocardial dysfunction. The presence of a gallop rhythm in a dog or cat is an indication for detailed cardiovascular evaluation, even in the absence of clinical signs. Care must be taken to differentiate a gallop from other transient sounds, such as splitting of the first or second heart sound and clicks (which usually occur during mid systole), and from arrhythmias.

9. What abnormalities are detected on electrocardiographic examination?

The electrocardiogram (EKG) provides information about heart rate, rhythm, and size. Elucidation of disturbances of cardiac rhythm is the primary use of EKG. In DCM, the EKG may reveal premature ventricular complexes, ventricular tachycardia, atrial premature complexes, atrial or junctional tachycardia, or atrial fibrillation. Sometimes there is evidence of ventricular hypertrophy, intraventricular conduction disturbances, such as left bundle-branch block, or left atrial enlargement. Broadening of the P-wave beyond 40 msec suggests left atrial enlargement. Concurrent P-wave notching may increase the specificity of P-wave broadening as a marker of left atrial enlargement.

10. Describe the expected radiographic findings in DCM.

Usually the cardiac silhouette is enlarged, with radiographic evidence of left atrial enlargement. When the left atrium is enlarged, pulmonary infiltrates indicate the presence of pulmonary edema and CHF. Initially, pulmonary edema results in an interstitial pulmonary infiltrate. With the accumulation of greater amounts of lung liquid, the small airways are flooded and an alveolar pulmonary infiltrate is observed. Often cardiogenic pulmonary edema has a symmetrical and central distribution. However, pulmonary edema of acute onset may have a patchy or generalized distribution. The ability of plain chest radiographs to resolve specific cardiac chambers is limited, and the radiographic appearance of DCM is variable. Some Doberman pinschers, for example, have minimal radiographic evidence of cardiac enlargement, showing only loss of the caudal cardiac waist, indicating left atrial enlargement, and alveolar pulmonary infiltrates of edema.

11. When is echocardiography indicated?

Echocardiography provides a noninvasive assessment of cardiac chamber dimensions and myocardial function. It is the means by which to obtain a definitive noninvasive diagnosis of DCM and should be considered in all patients suspected of myocardial disease. Echocardiography is indicated when the cause of dyspnea remains unclear after radiographic examination. In some instances, echocardiography can be performed with the patient standing or in sternal recumbency with minimal restraint and, therefore, less stress to the patient. When available, echocardiography should be considered before radiography in dyspneic patients with physical findings that suggest DCM. Although echocardiography cannot provide a diagnosis of CHF, it can be used to determine whether the patient has structural cardiac abnormalities that may reasonably represent a substrate for development of CHF.

12. What echocardiographic findings typify dilated cardiomyopathy?

In DCM, echocardiography demonstrates atrial and ventricular dilation with hypokinesis. Usually, there is left ventricular or biventricular dilation; occasionally, the right ventricle is preferentially affected. Shortening fraction (SF), a measure of systolic myocardial function, is low, often in the range of 5–15%. Extracardiac disorders, such as sepsis, also may impair myocardial function and result in a decrease in SF. Despite what may be a rapid clinical course, the development of DCM is usually a gradual process. Therefore, diminished SF in the absence of ventricular and atrial dilation may be related to extracardiac disease or method of measurement; it is unlikely to explain signs of CHF. In DCM, the valves are structurally normal, although Doppler studies often demonstrate mitral and tricuspid valve regurgitation.

13. What are the goals in the management of acute CHF?

In CHF the intravascular volume is increased, and elevated ventricular filling pressures are reflected in venous congestion and the resultant accumulation of tissue fluid in the associated capillary bed. Pulmonary edema, the consequence of left ventricular failure, is immediately life-threatening. Right ventricular failure results in ascites and sometimes pleural effusion; it is generally better tolerated than pulmonary edema. The goals of acute CHF management are urgent restoration of normal pulmonary gas exchange and preservation or augmentation of tissue perfusion. These goals are accomplished largely through pharmacologic manipulation of three of the main determinants of cardiac output—preload, afterload, and contractility.

14. How is preload manipulated in acute CHF?

In fulminant pulmonary edema, a diuretic is administered intravenously. Loop diuretics are potent, act quickly, and may be effective in patients with renal dysfunction. Furosemide is used most commonly. In severe pulmonary edema, it may be administered at doses of 1–6 mg/kg; dosage intervals should be determined by clinical response. Furosemide affects the transport of electrolytes across the walls of the nephron and favors the production of large volumes of dilute urine. The resulting diuresis reduces intravascular volume and, therefore, ventricular filling pressures. When ventricular filling pressures are reduced, the lymphatic vessels can clear the accumulated tissue fluid.

Nitroglycerin (NG) may be administrated transdermally. Controlled dosing patches and a cream are commercially available. Nitrates cause vasodilation through a pathway that increases intracellular cyclic guanosine monophosphate (cGMP). The effect of nitroglycerin is most pronounced in the venous circulation and in specific arteriolar beds such as the epicardial coronary vasculature. Pulmonary venous dilation lowers ventricular filling pressures and therefore decreases venous congestion. The NG patch or cream may be applied to any hairless area of skin. Application to the inguinal area or trunk may result in more predictable absorption than application to the pinnae of the ear. In severe, fulminant edema phlebotomy may be used for rapid reduction of ventricular filling pressures.

Interventions that reduce preload are necessary and may resolve pulmonary edema rapidly. However, except in special circumstances, such measures do not have a salutary effect on cardiac output. When the ventricle is dilated, the reduction of preload has favorable clinical effects but little effect on stroke volume. Excessive diuresis, however, may reduce cardiac output and tissue perfusion.

15. How is afterload manipulated in acute CHF?

CHF due to systolic myocardial dysfunction is associated with a mismatch of afterload and contractility. It is useful to consider the relationship among perfusion pressure, vascular resistance, and cardiac output. By analogy to Ohm's law, $BP = SVR \times Q$, where Q = cardiac output, BP = blood pressure, and SVR = systemic vascular resistance. Peripheral vascular resistance is an important determinant of afterload, and pharmacologic dilation of arterioles may have a beneficial effect in patients with CHF. In CHF due to DCM, judicious vasodilation reduces afterload and thus increases stroke volume with minimal effects on perfusion pressure.

Nitroprusside is a balanced vasodilator that has a pronounced effect on the systemic arterioles. Metabolism of nitroprusside is rapid and results in the release of cyanide and nitric oxide. The nitrate metabolite possesses vasodilatory properties. Nitroprusside is infused intravenously at doses of 1–10 μg/kg/min. It is a potent vasodilator and should be used only in carefully controlled circumstances. Measurement of systemic blood pressure is recommended, and the dose should be titrated based on serial blood pressure measurements and indices of peripheral perfusion. Because cyanide toxicosis is a potential adverse side effect, the use of nitroprusside should be limited to less than 48 hours.

16. Is inotropic support indicated?

In DCM impaired systolic myocardial function is the primary pathophysiologic basis for CHF. Pharmacologic inotropic support is indicated in patients with low cardiac output and congestive signs.

17. Compare and contrast the available positive inotropes.

Essentially all of the positive inotropes act by increasing the availability of calcium within the sarcomere. The available positive inotropes fall in one of three pharmacologic categories: (1) digitalis glycosides (digoxin, digitoxin); (2) phosphodiesterase inhibitors (the bipyridine derivatives, amrinone and milrinone); and (3) cathecholamines or synthetic analogs (dopamine, dobutamine, epinephrine).

Digoxin can be administered intravenously or orally. The cardiac glycosides bind to and inhibit the sodium-potassium pump of the cardiomyocyte. The resultant change in cellular tonicity leads to an increase in intracellular calcium concentration, which, in turn, increases the inotropic state. The digitalis glycosides also have autonomic effects that are likely favorable in patients with CHF as well as antiarrhythmic properties. However, the glycosides are relatively weak inotropes, and their therapeutic index is low. They are indicated in the chronic therapy of CHF but have a relatively limited role in the critical care setting.

Amrinone and milrinone are relatively potent positive inotropes that also exert a vasodilatory effect. Their action is mediated through inhibition of phosphodiesterase, an enzyme that catalyzes the breakdown of cyclic adenosine monophosphate (cAMP). Inhibition of phosphodiesterase results in an increase in cAMP, an intracellular second messenger that has many effects, including elevation of the intracellular calcium concentration. Clinical trials in people have not shown that inotropes, other than digitalis and possibly vesnarinone, have a beneficial effect when given chronically. Consequently, the phosphodiesterase inhibitors are not available for oral administration and must be administered by intravenous infusion. The increase in intracellular calcium concentration is potentially arrhythmogenic, and EKG monitoring is recommended during administration.

Dobutamine and other catecholamine derivatives or analogs stimulate adrenergic receptors. Adrenergic receptors are coupled by G-proteins to adenylate cyclase, an enzyme that catalyzes the release of cAMP. Increases in cAMP levels result in increased intracellular calcium concentration. Catecholamines must be administered by intravenous infusion. Dobutamine is a relatively selective agonist of beta-adrenergic receptors. In contrast, dopamine is a flexible molecule and can stimulate beta-adrenergic receptors, dopaminergic receptors, and alpha-adrenergic receptors. All catecholamine analogs lose receptor specificity at higher doses. Consequently, their use may increase peripheral vascular resistance to the patient's detriment. The administration of dobutamine results in greater increases in stroke volume relative to increase in heart rate; for this and other reasons, dobutamine is superior to dopamine. EKG monitoring is recommended during infusion of adrenergic agents.

18. Is supplemental oxygen administration indicated? If so, what routes of oxygen administration should be used?

Oxygen should be administered to dyspneic patients with CHF. An oxygen cage is probably the most convenient method, although the use of a nasal cannula is appropriate if tolerated by the patient. Mechanical ventilation using positive end-expiratory pressures may be considered in cases of severe, fulminant pulmonary edema. However, when the patient with DCM and CHF presents for the first time, the resolution of dyspnea and pulmonary edema is often surprisingly rapid even with conservative measures; thus the need for mechanical ventilation is obviated.

19. What agents are appropriate for the chronic management of DCM?

A regimen that includes digoxin, an ACE inhibitor, and furosemide has become accepted for the management of CHF due to DCM. ACE inhibitors, which include captopril, enalapril, and benazepril, inhibit the enzyme that catalyzes the conversion of angiotensin I to angiotensin II (AII). AII is a vasoconstrictor that has numerous other effects, including modulation of the adrenergic nervous system, stimulation of antidiuretic hormone and aldosterone release, and trophic effects on myocardium. The administration of enalapril to dogs with CHF due to DCM improves quality of life and has a favorable effect on mortality.

20. What is the role of digitalis in DCM?

Digitalis compounds have a positive inotropic effect and modulate the function of the adrenergic nervous system. They are unique in that they exert a positive inotropic effect yet lower heart rate and control the ventricular response rate in atrial fibrillation.

21. How is atrial fibrillation managed in the setting of DCM?

Experimentally, a critical mass of atrial myocardium is required to support the arrhythmia of atrial fibrillation (AF). Only a few breeds of dog are sufficiently large to develop AF in the absence of cardiac disease. In dogs, AF usually signifies the presence of marked and possibly irreversible atrial enlargement. Because the predisposing cause of AF generally cannot be corrected in DCM, attempts to effect conversion to sinus rhythm are seldom successful. Furthermore, the risk of thromboembolism, which often complicates AF in people, seems to be low in dogs. Therefore, conversion to sinus rhythm is not generally attempted. Therapy of AF in the setting of DCM is directed toward optimizing stroke volume and myocardial oxygen demand through slowing of the ventricular response rate.

22. What drugs are available for slowing ventricular response rate in AF due to DCM?

Digoxin is used initially to control heart rate in AF or other supraventricular tachycardias that complicate DCM. Digoxin has a relatively long elimination half-life and a narrow therapeutic index. For these reasons, the use of loading doses is not generally recommended. It may take 4–7 days to achieve therapeutic plasma levels when maintenance doses are administered. Other drugs can be considered when the urgent control of heart rate is indicated.

It is important to consider several factors before negatively chronotropic drugs are used in the critical care setting. Other than digitalis, all of the currently available drugs that slow the heart are negative inotropes. The rapid ventricular response to AF that can be observed in DCM is a compensatory mechanism; some patients with severe CHF are critically dependent on elevated heart rate and diminished contractile response to maintain cardiac output. Furthermore, unlike some pathologic tachycardias, the rate that the heart in AF adopts is at least partly subject to physiologic influence. Often control of congestive signs reduces anxiety, and a decrease in the ventricular rate in AF is likely to accompany the resolution of pulmonary edema. Rapid slowing of rapid ventricular rate in AF, therefore, must be undertaken only with caution.

Given these caveats, it is likely that irregular ventricular rhythms with rates greater than 240 beats/min are deleterious because they are associated with diminished stroke volume and high myocardial oxygen demand. The cautious use of calcium channel blockers or beta-adrenergic antagonists may be considered. Injectable or oral diltiazem is the author's first choice in this scenario. Diltiazem has a restraining effect on the AV node but a relatively weak negative inotropic effect. A beta-adrenergic antagonist such as esmolol may be considered, although the potent negative inotropic properties of beta blockers must be recognized. The optimal heart rate in AF with overt CHF is not known, although reducing the rate to 180–200 beats/min may be reasonable. The optimal ventricular response rate after congestive signs have been controlled is probably lower.

23. What are the roles of calcium channel antagonists, beta blockers, and digitalis in AF due to DCM?

Digoxin is used to control the ventricular response rate in AF associated with DCM. In some patients with DCM slowing of the heart rate does not occur despite control of congestive signs. The cautious use of diltiazem, a calcium channel blocker, or a beta-adrenergic antagonist such as atenolol or propranolol may be considered as adjunct therapy. Recent evidence suggests that the long-term use of beta-adrenergic antagonists in CHF related to systolic myocardial dysfunction may have a beneficial effect on hemodynamics and survival. For this reason, these agents may be preferred when it is necessary to use drugs in addition to digoxin for slowing of heart rate in AF associated with DCM.

24. What monitoring is appropriate for patients with CHF due to DCM?

Patients with CHF are fragile. The relative risk-to-benefit ratio of manipulation for diagnostic procedures must be carefully considered. Invasive monitoring, including placement of a Swan-Ganz catheter and cannula for direct measurement of systemic blood pressure, provides nearly complete hemodynamic information that can be used to modify therapy. However, such complete instrumentation requires intensive nursing care, is difficult to maintain, and is not inexpensive.

Devices that measure blood pressure indirectly provide useful information if their limitations are recognized. Systemic blood pressure is a valuable measure because a perfusion pressure of about 60 mmHg is necessary to maintain glomerular filtration rate and viability of vital capillary beds. However, most veterinary patients with CHF are normotensive at presentation. Furthermore, blood pressure is not a measure of flow, and it is possible for blood pressure to be maintained at the expense of cardiac output. The measurement of central venous pressure (CVP) provides useful information, and the technique is relatively easy. CVP is a measure of right ventricular filling pressure; it does not provide information about pulmonary venous pressure in the setting of left ventricular dysfunction.

When available, the measurement of blood gases provides information about ventilation and tissue oxygenation. The calculation of the alveolar–arterial oxygen gradient estimates the degree of ventilation/perfusion mismatch due to pulmonary edema. Estimation of oxyhemoglobin saturation with pulse oximetry is noninvasive and serves as a worthy substitute for measurement of blood gases when the patient cannot tolerate the stress of arterial puncture.

Despite the availability of numerous relatively elaborate monitoring techniques, most patients with CHF due to DCM can be managed with careful attention to vital signs. Monitoring of heart rate and respiratory rate and character, assessment of femoral arterial pulse, and observation of mucous membranes provide invaluable information about response to therapy and short-term prognosis.

25. What is the prognosis of CHF due to DCM?

The prognosis of CHF due to DCM is generally poor. If the patient survives beyond the initial presentation, survival of 6–12 months and occasionally longer is possible with careful medical management. A few patients may respond favorably to supplementation with nutrients such as carnitine or taurine. However, DCM in dogs is usually terminal.

CONTROVERSY

26. Are beta-adrenergic antagonists indicated in the therapy of CHF due to DCM?

The beta-adrenergic antagonists have effects that are negatively inotropic, dromotropic, and chronotropic. Intuitively, the use of a negative inotrope seems contraindicated in the setting of DCM, in which the primary pathophysiologic mechanism is a deficit of systolic myocardial function. However, recent evidence from studies of experimentally induced cardiac disease in dogs and clinical studies of people with myocardial disease suggests that beta-adrenergic antagonists have a role in the therapy of CHF due to systolic dysfunction. The long-term use of beta-adrenergic antagonists in people with myocardial disease has improved hemodynamics, exercise tolerance, and longevity. Beta-adrenergic antagonists seem to preserve myocardial function in dogs with induced CHF. These findings are consistent with the currently accepted notion that CHF is a neurohumeral syndrome associated with activation of the adrenergic nervous system and RAAS. It is likely that these compensatory mechanisms have favorable effects in the short term. However, with chronicity they have a detrimental effect on cardiac function and contribute to the inexorable decline in myocardial function that is characteristic of heart failure. The reason that beta-adrenergic antagonists are helpful in CHF is unknown, although they probably protect the heart from the adverse consequences of unopposed adrenergic activation. A favorable effect on myocardial oxygen consumption resulting from effects on heart rate also may be important. Upregulation of beta receptors, which are known to be dysfunctional (downregulated) in heart failure, also may contribute to the beneficial effects, although this mechanism is likely of lesser importance.

BIBLIOGRAPHY

1. Calvert CA, Chapman WL, Toal RL: Congestive cardiomyopathy in Doberman pinscher dogs. J Am Vet Med Assoc 191:598–602, 1982.
2. Cleland JGF, Bristow MR, Erdmann E, et al: Beta-blocking agents in heart failure: Should they be used and how? Eur Heart J 17:1629–1639, 1996.
3. Cobb MA: Idiopathic dilated cardiomyopathy: Advances in aetiology, pathogenesis and management. J Small Animal Pract 33:113–118, 1992.
4. COVE Study Group: Controlled clinical evaluation of enalapril in dogs with heart failure: Results of the Cooperative Veterinary Enalapril Study Group. J Vet Intern Med 9:243–252, 1995.
5. Harpster NK: Boxer cardiomyopathy. In Kirk RW (ed): Current Veterinary Therapy VII—Small Animal Practice. Philadelphia, W.B. Saunders, 1983, pp 329–337.
6. Keene BW: Canine cardiomyopathy. In Kirk RW (ed): Current Veterinary Therapy X—Small Animal Practice. Philadelphia, W.B. Saunders, 1989, pp 240–251.
7. Keene BW, Panciera DP, Atkins CE, et al: Myocardial L-carnitine deficiency in a family of dogs with dilated cardiomyopathy. J Am Vet Med Assoc 198:647–650, 1991.
8. Knight DH: Efficacy of inotropic support of the failing heart. Vet Clin North Am Small Animal Pract 21:879–904, 1991.
9. Sabbah HN, Shimoyama H, Kono T, et al: Effects of long-term monotherapy with enalapril, metoprolol, and digoxin on the progression of left ventricular dysfunction in patients with heart failure. Circulation 89:2852–2859, 1994.

52. CARDIAC ARRHYTHMIAS

Andrew Beardow, B.V.M.&S., M.R.C.V.S.

1. What are the fundamental mechanisms of arrhythmogenesis?

Three mechanisms are commonly described in the induction of arrhythmias: (1) reentry, (2) enhanced automaticity, and (3) triggered activity.

Reentry. Loops of cells or tissues with differing conduction properties are established, and disparities of conduction within the loop allow perpetuation of an impulse that otherwise would be extinguished. If the timing is right, such impulses trigger ectopic depolarizations in nonrefractory tissue. The loops may occur at the microscopic, cellular level or the macroscopic level. The microscopic loop consists of Purkinje cells and myocytes and a region of diseased tissue that acts as a unidirectional block in one limb of the loop. As an impulse passes down the conduction pathway, it is blocked from antegrade conduction through the diseased pathway. The impulse continues past this region in other portions of the loop and is then conducted in a retrograde direction in the diseased portion because this limb of the loop was not depolarized and therefore is not refractory. If the timing is correct, the tissue beyond the block is ready to conduct another impulse, setting up a reentry loop.

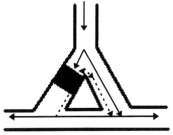

Area of unidirectional block.

Macroreentry loops use larger circuits composed of existing conduction pathways, i.e., reentry loops within the the the atrioventricular (AV) node or by an accessory pathway, as in Wolff-Parkinson-White (WPW) syndrome. In humans up to 85% of supraventricular tachyarrhythmias (SVTs) may be due to macroreentry loops utilizing disparity of conduction velocities in the fast and slow pathways through the AV node. These pathways also exist in the canine AV node, but it is unclear how many SVTs in dogs are generated through this mechanism.

Enhanced automaticity. In this mechanism of arrhythmogenesis, either normal pacemaker tissues show abnormal activity or cells that are not usually automatic become so. Automaticity is a property of phase 4 of the action potential. In automatic cells a leakage of ions allows the resting membrane potential to change, moving it toward threshold. When the threshold is reached, depolarization is triggered. The rate of change of this potential determines the rate at which it reaches threshold and hence how frequently the pacemaker will fire. Changes in the membrane or the prevailing autonomic tone may affect this mechanism and hence enhance automaticity. Diseased cells that normally do not show automaticity may start to do so. For example, the membranes of diseased myocardial cells may develop an abnormal permeability to calcium ions. This leak allows the membrane to depolarize spontaneously, reach threshold, and trigger a premature beat.

Triggered activity. As the name indicates, triggered activity does not occur spontaneously but requires one wave of depolarization to trigger another. It is believed that oscillations in the membrane potential following an action potential are responsible for this activity. Disease states or, in some cases, drugs render the membrane unstable and likely to allow such oscillations. Described as afterdepolarization, these oscillations are further classified, depending on their relationship to the action potential, as either early or late. Late afterdepolarizations are typically cited as causing the arrhythmias induced by digoxin intoxication.

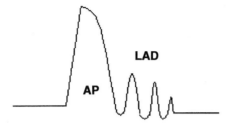

Triggered activity. AP = action potential, LAD = late afterdepolarization.

2. What steps are taken to determine the focus of an arrhythmia?

1. Try to identify a normal PQRST, i.e., a complex that originated from the sinoatrial (SV) node, was conducted through the AV node, and depolarized the ventricle with a normal timing and conduction pattern. A normal PQRST may show some abnormalities because of underlying disease, such as abnormal AV nodal conduction, aberrant ventricular conduction, or an abnormally shaped P-wave due to atrial changes. If you are in doubt, try to identify several complexes that look the same; all of them may have the same abnormality, but in each a P-wave is followed after an appropriate interval by a QRS complex and a T-wave.

2. Compare the normal complex with others on the strip. If the abnormal complexes have only a QRS complex and a T-wave, do they look like the normal QRS-T complex? If so, the arrhythmia most likely arises at or above the AV node and is therefore supraventricular in origin. If not, the arrhythmia is probably ventricular in origin.

3. Try to identify any P-waves on the strip. Do they have a temporal relationship to the abnormal QRS complexes? The answer may help to determine whether the source of a supraventricular arrhythmia is atrial or junctional.

3. Arrhythmias are common in emergency patients. Clinical signs compatible with arrhythmia, such as syncope or weakness, may be described. What techniques help to correlate clinical signs with arrhythmia?

1. **Observation of clinical signs** while the patient is monitored in hospital. If you are lucky, you may be monitoring the EKG when clinical signs develop.

2. **Event recording.** A small device, about the size of a pager, is attached to the patient and records the EKG continuously in a 5-minute electronic loop memory. The owner activates the unit when the patient has an episode, and the unit locks the EKG into memory. Because the unit is programmable, the amount of EKG recorded before and after activation may be varied. The batteries typically last up to 7 days, and some units record up to 5 events. Such devices are useful if an episode typically occurs once weekly. The major disadvantage is that the owner must witness the event.

3. **Holter monitoring.** Holter monitors record the EKG for 24 or 48 hours. The recording is made either on a cassette tape or with solid-state technology. However the data are recorded, the entire 24-hour EKG is analyzed by a computer, allowing documentation of the frequency as well as the presence of arrhythmia. Holter monitors often have an event button that can be activated by the owner, thus allowing correlation of the EKG with the event. The owner need not be present, however, for the device to record an arrhythmia that may be judged serious enough to cause clinical signs. The major disadvantages of Holter monitors are the size of the unit, which tends to limit their use to patients weighing over 10 kg, and the fact that only 24 hours of recording time are available, which limits their use when clinical signs occur infrequently.

    4. **Response to therapy.** Although frequently the method of choice, observation of response to therapy is the least satisfactory method of establishing a cause-and-effect relationship between arrhythmias and clinical signs. Both clinical signs and arrhythmias may resolve spontaneously, independently of therapy. Conversely, use of a single EKG to measure response to therapy may give false evidence of efficacy; for example, the EKG may have been recorded during the 2 minutes when the arrhythmia was temporarily quiescent. In either circumstance, the patient may be condemned to a prolonged course of inappropriate therapy.

4. In examining the EKG of a patient with tachyarrhythmia, what is the most important first step?

    Try to establish whether the arrhythmia is supraventricular or ventricular in origin. Broadly speaking, this distinction, above all others, is the most useful first step in choosing the most appropriate therapy. Even if you cannot definitively categorize the arrhythmia, first-line therapy stands a better chance of success if it is based on your best guess. It is not unusual to have to reassess your diagnosis frequently throughout the management of tachyarrhythmias because of inappropriate therapeutic response or a change in the underlying arrhythmia.

5. Describe the classification system for antiarrhythmic drugs. To which class(es) do lidocaine, procainamide, diltiazem, and propranolol belong?

    The Vaughan-Williams classification for antiarrhythmic drugs is based on their effect on the action potential of the cardiac myocyte:

    Class I drugs, frequently described as membrane stabilizers, block the fast sodium channel. Class I drugs are subdivided according to their effect on the action potential in terms of automaticity, conductivity, contractility, AV conduction, and fibrillation threshold.

Class IA	Decreased automaticity	Procainamide	SVT
	Decreased conductivity	Quinidine	VT
	Decreased contractility		WPW
Class IB	Decreased automaticity	Lidocaine	VT
	Decreased contractility	Tocainide	
	Increased AV conduction	Mexiletine	
	Increased fibrillation threshold		
Class IC	Decreased automaticity	Flecainide	VT
	Decreased conductivity	Encainide	WPW
	Decreased contractility		
	Decreased AV conduction		

    Class II drugs are the beta blockers, which decrease automaticity and conductivity. They cause variable degrees of depression of both contractility and AV node conduction, depending on the drug in question. Beta blockers are used to manage supraventricular tachycardia (SVT), ventricular tachycardia (VT), and Wolff-Parkinson-White syndrome (WPW).

    Class III drugs are the neural adrenergic antagonists, which recently have received a great deal of attention in management of arrhythmias refractory to class I drugs. Class III drugs decrease automaticity and conductivity and increase the fibrillation threshold. Many have significant side effects that must be taken into consideration. The most commonly used class III drugs are bretylium, amiodarone, and solotol.

    Class IV drugs, which block the slow calcium channel, have their most profound effects on AV node conduction. They also decrease automaticity, conductivity, and contractility, although the magnitude of these effects varies widely across the group. The most commonly used class IV drugs are verapamil and diltiazem.

6. How does the Vaughan-Williams classification help to determine the choice of antiarrhythmic drug?

    The ion that carries the action potential differs according to the location of the myocyte. For example, the action potential in the pacemaker cells of the SA and AV nodes is carried principally by the calcium ion. To treat arrhythmias arising from these tissues (SVTs), a class IV drug (calcium channel blocker) such as diltiazem is appropriate. Class I drugs act principally on the sodium channel and are therefore most useful for VTs because the sodium channel carries the depolarization phase of the action potential in ventricular myocytes.

7. What is proarrhythmia?

Proarrhythmia represents a change in or development of arrhythmias during treatment with antiarrhythmic drugs. This phenomenon was first galvanized into the minds of physicians when asymptomatic patients with arrhythmias began to die as a result of antiarrhythmic drugs. Proarrhythmia must be considered whenever antiarrhythmic drugs are used. All antiarrhythmic drugs affect the myocardial action potential. Although this effect is often beneficial, it may prove unpredictable, especially in diseased tissue. Hence drugs that suppress conduction velocity may affect the timing of conduction through reentrant loops in such way as to fine-tune the loop and exacerbate the arrhythmia. Clinicians must consider the risk/benefit ratio of such drugs before they are used. Asymptomatic patients with premature ventricular contractions (PVCs) do not invariably need antiarrhythmic therapy.

8. Which medications are often selected for management of acute SVTs in dogs?

The short-acting beta blocker esmolol, the unclassified agent adenosine, intravenous calcium channel blockers (diltiazem and verapamil), or intravenous digoxin is often selected.

Intravenous digoxin is the most difficult to manage and tends to be used less frequently. An exception is the patient with an SVT that may be atrial fibrillation and suspected dilated cardiomyopathy (DCM); beta blockers and calcium channel blockers are negative inotropes and should be used with extreme caution in such patients. Digoxin is also appropriate when dobutamine is indicated for the acute management of DCM in patients suspected of atrial fibrillation. Dobutamine increases the rate of conduction through the AV node and thus the ventricular response rate, thereby exacerbating tachycardia.

Of the calcium channel blockers, **diltiazem** may cause less myocardial depression than verapamil and thus may be the better choice.

Adenosine is a purine nucleotide found in every cell in the body. When exogenous adenosine is administered, it is presumed to bind to an extracellular purine receptor. It then decreases intracellular levels of the universal second messenger, cyclic adenosine monophosphate (cAMP), by blocking adenylate cyclase. Adenosine has profound inhibitory effects on AV node conduction and depresses SA node and ventricular automaticity. Cyclic AMP mediates many of the effects of catecholamines; therefore, adenosine ameliorates the arrhythmogenic properties of catecholamines.

9. When should a ventricular arrhythmia be treated?

Two major factors should be considered in deciding whether to treat a ventricular arrhythmia:

1. **Underlying disease process.** Certain emergency problems are often complicated by the onset of ventricular arrhythmias (e.g., gastric dilatation, volvulus). Frequently the ventricular rate is the same as the underlying sinus rhythm, and the patient is hemodynamically stable. Correction of underlying fluid deficit, acid–base disturbance, or pain may negate the need for antiarrhythmic therapy if the patient remains stable.

2. **Frequency and rate of arrhythmia.** There are no hard and fast rules about the need for therapeutic intervention in the management of arrhythmia. Typically therapy is indicated if the patient shows clinical signs associated with the arrhythmia or if the type of arrhythmia and signalment have a strong association with sudden death. For instance, boxer dogs with myocarditis and cardiomyopathy frequently die suddenly, presumably because of a fatal arrhythmia. Therefore, you may be more inclined to treat an asymptomatic boxer with frequent PVCs, especially if paroxysmal ventricular tachycardia is documented, than an otherwise healthy Labrador retriever with 18 single, uniform PVCs per minute.

10. How should an arrhythmia of ventricular origin be treated?

For immediate management of life-threatening arrhythmias, lidocaine is the drug of choice. Typically the initial dose is 2 mg/kg administered as an IV bolus. Lidocaine should be used without epinephrine. Diazepam may be given to control seizures. Cats invariably have seizures when given 2 mg/kg of lidocaine; therefore, in cats the dose is reduced to 0.2 mg/kg. Lidocaine is metabolized rapidly; for sustained effect, infuse 50–100 µg/kg/min. If there is any delay between the initial bolus and administration of the infusion, another bolus may be necessary.

Commonly used oral drugs include procainamide, mexiletine, and quinidine.

11. What concurrent problems affect the required dose of lidocaine?

Reduced blood flow to the liver decreases the required dose of lidocaine and may increase side effects, including mental depression. Low cardiac output and beta blockade decrease hepatic blood flow. Liver failure and administration of cimetidine also decrease hepatic clearance of lidocaine.

12. What if a bolus of lidocaine fails to convert the patient with ventricular arrhythmias?

- Combinations of antiarrhythmic drugs may help to convert patients who are refractory to monotherapy. Lidocaine may be combined with parenteral procainamide. In patients with no evidence of myocardial depression, beta blockers (e.g., propranolol, atenolol, esmolol) may be used.
- Class III antiarrhythmic drugs (amiodarone, sotolol, bretylium) also have been used in patients refractory to more conventional therapy, although experience with these drugs is limited.
- Reassess the patient, and correct fluid deficits, acid–base status, hypoxia, or any identifiable underlying disease.

BIBLIOGRAPHY

1. Lunney J, Ettinger SJ: Cardiac arrhythmias. In Ettinger SJ, Feldman EC (eds): Textbook of Veterinary Internal Medicine, 4th ed. Philadelphia, W.B. Saunders, 1995.
2. Miller MS, Tilley LP: Treatment of cardiac arrhythmias and conduction disturbances. In Miller MS, Tilley LP: Manual of Canine and Feline Cardiology, 2nd ed. Philadelphia, W.B. Saunders, 1995.
3. Tilley LP: Essentials of Canine and Feline Electrocardiography, 3rd ed. Philadelphia, Lea & Febiger, 1992.
4. Wall RE, Rush JE: Cardiac emergencies. In Murtaugh RJ, Kaplan PM (eds): Veterinary Emergency and Critical Care Medicine. St. Louis, Mosby, 1992.

53. CARDIAC PACEMAKERS

Eric Monnet, D.V.M., M.S.

1. What are the most common indications for pacemaker implantation in small animals?
• High-grade second-degree atrioventricular (AV) block
• Third-degree AV block
• Sick sinus syndrome
• Persistent atrial standstill with a slow ventricular escape rate

2. What are the clinical indications for a pacemaker?
Pacemaker implantation is indicated when clinical signs such as exercise intolerance, syncope, or congestive heart failure are related to bradycardia.

3. How do you stabilize a patient with clinically significant bradycardia before implantation of a permanent pacemaker?
It is necessary to increase the heart rate either with a temporary external pacemaker or pharmacologically. If a temporary external pacemaker is available, a flow-directed, ballon-tip bipolar electrode is introduced into the jugular vein and wedged in the trabeculae of the right ventricle under local anesthesia and light sedation. The EKG documents capture of the ventricle when the electrode is properly wedged in the trabeculae. Fluoroscopy also may be used to assist with placement of the electrode and to confirm its position. If a temporary external pacemaker is not available, constant intravenous infusion of a beta agonist (isoproterenol, 0.01 µg/kg/min) may be used during anesthesia to increase the rate of the escape rhythm, but this method is less reliable.

4. What techniques are available for permanent pacemaker implantation?
• Transvenous implantation through the jugular vein. The pulse generator is implanted in a subcutaneous pocket in the neck or thorax.
• Transdiaphragmatic implantation after celiotomy. The pulse generator is implanted in a pocket in the abdominal wall between the transverse abdominal and internal oblique muscles.

5. What are the three-letter codes on the pacemaker?
Pacemakers operate in different modes. A three-letter code has been developed to identify the different modes.

First Letter: Chamber Paced	*Second Letter:* Chamber Sensed	*Third Letter:* Response to Sensing
A (atrium)	A	I (inhibited)
V (ventricle)	V	T (triggered)
D (dual atrium and ventricle)	D	D (I and T)
	O (no sensing)	O (no response)

A pacemaker in VVI mode will pace and sense a ventricle and will not fire an impulse if a heart beat has been sensed (inhibited) (see figure at top of next page). VVI is the most commonly used mode in veterinary medicine.

6. What is sensing?
Sensing is the ability of the pacemaker generator to recognize intrinsic myocardial activity. Sensing is a function of the ability of the sensing amplifier to recognize a P or R wave. Sensing sensitivity is usually set at 1.0 mV. The P or R wave must be greater than 1.0 mV to inhibit the pacemaker generator.

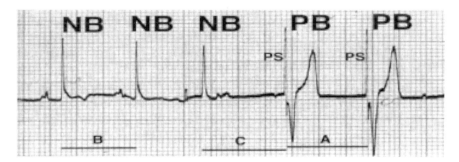

Electrocardiogram of a dog with sick sinus syndrome treated with a permanent pacemaker. This pacemaker was sensing and capturing appropriately. Each pacemaker spike is associated with a depolarization wave. **A** represents the normal time between two paced beats if no normal beats are sensed. Note that **B** < **A** and **C** = **A**. NB = normal beat, PB = paced beat, PS = pacemaker spike.

7. What type of electrodes may be used to pace the heart?

Electrodes may be unipolar or bipolar. With unipolar electrodes the electric current goes from the tip of the electrode (cathode) to the metallic box of the generator (anode). With bipolar electrodes, the anode and cathode are within the tip of the electrode. These leads may be further divided into endocardial or epicardial leads. Endocardial electrodes are usually bipolar, whereas epicardial electrodes are usually unipolar.

8. What is threshold to capture?

Threshold to capture is the minimal amount of energy required to induce a myocardial depolarization on the EKG (i.e., to capture the heart). Threshold to capture is determined by gradually decreasing the output of the generator until no QRS complex is seen on the EKG monitor. The output is then increased until the heart is captured again. For safety we set the output of the generator at 2 times the threshold. Threshold is measured in milliamperes (mA).

9. What are the major postoperative concerns?

- Continuous EKG monitoring for 24 hours to confirm proper function of the pacemaker.
- Heart rate should not drop below the preset rate of the pacemaker.
- Premature ventricular contractions (PVCs) often are seen after surgery because of the myocardial trauma from the lead implantation. Lidocaine may be used to suppress PVCs, but usually this is not necessary.
- The temporary transvenous lead is left in place for 24 hours as a back-up in case the permanent pacemaker has problems.

10. What are the most common causes of pacemaker failure?

- Failure to capture
- Failure to sense (oversensing and undersensing)
- Pulse generator failure

11. What is failure to capture?

Failure to capture occurs when the pulse generator fires an impulse at the appropriate time, but no depolarization of the myocardium is associated with the impulse (see figure at top of next page).

12. What causes failure to capture?

- Increased lead impedance 4–5 weeks after initial surgery due to fibrous tissue
- Lead fracture
- Lead dislodgment

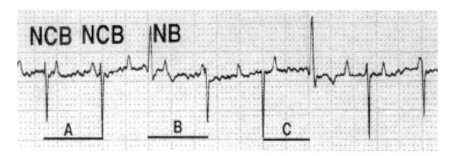

Electrocardiogram of a dog in third-degree AV block treated 4 weeks before this tracing with a permanent pacemaker demonstrates failure to capture. There are six pacemaker spikes (NCB = noncaptured beat) not associated with a depolarization wave, and two escape beats (NB = normal beat). Because **A** = **B** and **C** < **A**, the pacemaker is sensing appropriately. Correct sensing also implies that the lead is not broken.

13. What is failure to sense?

Failure to sense occurs when the pacemaker does not recognize appropriate myocardial electrical activity. Failure to sense is recognized on the EKG by the presence of a nonpaced heart beat between two normally timed paced beats or an absence of paced beats at the appropriate timing. Failure to sense places the animal at risk for competitive tachycardia and ventricular fibrillation. Failure to sense is caused by both oversensing and undersensing.

14. What are oversensing and undersensing?

Oversensing occurs when the sensing amplifier of the pulse generator detects inappropriate electrical activity and inhibits the pacemaker. It results from a high sensing sensitivity. Electrical activity may originate from extracardiac signals (myopotential, electromagnetic interference) or from intracardiac signals (lead problems, T-wave sensing, far-field sensing).

Undersensing occurs when the sensing amplifier of the pulse generator does not detect electrical activity and does not inhibit the pacemaker. It results from a low sensing sensitivity and is most commonly due to lead fracture or dislodgment.

16. What is generator failure?

Generator failure occurs most often when the battery runs out of power. Circuitry problems also may induce generator failure. A failing generator has erratic behavior; that is, it may fail to capture or to sense, or it may reset the pacing rate by itself.

17. What should be done if a dog with a pacemaker presents with sudden onset of syncope?

- Count the pulse rate, which should be higher than the preset pacing rate.
- Perform an EKG to differentiate failure to capture from failure to sense or generator failure.
- Evaluate cardiac function with echocardiography.
- Evaluate lead integrity with radiographs.
- Do exploratory surgery to evaluate the pulse generator and lead insertion in the generator and to measure lead impedance and R or P wave amplitude.

BIBLIOGRAPHY

1. Fox PR, Matthiesen DT, Purse D, Brown NO: Ventral abdominal, transdiaphragmatic approach for implantation of cardiac pacemakers in the dog. J Am Vet Med Assoc 189:1303–1308, 1986.
2. Fox PR, Moise NS, Woodfield JA, Darke PGG: Techniques and complications of pacemaker implantation in four cats. J Am Vet Med Assoc 199:1742–1753, 1991.
3. Orton EC: Pacemaker therapy. In Orton ED (ed): Small Animal Thoracic Surgery. Baltimore, Williams & Wilkins, 1995, pp 239–247.
4. Tilley LP: Special methods for treating arrhythmias: Cardiopulmonary arrest and resuscitation, pacemaker therapy. In Tilley LP (ed): Essentials of Canine and Feline Electrocardiography. Philadelphia, Lea & Febiger, 1992, pp 365–382.

54. PERICARDIAL EFFUSION

Dianne Dunning, D.V.M.

1. What is the pericardium?

The pericardium is a two-layer sac that envelopes and surrounds the heart. The outer layer (fibrous pericardium) is continuous at the heartbase with the great arteries and veins. At its apex, the fibrous pericardium forms the sternopericardial ligament, which attaches the pericardial sac to the ventral muscular diaphragm. The inner layer, which is formed by a single layer of mesothelial cells, adheres to the visceral or epicardial surface of the heart and turns back on itself to form the parietal layer, which is attached to the fibrous pericardium. Within the sac is 0.5–1.5 ml of serous fluid, which is an ultrafiltrate of serum. This fluid is maintained via osmosis, diffusion, and lymphatic drainage across the serosal surface.

2. What are the functions of the pericardium?

- Prevention of cardiac overdilation
- Myocardial lubrication
- Protection of the heart from infections or adhesions
- Maintenance of the heart in a fixed position within the chest
- Regulation of stroke volume between the two ventricles
- Prevention of right ventricular regurgitation when ventricular diastolic pressures are increased

Normal cardiac function may be maintained without the pericardium, as seen in dogs with congenital absence of the pericardium or dogs with pericardiectomy.

3. What are the causes of pericardial effusion?

The most common causes of pericardial effusion are neoplasia (58%) and benign idiopathic effusion (19%). Other less common causes of pericardial effusion are as follows:

- Infection
- Congestive heart failure
- Uremia
- Trauma
- Foreign bodies
- Coagulopathies
- Congenital or acquired peritoneopericardial hernias
- Pericarditis
- Left atrial rupture

4. What are the common tumors associated with pericardial effusion?

- Right atrial hemangiosarcoma (33%)
- Chemodectoma (12%)
- Metastatic adenocarcinoma (5%)
- Lymphoma (3%)
- Thymoma (3%)
- Undifferentiated carcinoma (3%)

5. What is benign idiopathic pericardial effusion?

Benign idiopathic pericardial effusion is a diagnosis of exclusion in patients with no evidence of underlying disease or bacterial infection. This syndrome is seen predominantly in large-breed male dogs, 8–9 years of age. The diagnosis is confirmed at surgery when no evidence of neoplasia is found. Pericardial histopathology reveals a chronic nonspecific, inflammatory, hemorrhagic pericarditis. The term *benign* is a misnomer and has fallen out of favor because pericardial effusion may be a life-threatening problem.

6. Which common organisms are associated with infectious pericardial effusion? What is their route of entry?

Actinomyces and *Nocardia* spp. are the two most common organisms isolated from animals with infectious pericardial effusion. These bacteria cause a chronic, suppurative tissue reaction with granuloma formation that is difficult to distinguish grossly from neoplasia. Granules within the tissue or exudate are characteristic but may not be present in all cases. The granules represent colonies of the organism. Differentiation between actinomycosis and nocardiosis can be confirmed only by culture of the organism. If antimicrobial therapy has been instituted before obtaining the samples for culture, as is often the case, the organisms may be difficult to culture. *Actinomyces* spp. generally respond best to penicillins, whereas *Nocardia* sp. responds best to potentiated sulfonamides. The route of entry is difficult to document but is usually from penetration of the pericardium by a foreign body via the trachea or esophagus. Actinomycocis and nocardiosis often are associated with plant awn penetrations and are a common problem in the western United States.

7. What is the pathophysiology of cardiac tamponade?
Pericardial effusion is the accumulation of fluid within the pericardial sac and may result in cardiac tamponade. Rate of fluid accumulation, volume of fluid, and characteristics of the pericardial sac play a role in determining signs associated with pericardial effusion. Rapid fluid accumulation, large quantities of fluid, and a diseased, noncompliant pericardial sac contribute to signs associated with cardiac tamponade. Cardiac tamponade occurs when intrapericardial pressure exceeds the ventricular diastolic pressure. The results are systemic venous congestion and decreased cardiac output. This is a life-threatening problem that must be quickly recognized and treated.

8. What are the most common findings in the clinical history of pericardial effusion?
- Lethargy (19.0%)
- Anorexia (14.3%)
- Dyspnea (16.7%)
- Collapse (14.3–32.6%)

9. Describe the most common clinical signs of pericardial effusion.
Clinical signs may be acute or chronic, depending on the rate and volume of pericardial fluid accumulation and characteristics of the pericardial sac. No pathognomonic signs of pericardial effusion exist. The most prevalent clinical signs associated with the disease are as follows:
- Muffled heart sounds (50.0%)
- Cachexia (28.6%)
- Weakness (40.5%)
- Tachycardia (heart rate > 150 bpm) (28.6–41.3%)
- Abdominal distention (35.7–58.7%)
- Weak arterial pulse (26.2%)

Jugular distention is the cardinal sign of cardiac tamponade in humans but appears to have a low prevalence in animals (2.4%), making it an unreliable indicator of disease. This may be due to lack of detection.

10. What is the diagnostic test of choice for pericardial effusion?
Echocardiograhy detects effusion in more than 90% of dogs. It is considered the diagnostic test of choice because of its accuracy and noninvasive nature. Up to 43% of tumors causing pericardial effusion are detected with two-dimensional echocardiography. Positive results are reliable with a specificity of 77%, but the absence of a visible mass on echocardiography does not rule out the presence of a mass lesion. Two-dimensional echocardiography has a greater sensitivity and specificity (66% and 100%, respectively) at detecting right atrial hemangiosarcoma. Right atrial hemangiosarcoma has a worse prognosis than other cardiac tumors. Diagnosis, prognosis, and therapeutic recommendations for dog with pericardial effusion are generally based on results of echocardiography.

11. Is the central venous pressure (CVP) useful in detecting pericardial effusion?
Absolutely. CVP > 12 cm H_2O is a consistent finding with pericardial effusion.

12. Describe the value of the EKG in diagnosing pericardial effusion.
EKG generally reveals normal sinus rhythm or sinus tachycardia. Electrical alternans is defined as a phasic alteration of the amplitude of the QRS complex from one cardiac beat to the next and is seen in 6.1–34.8% of cases with pericardial effusion. These phasic alterations are believed to be caused by the swinging of the heart within the pericardial sac. Small-amplitude complexes were once believed to be due to the poor conduction of the electrical impulses through the fluid, but they more likely result from decreased ventricular filling.

13. Are thoracic radiographs valuable in diagnosing pericardial effusion?

Thoracic radiographs are indicated as part of the minimal database to rule out metastatic disease or concurrent thoracic disease. The most common radiographic abnormalities in dogs with pericardial effusion are cardiomegaly (87.9%), pleural effusion (56%), and metastasis (68.8%).

14. What is the emergency treatment for an animal with significant pericardial effusion?

Pericardiocentesis.

15. How do you do a pericardiocentesis?

Clip and surgically prepare the skin on the right thoracic wall between the 4th and 6th intercostal spaces at the level of the costochondral junction. Connect the EKG leads to the animal. Inject ¼ ml of 2% lidocaine HCl at the insertion site and down to the pleural surface. Using an 8-French, 9-cm intravenous catheter (Safety Thoracocentesis System, Sherwood Medical, St. Louis), slowly insert the catheter and enter the pericardial space. Aspirate the fluid from the pericardial space.

16. How do you know whether the blood is from the pericardium or a cardiac chamber?

Blood within the pericardial space is defibrinated and will not clot. The first sample should be placed in a red-top collection tube and monitored for clotting. If a clot forms, remove the catheter and begin again.

17. What is the purpose of the EKG during pericardiocentesis?

As the catheter enters the pericardial space, it may touch the epicardium. If it does, the galvinometer in the EKG will detect the contact; you will see a bizarre QRS or even ventricular arrhythmias. These signs require that you back the catheter slightly outward as you continue to aspirate fluid.

18. Do you need to remove all of the fluid from the pericardial space to relieve the symptoms?

No. Removal of a small volume of fluid results in dramatic drops in intrapericardial pressure.

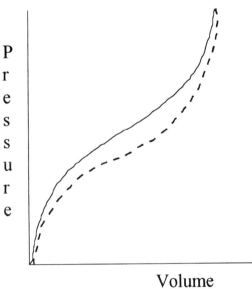

When fluid accumulates within the pericardial space *(solid line)*, there is a sigmoid-shaped pressure-volume curve. When fluid is removed from the pericardial space *(dotted line)*, the curve follows the hysteresis of the volume accumulation curve. Thus, when a small volume of fluid is removed, there is a dramatic drop in intrapericardial pressure.

Pressure

Volume

19. What laboratory data help to diagnose the cause of pericardial effusion?

Changes in laboratory data are variable and nonspecific. Recently, pericardial fluid pH has been explored as a test for discriminating between benign (inflammatory) and neoplastic (noninflammatory) origins of pericardial fluid. Inflammatory pericardial fluid has a markedly acidic pH value (6.5), whereas the pH of noninflammatory pericardial fluid is near the value of normal body fluid (7.5). Determination of pericardial fluid pH is inexpensive and simple to interpret but has not been evaluated in a large number of cases and therefore should be interpreted with caution.

20. Is cytology of the pericardial effusion of diagnostic value?

Cytologic examination of pericardial fluid is diagnostic for effusion due to infectious processes; however, it is of little benefit for differentiating between benign idiopathic and neoplastic effusions.

21. What are the treatment choices for pericardial effusion?

Historically, there have been multiple therapeutic approaches to dogs with pericardial effusion. Cases of probable idiopathic pericardial effusion are initially managed via multiple pericardiocentesis; surgery is used only if the effusion persists. Fifty percent of benign idiopathic pericardial effusions resolve with multiple pericardiocentesis. Patients with high probability of neoplasia usually undergo surgery for prevention of refractory cardiac tamponade and confirmation of diagnosis. Total pericardiotomy offers no advantage over subtotal pericardiotomy and is more time-consuming. Pericardiectomy is considered palliative for nonresectable cardiac tumors. Postoperative complications associated with pericardiectomy are uncommon.

22. What is the prognosis for dogs with pericardial effusion?

The prognosis of pericardial effusion in dogs depends on the etiology. Pericardial effusion secondary to neoplasia is reported to carry poor prognosis, whereas benign idiopathic pericardial effusion is thought to carry a better prognosis. However, few specific data about survival and prognostic indicators of survival of dogs with pericardial effusion are available.

BIBLIOGRAPHY

1. Aronsohn M: Cardiac hemangiosarcoma in the dog: A review of 38 cases. J Am Vet Med Assoc 187:922–926, 1985.
2. Aronsohn LR, Gregory CR: Infectious pericardial effusions in five dogs. Vet Surg 24:402–407, 1995.
3. Berg RJ, Wingfield W: Pericardial effusion in the dog: A review of 42 cases. J Am Animal Hosp Assoc 20:721–730, 1983.
4. Berg RJ, Wingfield W, Hoopes PJ: Idiopathic hemorrhagic pericardial effusion in eight dogs. J Am Vet Med Assoc 185:988–992, 1984.
5. Bouvy BM, Bjorlind DE: Pericardial effusion in dogs and cats. Part I: Normal pericardium and causes and pathophysiology of pericardial effusions. Comp Cont Educ Pract Vet 13:417–421, 1991.
6. Bouvy BM, Bjorlind DE: Pericardial effusions in dogs and cats. Part II: Diagnostic approach and treatment. Comp Cont Educ Pract Vet 13:633–641, 1991.
7. Edwards NJ: The diagnostic value of pericardial fluid pH determination. J Am Animal Hosp Assoc 32:63–67, 1996.
8. Hosgood G: Canine hemangiosarcoma. Comp Cont Educ Pract Vet 13:1065–1075, 1991.
9. Lorell BH, Braunwald E: Pericardial disease. In Braunwald E (ed): Heart Disease. Philadelphia, W.B. Saunders, 1992, pp 1485–1516.
10. Lorenzana R, Richter K, Ettinger SJ, et al: Infectious pericardial effusion in a dog. J Am Animal Hosp Assoc 21:725–728, 1985.
11. Mathiesen DT, Lammerding J: Partial pericardiectomy for idiopathic hemorrhagic pericardial effusion in the dog. J Am Animal Hosp Assoc 21:41–47, 1985.
12. Orton EC: Pericardium. In Orton EC (ed): Small Animal Thoracic Surgery. Baltimore, Williams & Wilkins, 1995, pp 177–184.
13. Reed JR: Pericardial diseases. In Fox PR (ed): Canine and Feline Cardiology. Philadelphia, W.B. Saunders, 1990, pp 495–518.
14. Richter KP, Jackson J, Hart JR: Thoracoscopic pericardiectomy in 12 dogs. Proceedings of the 14th Veterinary Medicine Forum, 1996, p 746.
15. Sisson D, Thomas WP, Ruehl WW, et al: Diagnostic value of pericardial fluid analysis in the dog. J Am Vet Med Assoc 184:51–55, 1984.

55. FELINE MYOCARDIAL DISEASE

Jonathan A. Abbott, D.V.M.

1. What is cardiomyopathy?

Cardiomyopathy is a disease of the myocardium that is unrelated to valvular disease, pericardial disease, coronary vessel disease, or anomalies of cardiac structure. The cardiomyopathies are classified according to etiology, when it is known, or according to functional or morphologic characteristics. Without other qualifiers, cardiomyopathy generally refers to primary myocardial disease—that is, myocardial disease that is etiologically independent of extracardiac factors. The term *secondary cardiomyopathy* or *specific heart muscle disease* is favored when the etiology is known or when the cardiomyopathy has an established association with environmental, metabolic, or infectious agents. For example, hypertrophic cardiomyopathy usually applies to an idiopathic myocardial disease characterized by concentric left ventricular hypertrophy. The term *thyrotoxic heart disease* or *thyroid-induced cardiomyopathy* is appropriate when myocardial disease occurs in the setting of hyperthyroidism.

2. What forms of myocardial disease occur in cats?

Three functional designations of primary myocardial disease are in widespread use:
- Hypertrophic cardiomyopathy
- Dilated cardiomyopathy
- Restrictive cardiomyopathy

Hypertrophic cardiomyopathy is probably the most common. In addition, secondary myocardial diseases, including hypertensive heart disease and thyrotoxic heart disease, are also recognized.

3. What characterizes each form of feline myocardial disease (FMD)?

Dilated cardiomyopathy. Dilated cardiomyopathy (DCM) is characterized by ventricular dilation and hypokinesis. Atrial dilation results from atrial myocardial disease, secondary atrioventricular (AV) valve incompetence, and elevation of ventricular filling pressures. The recognition of the association between nutritional taurine deficiency and DCM prompted supplementation of commercial cat food with this amino acid. Supplementation has reduced dramatically the prevalence of DCM in cats. Idiopathic DCM still occurs in cats, albeit uncommonly.

Hypertrophic cardiomyopathy. Hypertrophic cardiomyopathy (HCM) is characterized by hypertrophy of a nondilated ventricle in the absence of systemic hypertension, anatomic ventricular outflow tract obstruction, or metabolic derangements. Systolic ventricular performance in HCM is normal or hyperdynamic. Mitral valve regurgitation may complicate HCM because of distortion of the mitral valve apparatus related to hypertrophy, systolic anterior motion of the mitral valve leaflets, or papillary muscle dysfunction. Mitral valve regurgitation, together with elevation of ventricular filling pressures associated with diastolic dysfunction, contributes to the development of left atrial dilation.

Restrictive cardiomyopathy. Restrictive cardiomyopathy is characterized by atrial dilation and ventricular dimensions that are normal or nearly so and systolic myocardial function that is normal or only mildly diminished.

Expression of myocardial disease in cats is diverse. Although some cats have cardiomyopathies that fit easily into the above categories, in other cases the distinctions are less clear and the nature of the myocardial disease defies currently accepted methods of classification. For example, some feline cardiomyopathies have features of more than one morphologic or functional designation. Some of these cases may represent an intermediate phase of a progression in which the end result will conform more easily to current classification. The use of the term *intermediate cardiomyopathy* is probably appropriate in this setting. Alternatively, a functional and morphologic description based on echocardiographic findings is appropriate and perhaps superior to the use of a single term that, in a specific instance, may be inaccurate or lack specificity.

Thyrotoxic heart disease. The cardiovascular manifestations of thyrotoxicosis are varied. Some cats with hyperthyroidism develop a secondary myocardial disease that closely resembles idiopathic hypertrophic cardiomyopathy, whereas others have ventricular dilation with apparently preserved systolic function. Yet another subset of the hyperthyroid population is characterized by systolic myocardial dysfunction; dilated cardiomyopathy has been observed as a consequence of hyperthyroidism.

Hypertensive heart disease. Systemic hypertension results in concentric left ventricular hypertrophy in some cats.

4. The various forms of FMD differ in terms of pathophysiology. Contrast the mechanisms by which HCM and DCM result in cardiac dysfunction and congestive heart failure.

DCM is primarily a disorder of systolic myocardial dysfunction. When myocardial contractility is impaired, the stroke volume declines and the end-systolic ventricular volume is increased. This residual volume, augmented by pulmonary venous return, results in ventricular dilation. If ventricular filling pressures become sufficiently high, they are reflected onto the upstream capillary bed, resulting in the development of tissue edema or accumulation of effusions. Usually, the left ventricle is affected in DCM, and pulmonary edema is the expected consequence, although pleural effusions also may occur. Cardiogenic pleural effusion in cats is seldom associated with ascites and may result from diseases that, based on echocardiographic study, seem to affect primarily the left ventricle.

In contrast to DCM, the primary pathophysiologic mechanism in HCM is diastolic dysfunction. Diastolic function is difficult to quantify and perhaps less tangible than systolic function, which has an importance that is easily and intuitively grasped. Diastolic function is determined by the active, energy-requiring process of myocardial relaxation as well as a mechanical property of the ventricle known as compliance. Compliance is the relationship between a change in volume and the associated change in pressure. When primary diastolic dysfunction is present, ventricular filling pressures are elevated when diastolic volumes are normal or small. Congestive signs may result if elevated filling pressures are reflected onto the pulmonary venous circulation. Diastolic dysfunction also may explain signs of low-output failure because impaired ventricular filling reduces stroke volume.

5. What is feline endomyocarditis?

Recently, the clinical characteristics of a series of cats with histologic findings of endomyocarditis were described. A stressful event such as anesthesia for sterilization or declawing was noted in the history of many of these cats. The clinical presentation was characterized by sudden onset of severe dyspnea, radiographic pulmonary infiltrates, and echocardiographic evidence of minimal atrial enlargement. The echocardiographic finding of an abnormally echogenic endocardium was believed to be distinctive. The dyspnea was apparently associated with interstitial pneumonia. The cause of this syndrome is unknown. Recognition may be important, because the dyspnea is unlikely to be due to cardiogenic pulmonary edema; overly aggressive diuresis probably should be avoided when the diagnosis is suspected.

6. What historical findings are typically associated with FMD?

Clinical signs in FMD are generally related to congestive heart failure (CHF) or systemic thromboembolism. Dyspnea resulting from pulmonary edema or pleural effusion is the clinical sign that most commonly prompts owners to present the cat for veterinary evaluation. Onset of dyspnea of cats with myocardial disease may be surprisingly sudden; the owner may have been unaware of anything untoward in the cat's behavior before development of dyspnea. Possibly this is related to the fact that most cats lead a sedentary existence; they are able to conceal signs referable to the cardiovascular system until such signs are provoked by minimal stress or exertion.

7. What physical findings are expected in cats with FMD?

Vital signs. Often cats with FMD are presented for emergency evaluation of dyspnea. Typically, the respiratory rate is elevated and respiratory effort is increased. The patient may be distressed and anxious. Some cats with FMD and markedly reduced cardiac output become hypothermic. Elevated adrenergic tone is part of the syndrome of CHF; a consequent increase in heart rate is therefore expected. Indeed, tachycardia is evident on physical examination of some patients with FMD. However, even healthy cats have relatively high heart rates in the clinic due to an elevation in adrenergic tone, presumably related to anxiety. As a result, the heart rates of cats with CHF are often comparable to heart rates of healthy cats recorded in the veterinary clinic. Except when pathologic tachycardias such as ventricular tachycardia are present, the heart rate of cats with CHF seldom exceeds the upper limit of the range that is accepted for hospitalized cats. Indeed, bradycardia is sometimes noted on physical examination of cats with CHF. The bradycardia may result from conduction system disease or extracardiac factors. Bradycardia in cats with CHF may be associated with low cardiac output and hypothermia.

Auscultation. Auscultation may reveal crackles when pulmonary edema is present. A quiet thorax suggests pleural effusion. A systolic murmur is often but not invariably present. Some cats with FMD develop mitral valve regurgitation secondary to functional or structural changes of the mitral valve apparatus as a consequence of myocardial disease. A subpopulation of cats with HCM develops systolic anterior motion (SAM) of the mitral valve leaflets that may result in a murmur of dynamic outflow tract obstruction. More than one mechanism can explain the presence of a murmur in FMD; consequently, the systolic murmur associated with FMD is variable in intensity and character. The absence of a cardiac murmur should not exclude FMD from the differential diagnosis of cats with dyspnea. Audibility of the third or fourth heart sound or a gallop rhythm suggests myocardial dysfunction in many cats with FMD. The third heart sound (S_3) is associated with termination of the rapid ventricular filling phase of early diastole. It becomes audible when transmitral flow is increased, when the passive compliance of the ventricle is reduced, or when the end-systolic volume is high. In small animals, audibility of a third heart sound is most commonly associated with dilated cardiomyopathy. The fourth heart sound (S_4) is associated with the atrial contraction phase of diastole; it is accentuated and may be audible when ventricular relaxation is impaired. Distinction between the third and fourth heart sounds is not generally possible when the heart rate exceeds 150 bpm. An auscultated triple rhythm may represent a summation gallop resulting from fusion of the third and fourth heart sounds. The presence of a gallop rhythm in small animals is generally a specific sign of cardiac disease; therefore, recognition of the gallop is of much greater clinical importance than making the distinction between S_3 and S_4 gallop rhythms.

8. What is the role of electrocardiography in the diagnosis and management of FMD?

The electrocardiogram (EKG) provides information about heart rate, rhythm, and size. EKG evidence of ventricular hypertrophy is sometimes present in cats with myocardial disease. However, the primary utility of the EKG in evaluation of FMD is elucidation of disorders of rate and rhythm. Premature ventricular complexes and occasionally ventricular tachycardia may be detected. Because ventricular arrhythmia seldom complicates extracardiac disease in cats, this EKG abnormality provides useful diagnostic information in cats with signs of cardiovascular disease. Supraventricular arrhythmias, including atrial premature complexes, junctional premature complexes, and supraventricular tachycardia, also may occur in FMD. Bradyarrhythmias, including sinus bradycardia and various forms of atrioventricular (AV) dissociation related to AV block, also may complicate the presentation of FMD. AV block may result from structural disease of the conduction system, although sometimes the block is transient and associated with low cardiac output and hypothermia. When AV conduction disturbances are present, the rate of the idiojunctional or idioventricular rhythm often exceeds 100 bpm but is generally less than 150 bpm.

9. What is the role of thoracic radiography in the diagnosis of FMD?

Plain thoracic radiographs are invaluable because they allow assessment of cardiac size in relation to pulmonary vasculature and parenchyma. Usually, some degree of cardiac enlargement precedes the development of congestive heart failure. Therefore, the chest radiograph provides an indirect assessment of global cardiac performance. Unfortunately, however, thoracic radiography is relatively insensitive in the detection of chamber enlargement; furthermore, the ability to image specific chambers is limited. These shortcomings are particularly acute in feline thoracic radiography. In addition, the stress associated with restraint is poorly tolerated by feline patients in overt CHF. The risk-to-benefit ratio of restraint for diagnostic studies must be carefully assessed before radiographic studies are undertaken.

10. What is the role of echocardiography in the diagnosis of FMD?

Echocardiography is a noninvasive means by which to evaluate cardiac chamber dimensions and myocardial function. The cardiac septae can be visualized, allowing relatively precise assessment of specific cardiac chambers. Other diagnostic studies, including thoracic radiography, provide information that is not obtained by echocardiographic examination. However, echocardiography is required for noninvasive antemortem diagnosis of FMD. As stated previously, the expression of myocardial disease in cats is diverse and optimal therapy likely differs in the various forms of FMD. Echocardiography is therefore indicated to obtain a definitive diagnosis, which in turn provides information that guides therapy.

11. When should echocardiography be performed in patients suspected of FMD?

Echocardiography is recommended whenever FMD is suspected. In the emergency setting, the relative risk-to-benefit ratio of restraint for echocardiographic study must be carefully considered. When physical findings suggest CHF, it is often advisable to initiate treatment before undertaking diagnostic tests. However, it is sometimes possible to examine cats echocardiographically when they are in sternal recumbency and minimally restrained. Sometimes a cursory echocardiographic examination is better tolerated than restraint for radiographic examination. Cursory examination may be sufficient to establish that the patient has structural cardiac abnormalities that may reasonably have resulted in CHF. Respiratory signs in the absence of echocardiographic atrial enlargement are almost certainly due to extracardiac disease. As with any diagnostic test, there are limitations to echocardiography; however, if these limitations are understood, echocardiography is an appropriate initial diagnostic test in cats in whom history and physical findings suggest CHF.

12. How are congestive signs managed in cats with FMD?

Diuretics are used initially in the treatment of cardiogenic pulmonary edema. Furosemide, a potent loop diuretic, is administered intravenously. The fragility of feline patients with CHF should not be underestimated; if venous access is difficult to obtain, intramuscular administration is suggested. Diuretics act at the level of the nephron to increase urine volume. The consequent decrease in intravascular volume effects a decrease in ventricular filling pressures and favors the resolution of pulmonary edema.

When radiographic, sonographic, or physical findings suggest that signs of dyspnea are caused by pleural effusion, therapeutic thoracocentesis is recommended. Thoracocentesis is suggested before further diagnostic evaluation in patients with respiratory distress when physical findings indicate the presence of pleural effusion. Diuretics tend to mobilize body cavity effusions poorly, and the use of diuretics does not obviate the need for thoracocentesis when pleural effusion is the primary cause of dyspnea. Aggressive diuretic therapy without thoracocentesis may cause dehydration and signs of low cardiac output before causing a clinically apparent reduction in the volume of pleural effusion.

13. How is contractility manipulated in FMD?

Systolic myocardial dysfunction is seldom the primary cause of CHF in cats. Therefore, inotropic support is rarely indicated. However, catecholamines, including dobutamine, may be administered to cats with echocardiographic confirmation of systolic myocardial dysfunction. Careful monitoring is suggested because some cats develop adverse neurologic and gastrointestinal signs when receiving catecholamines.

14. How is supplemental oxygen administered?

The administration of supplemental oxygen is indicated when patients with FMD present in overt CHF and are short of breath. Cats with CHF are fragile and tolerate manipulation poorly. Usually, confinement in an oxygen cage is beneficial. An oxygen mask is generally tolerated only by moribund patients.

15. How are cats with FMD monitored?

Careful monitoring of body temperature is suggested because some patients with FMD and low cardiac output develop hypothermia. The noninvasive evaluation of blood pressure in cats is a challenging endeavor, although Doppler or oscillometric techniques may be considered if the patient tolerates the necessary degree of restraint. Cats, perhaps more than dogs, are apt to develop signs of low-output cardiac failure. Diuretics rarely have a salutary effect on cardiac output. In fact, a decrease in preload generally causes a decrease in stroke volume. This is usually well tolerated in patients with systolic dysfunction and dilated ventricles because the relationship between preload and stroke volume in this setting is not linear. A reduction in end-diastolic volume may relieve congestive signs with negligible effects on stroke volume. However, diseases of diastolic dysfunction are currently most prevalent in cats. In this setting, end-diastolic volumes are normal or small, and a relatively minor reduction in ventricular filling pressure may result in a clinically important decrease in stroke volume. Diuresis is certainly indicated when congestive signs are present. However, the adverse effects of excessive diuresis may be particularly acute in diseases characterized by diastolic dysfunction. When ventricular filling is impaired, the decrease in preload resulting from overly aggressive diuresis may have a noticeable and negative effect on cardiac output and result in clinical deterioration. Monitoring of the hematocrit and total protein is sometimes helpful in gauging the degree of hemoconcentration that has resulted from diuretic administration. Similarly, the blood urea nitrogen or, preferably, the creatinine level is monitored in patients with FMD.

16. Should intravenous fluids be administered to cats with FMD? If so, what kind of fluid?

The administration of intravenous fluid increases intravascular volume and, as a consequence, ventricular filling pressures. This has obvious benefit in hypovolemic patients. In CHF, ventricular filling pressures (preload) are already excessive. A clinical diagnosis of CHF means that ventricular filling pressures are elevated; in the setting of overt CHF, infusion of fluid does not effect an increase in stroke volume but is likely to contribute to the accumulation of edema fluid. The careful administration of maintenance volumes of crystalloid is considered when respiratory distress has resolved but the patient is slow to recover and unwilling or unable to take fluid and food by mouth. The use of a low sodium fluid, such as 5% dextrose in water or 0.45% saline with 2.5% dextrose in water, is recommended.

17. What are the roles of calcium channel blockers in FMD?

Calcium channel antagonists bind to the L-type calcium channels of myocardial and vascular smooth muscle cells. In general, the calcium channel antagonists act as negative inotropes, negative chronotropes, and vasodilators. Evidence also suggests that they increase the rate of myocardial relaxation—that is, they have a positive lusotropic effect. Based largely on the assumption that a positive lusotropic effect is helpful in HCM, they have found favor in treatment of HCM in cats.

Diltiazem is the calcium channel antagonist currently in widespread use for treatment of feline HCM. It is most often administered orally as chronic therapy and is used as an adjunct to diuretic therapy in patients with HCM and clinical signs due to CHF. In cats with HCM but no clinical signs, diltiazem is sometimes used in attempts to delay or prevent the onset of congestive signs. Its efficacy for this purpose is unknown. The author considers the use of diltiazem in cats with occult HCM if there is unequivocal echocardiographic evidence of left ventricular hypertrophy in the presence of left atrial dilation. Diltiazem also has a role as an antiarrhythmic agent when FMD is complicated by supraventricular arrhythmias. It is available in an injectable formulation that can be used in an attempt to terminate supraventricular tachycardia. In addition, injectable diltiazem may have a role in cats with overt CHF and normal or elevated heart rates that are unable to take medications orally.

18. What are the roles of beta-adrenergic antagonists in FMD?

The beta-adrenergic antagonists include propranolol, atenolol, carvedilol, and others. They bind competitively to the beta-adrenergic receptors and have negative inotropic, negative chronotropic, and negative dromotropic effects. Their effect on diastolic function is, for the most part, indirect and results from prolongation of ventricular filling time, although some evidence suggests that beta-adrenergic antagonists may increase ventricular distensibility. The negative inotropic effect may be beneficial in cats with HCM and systolic anterior motion (SAM) of the mitral valve. The results of a clinical trial suggest that diltiazem may be superior to propranolol for the treatment of CHF due to feline HCM. However, it is probably inappropriate to discard the use of beta-adrenergic antagonists completely in this setting. The effect of beta-adrenergic antagonists on heart rate is generally greater than the effect of diltiazem. Therefore, beta-adrenergic antagonists may have advantages over diltiazem in cases in which control of heart rate is an important objective, when SAM is present, or when HCM is complicated by ventricular tachyarrhythmia.

CONTROVERSIES

19. Are vasodilators indicated in HCM?

Vasodilators have proven efficacy in the treatment of patients with DCM and primary valvular disease. The rationale for their use is based on the premise that peripheral vascular resistance is inappropriately elevated in these disorders. The decrease in peripheral vascular resistance that results from vasodilation permits an increase in stroke volume, and the effect of judicious vasodilation is clearly beneficial.

Most cats with HCM have normal or hyperdynamic systolic ventricular performance. It is unlikely that a mismatch of systolic function and aortic impedance is present. Conceivably, treatment with vasodilators may result in systemic hypotension. An important hemodynamic consideration relates to the presence of SAM, a valve motion abnormality detected in some cats with HCM. Vasodilation may increase the pressure gradient associated with SAM, and vasodilators are believed to be contraindicated in human patients with HCM.

20. What is the role of angiotensin-converting enzyme (ACE) inhibitors in feline HCM?

The safety of the vasodilator enalapril has been investigated in a population of cats with HCM, and adverse effects related to the hemodynamic effects of the drug were not recognized. Mitral valve regurgitation occurs commonly in cats with HCM. In the setting of HCM complicated by mitral valve regurgitation, a decrease in peripheral vascular resistance may have favorable effects. Furthermore, the results of ACE inhibition are not limited to the mechanical effect of vasodilation. For example, experimental evidence suggests that ACE inhibitors have a positive lusotropic effect. In addition, ACE inhibition reduces aldosterone levels, an effect that is probably helpful in the setting of CHF. In addition, angiotensin II has trophic effects on myocardium. Although the relevance of these observations to spontaneous HCM in cats is unknown, it is possible that some of the neurohumoral effects of ACE inhibition are beneficial.

BIBLIOGRAPHY

1. Atkins CE, Gallo AM, Kurzman ID, Cowen P: Risk factors, clinical signs, and survival in cats with a clinical diagnosis of idiopathic hypertrophic cardiomyopathy: 74 cases (1985–1989). J Am Vet Med Assoc 201:613–618, 1992.
2. Bonagura JD, Fox PR: Restrictive cardiomyopathy. In Bonagura JD (ed): Current Veterinary Therapy XII—Small Animal Practice. Philadelphia, W.B. Saunders, 1995, pp 863–872.
3. Bossbaly MJ, Stalis I, Knight DH, VanWinkle T: Feline endomyocarditis: A clinical/pathological study of 44 cases [abstract]. J Vet Intern Med 8:144, 1994.
4. Bright JM, Golden AL, Gompf RE, et al: Evaluation of the calcium channel-blocking agents diltiazem and verapamil for treatment of feline hypertrophic cardiomyopathy. J Vet Intern Med 5:172–282, 1991.
5. Bright JM, Golden AL, Daniel GB: Feline hypertrophic cardiomyopathy: Variations on a theme. J Small Animal Pract 33:266–274, 1992.

6. Golden AL, Bright JM: Use of relaxation half-time as an index of ventricular relaxation in clinically normal cats and cats with hypertrophic cardiomyopathy. Am J Vet Res 51:1352–1356, 1990.
7. Hamlin RL: Heart rate of the cat. J Am Animal Hosp Assoc 25:284–286, 1989.
8. Kittleson MD: CVT update: Feline hypertrophic cardiomyopathy. In Bonagura JD (ed): Current Veterinary Therapy XII—Small Animal Practice. Philadelphia, W.B. Saunders, 1995, pp 854–863.
9. Opie LH, Poole-Wilson PA, Sonnenblick EH, Chatterjee K: Angiotensin-converting enzyme inhibitors and conventional vasodilators. In Opie LH (eds): Drugs for the Heart. Philadelphia, W.B. Saunders, 1995, pp 105–144.
10. Pion PD, Kittleson MD, Rogers QR, Morris JG: Myocardial failure in cats with low plasma taurine: A reversible cardiomyopathy. Science 237:764–768, 1987.
11. Rush JE, Freeman LM, Brown DJ, Smith FWK: The use of enalapril in the treatment of feline hypertrophic cardiomyopathy (HCM) [abstract]. J Vet Intern Med 9:202, 1995.

56. SYSTEMIC ARTERIAL THROMBOEMBOLISM

Steven L. Marks, B.V.Sc., M.S., M.R.C.V.S.

1. Define thromboembolism.

A thrombus is an intravascular deposit of fibrin and formed blood elements. Thromboembolism occurs when the entire thrombus or a piece of thrombus formed at one location travels in the vascular system and lodges in a distant site.

2. What is the basic pathophysiology of thromboembolism?

• Local endothelial or endocardial injury
• Altered blood flow or stasis
• Altered coagulability

3. List the factors that determine the clinical consequences of thromboembolism.

• Site of thrombus origin
• Degree of occlusion
• Collateral circulation

4. What are causes of arterial thromboembolism in cats?

The most common cause of thromboembolism in cats is myocardial disease. It may be seen with dilated cardiomyopathy, hypertrophic cardiomyopathy, and restrictive cardiomyopathy. Less common causes of arterial thromboembolism in cats include:

• Bacterial endocarditis   • Heartworm disease
• Neoplasia   • Idiopathic
• Sepsis

5. What are the most common anatomic sites for thromboembolism in cats?

The aorta and iliac bifurcation are the most common sites of thromboembolism in cats. Other sites include:

• Forelimbs   • Brain
• Kidney   • Gastrointestinal tract

6. What are causes of thromboembolism in dogs?

• Heartworm disease   • Neoplasia
• Hyperadrenocorticism   • Fractures
• Nephrotic syndrome   • Pancreatitis
• Disseminated intravascular coagulopathy • Myocardial disease

- Immune-mediated hemolytic anemia
- Sepsis
- Foreign body

7. What are the most common anatomic sites for thromboembolism in dogs?
- Aorta
- Pulmonary artery
- Lungs
- Kidney
- Forelimbs
- Gastrointestinal tract
- Brain

8. Describe the clinical signs of thromboembolism.
Clinical signs associated with thromboembolism are generally related to hypoperfusion of a specific area or organ system. The specific clinical signs are therefore related to the underlying disease or organ system involved. For example, clinical signs of pulmonary thromboembolism include hypoxemia and respiratory distress.

9. List clinical signs specific for thromboembolism of a limb.
- Lack of detectable pulses
- Decreased temperature compared with normal limb
- Cyanosis of nail beds or pads
- Neurologic deficits
- Pain

10. List diagnostic procedures that help to evaluate for the presence of thromboembolism.
The diagnostic tests should be directed toward finding the underlying disease that has led to thromboembolism:
- Complete blood count
- Biochemical profile
- Urinalysis
- Antithrombin III levels
- Adrenocorticotropic hormone stimulation test
- Heartworm antigen test
- Echocardiography
- Doppler ultrasound
- Thyroid profile
- Thoracic radiographs
- Blood gas analysis
- Ventilation/perfusion studies
- Coagulation profile
- Coombs test

11. Which tests are both specific and sensitive for thromboembolism?
- Selective or nonselective angiography
- Ultrasound to visualize thrombus
- Doppler studies to evaluate blood flow

12. What therapeutic options are available for thromboembolism?
Most therapy for arterial thromboembolism is directed toward correcting the underlying disease processes. Other therapy may be divided into supportive, preventive, or thrombolytic.

13. What supportive care is required for thromboembolism?
Supportive care is based on the system involved. For example, with pulmonary thromboembolism oxygen therapy is beneficial. For renal thromboembolism, surgical intervention and fluid therapy are suggested. Cats with arterial thromboembolism often require analgesia.

14. List therapies that may prevent further thromboembolism.
- Heparin
- Warfarin
- Aspirin

15. Which drugs may improve collateral circulation?
- Hydralazine
- Acepromazine

16. Which thrombolytic drugs are currently used?
- Streptokinase
- Urokinase
- Tissue plasminogen activator

17. Can heparin be used as an anticoagulant in all cases of thromboembolism?
No. Animals with protein-losing nephropathy often lose significant amounts of antithrombin III. Heparin requires antithrombin III as a cofactor. In such cases, fresh frozen plasma may be used as an antithrombin III source, or other anticoagulants such as warfarin may be considered.

18. What emergency therapy may be provided for thromboembolism?
Emergency therapy also should be directed toward the underlying disease process. Supportive care, including fluid therapy and analgesia, is generally indicated.

Pulmonary thromboembolism
- Oxygen
- Bronchodilators
- Vasodilators
- Calcium channel blockers
- Corticosteroids
- Thrombolytic drugs

Peripheral thromboembolism
- Vasodilators
- Aspirin
- Heparin
- Thrombolytic drugs

19. What is the prognosis of thromboembolic disease? How long should treatment be continued?
The prognosis for animals with thromboembolic disease is based on the underlying disease and how easily it can be managed. Overall the prognosis is guarded, especially for cats with myocardial disease, because recurrence is high. There is no time limit for medical management. Duration of treatment is usually based on the clinical condition of the animal and finances. Owners can provide good nursing care in their home.

CONTROVERSY

20. Is surgical therapy indicated for thromboembolic disease?
In most cases surgical therapy is not indicated because of instability due to the underlying disease process. If, however, aggressive medical management leads to no improvement, embolectomy may be considered. Unfortunately, recurrence of thromboembolism is nearly 100%.

BIBLIOGRAPHY

1. Baty CJ, Hardie EM: Pulmonary thromboembolism: Diagnosis and treatment. In Bonagura JD (ed): Current Veterinary Therapy XI. Philadelphia, W.B. Saunders, 1992, pp 137–142.
2. Dennis JS: Clinical features of canine pulmonary thrombus. Comp Cont Educ Pract Vet 15:1595–1603, 1993.
3. Feldman BF: Thrombosis: Diagnosis and treatment. In Kirk RW, Bonagura JD (eds): Current Veterinary Therapy IX. Philadelphia, W.B. Saunders, 1986, pp 505–508.
4. Harpster NK, Baty CJ: Warfarin therapy of the cat at risk of thromboembolism. In Bonagura JD (ed): Current Veterinary Therapy XII. Philadelphia, W.B. Saunders, 1995, pp 868–872.
5. Laste NJ, Harpster NK: A retrospective study of 100 cases of feline distal thromboembolism, 1977–1993. J Am Animal Hosp Assoc 31:492–500, 1995.
6. Klein MK, Dow SW, Rosychuk RAW: Pulmonary thromboembolism associated with immune-mediated hemolytic anemia in dogs: Ten cases (1982–1987). J Am Vet Med Assoc 195:246–250, 1989.
7. LaRue MJ, Murtaugh RJ: Pulmonary thromboembolism in dogs: 47 cases (1986–1987). J Am Vet Med Assoc 197:10, 1368, 1990.
8. MacDonald MJ, Kirby R: Feline cardiac emergencies. Semin Vet Med Surg 3:237–244, 1988.

VII. Oncologic and Hematologic Emergencies

Section Editor: Gregory K. Ogilvie, D.V.M.

57. NEUTROPENIA, SEPSIS, AND THROMBOCYTOPENIA IN PATIENTS WITH CANCER

Gregory K. Ogilvie, D.V.M.

1. How common are neutropenia and sepsis?

Sepsis is the most common cause of death in people with cancer, exceeding all other causes combined. Neutropenia secondary to malignancy or myelosuppressive effects of chemotherapy is a common predisposing factor for development of sepsis in dogs and cats. Because owners are demanding advanced care for their pets with cancer, the use of combination chemotherapy for treatment of a wide variety of malignancies in dogs and cats has increased; therefore, neutropenia and sepsis are emergencies of increasing prevalence and importance. Neutropenia and thrombocytopenia may occur in animals with many other diseases; the treatment is often the same for these patients as for animals with cancer.

2. Describe the pathogenesis and consequences of neutropenia and sepsis.

Neutropenia and sepsis may be transient problems that resolve when the animal's white blood cell count returns to normal, or they may progress to transient pyrexia or septic shock. Septic shock is the state of circulatory collapse secondary to overwhelming sepsis and/or endotoxemia. This syndrome frequently is fatal, with a mortality rate of 40–90% in humans. Although no data document the percentage of fatalities in pets with septic shock, it is believed to be at least as high as the percentage reported in people. The profound systemic effects of septic shock include cardiovascular effects, such as vasoconstriction leading to multiorgan failure; cardiac dysfunction, in part from lactic acidosis; and increased vascular permeability that leads to hyperviscosity and hypovolemia. Other systemic effects include liver dysfunction from splanchnic vascular pooling and tissue ischemia, acute renal failure, neutropenia, thrombocytopenia and coagulopathies, severe gastrointestinal damage, and various metabolic effects such as decreased insulin release and initial hyperglycemia followed by hypoglycemia.

3. What kinds of bacteria are most commonly involved in sepsis secondary to neutropenia?

Fortunately, the bacteria that most commonly cause morbidity and mortality in veterinary patients with cancer arise from the animal's own flora. Prolonged hospitalization and antibiotic use result in susceptibility to resistant strains of organisms. The increasing risk for fungal infections is an emerging problem in human oncology and probably will be recognized in the near future in veterinary medicine. Therefore, culturing for fungi will become an important issue.

4. What factors predispose patients with cancer to neutropenia and sepsis?

The most common factors that predispose patients to infections are granulocytopenia, cellular immune dysfunction, humoral immune dysfunction, splenectomy, indwelling vascular catheters, prolonged hospitalization, poor nutrition, neurologic dysfunction, and the effects of cancer itself.

5. What are the most common causes of granulocytopenia?

Granulocytopenia may result from leukemia or lymphoma caused by bone marrow destruction or from the myelosuppressive effects of chemotherapy. The myelosuppressive effects of chemotherapeutic agents can be categorized as high, moderate, and mild. These drugs cause a nadir (lowest part of the white blood cell count) at different times after administration. Infection early in the course of granulocytopenia typically is caused by endogenous bacteria that are relatively nonresistant. Frequent acquisition of blood samples greatly increases the risk of infection in cancerous animals. Other sites of entry of organisms include the skin, oral cavity, colon, and perianal area.

Myelosuppressive Effects of Chemotherapeutic Agents Used in Veterinary Medicine

HIGHLY MYELOSUPPRESSIVE	MODERATELY MYELOSUPPRESSIVE	MILDLY MYELOSUPPRESSIVE
Doxorubicin	Melphalan	L-Asparaginase*
Vinblastine	Chlorambucil	Vincristine*
Cyclophosphamide	5-Fluorouracil	Bleomycin
Carboplatin	Methotrexate	Corticosteroids

* Vincristine and L-asparaginase, if given at the same time, can be moderately myelosuppressive.
From Ogilvie GK, Moore AS: Managing the Veterinary Cancer Patient: A Practice Manual. Veterinary Learning Systems, Trenton, NJ, 1995, with permission.

Timing of Myelosuppression with Various Chemotherapeutic Agents

DELAYED MYELOSUPPRESSION (3–4 WEEKS)	MID-RANGE MYELOSUPPRESSION (7–10 DAYS)	EARLY MYELOSUPPRESSION (< 5 DAYS)
Carmustine	Cyclophosphamide	Paclitaxel
Mitomycin C	Doxorubicin	
	Mitoxantrone	

From Ogilvie GK, Moore AS: Managing the Veterinary Cancer Patient: A Practice Manual. Veterinary Learning Systems, Trenton, NJ, 1995, with permission.

6. Which specific bacteria are commonly associated with sepsis in patients with cancer?

The gram-negative bacteria most commonly associated with infection of patients with granulocytopenia include *Escherichia coli, Klebsiella pneumoniae, Pseudomonas* sp., and *Enterobacteriaceae* sp. The most common gram-positive bacteria often include *Staphylococcus epidermatidis* and *S. aureus*. The increase in the prevalence of gram-positive infection may be due to the chronic use of venous catheters.

7. What common causes or acquired conditions are associated with sepsis in patients with cancer?

Defects in cellular immunity are also a cause of sepsis in animals with cancer. Cellular immune dysfunction may be due to an underlying cause or antineoplastic agents and corticosteroids. It results in various bacterial, mycobacterial, fungal, and viral infections.

Humoral immune dysfunction is also associated with an increased prevalence of sepsis in human patients with cancer and may cause similar problems in animals with cancer. Agammaglobulinemic or hypogammaglobulinemic animals are susceptible to infections. Multiple myeloma and chronic lymphocytic leukemia are common neoplasms associated with humoral immune dysfunction.

Splenectomized animals are susceptible to overwhelming sepsis when infected with a strain of encapsulated bacteria against which they have not made antibodies. Dogs that have had routine splenectomy may have decreased long-term survival because they lack an intact immune system.

Indwelling vascular catheters have been associated with increased prevalence of sepsis. The longer a catheter is present, the higher the probability for infection, especially in neutropenic patients. The risk of catheter-induced sepsis can be minimized by using aseptic technique and by placing a new catheter in a new site every 2–3 days. Strict aseptic procedures should be used, especially with animals that are myelosuppressed. The use of semipermanent indwelling catheters in patients with cancer may be safe if strict aseptic procedures are followed by owners and health care professionals.

Other contributing factors include prolonged hospitalization, malnutrition, neurologic dysfunction, or a nonambulatory patient from any cause.

8. What is the best way to recognize the septic patient?

Physical examination may reveal an animal with hyperdynamic septic shock; hallmarks include brick-red mucous membranes, tachycardia, and short capillary refill times. These symptoms may be followed by gastrointestinal signs, altered mentation, and decreased blood pressure. End-stage signs (hypothermia, mucous membrane pallor, marked mental depression, bloody diarrhea, signs of multiorgan failure) reflect a hypodynamic state. Thrombocytopenia and neutropenia are often identified during the course of septic shock. Hyperglycemia is an early finding, followed in many instances by hypoglycemia. Although bacterial cultures may be deceptively negative, a positive culture is common. Metabolic acidosis is also common.

9. What is unusual about the results of diagnostic tests in a neutropenic patient with sepsis?

The absence of circulating neutrophils results in a urinalysis without pyuria and chest radiographs that are normal because of lack of neutrophilic infiltrates. Neutrophils are responsible for the early radiographic changes associated with pneumonia. Therefore, these conditions are often not identifiable by standard diagnostic tests.

10. What should be cultured in neutropenic, septic patients?

Quite simply, everything. Two, and preferably four, sets of blood cultures (aerobic and anaerobic) should be acquired. The timing of the sampling intervals is controversial; however, every 20–30 minutes before antibiotic therapy may be adequate. At least 5 ml of blood should be injected into appropriate culture containers. If central venous catheters are present, cultures of the port should be obtained. Ideally, culture bottles that contain an antibiotic-binding resin or other antibiotic-binding substance should be included with each culture for patients on antibiotics. A cystocentesis specimen for urine culture and analysis should be acquired in each case after the patient has been evaluated to ensure the presence of at least 60,000 platelets/µl. When neurologic signs are present, a cerebrospinal fluid (CSF) tap should be obtained and cultured appropriately. CSF should be sent for Gram stain, bacterial culture, cell count and differential, and glucose and protein determination. A cryptococcal antigen titer or India ink preparation should be performed in suspect cases. Acid-fast stains and culture probably are not indicated routinely. For animals with diarrhea, appropriate cultures should be done for clostridial bacteria, including appropriate assays for endotoxin. In addition, chest radiographs should be taken when a site for infection is not obvious.

11. Should other diagnostic tests be considered?

Other diagnostic imaging studies that should be considered include ultrasonography, especially echocardiography, to identify the presence of valvular endocarditis. Invasive tests that should be performed to identify specific sites of infection include bronchoscopy if pulmonary disease is suspected, skin biopsy if deep cutaneous infection is identified, and bone marrow biopsy, percutaneous liver biopsy, or exploratory laparotomy in select cases. In addition, a complete blood count with differential, biochemical profile, and urinalysis should be performed for each patient.

12. What are the overall goals of treating septic, neutropenic animals?

Treatment for septic, neutropenic animals is directed primarily at restoring adequate tissue perfusion, improving alterations in metabolism, and controlling systemic infection.

13. What type and how much fluid should be used to restore tissue perfusion?

Standard therapy includes crystalloid solutions and antibiotics. Although hypertonic solutions are currently under investigation for treatment of shock, crystalloid solutions such as lactated Ringer's solution are cited in most veterinary books as the first line of therapy, with an initial infusion rate for critical animals of 70–90 ml/kg IV for 1 hour, then 10–12 ml/kg/hr thereafter. The fluid rate then should be adjusted to meet the needs of each patient, as directed by monitoring of body weight, heart and respiratory rates, central venous pressure, ongoing losses such as vomiting and diarrhea, and urine output. Lactate-containing fluids may be contraindicated because septic animals are already hyperlactatemic and engaged in futile cycling throughout the course of septic shock; septic animals with cancer are even more likely to be detrimentally affected by lactate-containing fluids. The administration of lactate-containing fluids to hypermetabolic patients that are septic may further tax this energy-consuming system and result in further debilitation. Therefore, 0.9% NaCl or a balanced electrolyte crystalloid solution (e.g., Normosol R) should be used. Dextrose (2.5–5%) should be included in fluids when systemic hypoglycemia is identified during constant patient monitoring. In states of severe cardiovascular shock, 70–90 ml/kg for the first hour, followed by up to 10 ml/kg/hr thereafter, is recommended. When fluids are administered at this rate, the patient must be monitored closely and the rate changed to meet the needs of the animal.

14. What type of antibiotics are used in neutropenic patients, with or without sepsis?

Asymptomatic animals with less than 1,000–1,500 neutrophils/μl should be started on prophylactic antibiotics. Trimethoprim-sulfa (7.5 mg/kg twice daily orally) is often recommended for prophylactic therapy in neutropenic animals. Neutropenic animals in septic shock should be started on intravenous fluids and antibiotic therapy as soon as samples for bacterial cultures are acquired (see list below and table on next page). Reevaluation of an empiric antibiotic regimen is mandatory when the identity and sensitivity pattern of the bacteria become available. When a gram-negative infection is present, two antibiotics that are the most effective against the isolated organism are often recommended. Generally gram-positive infections are treated with a single appropriate antibiotic. When infection of a catheter is suspected, the infected device is removed and long-term antibiotic therapy is initiated. Approximately 70–80% of human patients are cured. Myelosuppressive chemotherapeutics should be withheld until the patient has recovered. Antibiotics used to treat septic patients with cancer include the following:

Gram-negative bacteria	**Gram-positive bacteria**
Gentamicin (1–3 mg/kg IV 3 times/day)	Na or K penicillin (25,000 U/kg IV 4 times/day)
Cephalothin (20–30 mg/kg IV 4 times/day)	Cephalothin (20–30 mg/kg IV 4 times/day)
Cefoxitin (22 mg/kg IV 3 times/day)	Cefoxitin (22 mg/kg IV 3 times/day)

Anaerobic bacteria
Metronidazole (15 mg/kg IV or IM 3 times/day)
Cefoxitin (22 mg/kg IV 3 times/day)

15. What other treatments can be used now or in the near future?

More advanced therapies include granulocyte transfusions; however, they have not been associated with beneficial responses in controlled trials. In addition, transfusion reactions and allosensitizations to specific antigens of the granulocytes may occur, and increased prevalence of severe pulmonary reactions may also be noted. Canine recombinant granulocyte colony-stimulating factor (rcG-CSF, 5 μg/kg/day SQ) and canine recombinant granulocyte-macrophage colony-stimulating factor (rcGM-CSF, 10 μg/kg/day SQ) have been associated with an increased rate of myeloid recovery in dogs and cats with neutropenia. These hematopoietic growth factors increase cell numbers and enhance neutrophil function but are not yet available commercially. Human recombinant G-CSF and GM-CSF are commercially available; however, long-term use may induce antibody formation to the protein. Of the two human recombinant proteins, rhG-CSF induces the most profound increase in canine and feline neutrophil numbers before development of antibodies is noted. Tumor necrosis factor antiserum, antibody to tumor necrosis factor, interleukin and interferon therapy, pooled immunoglobulin preparations, and monoclonal antibodies to neutralize endotoxin may be future treatments of choice.

Approach to the Febrile, Neutropenic Patient

1. Identify the site of infection.
   - Perform complete history and physical examination.
   - Acquire complete blood and platelet count, biochemical profile, and urinalysis.
   - 2–4 blood cultures, cystocentesis for culture and sensitivity, chest radiographs, and transtracheal wash and culture and sensitivity.
   - If indicated, culture and sensitivity for cerebrospinal fluid, catheters, joint fluid, feces.

2. Initiate supportive care.
   - Establish indwelling intravenous catheter aseptically, and initiate fluid therapy. For shock: 70–90 mg/kg for the first hour, followed by 10–12 ml/kg/hr. Adjust as needed thereafter.
   - Withhold chemotherapeutic agents.

3. Initiate intravenous antibiotic therapy after cultures.
   - If aminoglycosides are contraindicated (e.g., dehydration, renal disease)—cefoxitin (22 mg/kg 3 times/day).
   - If aminoglycosides not contraindicated—cefoxitin (22 mg/kg 3 times/day), gentamicin (2–3 mg/kg 3 times/day over 30 min). Monitor for nephrotoxicity.
   - Granulocyte colony-stimulating factor, if available (5 µg/kg/day SQ < 14 days if human recombinant product).

4. Redefine antibiotic therapy based on culture and sensitivity results.
   - Monitor fever and neutrophil count; give fluid therapy as needed for shock and support.

5. Discharge for home care (neutrophils > 1,500 µl and afebrile).
   - Appropriate antibiotic therapy (e.g., trimethoprim-sulfasalazine, 15 mg/kg orally 2 times/day).

6. Consider dose reduction with next course of chemotherapy (e.g., decrease by 25%).

From Ogilvie GK, Moore AS: Managing the Veterinary Cancer Patient: A Practice Manual. Veterinary Learning Systems, Trenton, NJ, 1995, with permission.

16. What can be done to prevent sepsis in neutropenic patients?

Sepsis can be prevented by altering the environment and by using surveillance cultures. Typical environmental manipulations include washing hands and changing protective gloves between each patient. This approach may prevent introduction of infections from patient to patient and from veterinarian to animal. Foods, objects, or specific materials (e.g., rectal thermometers) also may harbor bacteria. Prophylactic antibiotic therapy is recommended by some; however, it may result in increased bacterial resistance, especially in areas of high antibiotic use such as university hospitals. In humans, the most common prophylactic antibiotic therapy includes nonabsorbable agents, quinolones, trimethoprim-sulfamethoxazole, antifungal drugs, antiviral drugs, and antiparasitics. Immunization with appropriate viral vaccines may be of value; however, the vaccines must be initiated before starting chemotherapeutic agents.

17. What is the most common cause of thrombocytopenia?

A decreased platelet count is most commonly caused by the cytotoxic effects of chemotherapeutic agents, bone marrow infiltration by a malignant process, or consumption coagulopathy. If a chemotherapeutic agent induces bone marrow suppression that results in cytopenia, thrombocytopenia usually occurs a few days after neutropenia and before a decrease in red blood cells.

18. What factors predispose to thrombocytopenia?

Thrombocytopenia may occur in any patient with cancer that receives myelosuppressive chemotherapeutic agents. Drugs such as vincristine, bleomycin, and prednisone do not cause as significant a degree of thrombocytopenia as myelosuppressive agents such as doxorubicin. Compared with other myelosuppressive drugs, cyclophosphamide induces suppression in platelet numbers. Dogs or cats with bone marrow infiltration by a malignant process are more sensitive to the cytotoxic effects of chemotherapeutic agents that may result in thrombocytopenia. Other conditions that affect the bone marrow (e.g., ehrlichiosis, estrogen toxicity from exogenous supplementation or from a productive testicular tumor) are likely to make the marrow more sensitive to cytotoxic agents. Tumors that are frequently associated with coagulopathies (e.g., hemangiosarcoma, thyroid carcinoma) may cause consumptive thrombocytopenia. In addition, hypersplenism and chronic bleeding of any origin may cause a decrease in platelet numbers.

19. How is thrombocytopenia diagnosed?
Clinical signs include but are not limited to bleeding diatheses, melena, and weakness. The blood loss may occur into any organ and result in clinical signs related to the damaged tissues. An acute decline in platelet numbers may result in development of clinical signs at higher platelet counts than if the decline in platelets is much slower. Diagnosis is confirmed by obtaining platelet counts and doing bone marrow aspirate or biopsy. Bone marrow testing is essential and helps the clinician to determine whether decreased production is the problem. Clotting profiles (e.g., activated partial thromboplastin time, one-step prothrombin time, fibrin degradation products) may help to determine whether thrombocytopenia is due to coagulopathy, such as disseminated coagulopathy.

20. What is the treatment for thrombocytopenic patients?
Thrombocytopenia-related clinical signs may be exacerbated when drugs that affect platelet function are administered during overt or impending thrombocytopenia. Therefore, aspirin and aspirinlike drugs should be withheld. Obviously, the animal with thrombocytopenia should be kept quiet. Tranquilizers may be needed in some patients. In academic settings or large private practices, platelet transfusions may be administered to specific cases that are, or have a high likelihood of, bleeding uncontrollably. The amount of random donor platelet transfusion is generally about 3 U/m^2 body surface area or 0.1 U/kg body weight. It is often recommended that each unit be administered with 30–60 ml of plasma per unit of platelets. With acute bleeding that is not responsive to other treatments or procedures, epsilon aminocaproic acid (Amicar) may be given by the intravenous or oral route (250 mg/m^2 4 times/day). Vincristine (0.5 mg/m^2 body surface area) may be administered IV to induce premature release of platelets from megakaryocytes. Platelet count increases in approximately 4 days after vincristine is given.

BIBLIOGRAPHY

1. Couto CG: Management of complications of cancer chemotherapy. Vet Clin North Am 4:1037–1053, 1990.
2. Hardie EM, Rawlings CA: Septic shock. Compend Cont Educ Pract Vet 5:369–373, 1983.
3. Haskins SC: Shock. In Kirk RW (ed): Current Veterinary Therapy VIII. Philadelphia, W.B. Saunders, 1983, pp 2–27.
4. Hughes WT, et al: Infectious Diseases Society of America: Guidelines for the use of antimicrobial agents in neutropenic patients with unexplained fever. J Infect Dis 161:381–390, 1990.
5. Kirk RW, Bistner SL: Shock. In Handbook of Veterinary Procedures Emergency Treatment, 4th ed. 1985, pp 59–68.
6. Lazarus HM, Creger RJ, Gerson SI: Infectious emergencies in oncology patients. Semin Oncol 6:543–560, 1989.
7. Ogilvie GK, Moore AS: Neutropenia, sepsis and thrombocytopenia. In Managing the Veterinary Cancer Patient: A Practice Manual. Trenton, NJ, Veterinary Learning Systems, 1995, pp 149–156.
8. Parker MM, Parrillo JE: Septic shock, hemodynamics and pathogenesis. JAMA 250:3324–2230, 1983.
9. Wolfsheimer KJ: Fluid therapy in the critically ill patient. Vet Clin North Am 19:361–378, 1989.
10. Woodlock TJ: Oncologic emergencies. In Rosenthal S, Carignan JR, Smith BD (eds): Medical Care of the Cancer Patient, 2nd ed. Philadelphia, W.B. Saunders, 1993, pp 236–246.

58. ACUTE TUMOR LYSIS SYNDROME

Gregory K. Ogilvie, D.V.M.

1. What is acute tumor lysis syndrome?

Acute tumor lysis syndrome (ATLS) is a condition of acute collapse that may lead to death soon after administration of a chemotherapeutic agent to an animal with a chemosensitive tumor. In short, chemotherapy results in the acute death of large amounts of tumor and release of cellular contents that may be acutely toxic. This emergency situation is underrecognized in veterinary patients and is becoming more common with the widespread use of chemotherapeutic agents.

ATLS has been documented in humans with lymphoma, leukemia, and small cell lung cancer; in dogs it has been associated with lymphoma and leukemia. ATLS may occur after effective chemotherapy in animals with rapidly growing, bulky, chemosensitive tumors. The patient often presents with a history of acute decompensation over a short time, sometimes to the point of imminent death. Rapid diagnosis and therapy are essential to reduce mortality rates.

2. What factors predispose animals to ATLS?

In humans and animals, rapid tumor lysis may cause acute release of intracellular phosphate and potassium. This release of electrolytes causes hypocalcemia, hyperkalemia, and hyperphosphatemia. In humans with ATLS, hyperuricemia is also seen, but this is not a concern in veterinary patients. As noted earlier, ATLS is most common in patients with lymphoma or leukemia, partly because the intracellular concentration of phosphorus in human lymphoma and leukemic cells is 4–6 times higher than in normal cells.

ATLS is most common in animals with some degree of volume contraction and a large tumor mass that responds rapidly to cytolytic therapy. In addition, septic animals or animals with extensive neoplastic disease that infiltrates the parenchyma are predisposed to ATLS. Veterinary patients at highest risk are volume-contracted dogs with stage IV or V lymphoma that are treated with chemotherapy and undergo rapid remission. ATLS may be identified within 48 hours after the first treatment.

3. How is ATLS diagnosed?

When ATLS is suspected, rapid physical examination should be performed to identify telltale signs of cardiovascular collapse, vomiting, diarrhea, and ensuing shock. The hyperkalemia may result in a bradycardia and diminished P-wave amplitude, increased PR and QRS intervals, and, rarely, spiked T-waves on electrocardiogram. Biochemical analysis of blood may confirm the presence of hypocalcemia, hyperkalemia, and hyperphosphatemia. In the presence of elevated serum phosphate levels, hypocalcemia develops as a result of calcium and phosphate precipitation. Without effective treatment, renal failure may occur; therefore, concentrations of blood urea nitrogen and creatinine should be monitored closely.

4. What is the treatment for ATLS?

The ideal treatment is prevention. Identify predisposed patients that have heavy tumor burden, a chemoresponsive tumor, and volume contraction. Because the kidney is the main source of electrolyte excretion, metabolic abnormalities may be exacerbated in the presence of renal dysfunction. Identification of patients at risk and correction of volume depletion or azotemia may effectively reduce the risk of ATLS; chemotherapy should be delayed until metabolic disturbances such as azotemia are corrected. If ATLS is identified, the animal should be treated with aggressive crystalloid fluid therapy. Further chemotherapy should be withheld until the animal is clinically normal and all biochemical parameters are within normal limits.

Clinical Approach to Patients with Acute Tumor Lysis Syndrome

PROBLEM	APPROACH
1. Acute decompensation, shortly after chemotherapy	Evaluate the patient. Determine if tumor is responding rapidly. Do complete physical exam to evaluate for systemic disease, hydration status, and cardiac output. Rule in or out neutropenia, sepsis, coagulopathies, and organ failure with a hemogram, biochemical profile, urinalysis, and blood cultures.
2. Initiate specific support	Treat for shock, provide daily fluid needs, correct dehydration and electrolyte abnormalities, and compensate for external fluid losses. Consider non–lactate-containing fluids. In ATLS, 0.9% NaCl may be ideal until hyperkalemia and hyperphosphatemia are corrected. Some suggest that daily fluid needs are approximately 66 ml/kg; others estimate needs as closer to [30(kg) + 70]. Fluids can be administered in acute shock or shocklike states at a rate of up to 60–90 ml/kg for the first hour, followed by 10 ml/kg/hr, with close monitoring to adjust fluid rate as needed. If hypocalcemia secondary to hyperphosphatemia causes clinically significant signs (rare), exogenous parenteral calcium supplementation may be indicated.
3. Monitor patient	Monitor hydration, electrolytes, renal and cardiovascular function. Rate of fluid administration must be fine-tuned based on hydration, cardiovascular, renal, and electrolyte status.
4. Delay chemotherapy	Additional chemotherapy is withheld pending patient recovery.

From Ogilvie GK, Moore AS: Managing the Veterinary Cancer Patient: A Practice Manual. Veterinary Learning Systems, Trenton, NJ, 1995, with permission.

BIBLIOGRAPHY

1. Marcus SL, Einzig AI: Acute tumor lysis syndrome: Prevention and management. In Dutcher JP, Wiernik PH: Handbook of Hematologic and Oncologic Emergencies. New York, Plenum Press, 1987, pp 9–15.
2. Ogilvie GK, Moore AS: Acute tumor lysis syndrome. In Managing the Veterinary Cancer Patient: A Practice Manual. Trenton, NJ, Veterinary Learning Systems, 1995, pp 157–159.
3. Woodlock TJ: Oncologic emergencies. In Rosenthal S, Carignan JR, Smith BD (eds): Medical Care of the Cancer Patient. Philadelphia, W.B. Saunders, 1993, pp 236–246.

59. COAGULATION DISORDERS

Gregory K. Ogilvie, D.V.M.

1. What coagulation disorders occur in animals with cancer?

Disorders of hemostasis are a common cause of morbidity and mortality in animals and humans with cancer and may be loosely categorized as follows:

- Disseminated intravascular coagulopathy (DIC)
- Malignancy-associated fibrinolysis
- Platelet abnormalities
- Clinical syndrome of the hypercoagulable state of malignancy (e.g., hemangiosarcoma)
- Chemotherapy-associated thromboembolism (e.g., L-asparaginase, prednisone)

2. What is disseminated intravascular coagulation?

DIC is a consumptive coagulopathy that often is life-threatening. It should be considered an emergency and should be diagnosed and treated as soon as possible. DIC has been associated with several of the parameters noted above and occurs with many malignancies. The malignancy sometimes induces DIC when clotting factors are activated by tumor-induced procoagulants or when the tumor directly or indirectly stimulates platelet aggregation. The resultant formation of clots in the circulation consumes clotting factors and platelets and subsequently leads to widespread bleeding. In addition, deposition of fibrin throughout the body may result in concurrent microangiographic hemolytic anemia. To reduce morbidity and mortality, DIC must be identified and treated early. Best results are seen when at-risk patients are identified and supported with fluids and monitored for clotting coagulation disorders.

3. What factors predispose to coagulation defects?

DIC occurs with a wide variety of malignant conditions, including hemangiosarcoma, lymphoma, thyroid carcinoma, and inflammatory carcinoma. Treatment with chemotherapeutic agents or surgery or concurrent infection may induce or exacerbate DIC. Renal failure and loss of low-molecular-weight coagulation factors through glomeruli also may increase the risk of coagulation abnormalities. Thrombosis with or without DIC has been identified in dogs with hyperadrenocorticism and in dogs treated with high doses of glucocorticoids. The syndrome has been identified in dogs more often than in cats.

4. What is the best way to diagnose DIC?

Clinical signs supportive of a diagnosis of DIC include but are not limited to oozing from venipuncture sites, nosebleeds, oral bleeding, melena, ecchymoses and petechial hemorrhages anywhere on the body, and hematuria. Widespread thrombosis may cause multiorgan failure that results in various clinical signs, such as acute renal failure and acute onset of respiratory distress. The key is to identify the problem early in an emergency setting and to initiate therapy while the condition is clinically silent or before clinical signs become serious.

5. What laboratory abnormalities are associated with DIC?

Laboratory abnormalities associated with DIC vary, depending on the organs involved and whether the DIC is acute or chronic; the chronic form of DIC is rarely associated with clinical signs. In addition, red blood cell fragmentation may result from microangiographic events that are seen in DIC. Diagnosis is based on clinical findings and an elevated prothrombin time (PT), activated partial thromboplastin time (APTT), thrombocytopenia, prolonged activated clotting time (ACT), decreased antithrombin III concentrations, hypofibrinogenemia, and increased fibrin degradation products. Many emergency facilities routinely screen patients for DIC by performing ACTs.

Clinical and Laboratory Parameters Used to Diagnose
Disseminated Intravascular Coagulopathy

TESTS/OBSERVATIONS	ACUTE DIC	CHRONIC DIC
Clinical signs	Clinically evident coagulopathies	Few clinical signs evident
Onset and duration	Rapid onset, quick progression	Insidious, prolonged
Prothrombin time, activated partial thromboplastin time, activated clotting time	Prolonged	Normal to slightly decreased
Platelets	Decreased	Often normal
Fibrin degradation products	Very high	High
Fibrinogen	Decreased to normal	Normal
Antithrombin III	Reduced	Normal
Prognosis	Grave	Good

6. What are the causes of the coagulation disorders associated with DIC?

There are many causes for DIC-associated abnormalities. In each patient, identifying and specifically treating the underlying cause are the keys to successful treatment. Decreased platelet count may be caused by bone marrow failure, increased platelet consumption, or splenic pooling of platelets. Prolonged PT may be due to lack of one or more of the following clotting factors: X, VII, V, II (prothrombin), and I (fibrinogen). Increased APTT may be caused by a deficiency in one or more of the following clotting factors: XII, XI, IX, X, VIII, V, II, and I. Heparin and oral anticoagulant therapy prolong the APTT. Low fibrinogen levels are associated with decreased production or increased consumption of this protein.

7. What is the best treatment for DIC?

Specific treatment for DIC is controversial, but certain procedures are uniformly accepted despite the fact that few data document their efficacy. As mentioned earlier, the most important therapy for DIC is treatment of the underlying cause. Fluid therapy is essential to correct volume contraction and to reduce the possibility of ensuring renal failure and acid-base abnormalities. Increases in body weight, heart and respiratory rates, and central venous pressure may suggest volume overload. Volume overload is especially threatening when the patient is anuric secondary to acute renal shutdown.

In animals with a severe bleeding diathesis, fresh blood or plasma with clotting factors and platelets may be useful for replacing components of the blood that are consumed. If thrombosis appears to be the most clinically evident problem, heparin therapy may reduce the formation of thrombi. The amount of heparin to be used is controversial. One method is to administer heparin by intermittent subcutaneous or intravenous dosages or by constant-rate infusion to prolong the APTT by 1.5–2 times. Minidose heparin therapy (5–10 IU/kg/hr by constant-rate infusion or 75 IU/kg every 8 hours subcutaneously) may be helpful in some cases. Ten IU/kg SQ daily is also used by some.

Chemotherapeutic agents, including prednisone, should be withheld until all evidence of DIC is eliminated and the patient has recovered completely. Dogs and possibly cats that receive glucocorticoid therapy are at major risk for thromboembolic events that can initiate or perpetuate DIC.

Animals with acute DIC have a poor prognosis; therefore, identification of patients at high risk and prophylactic treatment are of great value. Routine monitoring of ACTs and platelet counts can identify animals in the early phases of DIC.

BIBLIOGRAPHY

1. Ogilvie GK, Moore AS: Disseminated intravascular coagulation. In Managing the Veterinary Cancer Patient: A Practice Manual. Trenton, NJ, Veterinary Learning Systems, 1995, pp 160–162.
2. Parry BW: Laboratory evaluation of hemorrhagic coagulopathies in small animal practice. Vet Clin North Am 4:729–742, 1989.
3. Smith MR: Disorders of hemostasis and transfusion therapy. In Skeel RT (ed): Handbook of Cancer Chemotherapy, 3rd ed. Boston, Little, Brown, 1991, pp 449–459.
4. Woodlock TJ: Oncologic emergencies. In Rosenthal S, Carignan JR, Smith BD (eds): Medical Care of the Cancer Patient. Philadelphia, W.B. Saunders, 1993, pp 236–246.

60. METABOLIC EMERGENCIES IN PATIENTS WITH CANCER

Gregory K. Ogilvie, D.V.M.

1. What are the most common metabolic emergencies in patients with cancer?

• Hypercalcemia (most common)
• Hypoglycemia (may result in nonspecific clinical signs and delayed diagnosis)
• Hyponatremia (underrecognized emergency)

HYPERCALCEMIA

2. What are the most common cancers associated with hypercalcemia of malignancy?

Lymphoma is the number-one cause of hypercalcemia in dogs and therefore should be eliminated as a diagnosis if a more obvious cause of hypercalcemia is not readily apparent. Other causes include apocrine gland/anal sac adenocarcinoma, mammary adenocarcinoma, and primary hyperparathyroidism. Parathyroid carcinomas and adenomas are rare malignancies, but intractable hypercalcemia may be caused by elevated parathormone levels.

3. What is the most common mechanism associated with hypercalcemia of nonparathyroid malignancies?

A parathormone-related peptide (PTH-rp) is most commonly associated with hypercalcemia of malignancy in dogs. Although it has been suggested that bone metastases may be associated with hypercalcemia, this mechanism is rare in veterinary medicine.

4. What are the most common clinical findings in animals with hypercalcemia of malignancy?

The oncologic emergency secondary to hypercalcemia of malignancy revolves around clinical signs associated with decreased sensitivity of the distal convoluted tubules and collecting ducts to antidiuretic hormone (ADH) and the vasoconstrictive properties of calcium, with decreases in renal blood flow and glomerular filtration rate. The epithelium undergoes degenerative changes, necrosis, and calcification. Progressive renal disease is noted clinically as polyuria and polydipsia, followed by vomiting, hyposthenuria, and dehydration. Calcium also may affect the gastrointestinal, cardiovascular, and neurologic systems directly and cause anorexia, vomiting, constipation, bradycardia, hypertension, skeletal muscle weakness, depression, stupor, coma, and seizures.

5. What other common differential diagnoses must be considered in dogs with hypercalcemia?

Other diagnoses that must be considered when an animal is evaluated for true hypercalcemia ($Ca^{++} > 12$ mg/dl) include laboratory error, error in interpretation (e.g., young growing dogs), hyperproteinemia from dehydration, acute renal failure, vitamin D and calcium toxicosis, granulomatous disorders, nonneoplastic disorders of bone, hypoadrenocorticism, true hyperparathyroidism, and chronic disuse osteoporosis.

6. Does serum protein or albumin influence serum calcium values?

Yes, in both cases. It is important to interpret calcium in relation to serum albumin and blood pH. The following correction formula for dogs takes albumin into account:

$$\text{Adjusted calcium (mg/dl)} = [\text{calcium (mg/dl)} - \text{albumin (gm/dl)}] + 3.5$$

Acidosis results in an increase in the free, ionized fraction of calcium and may magnify the observed clinical signs associated with hypocalcemia. Whenever possible, an ionized calcium value should be obtained so that the biologically active form of calcium can be assessed. The serum sample is taken anaerobically with a heparinized syringe. The blood in the heparinized syringe can then be placed on ice for subsequent analysis. An ionized calcium value does not have to be corrected for albumin or protein.

7. What is the ideal diagnostic plan for hypercalcemic animals?

All hypercalcemic patients should have serial serum calcium measurements and assessment of electrolytes, blood urea nitrogen, and creatinine levels. Elevated immunoreactive parathormone levels in association with hyperphosphatemia may suggest ectopic hormone production. Patients with multiple myeloma may have elevated calcium levels secondary to abnormal calcium binding to a paraprotein without elevation of ionized calcium, and malnourished patients with hypoalbuminemia may have symptoms of hypercalcemia with normal serum calcium levels.

8. What intravenous fluids should be used to treat hypercalcemic animals?

Treatment of an emergency secondary to hypercalcemia depends on the severity of clinical signs and presence of renal disease. Treatment entails use of intravenous 0.9% saline in volumes that exceed daily maintenance requirements. Many sources suggest that this amount of fluid is equal to or greater than 132 ml/kg$^{0.75}$/day (or approximately > 66 ml/kg/day plus exogenous losses from vomiting and diarrhea) plus replacement replacement fluids for dehydration. More recent data suggest that the correct amount of fluid is a more conservative [30(kg) + 70]. Potassium depletion should be prevented by addition of potassium chloride (KCl) to fluids based on serum potassium levels.

9. How should potassium depletion be treated?

Intravenous Potassium Supplementation to Correct Hypokalemia

SERUM POTASSIUM (mEq/L)	KCl ADDED TO EACH LITER OF FLUID (mEq)	MAXIMAL RATE OF INFUSION (ML/KG/HR)
< 2	80	6
2.1–2.5	60	8
2.6–3.0	40	12
3.1–3.5	28	16

When potassium is administered intravenously, the rate should not exceed 0.5 mEq/kg/hr. In addition, the patient should be watched carefully for signs consistent with overhydration and congestive heart failure, and effective antitumor therapy should be initiated as soon as possible.

10. How can drugs be used to treat patients with hypercalcemia?

Furosemide (1–4 mg/kg 2 times/day, IV or orally) and intravenous biphosphonates (e.g., etidronate, disodium palmidroate) also may be used in addition to saline diuresis. Intravenous biphosphonates have rapid hypocalcemic effects; they inhibit osteoclast activity.

Gallium nitrate produces concentration-dependent reduction in osteolytic response to parathormone and certain other types of lymphokines that cause hypercalcemia. Gallium nitrate infused at doses of approximately 100 mg/m^2 daily for 5 consecutive days successfully reduces high calcium levels in 86% of human patients.

Mithramycin, a chemotherapeutic agent that decreases bone resorption by reducing osteoclast number and activity, also has been shown to be effective in people. Because mithramycin is a sclerosing agent, it must be given as a bolus (25 µg/kg IV once or twice weekly) through a newly placed intravenous line. If extravasation occurs, ulceration and fibrosis will develop. Mithramycin has not been used extensively in dogs or cats; in refractory patients, it may require twice-weekly dosing.

Salmon calcitonin (4–8 MRC U/kg SQ) also may be used in refractory patients. Calcitonin inhibits bone resorption and thus causes a fall in serum calcium levels within hours of administration. When administered at approximately 40 U/kg, salmon calcitonin may result in hypocalcemia for several days.

Corticosteroids are effective for treatment of hypercalcemia. Corticosteroids block bone resorption caused by osteoclast-activating factor, increase urinary calcium excretion, inhibit vitamin D metabolism, and increase calcium absorption after long-term use. To be effective, high doses are generally required for several days. Steroids should not be used until tissue diagnosis is made, primarily because lymphomas are the primary cause of malignancy-associated hypercalcemia.

Most patients are effectively managed with hydration, mobilization, antitumor therapy, and treatment with hypocalcemia-inducing agents such as mithramycin, calcitonin, or corticosteroids. Serum calcium should be monitored at least twice weekly.

11. What drugs or vitamins are contraindicated in hypercalcemic animals?
Thiazide diuretics or vitamin A and D (which may elevate calcium levels) should not be used in hypercalcemic animals.

HYPOGLYCEMIA

12. What tumors are most commonly associated with hypoglycemia?
Fasting hypoglycemia in the face of hyperinsulinemia occurs most commonly with insulinomas; however, other tumors of the liver (e.g., hepatomas, carcinomas) also have been associated with hypoglycemia.

13. What other diagnoses are associated with hypoglycemia?
Liver disease (including glycogen storage diseases and sepsis) may mimic hypoglycemia of malignancy. In addition, because red blood cells metabolize glucose rapidly, delay in separating red blood cells from the serum may lead to spurious results.

14. What are the most common clinical signs associated with malignancy-induced hypoglycemia?
Before presenting with seizures, coma, and impending death, most animals have a history of fatigue, weakness, dizziness, and confusion associated with paroxysmal lowering of the blood glucose levels. Hypoglycemic dogs with neurologic signs present like any other patient with a central nervous system abnormality, such as brain tumor, brain trauma, meningitis, or metabolic encephalopathy.

15. What is the best diagnostic plan to confirm the presence of malignancy-associated hypoglycemia and to identify the underlying cause?
Insulin-producing tumors can be diagnosed by identifying elevated insulin levels in association with low blood glucose concentrations. In some cases, the identification of malignancy-associated hypoglycemia may require periodic sampling during a 72-hour fast. The diagnosis is made when the blood glucose is dramatically reduced but insulin levels are elevated. Although controversial, the amended insulin:glucose ratio has been advocated as a method to help diagnose insulin-producing tumors in domestic animals:

$$\frac{\text{Serum insulin } (\mu\text{U/ml} \times 100)}{\text{Serum glucose (mg/dl)} - 30} = \text{amended insulin:glucose ratio}$$

Values above 30 suggest a diagnosis of insulinoma or other insulin-producing tumor.

16. What is the treatment plan for animals with hypoglycemia of malignancy?

In an emergency setting, medical management is often necessary before, during, and after definitive therapy, especially in cases of insulinomas, which have a high metastatic rate. Glucose-containing fluids (2.5–5% dextrose in 0.9% NaCl or other isotonic crystalloid solution) should be administered to meet fluid requirements and to maintain blood glucose concentrations within acceptable limits. The administration of glucose, however, may trigger the tumor to release more insulin; therefore, a constant infusion of glucose to maintain normal serum glucose levels is preferred to intermittent high-dose bolusing.

Prednisone (0.5–2 mg/kg divided into 2 oral doses/day) is often effective in elevating blood glucose levels by inducing hepatic gluconeogenesis and decreasing peripheral utilization of glucose.

Diazoxide (10–40 mg/kg divided into 2 oral doses/day) may be effective in elevating blood glucose levels by directly inhibiting pancreatic insulin secretion and glucose uptake by tissues, enhancing epinephrine-induced glycogenolysis, and increasing the rate of mobilization of fatty acids. The hyperglycemic effects of diazoxide can be potentiated by concurrent administration of hydrochlorothiazide (2–4 mg/kg/day orally)

Propranolol (10–40 mg/kg 3 times/day orally), a β-adrenergic blocking agent, also may be effective in increasing blood glucose levels by inhibition of insulin release through the blockade of β-adrenergic receptors at the level of the pancreatic beta cell, inhibition of insulin release by membrane stabilization, and alteration of peripheral insulin receptor affinity.

Combined surgical and medical management of pancreatic tumors has been associated with remission times of 1 year or more. Once the patient is stable, surgical extirpation may be the treatment of choice for tumors that cause hypoglycemia. Because many tumors (including insulinomas) that induce hypoglycemia as a paraneoplastic syndrome are malignant, surgery alone often is not curative. In the case of insulinomas, partial pancreatectomy may be indicated; iatrogenic pancreatitis and diabetes mellitus are recognized complications.

HYPONATREMIA

17. What is the most common cause of hyponatremia that leads to an emergency?

An emergency condition related to the syndrome of inappropriate antidiuretic hormone secretion (SIADH) is a rare but underrecognized cause of true hyponatremia in patients with cancer.

18. What is SIADH?

SIADH is the presence of excessive quantities of antidiuretic hormone secondary to malignancy. The affected animal has low plasma osmolality despite inappropriate urine concentration (high sodium). Because this situation also may occur in renal disease, hypothyroidism, and adrenal insufficiency, these disorders must be excluded to confirm the diagnosis of SIADH.

19. What factors predispose an animal to hyponatremia due to SIADH?

The condition may be caused by a cancer or a drug that results in renal activation or enhanced release of antidiuretic hormone. SIADH has been identified in dogs with lymphoma. Drugs in veterinary medicine that may cause SIADH include but are not limited to chlorpropamide, vincristine, vinblastine, cyclophosphamide, opiates, thiazide diuretics, barbiturates, and isoproterenol.

20. What clinical signs are most commonly seen in animals with SIADH and hyponatremia?

When hyponatremia develops rapidly or sodium falls below 115 mg/dl, patients may develop mental status abnormalities, confusion, or coma. With profound hyponatremia, seizures also may occur. Serum and urine electrolytes, osmolality, and creatinine should be measured in suspect cases.

21. What is the best diagnostic plan to confirm SIADH?

The diagnosis of SIADH is initially made by the combination of hyponatremia on the biochemical profile and clinical signs. The diagnosis of SIADH is often missed. SIADH is associated with inappropriate sodium concentration in the urine for the level of hyponatremia in the serum. Urine osmolality is greater than plasma osmolality, but the urine specific gravity is not maximally dilute. With SIADH the urea nitrogen values in the serum are usually low because of volume expansion. Hypophosphatemia also may be noted. Adrenal and thyroid function should be normal.

22. What is the best treatment for animals with SIADH?

Initial treatment should be directed at resolution of the hyponatremia in an emergency setting. Fluids should be restricted to ensure that the patient receives only the amount needed to maintain normal hydration and to keep serum sodium concentration within normal levels. In an emergency setting, demeclocycline may correct hyponatremia to reduce ADH stimulus for free water reabsorption at the collecting ducts. The most common side effects of demeclocycline are nausea and vomiting. Lithium carbonate and phenytoin also have some use in treatment of SIADH. Hypertonic sodium chloride (3–5%) also may be used in an emergency situation; however, if not used carefully, it may result in fluid and circulatory overload. Furosemide may be used concurrently with the hypertonic saline to reduce volume overload. Rapid correction of hyponatremia may lead to neurologic damage. The following formula may help to determine approximate amounts of sodium to administer for correction of hyponatremia:

$$\text{Na for replacement (mEq)} = [\text{desired serum sodium (mEq/L)} - \text{observed serum sodium (mEq/L)}] \times \text{observed serum sodium (mEq/L)} \times \text{body weight (kg)} \times 0.6$$

BIBLIOGRAPHY

1. Besarb A, Caro JF: Mechanisms of hypercalcemia in malignancy. Cancer 41:2276–2285, 1978.
2. Felds ALA, Jese RG, Bergaagel DE: Metabolic emergencies. In DeVita VT, Hellman S, Rosenberg SA (eds): Cancer Principles and Practice of Oncology. Philadelphia, J.B. Lippincott, 1985, pp 1874–1876.
3. Franco-Saenz R: Endocrine syndromes. In Skeel RT (ed): Handbook of Cancer Chemotherapy. Boston, Little, Brown, 1991, pp 379–404.
4. Giger U, Gorman NT: Acute complications of cancer and cancer therapy. In Gorman NT (ed): Oncology. New York, Churchill Livingstone, 1986, pp 147–168.
5. Glover JH, Glick JH: Oncologic emergencies and special complications. In Calabrese P, Schein PJ, Rosenberg SA (eds): Medical Oncology: Basic Principles and Clinical Management of Cancer. New York, MacMillan, 1985, pp 1261–1326.
6. Kruger JM, Osborne CA, Polzin DJ: Treatment of hypercalcemia. In Kirk RW (ed): Current Veterinary Therapy IX. Philadelphia, W.B. Saunders, 1986, pp 75–90.
7. Leifer CE, Peterson ME, Matus RE, Patnaik AK: Hypoglycemia associated with nonislet cell tumors in 13 dogs. J Am Vet Med Assoc 186:53–62, 1985.
8. Meuten DJ: Hypercalcemia. Vet Clin North Am 14:891–899, 1984.
9. Ogilvie GK, Moore AS: Metabolic emergencies: Hypercalcemia, hyponatremia, and hypoglycemia. In Managing the Veterinary Cancer Patient: A Practice Manual. Trenton, NJ, Veterinary Learning Systems, 1995, pp 169–174.
10. Weir EC, Burtis WJ, Morris CA, et al: Isolation of a 16,000-dalton parathyroid hormone-like protein from two animal tumors causing humoral hypercalcemia of malignancy. Endocrinology 123:2744–2755, 1988.
11. Weir EC, Nordin RW, Matus RE, et al: Humoral hypercalcemia of malignancy in canine lymphosarcoma. Endocrinology 122:602–610, 1988.

61. CANCER TREATMENT-INDUCED CONGESTIVE HEART FAILURE

Gregory K. Ogilvie, D.V.M.

1. What chemotherapeutic agent is most commonly associated with development of cardiac disease?

Cardiac disease secondary to anthracycline or anthracyclinelike drugs is relatively common in dogs and may be life-threatening. Doxorubicin is the anthracycline commonly associated with development of cardiac disease. Cardiomyopathy is more common in pets that receive more than 8 standard doses of doxorubicin. Doxorubicin-induced cardiomyopathy is uncommon in cats.

2. What are the most common cardiac abnormalities associated with doxorubicin-induced heart disease?

Doxorubicin is associated with development of tachyarrhythmias and dilatative cardiomyopathy. Cardiomyopathy may occur in response to administration of any number of doses of doxorubicin, but the risk increases significantly after a dog receives a total cumulative dose exceeding 240 mg/m². The risk in cats appears to be minimal; however, histologic abnormalities have been found in cats that were given total cumulative doses between 130–320 mg/m².

3. Can radiation induce heart disease?

Yes. Radiation also can induce cardiomyopathy if the heart is in the radiation therapy field and if high enough doses are used. Histologic and clinically significant pericardial effusion develops approximately 3 months after completion of a 3-week radiation schedule. Radiation may include thinning of the myocardium and significant amounts of fibrosis 1 year after treatment.

4. What predisposing factors are associated with development of doxorubicin-induced cardiac disease?

Doxorubicin-induced cardiac disease may occur more frequently in animals with preexisting cardiac disease and in animals that cannot metabolize or eliminate the drug adequately after administration. Similarly, rapid infusion of the drug, which establishes high serum concentrations, may increase the prevalence of cardiac disease. Therefore, increased time for infusion of a dose of doxorubicin may reduce the prevalence of acute and chronic cardiac disease.

5. What are the most common clinical signs of doxorubicin-induced cardiomyopathy?

In an animal with cardiomyopathy and fulminant congestive heart failure, clinical signs vary from anorexia, lethargy, and weakness to more common signs associated specifically with decreased cardiac output and ensuing congestive heart failure. Owners may complain that their pet has exercise intolerance; coughing spells late at night, which may develop into a persistent cough at all times of day; abdominal distention; increased respiratory effort and rate; and generalized malaise.

The physical examination is helpful and may include identification of a jugular pulse, rapid heart and respiratory rates, ascites, cool extremities, cyanotic mucous membranes, delayed capillary refill, pitting edema of lower extremities, enlarged liver and spleen, and rapid, weak pulses. The chest may sound dull because of pleural effusion, or pulmonary edema may cause crackling lung sounds. Heart murmurs or an abnormal rhythm is frequently auscultated; the heart sounds in dogs with atrial fibrillation may sound like jungle drums (i.e., irregularly irregular) on auscultation. Electrocardiography may suggest heart chamber enlargement or reveal arrhythmias, which may be supraventricular or ventricular in origin.

6. What are the most rewarding tests for diagnosis of doxorubicin-induced cardiac disease?

In a recent study, 32 of 175 dogs treated with doxorubicin developed clinically evident cardiac disease. Thirty-one had electrocardiographic abnormalities, including arrhythmias (premature atrial complexes, atrial fibrillation, paroxysmal atrial and sinus tachycardia, ventricular arrhythmias, bundle branch blocks, atrioventricular dissociation) and nonspecific alterations in R wave, ST segment, or QRS durations. Seven dogs had overt congestive heart failure that resulted in death within 90 days despite supportive therapy. Arrhythmias may occur at the time of treatment or within a variable period after treatment is complete. In people with doxorubicin-induced cardiac diseases, significant dysrhythmias often are present without other physical or historical abnormalities.

Chest and abdominal radiographs are valuable in identifying evidence of cardiac disease, including pericardial or pleural effusions; enlargement of the heart, liver, spleen, and pulmonary veins; and pulmonary edema, which usually is first noted around the hilar region. Echocardiography is extremely valuable for confirmation of pericardial effusion and documentation of chamber size, myocardial wall thickness, and parameters such as ejection fraction, cardiac output, and contractility. Blood pressure measurements may assist in documentation of hyper- or hypotension. An elevated central venous pressure aids diagnosis of cardiac insufficiency. Finally, more specific tests may further clarify a diagnosis of drug- or radiation-induced cardiac disease. Examples include fluid analysis of thoracic or abdominal effusion (usually a modified transudate with reactive mesothelial cells and macrophages) and contrast radiography. Unfortunately, no evaluation can be performed routinely in veterinary practice to predict whether cardiotoxicity will occur in dogs that receive anthracycline agents or radiation therapy. This precludes withdrawal of therapy before overt signs of cardiac insufficiency occur. In people, nuclear medicine imaging techniques may be able to predict the development of doxorubicin cardiomyopathy before it becomes clinically evident.

7. If doxorubicin-induced cardiomyopathy is identified, can doxorubicin treatment be reinitiated in the future?

The simple answer is no. Work at Colorado State University suggests that development of cardiomyopathy may be associated with a profound decrease in contractility without substantial alterations in quality of life. Once alterations in cardiovascular performance are documented, the administration of doxorubicin should be discontinued indefinitely. The important lesson from these data is that the animal's quality of life rather than results of diagnostic tests should dictate whether therapy should be initiated.

8. How does one prevent doxorubicin-induced cardiac disease (other than not giving the drug)?

The hallmark of doxorubicin-induced heart disease is development of dilatative cardiomyopathy. Many methods to prevent its development have been explored. Vitamin E, thyroxine, and selenium treatments are ineffective for prevention of cardiomyopathy. In people, low-dose doxorubicin therapy reduces the prevalence of cardiomyopathy. The compound ICRF-187 is more effective; it substantially reduces the occurrence of cardiomyopathy in dogs treated concurrently with doxorubicin.

9. What is the preferred treatment for dogs with anthracycline-induced cardiomyopathy?

Treatment of cardiomyopathy begins with indefinite discontinuation of the inciting cause (e.g., radiation or doxorubicin). Evidence suggests that in some humans with doxorubicin-induced cardiomyopathy clinical signs gradually resolve and cardiac function improves. Studies are needed to determine whether this is also true in pets. Diuretics, a low salt diet, rest, oxygen therapy, positive inotropes, and vasodilators should be used as dictated by the clinical status of the patient. For example, furosemide may be used 2–3 times/day in a compensated animal, whereas in a patient in respiratory distress from severe, fulminant pulmonary edema, it may be used every few hours, if necessary. Digoxin, a positive inotrope, may be given orally or parenterally in combination with a preload or afterload reducer; therapeutic levels of digoxin, when given orally, are generally not achieved for a few days, which may be adequate for an animal that is relatively stable. Factors such as dehydration and electrolyte disturbances may promote development of digoxin toxicoses. Because digoxin toxicity is a serious problem that occurs frequently, intravenous loading doses should not be used unless absolutely necessary. Regardless of the method of digitalization, periodic determination of serum digoxin concentrations is essential for adjustment of drug dosage to maintain therapeutic levels.

In an acutely decompensated, dying dog with cardiomyopathy, a constant-rate infusion of dobutamine combined with intravenous furosemide and an intravenous (e.g., nitroprusside) or transdermal (e.g., 2% nitroglycerin, enalapril) pre- or afterload reducer may be more logical than oral treatment. The dobutamine may increase cardiac output within minutes to hours compared with days before improvement of cardiac output with oral digoxin therapy. More detailed treatment of cardiomyopathy is outlined in the table below.

Therapeutic Approach for Dog or Cat with Drug- or Radiation-induced Dilatative Cardiomyopathy

GENERAL PRINCIPLE	SPECIFIC DETAILS, DRUG DOSAGES, AND TOXICITIES
1. Discontinue cardiotoxic agents.	All cardiotoxic drugs should be discontinued indefinitely. Additional radiation therapy to the heart should be avoided.
2. Enforce complete rest.	Avoidance of excitement is essential. Consider cage rest in or out of an oxygen-enriched environment.
3. Oxygenate.	Acquire and maintain a patent airway. Provide supplemental oxygen if needed; 50% oxygen should not be used for more than 24 hr to avoid pulmonary toxicity. Perform thoracocentesis to reduce pleural effusion. Initiate diuretic therapy for pulmonary edema (see below).
4. Reduce pulmonary edema.	Furosemide (drug of choice; monitor for dehydration, hypokalemia) Dogs: 2–4 mg/kg IV or IM every 2–12 hr, depending on severity of edema; decrease to 1–4 mg/kg 1–3 times/day orally for maintenance therapy. Cats: 1–2 mg/kg IV or IM every 4–12 hr, depending on severity of edema; decrease to 1–2 mg/kg 1–3 times/day orally for maintenance therapy. Hydrochlorothiazide/spironolactone combination (use with furosemide or as maintenance therapy; monitor for dehydration, electrolyte abnormalities) Dogs: 2–4 mg/kg orally twice daily. Cats: 1–2 mg/kg orally twice daily.
5. Increase contractility.	Perform pericardiocentesis if pericardial effusion is present in significant amounts to reduce contractility. Digoxin (monitor blood levels to acquire and maintain therapeutic blood levels [1–2 ng/ml]; watch for anorexia, vomiting, diarrhea, and EKG abnormalities suggestive of digoxin toxicity): Dogs: < 22 kg, 0.011 mg/kg orally twice daily; > 22 kg, 0.22 mg/m² orally twice daily. Cats: < 3 kg, ¼ of 0.125 mg tablet every other day; 3–6 kg, ¼ of 0.125 mg tablet daily. Dobutamine (monitor for tachycardia and arrhythmias): Dogs and cats: 1–10 µg/kg/min constant-rate infusion, usually in combination with pre- or afterload reducer and furosemide in severe, fulminant congestive heart failure. Milrinone (monitor for GI toxicity, hypotension): Dogs and cats: 0.5–1 mg/kg orally twice daily.

Table continued on next page.

Therapeutic Approach for Dog or Cat with Drug- or Radiation-induced Dilatative
Cardiomyopathy (Continued)

GENERAL PRINCIPLE	SPECIFIC DETAILS, DRUG DOSAGES, AND TOXICITIES
6. Redistribute blood volume.	Vasodilators 2% nitroglycerin ointment; watch for hypotension. Dogs: $\frac{1}{4}$–$\frac{3}{4}$ inch on skin or in ear 4 times/day Cats: $\frac{1}{8}$–$\frac{1}{4}$ inch on skin or in ear 4 times/day Sodium nitroprusside (5–20 µg/kg/min constant-rate infusion); watch for hypotension; prolonged use may result in cyanide toxicity. Miscellaneous: Morphine for dogs only (0.05–0.5 mg/kg IV, IM, or SQ) to reduce apprehension and to redistribute blood volume.
7. Reduce afterload.	Enalapril: dogs and cats: 0.25–0.5 mg/kg orally once or twice daily (do not use in conjunction with nitroprusside; monitor for hypotension). Hydralazine: dogs: 0.5–2 mg/kg orally twice daily (do not use in conjunction with nitroprusside; monitor for hypotension).
8. Control arrhythmias.	See following table.
9. Monitor response to therapy.	Pulse, respiratory rate, EKG, body weight, central venous pressure, urine output, hydration, electrolytes, blood urea nitrogen, creatinine, blood gases, quality of life. Adjust therapy as indicated.

From Ogilvie GK, Moore AS: Managing the Veterinary Cancer Patient: A Practice Manual. Veterinary Learning Systems, Trenton, NJ, 1995, with permission.

Arrhythmias may occur during infusion of a chemotherapeutic agent. If they persist, interfere with an animal's quality of life, or serve as a serious threat to survival, therapy should be instituted and the underlying cause identified and eliminated. In each case, the potential adverse effects of the antiarrhythmic agents must be evaluated and considered before therapy is initiated.

Drugs Used to Treat Supraventricular and Ventricular Arrhythmias Induced by Anthracycline
Antibiotics or Radiation Therapy

DRUG	SPECIFIC DETAILS, DRUG DOSAGES, AND TOXICITIES
Bradyarrhythmias	
Atropine (sinus bradycardia, sinoatrial arrest, atrioventricular [AV] block)	Dogs and cats: 0.01–0.02 mg/kg IV; 0.02–0.04 mg/kg SQ; short-acting. (Monitor for sinus tachycardia, paradoxic vagomimetic effects.)
Glycopyrrolate (sinus bradycardia, sinoatrial arrest)	Dogs and cats: 0.005–0.01 mg/kg IV; 0.01–0.02 mg/kg SQ. (Monitor for sinus tachycardia, paradoxic vagomimetic effects.)
Isoproterenol (sinus bradycardia, sinoatrial arrest, complete AV block	Dogs: 1 mg in 250 ml 5% dextrose; administer IV at rate of 0.01 µg/kg/min. Cats: 0.5 mg in 250 ml 5% dextrose; administer IV to effect. (Monitor for CNS stimulation, arrhythmias, emesis.)
Tachyarrhythmias	
Digoxin (supraventricular premature complexes, supraventricular tachycardia, atrial fibrillation)	Dogs: < 22 kg, 0.011 mg/kg orally twice daily; > 22 kg, 0.22 mg/m^2 orally twice daily. Cats: < 3kg, $\frac{1}{4}$ of 0.125 mg tablet every other day; 3–6 kg, $\frac{1}{4}$ of 0.125 mg tablet daily. (Monitor blood levels to acquire and maintain therapeutic blood levels [1–2 ng/ml]; watch for anorexia, vomiting, diarrhea, and EKG abnormalities suggestive of digoxin toxicity.)

Table continued on next page.

Drugs Used to Treat Supraventricular and Ventricular Arrhythmias Induced by Anthracycline Antibiotics or Radiation Therapy (Continued)

DRUG	SPECIFIC DETAILS, DRUG DOSAGES, AND TOXICITIES
Lidocaine (premature ventricular contractions, ventricular tachycardia)	Dogs: 2–4 mg/kg IV slowly as bolus (maximum of 8 mg/kg) followed by 25–75 mg/kg/min constant-rate infusion. Cats: 0.25–1 mg/kg IV over 4–5 minutes. (Monitor for CNS excitation, seizures, vomiting, emesis, lethargy, arrhythmias.)
Tocainide (premature ventricular contractions, ventricular tachycardia)	Dogs: 5–20 mg/kg 3 or 4 times/day orally. (Monitor for CNS signs or GI toxicity.)
Procainamide (premature ventricular contractions, ventricular tachycardia)	Dogs: 20–40 mg/kg 4 times/day orally, IM; 8–20 mg/kg IV; 25–50 µg/kg/min constant-rate infusion.
Propranolol (supraventricular premature complexes and tachyarrhythmias, atrial fibrillation, ventricular premature complexes)	Dogs and cats: 0.04–0.06 mg/kg IV slowly or 0.2–1.0 mg/kg orally 2 or 3 times/day, often in combination with digoxin for supraventricular arrhythmias. (Monitor for decreased contractility, bronchoconstriction.)
Diltiazem (supraventricular premature complexes and tachyarrhythmias, atrial fibrillation)	Dogs: 0.5–1.5 mg/kg 3 times/day orally. Cats: 1.75–2.4 mg/kg 2 or 3 times/day orally. (Monitor for bradyarrhythmias and hypotension.)

From Ogilvie GK, Moore AS: Managing the Veterinary Cancer Patient: A Practice Manual. Veterinary Learning Systems, Trenton, NJ, 1995, with permission.

BIBLIOGRAPHY

1. Cotter SM, Kanki PJ, Simon M: Renal disease in five tumor-bearing cats treated with Adriamycin. J Am Animal Hosp Assoc 21:405–411, 1985.
2. Couto CG: Management of complications of cancer chemotherapy. Vet Clin North Am 4:1037–1053, 1990.
3. Jakacki RI, Larsen RL, Barber G, et al: Comparison of cardiac function tests after anthracycline therapy in childhood. Cancer 72:2739–2745, 1993.
4. Maulin GE, Fox PR, Patnaik AK, et al: Doxorubicin-induced cardiotoxicosis: Clinical features of 32 dogs. J Vet Intern Med 6:82–88, 1992.
5. McChesney SL, Gillette EL, Powers BE: Radiation-induced cardiomyopathy in the dog. Radiat Res 113:120–132, 1988.
6. Ogilvie GK, Moore AS: Chemotherapy or radiation-induced congestive heart failure. In Managing the Veterinary Cancer Patient: A Practice Manual. Trenton, NJ, Veterinary Learning Systems, 1995, pp 175–181.

62. CHEMOTHERAPY-INDUCED ANAPHYLAXIS

Gregory K. Ogilvie, D.V.M.

1. What chemotherapeutic agent is most commonly associated with development of anaphylaxis?

L-Asparaginase is the drug most commonly associated with development of anaphylaxis, although anaphylaxis or an anaphylaxislike reaction may occur after administration of any drug. Anaphylaxis most commonly occurs within minutes to a few hours after administration of the inciting drug. Hypersensitivity reactions may occur with any drug, but they occur most commonly with doxorubicin, paclitaxel, and etoposide.

2. How common is anaphylaxis in dogs or cats receiving L-asparaginase?

L-Asparaginase is well known for inducing anaphylaxis, hemorrhagic pancreatitis, diabetes mellitus, and coagulopathies in dogs and people. In one study, 48% of dogs given L-asparaginase intraperitoneally developed adverse effects; 30% of these dogs exhibited signs of anaphylaxis, similar to reports in children that were given L-asparaginase intravenously. The same study showed that intramuscular administration completely eliminated signs associated with anaphylaxis but did not reduce remission rates. Dogs given L-asparaginase subcutaneously had a longer time until remission compared with dogs given the drug intramuscularly. Until more information is known, the drug should be given intramuscularly to minimize adverse effects and to maximize efficacy.

3. What is the mechanism of L-asparaginase-induced anaphylaxis?

L-Asparaginase-induced anaphylaxis and hypersensitivity are common because of enzyme immunogenicity. Anaphylaxis usually is caused by IgE-mediated mast cell degranulation; however, certain substances (e.g., bacterial and fungal cell walls) may trigger anaphylaxis by activating the alternate complement pathway. During activation of this alternate pathway, C3a and C5a are formed; both are potent anaphylatoxins capable of degranulating mast cells and basophils. Although the exact mechanism of L-asparaginase-induced anaphylaxis is largely unexplored in dogs, anaphylaxis in children with acute lymphoblastic leukemia is thought to be induced by complement activation due to formation of immune complexes of L-asparaginase and specific antibodies. Anaphylaxis usually occurs within seconds to minutes after administration of L-asparaginase.

4. What is the mechanism of action associated with anaphylaxis due to other chemotherapeutic agents?

The hypersensitivity reaction secondary to doxorubicin is thought to be related to mast cell degranulation. Cremophor El and polysorbate 80 carriers are responsible for the hypersensitivity reaction induced by paclitaxel and etoposide, respectively.

5. What predisposing factors are associated with chemotherapy-induced anaphylaxis?

One predisposing factor related to anaphylaxis secondary to L-asparaginase or other drug therapy is a history of prior exposure. Because L-asparaginase is a bacterial product that is ubiquitous in mammalian systems, prior exposure may be an uncontrollable risk factor. In addition, anaphylactic and hypersensitivity reactions are worse in animals with a prior condition such as atopy, which results in a build-up of mast cells and eosinophils before drug treatment. As mentioned earlier, the route of administration also may be a contributing factor to development of an anaphylactic or hypersensitivity reaction.

6. What are the best diagnostic methods for identifying chemotherapy-induced anaphylaxis?

The most common clinical signs of drug-induced anaphylaxis are acute collapse and cardiovascular failure, which lead to shock and death. The event usually occurs within minutes after parenteral injection of the offending drug, although some anaphylactic reactions have been reported hours to days after drug therapy. The patient generally is pale and weak, with bradycardia or tachycardia and rapid, thready pulse. Mucous membranes are generally pale to cyanotic. Peripheral extremities are often cool to the touch, and blood pressure is low.

Hypersensitivity reactions may result in profound pruritus during and after administration of the drug. Pruritus may result in head shaking and swelling of the ears, lips, paws, or near the vein or area being treated. The erythematous reaction usually lasts for the duration of treatment. Occasionally, the edematous and erythematous reaction may last for hours after treatment is finished.

7. Can chemotherapy-induced anaphylaxis be prevented?

Yes. For example, 81 dogs with histologically confirmed, measurable malignant tumors were used in a prospective study to determine the prevalence of anaphylaxis associated with intramuscular administration of 232 doses of L-asparaginase (10,000 U/m²). None of the dogs exhibited clinical signs associated with anaphylaxis. Therefore, to reduce the probability of anaphylaxis, L-asparaginase should be given IM rather than IV or interperitoneally. In addition, because L-asparaginase is a potent inducer of anaphylaxis, administration of a test dose is advised.

Hypersensitivity reactions secondary to the administration of doxorubicin can be eliminated almost completely by dilution in 250–500 ml of 0.9% NaCl and administration over 20–40 minutes. Hundreds of doses of doxorubicin have been administered at the Comparative Oncology Unit at Colorado State University, and only 1–3 dogs have shown hypersensitivity reactions. Some advocate pretreatment with diphenhydramine and glucocorticoids to reduce the prevalence of hypersensitivity reactions.

The reactions secondary to the carriers in paclitaxel and etoposide can be reduced by slowing the rate of infusion and by pretreatment with dexamethasone (1–2 mg/kg IV), diphenhydramine (2–4 mg/kg IM), and cimetidine (2–4 mg/kg IV slowly) 1 hour before infusion of the chemotherapeutic agent. If a reaction is noted, the infusion can be discontinued temporarily until the animal is more comfortable.

8. What is the treatment of chemotherapy-induced anaphylaxis?

Anaphylaxis is a potentially fatal condition and should be treated immediately with supportive care, fluids, glucocorticoids, H_1 receptor antagonists, and epinephrine. Treatment is detailed in the table below.

General Approach to Treatment of an Animal with Drug-induced Anaphylaxis

GENERAL PRINCIPLE	SPECIFIC DETAILS
1. Evaluate the patient.	Do physical examination; ascertain temporal relationship to drug treatment; discontinue drug infusion or injection indefinitely.
2. Ensure a patent airway and cardiac output.	Initiate CPR if indicated; establish airway; breathe for patient after endotracheal intubation; initiate cardiac compressions; initiate drug therapy.
3. Establish vascular access; initiate fluid and drug therapy	Establish indwelling IV catheter aseptically; initiate fluid therapy: For shock: ≤ 70–90 ml/kg for first hour followed by 10–12 ml/kg/hr; adjust as needed thereafter. Concurrently, initiate drug therapy: Dexamethasone NaPO₄ (2 mg/kg IV) Diphenhydramine (2–4 mg/kg IM; watch for toxicoses, especially in cats) Epinephrine (0.1–0.3 ml of a 1:1,000 solution IV or IM for severe reactions)

From Ogilvie GK, Moore AS: Managing the Veterinary Cancer Patient: A Practice Manual. Veterinary Learning Systems, Trenton, NJ, 1995, with permission.

Hypersensitivity reactions are treated by terminating drug therapy. Reactions usually subside within minutes. The patient can then be treated with H_1 receptor antagonists (see table) before reinitiating drug treatment at a much slower rate.

BIBLIOGRAPHY

1. Degen MA: Acute hypersensitivity reactions In Kirk RW (ed): Current Veterinary Therapy X. Philadelphia, W.B. Saunders, 1989, pp 537–542.
2. Fabry U, Korholz D, Jurgens H, et al: Anaphylaxis to L-asparaginase during treatment for acute lymphoblastic leukemia in children. Evidence of a complement-mediated mechanism. Pediatr Res 19:400–408, 1985.

3. Nesbit M, Chard R, Evans A, et al: Evaluation of intramuscular versus intravenous administration of L-as-paraginase in childhood leukemia. Am J Pediatr Hematol Oncol 1:9–13, 1979.
4. Ogilvie GK, Atwater SW, Ciekot PA, et al: Prevalence of anaphylaxis associated with the intramuscular administration of L-asparaginase to 81 dogs with cancer: 1989–1991. J Am Animal Hosp Assoc 1994.
5. Ogilvie GK, Cockburn CA, Tranquilli WJ, Reschke RW: Hypotension and cutaneous reactions associated with etoposide administration in the dog. Am J Vet Res 49:1367–1370, 1988.
6. Ogilvie GK, Curtis C, Richardson RC, et al: Acute short term toxicity associated with the administration of doxorubicin to dogs with malignant tumors. J Am Vet Med Assoc 195:1584–1587, 1989.
7. Ogilvie GK, Moore AS: Chemotherapy-induced anaphylaxis and hypersensitivity. In Managing the Veterinary Cancer Patient: A Practice Manual. Trenton, NJ, Veterinary Learning Systems, 1995, pp 182–185.
8. Ogilvie GK , Walters LM, Powers BE, et al: Organ toxicity of NBT Taxol in the rat and dog: A preclinical study. Proceedings of the 13th Annual Veterinary Cancer Society Conference, 1993, pp 90–91.
9. Teske E, Rutteman GR, van Heerde P, Misdorp W: Polyethylene glycol-L-asparaginase versus native L-as-paraginase in canine non-Hodgkin's lymphoma. Eur J Cancer 26:891–895, 1990.

63. EXTRAVASATION OF CHEMOTHERAPEUTIC DRUGS

Gregory K. Ogilvie, D.V.M.

1. What chemotherapy agents may cause a perivascular reaction or slough?

Many chemotherapeutic agents are known to induce significant tissue injury after extravasation. Some are severe, irreversible vesicants; others are irritants. The agents commonly used in veterinary medicine include the following:

Actinomycin D	Mithromycin
Daunorubicin	Vinblastine
Doxorubicin	Vincristine
Epirubicin	Mitoxantrone
Etoposide	Cisplatin

Management of extravasation in human and veterinary medicine is anecdotal and extremely controversial. Despite this controversy, guidelines have been established for clinical use (see question 4).

2. How can perivascular reactions or slough be prevented?

As expected, accurate and secure first-stick catheter placement is absolutely essential in administering drugs that can cause tissue damage if extravasated perivascularly. Generally, only small (22–23 gauge) indwelling intravenous catheters should be used when treatment volumes exceed 1 ml; 23–25-gauge butterfly needles are used for administering small volumes of drugs such as vincristine. All persons involved in patient care should note when and where blood samples are taken by venipuncture and where catheters have been placed previously. This practice prevents administration of chemotherapeutic agents through veins that may leak because of previous procedures. Only recently placed catheters should be used for administration of chemotherapeutic agents. Extreme care should be taken in administering drugs to animals with fragile veins (e.g., diabetics and some aged animals). The catheter should be checked for patency with a large injection of saline (e.g., 12–15 ml) before and after administration of the drug. In addition, the catheter must be checked for patency during infusion, and the injection site must be checked during treatment.

3. What is the best method to diagnose a chemotherapy-induced extravasation?

Usually there is no doubt whether an extravasation has occurred. Some agents are highly caustic if given perivascularly; animals may vocalize or physically react to pain at the injection site. Treatment for extravasation must begin immediately. Evidence of tissue necrosis generally does not appear for 1–10 days after injection and may progress for 3–4 weeks. Lesions may start as mild erythema and progress to an open, draining wound that will not heal without extensive debridement and plastic surgery weeks to months after the perivascular slough begins when all damage is evident. The lesions occur early with vinca alkaloids and late with anthracycline antibiotics such as doxorubicin.

4. What is the treatment of choice for perivascular injection of a chemotherapeutic agent?

Every person involved with the administration of chemotherapeutic agents should be aware of procedures for treatment of extravasation. The procedures should be posted in a common area, and all materials needed to treat extravasation should be readily accessible. Because of extensive use in veterinary practice, doxorubicin and vinca alkaloids are the most common cause of perivascular sloughs. Unfortunately, no method effectively eliminates tissue necrosis. For example, sodium bicarbonate, corticosteroids, dimethyl sulfide (DMSO), alpha tocopherol, N-acetylcysteine, glutathione, lidocaine, diphenhydramine, cimetidine, propranolol, and isoproterenol are not effective for treatment of doxorubicin extravasations.

General Outline for Immediate Treatment of Extravasation of Drugs
Commonly Used in Veterinary Medicine

GENERAL PROCEDURE/ SPECIFIC DRUGS	SPECIFIC DETAILS
Minimize amount of drug at site.	Do *not* remove the catheter or needle.
	With a syringe, immediately withdraw as much drug as possible from the tissue, tubing, and catheter.
	Administer antidote (see below) or sterile saline to neutralize or dilute the drug.
Doxorubicin, daunorubicin, epirubicin, idarubicin, actinomycin-D	Apply ice or cold compresses for topical cooling for 6–10 hr to inhibit vesicant cytotoxicity. *Do not apply heat.*
	Doxorubicin: inactivate by infiltrating site with bi(3,5-dimethyl)-5-hydromethyl-2-oxomorpholin-3-yl (also known as DHM3), if available.
	Controversial:
	Topical DMSO
	Infiltrate area with 1 mg/kg hydrocortisone.
	Surgical debridement or plastic surgery may be indicated in rare cases.
Vincristine, vinblastine, etoposide	Infiltrate area with 1 ml of hyaluronidase (150 U/ml) for every ml extravasated to enhance absorption and to disperse the drug.
	Apply warm compresses to the site for several hours to enhance systemic absorption.
	Controversial:
	Topical DMSO
	Infiltrate area with 1 mg/kg hydrocortisone.
Cisplatin	Inject 1 ml of ⅙ molar isotonic sodium thiosulfate for each ml of cisplatin extravasated to inactivate the drug. Treatment is recommended for extravasation of large quantities of cisplatin.

From Ogilvie GK, Moore AS: Managing the Veterinary Cancer Patient: A Practice Manual. Veterinary Learning Systems, Trenton, NJ, 1995, with permission.

Once tissue damage is identified, an Elizabethan collar and bandages with a nonstick pad are essential to allow the area to heal without self-trauma. The bandage should be changed daily as long as the area is draining or has the potential for infection. If a bacterial infection is noted, culture and sensitivity testing and appropriate use of antimicrobials are essential. Frequent cleansing and debridement may be necessary. In some cases, reconstructive surgical repair is essential.

BIBLIOGRAPHY

1. Hubbard S, Duffy P, Seipp C: Administration of cancer treatments: Practical guide for physicians and nurses. In DeVita VT Jr, Hellman S, Rosenberg S (eds): Cancer: Principles and Practice of Oncology, 3rd ed. Philadelphia, J.B. Lippincott, 1989, pp 2369–2402.
2. Hubbard S, Jenkins JF: Chemotherapy administration: Practical guidelines. In Chabner BA, Collins JM (eds): Cancer Chemotherapy: Principles and Practice. Philadelphia, J.B. Lippincott, 1990, pp 449–464.
3. Ogilvie GK, Moore AS: Extravasation of chemotherapeutic agents. In Managing the Veterinary Cancer Patient: A Practice Manual. Trenton, NJ, Veterinary Learning Systems, 1995, pp 137–141.
4. Wittes RE, Hubbard SM: Chemotherapy: The properties and uses of single agents. In Wittes RE (ed): Manual of Oncologic Therapeutics, 1991/1992. Philadelphia, J.B. Lippincott, 1991, pp 116–121.

64. CHEMOTHERAPY-INDUCED ACUTE RENAL FAILURE

Gregory K. Ogilvie, D.V.M.

1. What drugs are most commonly associated with development of renal failure?

Cisplatin, piroxicam, and methotrexate are commonly associated with renal failure in veterinary patients. Doxorubicin has been shown to induce renal disease in some dogs and cats. In addition, renal failure is induced by a wide variety of malignant conditions, including transitional cell carcinoma.

2. How does cisplatin induce renal damage?

The most nephrotoxic chemotherapeutic agent is cis-diamminedichloroplatinum II (cisplatin), a heavy metal coordination compound that has antineoplastic activity against various malignant tumors in dogs. In dogs, 80–90% of the drug is eliminated in the urine within 48 hours. Nephrotoxicosis, characterized by reduced glomerular filtration rate and tubular injury, is the major dose-limiting toxicosis. Renal toxicosis may range from brief increases in serum urea nitrogen and creatinine concentrations to irreversible renal failure. However, renal damage generally is not a clinical problem if adequate hydration is maintained. Various administration protocols have been suggested to limit or eliminate cisplatin nephrotoxicosis in dogs. Each protocol includes the use of intravenous saline solution during the 1- to 24-hour diuresis period (see question 8).

3. Do other chemotherapeutic agents induce renal disease?

Doxorubicin also induces acute and chronic renal failure in dogs and cats. One study suggests that the renal damage in cats is dose-dependent; however, this observation has not been repeated. Renal failure in dogs also has been induced with variable cumulative doses of doxorubicin. Another unrelated drug, methotrexate, is eliminated primarily from the kidneys and also has been associated with development of nephrotoxicity. Piroxicam, a nonsteroidal antiinflammatory agent, has been shown to be effective for treating dogs with transitional cell carcinoma of the bladder and squamous cell carcinomas of the head and neck.

4. Can the physical presence of a tumor result in kidney damage?

Dogs with transitional cell carcinoma of the bladder, urethra, or prostate commonly have urethral obstruction that may lead to hydroureter and hydronephrosis. The concurrent septic cystitis seen in most patients with bladder tumors may induce secondary pyelonephritis. The end result is acute and chronic renal failure.

5. What factors predispose to development of chemotherapy-induced kidney damage?

In veterinary medicine, two of the most common predisposing factors associated with development of acute renal failure are cancer and nephrotoxic drugs, including chemotherapeutic agents. Therefore, when chemotherapeutic agents are used in veterinary patients, other nephrotoxic drugs such as aminoglycosides should be avoided. Other risk factors associated with development of acute and chronic renal failure in dogs and cats are decreased cardiac output, urinary tract infection, sepsis, preexisting renal disease, advanced age, dehydration, fever, liver disease, hypokalemia, and hypercalcemia. Several studies have shown that preexisting renal disease may be one of the most important predisposing factors for development of cisplatin-induced acute renal failure.

6. What are the best ways to diagnose kidney damage induced by chemotherapeutic agents?

Acute or chronic renal failure results from decreased glomerular filtration rate with or without tubular damage; therefore, the parameters used for diagnosis are related to damage to these structures. Renal disease may have been significant for variable periods before clinical, hematologic, and biochemical abnormalities were identified, because at least two-thirds of kidney function must be abnormal before overt evidence of renal disease develops.

Acute renal failure may occur with nonoliguria, oliguria, or anuria. Regardless of the amount of urine, it is usually isothenuric or minimally concentrated with a high sodium content (> 40 mEq/L). Glucose, protein, and renal epithelial cells also may be noted in the urine, along with an acute rise in serum urea nitrogen, creatinine, and phosphorus concentration. In oliguric or anuric renal failure, body weight, heart rate, and central venous pressure may increase if fluids are administered before urine flow is reestablished.

7. What is the best treatment for dogs with chemotherapy-induced renal failure?

The best treatment for acute or chronic renal failure is prevention. Substantial data show that cisplatin nephrotoxicity can be reduced and almost eliminated with adequate hydration. The incidence of doxorubicin- and methotrexate-induced renal failure can be reduced by eliminating dogs with preexisting renal disease and by increasing the duration of time the drug is administered. Because cisplatin is a profound nephrotoxin, a brief discussion of hydration schemes to reduce kidney damage is followed by a review of treatment for acute renal failure.

8. How does the method of administering cisplatin influence the induction of renal failure?

The duration of saline diuresis may influence the induction of renal failure in dogs. For example, 24-, 6-, and 4-hour diuresis protocols have been shown to be effective for administering cisplatin with a low probability of inducing renal failure. Shorter diuresis protocols have been shown to be detrimental. For example, a 1-hour diuresis protocol was evaluated for safety and effectiveness. Four doses of cisplatin (70 mg/m^2 of body surface every 3 wk) were administered intravenously to 6 healthy dogs over a 20-minute period after 0.9% NaCl solution (saline) was administered intravenously for 1 hour at a volume of 132 ml $(kg)^{0.75}$. Each dog vomited at least once within 8 hours after each treatment. Clinical status, body weight, and food consumption were normal throughout the 12-week study for 5 of the 6 dogs. The sixth dog developed acute renal failure and became acutely blind and deaf within 3 days after the fourth dose of cisplatin. Electrolyte, creatinine, and serum urea nitrogen values remained within normal limits in all dogs immediately before each treatment and in 5 of 6 dogs evaluated 3 weeks after the final treatment. The serum creatinine value (3.3 mg/dl) obtained from the beagle euthanized 2 weeks after the fourth treatment was above normal. Despite the normality of all but one of the creatinine values, the serum creatinine concentrations obtained 3 weeks after the final treatment with cisplatin were higher than pretreatment values. Glomerular filtration rate, as determined by exogenous and endogenous creatinine clearance tests, was significantly decreased 3 weeks after the fourth treatment of cisplatin compared with data from all other evaluation periods. Neutrophil counts decreased below pretreatment values at the third, fourth, and fifth evaluation periods. Therefore, this protocol cannot be recommended.

9. What is the best treatment for chemotherapy-induced renal failure?

The initial goals for treating drug- and tumor-related acute renal failure in dogs and cats are to discontinue all drugs that may be nephrotoxic, to document prerenal or postrenal abnormalities, and to initiate fluid therapy. The primary objectives of fluid therapy are to correct deficits such as dehydration and excesses such as volume overload, as seen in oliguric renal failure; to supply maintenance needs; and to supplement ongoing losses, such as those due to vomiting and diarrhea. Each patient must be assessed carefully, and a treatment plan must be based on hydration status, cardiovascular performance, and biochemical data. Maintenance requirements vary from 44–110 ml/kg body weight; smaller animals require the larger amount. A simpler formula is to use 66 ml/kg/day. The amount of fluid that is needed daily for maintenance must be supplemented by an amount equal to external losses due to vomiting and diarrhea. In patients with renal failure, 1.5–3 times this amount of fluid is administered daily to achieve diuresis. The success of diuresis can be monitored by documenting adequate urine output (> 2 ml/kg/hr). Fluid therapy should meet daily needs, replace excessive losses, and correct dehydration. The percentage of dehydration should be determined; approximately 75% of the fluids needed to correct dehydration should be administered during the first 24 hours. Fluid therapy should be altered to correct electrolyte and acid-base abnormalities. In acute renal failure, potassium-containing fluids generally are not ideal because systemic hyperkalemia is often present. Until more is known about the systemic effects of sepsis, lactate-containing fluids should be avoided because sepsis and cancer are associated with hyperlactatemia, which worsens with administration of lactate-containing fluids.

Fluid Therapy for a 10-kg Dog with 5% Dehydration and Diarrhea

TASK	CALCULATION
1. Correct dehydration.	5% (0.05) × 10 kg body weight = 0.5 kg of water needed to correct dehydration 1000 ml/kg of water × 0.5 kg = 500 ml of water needed to correct dehydration 75% (0.75) × 500 ml = 375 ml of fluid should be administered to replace 75% of dehydration
2. Administer fluids to meet daily needs.	66 ml/kg (daily requirement) × 10 kg body weight = 660 ml needed on daily basis. Others believe that daily requirements are best estimated as [30 (kg) + 70]. Increase this amount by 1.5–3 times to induce mild-to-moderate diuresis in patients with renal failure, ensuring urine output > 2 ml/kg/hr.
3. Replace ongoing losses.	Estimated losses through diarrhea = 200 ml
4. Fluids needed, first 24 hr.	375 ml + 660 ml + 200 ml = 1,235 ml; increase fluid therapy judiciously to increase urine output to sustain mild-to-moderate diuresis.

From Ogilvie GK, Moore AS: Managing the Veterinary Cancer Patient: A Practice Manual. Veterinary Learning Systems, Trenton, NJ, 1995, with permission.

General Approach for a Dog in Renal Failure

GENERAL PRINCIPLE	SPECIFIC DETAILS
1. Stop administration of nephrotoxins.	Discontinue cisplatin, methotrexate, doxorubicin, and aminoglycosides; avoid anesthesia.

2. Assess patient status.	Complete blood count, blood chemistry profile
	 Specifically determine:
	    % dehydration
	    Amount of ongoing losses (e.g,. vomiting, diarrhea, blood loss)
	    Maintenance of fluid requirements
	    Electrolyte and biochemical abnormalities
	    Cardiovascular performance
	    Urine output

Table continued on next page.

General Approach for a Dog in Renal Failure (Continued)

GENERAL PRINCIPLE	SPECIFIC DETAILS
3. Select and administer specific fluids.	Tailor therapy to needs of each patient: Isotonic polyionic fluid initially, preferably postassium-free (e.g., NaCl). Correct dehydration first over 6–8 hr to prevent further renal ischemia while watching carefully for pathologic oliguria and subsequent volume overload. Meet maintenance requirements (approximately 66 ml/kg/day). Meet ongoing losses (vomiting, diarrhea). Induce mild-to-moderate diuresis.
4. Monitor urine output, ensure adequate output.	Metabolism cage or indwelling catheter For inadequate output (< 0.5–2 ml/kg/hr): Mannitol or dextrose, 0.5–1.0 gm/kg in slow IV bolus Furosemide, 2–4 mg/kg IV every 1–3 hr as needed Dopamine, 1–3 µg/kg/min IV (50 mg dopamine in 500 ml of 5% dextrose = 100 µg/ml solution)
5. Correct acid-base and electrolyte abnormalities.	Rule out hypercalcemia of malignancy; treat specifically for that if identified.
6. Provide mild-to-moderate diuresis.	Urine output: 2–5 ml/kg/hr; monitor body weight, heart and respiratory rate, and central venous pressure for signs of overhydration.
7. Consider peritoneal dialysis if not responsive.	Temporary or chronic ambulatory peritoneal dialysis with specific dialysate solution may be helpful.
8. Initiate long-term plans.	Continue diuresis until blood urea nitrogen and creatinine normalize or until values stop improving despite aggressive therapy and clinically stable patient; then gradually taper fluids. Control hyperphosphatemia if indicated (e.g., aluminum hydroxide, 500 mg at each feeding). Treat gastric hyperacidity if indicated (cimetidine, 5–10 mg/kg every 6 hr IV or orally).

From Ogilvie GK, Moore AS: Managing the Veterinary Cancer Patient: A Practice Manual. Veterinary Learning Systems, Trenton, NJ, 1995, with permission.

If oliguric renal failure is present, a diligent and aggressive approach should be made to increase urine output, first by increasing glomerular filtration rate and renal blood flow. In addition, osmotic diuresis can be used to increase urine flow. If urine output is less than 0.5–2 ml/kg/hr despite aggressive fluid therapy, furosemide should be administered every 1–3 hours. Furosemide increases glomerular filtration rate and enhances diuresis in many patients. If furosemide is not effective, mannitol or 50% dextrose may be used as an osmotic diuretic to enhance urine production. The advantage of dextrose over mannitol is that dextrose can be detected on a urine glucose test strip. If furosemide and osmotic diuretics are not effective, dopamine may be administered as a constant-rate infusion. Dopamine enhances renal blood flow and increases urine output secondarily.

Treatment for acute renal failure should be continued until the patient is substantially improved and until abnormal biochemical parameters have been corrected or at least stabilized. Therapy then should be tapered over several days and a home treatment plan developed, including avoidance of nephrotoxic drugs, high-quality, low-quantity protein diet, maintenance of a low stress environment, and provision of fresh, clean water at will.

BIBLIOGRAPHY

1. Chiuten D, Vogel S, Kaplan B, et al: Is there cumulative or delayed toxicity for cis-platinum? Cancer 52:211–214, 1983.
2. Cotter SM, Kanki PJ, Simon M: Renal disease in five tumor-bearing cats treated with Adriamycin. J Am Animal Hosp Assoc 21:405–412, 1985.

 3. Cvitkovic E, Spaulding J, Bethune V, et al: Improvement of cis-dichlorodiammineplatinum (NSC 119875): Therapeutic index in an animal model. Cancer 39:1357–1361, 1977.
 4. Himsel CA, Richardson RC, Craig JA: Cisplatin chemotherapy for metastatic squamous cell carcinoma in two dogs. J Am Vet Med Assoc 89:1575–1578, 1986.
 5. Kirby R: Acute renal failure as a complication of the critically ill animal. Vet Clin North Am 19:1189–1208, 1989.
 6. LaRue SM, Withrow SJ, Powers BE, et al: Limb-sparing treatment for osteosarcoma in dogs. J Am Vet Med Assoc 195:1734–1744, 1989.
 7. Mehlhaff CJ, Leifer CE, Patnaik AK, et al: Surgical treatment of pulmonary neoplasia in 15 dogs. J Am Vet Med Assoc 20:799–803, 1984.
 8. Ogilvie GK, Fettman MJ, Jameson VJ, et al: Evaluation of a one hour saline diuresis protocol for the administration of cisplatin to dogs. Am J Vet Res 53:1666–1669, 1992.
 9. Ogilvie GK, Krawiec DR, Gelberg HB, et al: Evaluation of a short-term saline diuresis for the administration of cisplatin. Am J Vet Res 49:1076–1078, 1988.
10. Ogilvie GK, Moore AS: Chemotherapy induced acute renal failure. In Managing the Veterinary Cancer Patient: A Practice Manual. Trenton, NJ, Veterinary Learning Systems, 1995, pp 189–196.
11. Ogilvie GK, Straw RC, Jameson VJ, et al: Prevalence of nephrotoxicosis associated with a four hour saline solution diuresis protocol for the administration of cisplatin to dogs with sarcomas: 64 cases (1989–1991). J Am Vet Med Assoc 202:1845–1848, 1993.
12. Page R, Matus RE, Leifer CE, et al: Cisplatin, a new antineoplastic drug in veterinary medicine. Am Vet Med Assoc 186:288–290, 1985.
13. Shapiro W, Fossum TW, Kitchell BE, et al: Use of cisplatin for treatment of appendicular osteosarcoma in dogs. Am Vet Med Assoc 192:507–511, 1988.

65. ANEMIA, THROMBOCYTOPENIA, AND HYPOPROTEINEMIA

Gregory K. Ogilvie, D.V.M.

1. When are transfusions needed?

Transfusions are frequently needed for veterinary patients as a result of various problems, including blood loss, disseminated intravascular coagulation (DIC), clinical syndromes associated with the hypocoagulable state of malignancy and other diseases, and other hematologic abnormalities. In general, transfusions and specific blood components should be given only when specifically indicated. Other emergency support procedures, such as fluid therapy, should be used concurrently. The recent availability of blood components commercially makes this form of therapy practical for general practitioners.

2. When should blood component therapy be used? How long can blood components be stored?

Blood components should be administered when clinically indicated to either dogs or cats, especially in an emergency setting. Because blood component therapy takes time to prepare and to administer, forethought is essential. Blood component therapy should be initiated early in the management of critical patients but only when indicated. Whole blood or packed red blood cells may be administered immediately or stored for at least 21 days. Fresh frozen plasma has adequate levels of clotting factors for up to 1 year. Frozen plasma stored for longer than 1 year may have a diminished amount of clotting factors V and VII and von Willebrand's factor. Dog blood can be drawn into human unit bags, holding approximately 450 ml of blood and 50 ml of anticoagulant. The plasma can be decanted to make packed cells. In cats a unit is frequently defined as 50 ml, which is the maximal amount that can be drawn safely from average adult cats.

3. What type of blood should be used to transfuse dogs or cats with acute blood loss?

Although there is a theoretical advantage to transfusing fresh whole blood, packed red blood cells may be administered with excellent results. Red blood cells stored for more than 2 weeks may have a depletion of 2,3 DPG (diphosphoglycerate), which may diminish red blood cell oxygen-carrying capacity. Transfusion should be performed to keep the hematocrit above 15% in dogs and above 10% in cats, when possible. In each case, the patient's response to transfusion should be just as important a determinant as the hematocrit or amount to be transfused. Dogs and cats with acute blood loss are less tolerant of low hematocrit values, whereas those with a gradual reduction in red blood cell numbers are able to adapt to extremely low red blood cell numbers, especially cats.

4. What are the indications to transfuse a dog with immune-mediated hemolytic anemia?

Immune-mediated hemolytic anemia may require the administration of red blood cells, even if it results in lysis in some of the transfused blood. An immune-mediated hemolytic event may result in acute or gradual onset of a low hematocrit. Therefore, the patient may present like an animal with either acute or chronic blood loss. Adjunctive therapy with glucocorticoids, azathioprine, and cyclosporine is often essential to treat the underlying disease. Dogs and cats with hemolytic anemia cannot be cross-matched adequately because of the presence of antibodies. Frequent evaluation of packed cell volume is essential.

5. What are the indications to transfuse a dog with nonregenerative anemia?

Generally nonregenerative anemia is relatively mild and often does not require transfusion. However, in some cases nonregenerative anemia is quite severe and requires either fresh whole blood or packed red blood cells. Some dogs and cats with nonregenerative anemia do quite well clinically until they are stressed for any reason. Stresses include but are not limited to unexpected confinement or kenneling, disease of any kind, or presentation to the veterinarian for routine evaluation. In addition, the administration of erythropoietin may be of value; however, antibodies directed to the erythropoietin are possible.

6. What are the indications to treat a patient with thrombocytopenia?

Platelet counts greater than 30,000–40,000 are rarely associated with bleeding disorders. Indeed, a gradual reduction in platelet counts may result in healthy-appearing patients with only 2,000–3,000 platelets. Recently released platelets have much greater function than older platelets. Platelet transfusion should be used only in dogs or cats that exhibit clinical signs. Platelet-rich plasma may be considered in such patients; however, the half-life of platelets may last for only days or weeks or less, especially in the presence of immune-mediated conditions. One unit per 20 kg body weight of platelet-rich plasma or fresh whole blood should be administered and repeated every hour until an adequate platelet count is reached.

7. What drug can be used to increase platelet numbers, assuming adequate megakaryocytes are present?

Vincristine (0.5 mg/m^2 IV every 1–3 weeks) may be administered to induce premature release of platelets from the bone marrow at other sites during this time. The platelet count usually increases 3–5 days after vincristine is administered.

8. What is disseminated intravascular coagulation?

DIC is a syndrome with severe bleeding and consumption of clotting factors and platelets.

9. How is DIC treated?

Approximately one unit of fresh frozen plasma can be used and repeated as needed to maintain prothrombin and partial thromboplastin time at 1–1.5 times the normal bleeding time. Use of heparin is controversial; however, if used in conjunction with platelets, it may have beneficial results. When all cell lines (red blood cells and platelets) are decreased, fresh whole blood also can be used.

10. When are plasma transfusions used to treat dogs with hypoproteinemia?

Plasma transfusions may be of value in patients with decreased albumin levels. Administration of protein may cause a slow increase in plasma proteins because only 40% of the body albumin is in the intravascular space, whereas 60% resides within the interstitial space. Therefore, the administration of fresh frozen plasma must increase the albumin not only within the circulating space but also within the interstitial spaces, which may require repeated administration of proteins. Obviously, the administration of fresh frozen plasma from various donors may result in the development of antibodies. Colloidal solutions such as dextrans or hetastarch also may be useful despite the fact that their half-life may be quite short.

11. How do you determine how much blood or blood components to administer?

Animals with significant acute blood loss should be treated first for shock with crystalloid solutions. Hypertonic saline is also a reasonable choice in select patients. Packed red blood cells may be given with crystalloid fluids or whole blood. As a general rule, one unit of packed red blood cells is administered per 20 kg body weight with close adjustments to maintain the hematocrit above 15%. Dogs that require whole blood for either acute or chronic anemias should be transfused using the general guidelines below:

General rule: amount to transfuse

$$\text{ml donor blood} = [(2.2 \times wt_{kg}) \times (40_{dog} \text{ or } 30_{cat}) \times PCV_{desired} - PCV_{recipient})]PCV_{donor}$$

where PCV = packed cell volume; 2.2 ml of blood/kg raises PCV by 1% when transfused blood has a PCV of 40.

General rule: rate of transfusion

Dogs: 0.25 ml/kg/30 min or faster (22 ml/kg/day) with close patient monitoring
Cats: 40 ml/30 min with close patient monitoring

Whenever plasma transfusions are considered, it should be remembered that 60% of the blood volume is plasma. In addition, only 40% of the albumin in an animal is in the plasma. Therefore, it takes half a dozen units of plasma to raise the albumin of a 66-pound dog from 1.8 gm/dl to 3 gm/dl.

12. What are the possible complications after transfusion?

Hemolysis is probably the most serious adverse effect; however, it is relatively rare. An acute hemolytic reaction may result in elevated temperature, heart rate, and respiration rate; tremors; vomiting; and collapse. When this occurs, blood component transfusion should be stopped, and the patient's plasma should be checked for hemoglobinemia. Crystalloid fluids should be initiated, and urine output should be monitored. Delayed hemolysis is also possible in some patients.

Fever that develops during transfusion may indicate bacterial contamination of the blood, or the fever may be related to leukocyte antigens that cause an elevation of endogenous pyrogens. Elevation in body temperature is more commonly seen in cats than in dogs.

Allergic reactions may manifest as urticaria and angioneurotic edema. If such signs are noted, the transfusion should be discontinued, and glucocorticoids should be administered.

When large volumes of blood are administered, **volume overload** should be monitored and treated appropriately

Citrate toxicity, another possible complication of stored blood transfusion, may cause an acute decrease in serum ionized calcium. Citrate toxicity may induce muscle tremors, facial twitches, and seizures as a result of hypocalcemia. Intravenous calcium gluconate and cessation of transfusion are the treatments of choice.

Rarely, **blood ammonia levels** may rise and cause associated clinical signs, such as mental dullness or seizures. This is usually seen in blood that is stored over a prolonged period and is usually associated with packed red blood cells. Treatment should be the same as for hepatoencephalopathy.

BIBLIOGRAPHY

1. Giger U: The feline AB blood group system and incompatibility reactions. In Kirk RW, Bonagura JD (eds): Current Veterinary Therapy XI—Small Animal Practice. Philadelphia, W.B. Saunders, 1992, pp 470–474.
2. Ogilvie GK, Moore AS: Transfusion support. In Managing the Veterinary Cancer Patient: A Practice Manual. Trenton, NJ, Veterinary Learning Systems, 1995, pp 137–141.
3. Stone MS, Cotter SM: Practical guidelines for transfusion therapy. In Kirk RW, Bonagura JD (eds): Current Veterinary Therapy XI—Small Animal Practice. Philadelphia, W.B. Saunders, 1992, pp 479, 645.

VIII. *Neurologic Emergencies*

Section Editor: Wayne E. Wingfield, D.V.M., M.S.

66. INTERVERTEBRAL DISK DISEASE

Wayne E. Wingfield, D.V.M., M.S.

1. Describe the anatomy of an intervertebral disk.
Intervertebral disks are circular gelatinous cushions located between each pair of vertebral bodies, with the exception of the first and second cervical vertebrae. Each disk consists of two parts:
- Nucleus pulposus: a central gelatinous area
- Annulus fibrosus: an outer fibrous ring that is approximately twice as thick dorsally as ventrally

From the second to the tenth thoracic vertebrae, each disk is overlaid by a band of ligamentous tissue known as the intercapital ligament.

2. How does the anatomy of the intervertebral disk relate to disk extrusions?
Most disk extrusions occur in a dorsal direction (the thinner part of the annulus fibrosus), and the presence of the intercapital ligament explains the relative paucity of dorsal disk herniations in all but the cervical, caudal thoracic, and lumbar vertebrae.

3. What is the difference between extrusion and propulsion of intervertebral disk displacement?
Extrusion. The annulus fibrosus is ruptured, and all or part of the nucleus pulposus is displaced into the vertebral canal.
Protrusion. The annulus fibrosus is intact, but the nucleus pulposus causes a dorsal displacement into the vertebral canal.

4. Describe Hansen's classification of intervertebral disk herniation.

Hansen's type 1	Degenerative changes (premature chondroid metaplasia associated with mineralization, necrosis, and dissecation) leading to a rapid expulsion of a nucleus pulposus through a weakened dorsal annulus fibrosus.
Hansen's type 2	Gradual protrusion of disk material contained within an intact but degenerate (fibroid metaplasia) annulus.

5. Which breeds are associated with the two classes of intervertebral disk herniation?

Hansen's type 1	Chondrodystrophoid breeds (e.g., dachshunds, Lhasa apso, Shih Tzu, Welsh corgi, beagles, cocker spaniels, Pekinese) with disk extrusion
Hansen's type 2	Nonchondrodystrophoid breeds (e.g., German shepherds, Labrador retrievers) with disk protrusion

6. What is a type 3 intervertebral disk lesion?
The type 3 disk lesion also has been called a "gunshot" disk lesion. A small fragment of nucleus pulposus is ejected into the vertebral canal with high velocity. Often there is direct penetration

of the spinal cord, which results in peracute or acute onset of rapidly progressive paralysis, frequently with loss of pain sensation.

7. What accounts for the predilection of different breeds for intervertebral disk disease?
Most likely, genetic predisposition.

8. Describe the pathogenesis of spinal injury subsequent to intervertebral disk extrusion or protrusion.
The spinal cord injury is due to a combination of vascular and mechanical effects. The contribution of each is controversial.

Mechanical effects. Spinal cord compression results from disk fragments and extradural hemorrhage caused by tearing of the venous sinuses (acute disk extrusions). Both vascular occlusion and mechanical distortion result.

Vascular effects. Acute disk extrusion is associated with an assortment of vascular changes that may progress to central hemorrhagic necrosis and myelomalacia. Vascular changes include vasospasm, endothelial cell swelling, thrombi, and vascular tears. Implicated endogenous chemicals include norepinephrine, dopamine, endorphins, prostaglandins, oxygen free radicals, and calcium. The resultant central hemorrhagic necrosis is most pronounced in the gray matter, because its blood supply is 5 times that of white matter.

9. Identify the neurologic signs associated with an intervertebral lesion in each of the following spinal cord segments:

C1–C5	Upper motor neuron (UMN) to all limbs
C6–T2	Lower motor neuron (LMN) to thoracic limbs and UMN to pelvic limbs
T3–L3	Normal thoracic limbs, UMN to pelvic limbs
L4–S2	Normal thoracic limbs, LMN to pelvic limbs
S1–S3	Partial LMN to pelvic limbs, absent perineal reflex, atonic bladder
Caudal nerves	Atonic tail

10. What radiographic signs are associated with intervertebral disk protrusion or extrusion?
• Narrowing and dorsal wedging of the intervertebral disk space
• Reduction in size and opacification of the intervertebral foramen
• Narrowing of the interarticular facet space

11. Is the calcified disk in situ the likely site of the offending lesion?
No. Calcified disks in situ are rarely the cause of paresis or paralysis.

12. What is the role of myelography in intervertebral disk disease?
If surgery is contemplated, myelography helps to select the appropriate surgical procedure. The contrast column usually deviates at the site of the disk lesion. When spinal cord edema is present, compression often extends over several segments, but the lesion is usually centered in the area of the myelographic column impingement.

13. Describe the treatment of animals with intervertebral disk disease.
Few prospective studies assess the benefits of medical vs. surgical therapy. In addition, questions remain about fenestration, hemilaminectomy, dorsal laminectomy, and combinations of these surgical procedures. Usually the decision is based on the following factors:
• Patient's neurologic status
• Experience of the veterinarian
• Available surgical expertise
• Financial considerations and concerns of the pet owner.

CONTROVERSIES

14. What are the indications for medical management of intervertebral disk disease?
- First episode of ataxia, pain, or mild paresis
- Paralysis for more than 24 hours with no deep pain perception
- Owner's refusal of surgical option

15. Should corticosteroids be administered to patients with intervertebral disk disease?
Corticosteroids given to animals with intervertebral disk disease are most beneficial during the first 12–24 hours; their effect wanes thereafter.

16. What benefits do corticosteroids offer to patients with intervertebral disk disease?
- Antiinflammatory effects
- Inhibition of lipid peroxidation by oxygen free radicals
- Increase in blood flow
- Enhancement of neuronal excitability
- Preservation of neurofilament proteins

17. Which corticosteroid should be used to treat intervertebral disk disease?
Currently two corticosteroids are used:
- **Methylprednisolone.** Studies in humans and cats showed improved outcome after spinal injury. Response appears to be biphasic. Doses of 15 mg/kg show a suboptimal response, whereas at 60 mg/kg deleterious effects result from decreased spinal blood flow. Currently no studies in dogs show benefits of this drug. The positive results do not restore the ability to walk in tetraplegic patients, and in chronic studies the effects may not be sustained.
- **Dexamethasone.** Although less expensive, dexamethasone causes significant gastrointestinal complications.

18. When is surgery indicated in animals with intervertebral disk disease?
- More than one episode of pain, ataxia, or mild paraparesis
- Severe paraparesis or paraplegia with intact deep pain perception
- Deterioration of neurologic status with medical therapy
- Paralysis without perception of deep pain for less than 24 hours

BIBLIOGRAPHY

1. Bracken MB, Shephard MJ, Collins WF Jr, et al: A randomized, controlled trial of methylprednisolone or naloxone in the treatment of acute spinal cord injury: Results of the Second National Acute Spinal Cord Injury Study. N Engl J Med 322:1405–1411, 1990.
2. Bracken MB, Shephard MJ, Collins WF Jr, et al: Methylprednisolone or naloxone treatment after acute spinal cord injury: 1-year follow-up data. Results of the Second National Acute Spinal Cord Injury Study. J Neurosurg 76:23–31, 1992.
3. Brown SA, Hall ED: Role of oxygen-derived free radicals in the pathogenesis of shock and trauma, with focus on central nervous system injuries. J Am Vet Med Assoc 200:1849–1858, 1992.
4. Fingeroth JM: Treatment of canine intervertebral disk disease: Recommendations and controversies. In Bonagura JD (ed): Current Veterinary Therapy XII. Philadelphia, W.B. Saunders, 1995, pp 1146–1153.
5. Kornegay JN: Intervertebral disk disease—Diagnosis and surgical management. Proceedings of the IVECCS V, San Antonio, TX, 1996, pp 274–278.
6. Shell LG: Differential diagnosis for acute-onset paraparesis. Vet Med 91:230–239, 1996.

67. SEIZURES

Wayne E. Wingfield, D.V.M., M.S., and J. Michael McFarland, D.V.M.

1. What is a seizure?
A seizure is a paroxysmal, transitory disturbance of brain function that has sudden onset, ceases spontaneously, and is likely to recur. Although most veterinarians call the resulting effects (e.g., jerky movements, staring) a "seizure," the seizure is the neuronal event itself. The observable manifestation is called "seizure activity."

2. Why are seizures an important emergency?
Something is interfering with normal functioning of a group of neurons. The hyperactivity of the neurons causes a build-up of metabolic byproducts, resulting in a harmful effect on the neurons. Neurons depend on aerobic metabolism. When the need for oxygen outstrips the availability, the neuron is injured. If this situation is prolonged, cell death results.

3. Describe the general pathophysiology of seizures.
Seizures are the result of disturbances in normal electrical activity in the brain. Anything that alters neuronal function may lead to a lower threshold of excitability and spontaneous depolarization. If the depolarization wave spreads to other areas of the brain or the entire nervous system, seizures result. The basic pathophysiologic processes that result in seizures are excessive cellular excitation and loss of cellular inhibition.

4. How are seizures classified?
In veterinary medicine, objective evidence for the following human classification is lacking, but the classification is useful:
1. Partial seizures
   • Simple partial seizures (consciousness preserved)
   • Complex partial seizures (consciousness impaired)
   • Partial seizures with secondary generalization
2. Generalized-onset seizures
   • Idiopathic epilepsy
   • Psychomotor seizures (temporal lobe epilepsy)

5. What is the difference between focal and generalized seizures?
Focal seizures remain localized to one body region. They may become generalized and are more often associated with structural brain disease.

Generalized seizures affect the entire body simultaneously.

6. What is the most common seizure in animals?
Generalized, tonic-clonic seizures.

7. Define status epilepticus.
Status epilepticus is defined as more than two seizures without recovery between or a single seizure lasting more than 30 minutes. Most seizures last less than 2 minutes; therefore, any seizure longer than 10 minutes should be considered status epilepticus.

8. Give examples of bizarre behaviors that may be manifestations of seizure disorders in animals.
• Fly-biting
• Flank-sucking
• Tail-biting

9. What are the common causes of seizures?
1. Idiopathic epilepsy
2. Metabolic disease
   - Hypoglycemia
   - Hypocalcemia
   - Hyperkalemia
   - Hypoxia
   - Renal or hepatic disease
3. Infection
   - Feline infectious peritonitis
   - Canine distemper
   - Toxoplasmosis
   - Rabies
   - Other fungal or bacterial causes
4. Inflammation (noninfectious)
   - Trauma
   - Granulomatous meningoencephalitis
5. Neoplasia
6. Malformation
   - Hydrocephalus
   - Lissencephaly
   - Lysosomal storage disorders
7. Toxicities

10. How can the signalment aid in the initial diagnosis of seizures?
1. **Age**
   - < 1 year
     Congenital: hydrocephalus, lissencephaly
     Inflammatory: meningitis
     Metabolic: portosystemic shunts
     Toxic: lead, ethylene glycol, organophosphates
   - 1–5 years: primary epilepsy
   - > 5 years
     Neoplasia
     Metabolic: hepatic or renal dysfunction, hyperadrenocorticism, hypoadrenocorticism
2. **Breed**
   - Beagle, German shepherd, Keeshond, collie, Belgian Tervuren: genetic or inherited primary epilepsy
   - Miniature/toy breeds: hypoglycemia
   - Yorkshire terrier, schnauzer: portosystemic shunts
3. **Sex:** epilepsy affects males more often than females.

11. Is a neurologic examination helpful in animals with seizures?
Certainly. You need to examine carefully the cranial nerves, comparing right to left and completing the examination with assessment of motor function and reflexes of the extremities. Idiopathic seizures are not commonly associated with interictal neurologic deficits. The caveat is that some dogs may have neurologic deficits in the postictal period that last for days after the seizure. Metabolic causes of seizures may be associated with persistent neurologic deficits, which are most commonly symmetrical.

12. What diagnostic testing should be done to localize the lesion?
- Laboratory studies: complete blood count, serum biochemical profile, urinalysis, and heartworm or FELV/FIV testing
- Electrocardiogram
- Specialized testing: blood lead, ethylene glycol
- Radiography: thoracic, abdominal
- Computed tomography and magnetic resonance imaging

13. How should status epilepticus be treated initially?

Status epilepticus is a true emergency and must be managed quickly. The ABCs (airway, breathing, circulation) must be attended to immediately. Supplemental oxygen should be supplied. If the airway and breathing are compromised, an endotracheal tube is inserted and ventilation is assisted. Venous access should be established and crystalloid fluids administered. If the severity of the seizure or the size of the animal prevents quick venous access, diazepam may be administered rectally at 0.5–2 mg/kg. Intravenous diazepam is delivered to effect (up to 2 mg/kg). If diazepam is not effective, phenobarbital is administered intravenously up to to 16 mg/kg. You may not see an effect with phenobarbital for 20 minutes if the animal has not taken the drug previously. Constant-rate infusions of phenobarbital may be given at 2–4 mg/kg/hr. If all else fails, anesthetize the animal with pentobarbital at 3–5 mg/kg intravenously to effect. Body temperature may be quite high if the patient has been seizing for more than 10 minutes. Seizure control and intravenous fluids are usually adequate to correct hyperthermia. Use caution if cold water bathing is necessary (temperature > 105° F after 10 min); hypothermia is frequently a problem in patients requiring long-term sedation.

14. How are seizures treated pharmacologically?

Drug	Pharmacokinetics	Metabolism	Dosage	Interactions, Side Effects, Toxicity
Diazepam	Half-life = 3.2 hr	Hepatic	0.5–2 mg/kg IV or rectally	CNS depression
Phenobarbital	Half-life = 47–74 hr (dogs); 34–43 hr (cats)	Renal excretion	Up to 16 mg/kg IV; 2–4 mg/kg orally 2 times/day	CNS depression/excitability; PU, PD, PP
Primidone	Half-life = 10–14 hr	Hepatic	15–30 mg/kg/day divided into 3 doses	Sedation, PU, PD, nystagmus, anorexia, hepatotoxicity, dermatitis
Phenytoin	Half-life = 4 hr	Hepatic	35–50 mg/kg 3 times/day	Sedation, PU, PD, nystagmus, tachycardia, hepatopathy, coagulation defects, toxic to cats
Clonazepam	Half-life = 1.4 hr	Hepatic	0.5 mg/kg orally 2 or 3 times/day	Sedation; after prolonged treatment may see withdrawal signs
Cloazepate	Half-life = 41 hr (humans)	—	2 mg/kg orally 2 times/day	?
Potassium bromide	Half-life = 25 days	Renal excretion	Loading dose = 400–600 mg/kg orally over 30–60 min; 20–60 mg/kg/day orally or divided into 2 doses	Vomiting, sedation, diarrhea, constipation

CNS = central nervous system, PU = polyuria, PD = polydipsia, PP = polyphagia.

15. What is a toxic blood level of phenobarbital?

40 µg/ml.

BIBLIOGRAPHY

1. Cunningham JC: Inheritance and idiopathic canine epilepsy. J Am Animal Hosp Assoc 24:421–424, 1988.
2. Farnbach GC: Seizures in the dog. Part I: Basis, classification, and predilection. Comp Cont Educ Pract Vet 6:569–574, 1984.
3. Oliver JE: Seizure disorders in companion animals. Comp Cont Educ Pract Vet 2:77–85, 1980.
4. Podell M, Fenner WR, Powers JD: Seizure classifications in dogs from a nonreferral-based population. J Am Vet Med Assoc 206:1721–1728, 1995.
5. Scheuer ML, Pedley TA: The evaluation and treatment of seizures. N Engl J Med 323:1468–1474, 1990.
6. Service FJ: Hypoglycemic disorders. N Engl J Med 332:1144–1152, 1995.
7. Shell LG: Canine distemper. Comp Cont Educ Pract Vet 12:173–179, 1990.

68. MENINGITIS AND ENCEPHALITIS

Michael S. Lagutchik, D.V.M.

1. Define meningitis and encephalitis.

Meningitis and encephalitis refer to inflammatory conditions of the meninges and brain parenchyma, respectively. Meningitis is characterized by inflammation of the meninges with involvement of the subarachnoid space—by strict definition, inflammation of nonneural tissue. Because of the close association of structures in the cranium, meningitis and encephalitis often occur simultaneously, a condition termed **meningoencephalitis**.

2. What are the causes of meningitis and encephalitis?

Inflammatory diseases of the central nervous system (CNS) are usually divided into infectious and noninfectious causes. Infectious causes include bacterial, fungal, protozoal, parasitic, rickettsial, and viral organisms. Noninfectious causes include steroid-responsive meningitis, granulomatous meningoencephalitis/reticulosis (GME), polioencephalomyelitis of cats, and several breed-specific disorders.

3. How common is infectious meningitis?

In general, infectious meningitis, regardless of the exact agent involved, is extremely uncommon in dogs and cats.

4. If infectious meningitis is not common, why bother with rapid recognition and treatment?

Failure to recognize rapidly, diagnose definitively, and institute therapy for cases of infectious meningitis frequently leads to high mortality rates. In fact, in people with suspected acute meningitis, intravenous antibiotic therapy is indicated even before culture and sensitivity testing of a cerebrospinal fluid (CSF) sample.

5. What is a brain abscess?

A brain abscess is a focal accumulation of pus in the CNS. Clinical signs reflect a steadily progressive mass lesion that usually presents subacutely. Brain abscesses are uncommon. Brain abscesses are usually focal, with signs referable to the affected site in the CNS. Most patients have a history of recent ear, respiratory, or oral infection, which is the usual source of CNS infection. Most abscesses are cerebellopontine, from otic infections, and thus are usually unilateral. Abscesses progress steadily and are usually fatal unless (and even if) prompt treatment is initiated. Diagnosis is made by CSF analysis and enhanced imaging (CT/MRI) to differentiate from neoplasms or GME. Treatment involves appropriate antibiotic therapy, surgical drainage (ideal, but not practical in most cases), and supportive care.

6. List the most common agents that cause infectious meningitis.
- Bacterial: *Staphylococcus* spp., *Pasteurella multocida, Actinomyces* spp., *Nocardia* spp., *Listeria monocytogenes*
- Fungal: *Cryptococcus neoformans, Aspergillus* spp.
- Parasitic: *Dirofilaria immitis, Cutereba* spp., *Toxascaris* spp., *Ancylostoma* spp., *Taenia* spp., and *Angiostrongylus* spp.
- Viral: rabies virus, feline infectious peritonitis (FIP), canine distemper virus, pseudorabies, and parvovirus and herpes viruses in puppies
- Rickettsial: *Ehrlichia* spp., *Rickettsia rickettsii* (RMSF), *Neorickettsia helminthoeca* (salmon-poisoning fluke), *Borrelia burgdorferi* (Lyme disease)
- Protozoal: *Toxoplasma gondii, Neospora caninum, Babesia* spp.

Viral, protozoal, and parasitic infections usually cause parenchymal signs (encephalitis), whereas bacterial infections usually cause meningeal signs (meningitis). Fungal and rickettsial agents may cause either meningeal or parenchymal signs or both.

7. Describe the most common noninfectious cause of meningitis.
The most common noninfectious cause of meningitis is termed **steroid-responsive meningitis**, which is a breed-related (see question 9) and non–breed-associated multisystemic polyarteritis and necrotizing vasculitis involving the meninges. Affected breeds include the weimaraner, German short-haired pointer, boxer, Bernese mountain dog, beagle, and Japanese akita. It is rarely reported in cats. Animals display classic signs of pyrexia, pain, and cervical rigidity. Most dogs are young. An immune-mediated cause is suspected, because most dogs respond to some degree to immunosuppressive doses of glucocorticoids. CSF analysis reveals a neutrophilic pleocytosis and elevated protein count.

8. Describe the most common noninfectious cause of encephalitis.
Granulomatous meningoencephalitis (GME) is a nonsuppurative inflammatory disease with focal or diffuse CNS lesions. Three forms are recognized: (1) focal GME usually involves the brainstem; (2) disseminated GME is widespread, involving the cerebrum, lower brainstem, cerebellum, and cervical cord; and (3) ocular GME involves the eyes and optic nerves. The cause of GME is unknown, although an immunologic basis is suspected. Signs are nonspecific but usually resemble typical signs of encephalitis. The disease may have acute and chronic presentations. CSF analysis usually shows mild-to-moderate increases in protein (40–110 mg/dl) and moderate-to-marked pleocytosis, primarily mononuclear cells (50–660 WBC/cm^3). Treatment usually consists of immunosuppressive doses of steroids; success is variable, especially in the long term.

9. Are meningitis and encephalitis associated with specific breeds of dogs?
Yes. Three breed-specific conditions are reported:
1. The so-called beagle pain syndrome is a severe form of steroid-responsive meningitis with polyarthritis causing cervical pain. A genetic disposition is assumed, and an immunologic basis is suspected. Prednisone therapy is associated with complete remission.
2. Bernese mountain dogs are reported to be susceptible to severe necrotizing vasculitis and polyarteritis (Bernese mountain dog aseptic meningitis). Although the cause is undetermined, clinical signs in most dogs resolve with steroid therapy.
3. Pug meningoencephalitis is common, and affected dogs usually present with sudden onset of seizures and signs referable to meningitis and cerebral involvement. In contrast to the first two disorders, therapy with steroids and anticonvulsants is usually unrewarding.

10. How do patients with meningitis or encephalitis usually present?
Most CNS inflammatory diseases present in an acute manner, but some are chronic and insidious (GME, fungal infections). Meningitis and encephalitis should be considered whenever the clinician is presented with rapidly developing and spreading CNS dysfunction. Clinical signs are highly variable, depending on the site and degree of involvement; signs may be focal, multifocal, or diffuse and may rapidly spread from focal to diffuse.

11. Describe the clinical signs of encephalitis.

Signs of encephalitis usually suggest diffuse parenchymal involvement, often slightly asymmetric. Hallmark findings are altered state of consciousness (e.g., depression, stupor, coma), behavioral changes, visual impairment despite normal pupillary light reflexes, incoordination, voluntary motor dysfunction, CNS dysfunction, and seizures. If encephalomyelitis is present, sensory ataxia, postural deficits, motor dysfunction, and cranial nerve dysfunction may be seen.

12. Describe the clinical signs of meningitis.

Classic findings in meningitic patients are pain (usually cervical) and fever. Animals are reluctant to be handled around the neck and show cervical hyperesthesia and muscle rigidity. In severe cases, opisthotonus and forelimb hyperextension may be present. Animals also may have generalized hyperesthesia and signs of encephalitis.

13. If you think a patient has either meningitis or encephalitis, what diagnostic tests should be considered?

The most important diagnostic test is analysis of cerebrospinal fluid, including measurement of opening pressure, gross visual examination, cytologic and biochemical analyses, microbial culture and sensitivity testing, and serologic testing. Other tests that should be performed include a minimal database and otic and ophthalmic examinations. Tests that may be required include blood and urine cultures, skull radiographs, electroencephalography, and enhanced imaging procedures (CT/MRI).

14. What are the risks of CSF collection in patients with meningitis and encephalitis?

Three factors in meningitic and encephalitic patients make CSF collection more difficult to manage:

1. Anesthesia, although always potentially dangerous, presents added risk because of the underlying degree of altered states of consciousness and potential involvement of the midbrain, especially the respiratory center.

2. Encephalitic patients have some degree of cerebral edema. When CSF is removed, further parenchymal swelling may result, with the risk of midbrain and medullary brainstem compression (tentorial herniation).

3. Alterations in CSF flow dynamics increase the risk of spread of infection.

15. What results on CSF analysis support a diagnosis of meningitis or encephalitis?

The pressure reading first measured on tapping the CSF space (opening pressure) is usually moderately to severely elevated in inflammatory diseases secondary to impaired CSF resorption. Brain tumors are the primary differential for increased CSF pressure and typically have massive pressure increases. On gross CSF evaluation, turbidity and an off-white to grayish color suggest meningitis due to increased cell and protein contents.

16. What cytologic findings are consistent with meningitis or encephalitis?

The characteristic cytologic finding in meningitis and encephalitis is increased total cell count. The differential count helps to identify the underlying cause. Suppurative meningitis reveals elevated polymorphonuclear neutrophil (PMN) counts (> 5 neutrophils/hpf), typically seen in bacterial infections. Mixed cell types (macrophages, lymphocytes, PMNs, and plasma cells) suggest mixed inflammation characteristic of fungal, protozoal, and idiopathic meningitis and encephalitis. Predominantly mononuclear cells, especially lymphocytes, suggest viral and rickettsial infections and neoplasms. Increased eosinophils suggest parasitic infection.

17. What biochemical findings are consistent with encephalitis or meningitis?

The characteristic biochemical finding in meningitis and encephalitis is an increased total protein count. Protein electrophoresis usually shows this increase to be due predominantly to an increase in globulin count. Albumin is increased in most cases of CNS disease, but globulin is typically increased only in inflammatory diseases.

18. What is the appropriate therapy for bacterial meningitis?
Obviously, the ideal therapy consists of antibiotic administration based on CSF culture and susceptibility testing. However, empirical therapy should be instituted immediately if bacterial meningitis is suspected. Antibiotics with good penetration of CNS barriers—and thus good first choices—include chloramphenicol, isoniazid, metronidazole, trimethoprim-sulfamethoxazole, and rifampin. Acceptable choices with intermediate penetration that is probably improved in the face of inflammation include amoxicillin, ampicillin, and penicillin G. Drugs to avoid because of poor penetration include cephalosporins and aminoglycosides.

BIBLIOGRAPHY

 1. Fenner WR: Diseases of the brain. In Ettinger SJ, Feldman EC (eds): Textbook of Veterinary Internal Medicine, 4th ed. Philadelphia, W.B. Saunders, 1995, pp 604–629.
 2. Kolson DL, Gonzalez-Scarano F: Viral encephalitis. In Carlson RW, Geheb MA (eds): Principles and Practice of Medical Intensive Care. Philadelphia, W.B. Saunders, 1993, pp 687–698.
 3. Luttgen PJ: Inflammatory disease of the central nervous system. Vet Clin North Am Small Animal Pract 18:623–640, 1988.
 4. Meric SM: Breed-specific meningitis in dogs. In Kirk RW, Bonagura JD (eds): Current Veterinary Therapy XI. Philadelphia, W.B. Saunders, 1992, pp 1007–1009.
 5. Reves R: Meningitis. In Parsons PE, Wiener-Kronish JP (eds): Critical Care Secrets. Philadelphia, Hanley & Belfus, 1992, pp 174–178.
 6. Sarfaty D, Carrillo JS, Greenlee PG: Differential diagnosis of granulomatous meningoencephalomyelitis, distemper, and suppurative meningoencephalitis in the dog. J Am Vet Med Assoc 188:387–392, 1986.
 7. Tipold A, Jaggy A: Steroid responsive meningitis-arteritis in dogs: Long-term study of 32 cases. J Small Animal Pract 35:311–316, 1994.
 8. Trenholme GM, Goodman LJ: Specific infections with critical care implications. In Parrillo JE, Bone RC (eds): Critical Care Medicine: Principles of Diagnosis and Management. St. Louis, Mosby, 1995, pp 1011–1027.
 9. Tunkel AR, Scheld WM: Bacterial meningitis. In Carlson RW, Geheb MA (eds): Principles and Practice of Medical Intensive Care. Philadelphia, W.B. Saunders, 1993, pp 454–466.
10. Ziller A: Meningitis. In Markovchick VJ, Pons PT, Wolfe RE (eds): Emergency Medicine Secrets. Philadelphia, Hanley & Belfus, 1993, pp 75–78.

69. COMA

Tim Hackett, D.V.M., M.S.

1. Define coma. How is it different from stupor or obtundation?
Coma is a disorder of consciousness defined by absence of awareness. The comatose animal appears asleep but is unable to respond to external stimuli or physiologic needs except by reflex activity. **Stupor** implies a state of depressed consciousness responsive to some stimuli, even though it may lapse back into unconsciousness when the stimulus is withdrawn. An animal is considered **obtunded** when it is not alert, when it is disinterested in its environment, or when it has a less than normal response to external stimuli.

2. What parts of the brain must be affected to produce coma?
Consciousness is maintained by sensory stimuli passing through the ascending reticular activating system (ARAS) of the rostral brainstem to the cerebral cortex. Decreased consciousness results from either global lesions of both central hemispheres or a lesions affecting the ARAS.

3. How does coma change emergency management?
With any emergency, ensuring a patent airway, providing adequate ventilation, and restoring circulating blood volume are necessary to prevent irreversible organ damage. The danger with

animals suffering coma from increased intracranial pressure is that any therapeutic maneuver or drugs that increase brain blood volume may lead to irreversible brainstem herniation. In administering fluids and analgesics and in handling such patients, care must be taken to prevent iatrogenic increases in intracranial pressure.

4. Describe the initial treatment of comatose patients.

1. Check for a patent airway and ensure that ventilation is adequate. The $PaCO_2$ should be kept below 35 mmHg to reduce cerebral blood flow and minimize cerebral edema.

2. Ensure adequate perfusion and cardiovascular function. Fluid therapy should be individualized because supernormal blood volume and pressure contribute to increased intracranial pressure.

3. Elevate the head and avoid compressing the jugular veins with catheters, bandages, or positioning.

4. Following volume restoration, give corticosteroids: methylprednisolone sodium succinate, 30 mg/kg IV, or dexamethasone sodium phosphate, 0.25 mg/kg IV.

5. Maintain body temperature between 99° F and 102° F.

6. Control seizures with diazepam and, if necessary, phenobarbital.

7. Supply glucose as needed to maintain blood levels between 100 and 200 mg/dl.

8. Supplemental oxygen is important to ensure that the PaO_2 is above 60 mmHg. To avoid handling the animal's head, an oxygen cage is preferable to face mask or nasal insufflation. Supplemental oxygen is not a substitute for ventilatory support and does not prevent hypercarbia. If the animal becomes hypercarbic, ventilatory support is necessary to prevent increased intracranial pressure.

5. How does a history of trauma affect emergency management of coma?

Trauma causes structural damage to the brain through contusion, laceration, and hemorrhage. The presence of hemorrhage within the calvarium complicates therapy because aggressive fluid administration and oncotic agents such as mannitol may worsen intracranial hemorrhage. Patients with head trauma should be evaluated carefully for signs of focal neurologic deficits, which may indicate a space-occupying hemorrhage. The therapeutic goals in cases of head trauma include normalizing blood pressure with as little crystalloid fluid as possible; lowering the PCO_2 to 35–40 mmHg, and frequently repeated neurologic examinations. Patients with progressive neurologic deficits may require aggressive therapy and even surgery if intracranial pressure continues to rise.

6. When should mannitol be used in patients with increased intracranial pressure? What are the contraindications?

Mannitol, an osmotic diuretic, dehydrates tissues and is effective in reducing brain tissue volume. In the presence of diffuse cerebral edema, it is the most effective agent to decrease intracranial hypertension. Its effects depend on an intact blood–brain barrier. Mannitol may cause a dramatic elevation in intracranial pressure before it exerts its action and reduces tissue volume. Furosemide may be given first to diminish this response. Mannitol is contraindicated in patients with hypovolemic shock, active bleeding, or cardiovascular compromise. It may lead to volume overload and continued hemorrhage. If mannitol leaks into tissues, it may draw excessive fluids with it. This is a major concern with space-occupying intracranial hemorrhage. Mannitol may leak into the hematoma, bringing with it more fluid and further compressing the cerebrum.

7. What are the general pathophysiologic categories of coma?
• Bilateral, diffuse cerebral disease
• Compression of the rostral brainstem (midbrain, pons)
• Destructive lesions of the rostral brainstem
• Metabolic or toxic encephalopathies

8. Describe the diagnostic approach to comatose patients.

Potential brain disease first should be classified according to location of the lesion and clinical course over time. History, physical examination, and serial neurologic examinations are the most useful tools. The clinician should assume increased intracranial pressure (ICP) in any animal with altered consciousness. Care should be taken to avoid anything that would further increase ICP. Neurologic examination of the comatose patient should determine whether the lesion is focal, multifocal, or diffuse. The examination should be repeated frequently to determine whether the patient is improving, unchanged, or worsening. Primary CNS disease causing coma and stupor should be considered when lateralizing signs or cranial nerve deficits are noted. Generalized disease of the cortex, cerebellum, or brainstem suggests a primary process outside the central nervous system. Diagnostic tests to look for evidence of toxic or metabolic disease or organ dysfunction help to differentiate primary CNS disease from other causes.

9. What initial laboratory evaluations should be performed in comatose patients?

Acute coma without a history of trauma suggests a toxic or metabolic disorder. Owners should be questioned about access to various drugs and poisons, including antidepressants, tranquilizers, alcohol, and ethylene glycol. Blood should be drawn immediately for serum chemistries, looking for evidence of organ dysfunction. Blood glucose can be tested easily on admission. Hypoglycemia may be treated quickly while its cause is investigated. A complete blood count may reveal signs of systemic infectious disease or thrombocytopenia. Urinalysis may reveal calcium oxalate crystals in cases of ethylene glycol intoxication or casts and isosthenuria with acute renal failure. Activated clotting time (ACT) can be tested quickly to assess the intrinsic and common coagulation pathways; ACT is markedly prolonged in patients with acquired coagulopathies. Once the results of the screening tests have ruled out organ dysfunction and metabolic disease, cerebral spinal fluid analysis and either computed tomography or magnetic resonance imaging should be performed.

10. What are the major causes of coma?

Causes of Coma

Trauma	Metabolic diseases
Intracranial mass lesions	Diabetes mellitus
Abscess	Hypoglycemia
Granuloma	Hepatic encephalopathy
Neoplasia	Myxedma coma
Hemorrhage	Uremic encephalopathy
Vascular disease	Drugs
Coagulopathy	Barbiturates
Hypertension	Opiates
Embolism	Alcohol
Inflammatory diseases	Tranquilizers
Canine distemper	Bromides
Granulomatous meningoencephalitis	Toxins
Bacterial and fungal meningitis	Ethylene glycol
Protozoal infections	Lead
	Carbon monoxide
	Arsenic

11. Describe changes in pupil size, position, and reaction to light that help to determine location and severity of disease.

Symmetric pupils with normal direct and consensual response to light require a functional ventrorostral brainstem, optic chiasm, optic nerves, and retinas. Increased intracranial pressure and herniation of the cerebellum under the tentorium cerebelli stimulate the nuclei of the oculomotor (third cranial) nerve, causing brief miosis of both pupils. As the pressure increases and the nuclei are irreversibly damaged, the pupils become fixed and dilated.

Anisocoria suggests primary CNS disease. If the pupils are unequal at rest but both respond normally to light and darkness, a unilateral cerebrocortical lesion contralateral to the larger pupil is likely. If the dilated pupil does not respond to light or darkness, a unilateral oculomotor nerve III lesion is present.

Metabolic diseases may cause symmetric miosis, whereas increased sympathetic tone may cause symmetric mydriasis. However, both respond normally to light and darkness. Symmetric miosis with no response to light or darkness is seen with damage to the pons, iridospasm, or bilateral sympathetic denervation (Horner's syndrome).

12. What abnormal breathing patterns may be seen in comatose patients?

Lesions of the medulla may damage the basic rhythmic control of inspiration and expiration. Functional transection of the brainstem cranial to the medulla allows ventilation to continue but in gasps rather than smooth inspiration and expiration. Damage to the midpons cranial to the apneustic area results in apneustic respiration, characterized by prolonged inspiration and short expiration. Cheyne-Stokes respiration is characterized by deep breathing followed by periods of apnea or shallow respirations and indicates that normal feedback mechanisms no longer function. With normal control of ventilation impaired, the deep breathing causes a drop in CO_2 of arterial blood. This drop is detected by the respiratory center in the brainstem, and respiration is inhibited. Progressive deterioration or compression of the brainstem often causes a slowing of respirations associated with rapid progression toward death.

13. What is the oculovestibular reflex? How can it be used to assess comatose patients?

Infusion of cold water into an ear canal normally induces horizontal nystagmus with the fast phase opposite the direction of the infused ear. Infusion of warm water induces horizontal nystagmus with the fast phase toward the infused ear. This caloric test of the oculovestibular reflex requires integrity of the brainstem, medial longitudinal fasciculus, and cranial nerves III, IV, VI, and VIII.

14. What is hepatic encephalopathy?

Hepatic encephalopathy is a clinical syndrome characterized by abnormal mentation, altered consciousness, and impaired neurologic function in patients with advanced liver disease and severe portosystemic vascular shunts. Hepatic encephalopathy results when the liver fails to remove toxic products of gut metabolism from the portal blood. Ammonia, mercaptans, short-chain fatty acids, and gamma-aminobutyric acid (GABA) agonists have been implicated in the pathogenesis of hepatic encephalopathy.

15. How is hepatic encephalopathy diagnosed?

Hepatic encephalopathy is suspected in patients with bizarre behavior after eating or with altered mentation and elevated liver enzymes. With hepatocellular damage both alanine transferase (ALT) and aspartate transferase (AST) are elevated. With congenital portosystemic shunts or end-stage liver failure, ALT and AST may be normal. Chemical parameters that suggest poor liver function include low blood urea nitrogen, low blood glucose, low albumin, lower serum cholesterol, and elevated serum bilirubin. Fasting and postprandial serum bile acids are markedly abnormal. Blood ammonia levels may be normal or elevated. Nuclear scintigraphy may be used to quantitate blood flow around the liver with portosystemic shunts.

16. What treatments are available for patients with hepatic encephalopathy?

Withdrawal of dietary protein is necessary to prevent production of intestinal ammonia. A 10% povidone iodine enema solution rapidly suppresses colonic bacteria and impairs ammonia production. Lactulose (1-4-beta-galactosidofructose; Cephulac, Merrell-Dow) is hydrolyzed by intestinal bacteria to lactic, acetic, and formic acid. With the lower intestinal pH, ammonia (NH_3)

accepts an additional H+ proton to form the less diffusible ammonium ion (NH_4), effectively trapping ammonium within the colon. Lactulose is an unabsorbed solute and also causes an osmotic diarrhea, decreasing intestinal transit time and absorption. Lactulose may be given orally but should be given rectally in patients with altered mentation.

BIBLIOGRAPHY

1. Chrisman CL: Coma and disorders of consciousness. In Proceedings of the Fourth International Veterinary Emergency and Critical Care Symposium, San Antonio, TX, 1994, pp 110–114.
2. Dayrell-Hart B, Kilde A: Intracranial dysfunctions: Stupor and coma. Vet Clin North Am Small Animal Pract 19:1209–1222, 1989.
3. De Lahunta A: Veterinary Neuroanatomy and Clinical Neurology. Philadelphia, W.B. Saunders, 1983, pp 349–352.
4. Kirby R: Approach to medical management of head trauma. Proceedings of the Fifth International Veterinary Emergency and Critical Care Symposium, San Antonio, TX, 1996, pp 263–267.
5. Oliver JE, Lorenz MD: Handbook of Veterinary Neurology. Philadelphia, W.B. Saunders, 1993, pp 272–295.

70. ACUTE PROGRESSIVE LOWER MOTOR NEURON DISEASE

Ronald S. Walton, D.V.M.

1. What are the four primary differential diagnoses for acute progressive lower motor neuron disease in dogs?
- Tick paralysis
- Botulism
- Acute idiopathic polyradiculoneuritis (coon hound paralysis)
- Aminoglycoside toxicity

2. Coon hound paralysis (CHP) is similar to which acute polyneuritis in humans?
Landry-Guillain-Barré syndrome.

3. Describe the pathophysiology of CHP.
CHP attacks primarily the ventral nerve roots and spinal nerves. The primary features are immune-mediated segmental demyelination and axonal degeneration. The neurologic signs are due to failure of motor impulse conduction from the spinal cord to the muscle fiber. Pain perception is usually normal because the dorsal root structures are affected only mildly.

4. Describe the clinical signs of CHP.
The neurologic signs develop suddenly. The onset of clinical signs has been associated with exposure to a raccoon 7–14 days previously. However, CHP also is seen in dogs with no known raccoon exposure. The neurologic signs typically begin as pelvic limb paresis and hyporeflexia, which quickly progress to tetraparesis in 24–48 hours after the first neurologic signs develop.

5. What are the treatment and prognosis for CHP?
No specific treatment is available for CHP. The underlying pathophysiology supports an immune-mediated reaction; however, no evidence currently supports the use of glucocorticoid therapy. The only therapy is supportive with good general nursing care. The prognosis is usually good.

6. What two species are implicated primarily in tick paralysis in the United States?
Dermacentor andersoni and *D. virabilis.*

7. Describe the pathophysiology of tick paralysis.
A salivary neurotoxin secreted by the engorged female tick acts at the neuromuscular junction. This toxin either blocks the release of acetylcholine or inhibits depolarization at the terminal portion of the motor nerve. The toxin may alter the ionic flux that mediates action potential production in both motor and sensory nerves.

8. Describe the typical clinical signs of tick paralysis.
Neurologic signs develop 7–10 days after attachment of the tick. The early signs manifest as ataxia, which rapidly progresses to paresis. Paralysis soon follows, with areflexia and hypotonus as prominent features. In cases in the United States, cranial nerve involvement is rare. Respiratory paralysis may occur if the tick is not removed. In Australia a more severe form of tick paralysis is seen, with autonomic nervous system and respiratory dysfunction or failure as common features.

9. Are dogs and cats equally affected by tick paralysis?
No. Cats appear to be resistant to tick paralysis as it is seen in the United States. However, in Australia, where cases of tick paralysis are much more severe, cats and dogs appear to be equally affected. Respiratory failure and autonomic dysfunction occur much more frequently with the *Ixodes holocyclus*-induced paralysis seen in Australia. In addition, the symptoms often persist with tick removal.

10. How do you treat a case of tick paralysis?
In the United States removal of the tick causes rapid improvement in the clinical signs. The typical patient shows complete recovery within 72 hours. The tick must be removed carefully. Failure to remove the entire head may actually worsen the clinical signs. The entire animal should be checked carefully, paying particular attention to the interdigital spaces and ear canal. A topical insecticide solution should be applied to the entire surface of the animal's body. In Australia, a much more severe form of the disease is seen. Clinical signs may worsen even when the *Ixodes* tick is removed. The use of mechanical ventilation and hyperimmune serum has been advocated in such cases to treat the profound respiratory failure that may occur.

11. Which North American snake's venom can induce acute progressive and diffuse lower motor neuron signs?
Coral snake.

12. In an acutely tetraparetic dog or cat, which system should you monitor most closely while you are determining an etiologic diagnosis?
The respiratory system should be monitored closely. Acute lower motor neuron disorders may progress to the respiratory musculature and respiratory insufficiency. Severe cases may require mechanical ventilation. Respiratory function is evaluated with arterial blood gas measurement.

13. Which class of antibiotics may induce signs of acute diffuse lower motor neuron disorders? What is the underlying mechanism?
Aminoglycoside antibiotics can induce neuromuscular paralysis secondary to their neuromuscular blocking action. The effects are similar to those of curare. The aminoglycosides may show dramatic effects, particularly if injected into a body cavity (e.g., the thorax). Intrathoracic administration of gentamicin has been associated with paralysis of the diaphragm secondary to blockade of the phrenic nerves. These signs typically resolve rapidly when the drug is withdrawn.

14. Describe the pathophysiology of botulism.

The clinical signs of botulism develop after ingestion of preformed toxin of *Clostridium botulinum*. The toxin produces a neuromuscular blockade inhibiting the release of acetylcholine from the terminals of cholinergic fibers. Nerve conduction velocities may be slowed in some patients, indicating an interference with impulse transmission as well. The clinical signs develop after an incubation period of 6 days or less.

15. Describe the typical clinical signs of botulism.

The signs indicate an acute progressive lower motor neuron disorder; they vary with the amount of toxin ingested from vague generalized weakness to tetraplegia and respiratory failure. A patient with botulism may show involvement of both spinal and cranial nerves. Cranial nerve involvement is typically not seen with either tick paralysis or CHP.

16. How can electromyographic (EMG) studies help to differentiate an acute lower motor neuron disorder?

In **polyradiculoneuritis** EMG findings include diffuse denervation of affected muscles. Fibrillation potentials and positive sharp waves are the prominent features. The evoked potentials are slightly reduced in amplitude and may even be polyphasic. However, they are not as severely affected as in cases of botulism or tick paralysis.

Tick paralysis shows no signs of denervation. However, there is marked reduction in amplitude of evoked motor potentials. The nerve conduction velocities may be slightly slower than normal, and the terminal conduction times also may be prolonged.

Botulism shows signs of spontaneous activity, including fibrillation waves and positive sharp waves. The typical case also shows a small muscle action potential in response to a single supramaximal stimulus. Nerve conduction velocities range from normal to slightly slowed.

17. Which of the three–polyradiculoneuritis, tick paralysis, or botulism—typically has cranial nerve involvement as a clinical feature?

Botulism.

BIBLIOGRAPHY

1. Barsanti JA: Botulism. In Greene CE (ed): Infectious Diseases in the Dog and Cat. Philadelphia, W.B. Saunders, 1990, p 518.
2. Braund KG: Peripheral nerve disorders. In Ettinger, Feldman (eds): Textbook of Veterinary Internal Medicine. Philadelphia, W.B. Saunders, 1995, pp 701–726.
3. Cuddon PA: Electrophysiological and immunological evaluation in coon hound paralysis. In Proceedings of the Eighth Annual Veterinary Internal Medicine Forum, Washington, DC, 1990, pp 1009–1912.
4. Duncan ID: Canine and feline peripheral polyneuropathies. In Wheeler SJ (ed): Manual of Small Animal Neurology, 2nd ed. Gloucestershire, UK, 1995, pp 208–218.
5. Herratage ME, McKerrell: Episodic weakness and collapse. In Wheeler SJ (ed): Manual of Small Animal Neurology, 2nd ed. Gloucestershire, UK, 1995, pp 189–207.
6. Marks SL, Mannella C, Schaer M: Coral snake envenomation in the dog. J Am Animal Hosp Assoc 26:629–634, 1990.
7. Oliver JE, Lorenz MD: In Handbook of Veterinary Neurology, 2nd ed. Philadelphia, W.B. Saunders, 1993, pp 185–189.
8. Oliver JE: Generalized weakness. In Proceedings of the Twelfth Annual Veterinary Internal Medicine Forum, San Francisco, 1994, pp 935–941.

71. BRAIN DEATH

Wayne E. Wingfield, M.S., D.V.M.

1. Define brain death.

Brain death is the irreversible cessation of all functions of the brain, including the brainstem.

2. Why is brain death important in veterinary emergency and critical care medicine?

For centuries animals were deemed dead when they stopped breathing and their hearts stopped beating. With the era of critical care, cessation of brain functions began to be considered the main reason for diagnosing death. Medical concern over making safe and appropriate diagnosis of brain death in respirator-supported animals led to elaboration of criteria.

3. What combination of factors has been shown to result in inability to survive?

- Irreversible coma with apnea
- Absence of brainstem reflexes
- No blood flow above the foramen magnum
- Isoelectric electroencephalogram 6 hours after onset of coma and apnea

4. What are common synonyms for brain death?

- Cerebral death
- Irreversible coma
- Persistent vegetative state
- Death

5. What are the essential components of brain death?

- Rule-out of contributing causes
- Irreversibility
- Lack of cerebral function
- No brainstem reflexes

6. What are the possible contributing factors to brain death?

- Hypothermia (core temperature < 32.2° C [90° F])
- Electrolyte disturbances (hyperkalemia, hyponatremia)
- Metabolic and acid–base disturbances (hypoglycemia, metabolic acidosis)
- Continuing neuromuscular blockade after administration of neuromuscular blocking drugs
- Central nervous system depressant drugs (barbiturates, narcotics, benzodiazepines)

7. How do you check for lack of cerebral function?

- No spontaneous movements, seizures, or motor posturing (remember: spinal reflexes may persist after death)
- No response of any kind in the cranial nerve distribution to painful stimuli
- Isoelectric electroencephalogram

8. How do you check for absence of brainstem reflexes?

1. Fixed, dilated pupils with no direct or consensual response to light
2. Pupils are mid-sized to larger (make sure that no atropine or catecholamines are blocking the pupillary response to light)
3. No corneal reflex
4. No vestibulo-ocular responses to cold water stimulation
5. No gag reflexes
6. No response to suction catheter placed down the endotracheal tube into the trachea
7. No "doll's eye" phenomena

9. What is the apnea test?

1. Place an arterial line, connect a pulse oximeter, and have at hand facilities for blood gas measurement.

2. Adjust the ventilator to an FIO_2 of 1.0 (100% oxygen).

3. Adjust the ventilator, if necessary, to achieve a PaO_2 of 40–50 mmHg.

4. Draw an arterial blood gas sample.

5. Start a stopwatch, disconnect the ventilator, and insufflate at 2–6 L/min through the tracheal catheter to help prevent hypoxemia. Watch for any movements suggestive of respiratory effort.

6. After the animal is disconnected from the ventilator for 10 minutes, draw a second arterial blood gas sample and reconnect the ventilator.

7. Compute the rise in $PaCO_2$ during the apneic period. The rise should exceed 10 mmHg, and no respiratory effort should be present for the apnea test to indicate that no spontaneous respiratory activity is present.

10. How is doxapram hydrochloride used to verify apnea?

Doxapram HCl is a central respiratory stimulant. We have used it to verify apena in animals after cardiopulmonary arrest. If an animal does not respond to the injection, the electroencephalogram is consistently isoelectric.

11. What are the two determinants of consciousness?

Arousal and awareness.

12. How is death defined?

Consciousness characterizes an animal's existence, and the irreversible loss of consciousness defines death. Consciousness is the most integrative function in the body and results in the functioning of the animal as a whole.

BIBLIOGRAPHY

1. Kinney HC, Samuels MA: Neuropathology of the persistent vegetative state. N Engl J Med 330:1499–1508, 1994.
2. Pallis C: ABC of brain stem death: From brain death to brain stem death. BMJ 28:1487–1490, 1982.
3. Truog RD, Flacker JC: Rethinking brain death. Crit Care Med 20:1705–1713, 1992.

IX. *Metabolic Emergencies*

Section Editor: *Michael R. Lappin, D.V.M., Ph.D.*

72. DIABETES MELLITUS

Lynda D. Melendez, D.V.M.

1. What are the most common medical emergencies associated with diabetes mellitus?

The most common medical emergencies associated with diabetes mellitus are diabetic ketoacidosis (DKA), hyperosmolar diabetes mellitus (HDM), and insulin overdose causing severe hypoglycemia. These three syndromes may present in much the same manner but are distinguishable with initial blood work. Often they are precipitated by underlying disease processes such as pyelonephritis, pancreatitis, pyometra, prostatitis, hyperadrenocorticism, renal failure, and heart failure.

2. List the primary metabolic abnormalities that characterize DKA.
- Hyperglycemia
- Metabolic acidosis
- Ketonemia
- Dehydration
- Electrolyte deficiencies

3. List the ketoacids of DKA.
- Acetoacetate
- β-Hydroxybutyrate
- Acetone

4. What is the pathogenesis of DKA?

DKA results from an imbalance in concentrations of insulin and its counterregulatory hormones, glucagon, catecholamines, cortisol, and growth hormone; an absolute or relative deficiency of insulin is accompanied by a relative excess of counterregulatory hormones, especially glucagon. This shift in the glucagon:insulin ratio eventually results in hyperglycemia because of increased hepatic glycogenolysis and gluconeogenesis as well as decreased uptake of serum glucose by insulin-dependent tissues. Once serum glucose concentration exceeds the renal threshold of 180 mg/dl (dogs) or 230 mg/dl (cats), glucosuria ensues, resulting in osmotic diuresis, significant calorie loss, and polyuria with compensatory polydipsia.

The loss of calories and the lack of availability of glucose for insulin-dependent tissues stimulate the mobilization of adipose for an energy source. Mobilization of adipose is mediated by hormone-sensitive lipase, which is activated by the increased glucagon:insulin ratio. Fat is transported to the liver in the form of long-chain free fatty acids (FFAs); in the liver ketone formation is favored over esterification into triglycerides because of the increased glucagon. The ketone bodies produced by oxidation of FFAs include β-hydroxybutyrate, some of which undergoes decarboxylation into acetone, and acetoacetate. In normal animals, ketones are metabolized by peripheral tissues and form carbon dioxide and water, which in turn are used to produce bicarbonate; in diabetics, the production of ketones exceeds utilization. Ketones are acids that are generally buffered by bicarbonate in the extracellular fluid. Decreased production of bicarbonate and excessive production of ketones result in the development of ketonuria and metabolic acidosis.

5. What causes the dehydration and electrolyte disturbances in DKA?

Osmotic diuresis causes a secondary medullary wash-out and significant loss of water and electrolytes, primarily sodium and potassium. Additional sodium and potassium ions are excreted in the urine, combined with the negatively charged ketone bodies, to maintain electrical neutrality. In addition, sodium is lost through the kidney, primarily from lack of insulin. Vomiting and diarrhea occur in some animals with DKA and contribute to fluid and electrolyte deficits. Total body water is significantly decreased as water moves from intracellular into extracellular space in response to the increased serum osmolality created by hyperglycemia and then is lost through either the renal or gastrointestinal system.

If severe enough, dehydration results in decreased renal perfusion and prerenal azotemia. Total body potassium is often deficient, although the animal may have normal or even elevated serum potassium concentrations. Metabolic acidosis results in the exchange of hydrogen ions for intracellular potassium (see chapter 77). Because insulin drives potassium into the intracellular compartment, the net effect is an efflux of potassium from its intracellular stores to extracellular space. Because serum biochemistry profiles measure only extracellular potassium, total body concentrations are usually underestimated.

6. What are the common clinical signs and physical findings for an animal with DKA?

Clinical signs are often nonspecific but include lethargy, weakness, anorexia, vomiting, and diarrhea. Polyuria, polydipsia, and weight loss with ravenous appetite often precede the development of presenting signs. Dehydration, hepatomegaly, cataracts, hyperventilation, and a fruity odor to the breath may be detected on physical examination.

7. Which laboratory tests are useful in assessing an animal with DKA?

Serum biochemistry profile, complete blood count, and urinalysis are the minimal diagnostic procedures to confirm DKA and to evaluate other potentiating problems. However, while you are waiting for these results, determination of blood glucose by using a glucose reagent strip or glucometer helps to distinguish a hyperglycemic diabetic crisis from hypoglycemia. Urinalysis reagent strips identify glucosuria and often ketonuria. However, β-hydroxybutyrate, which predominates in dehydrated patients, does not react well with reagent strips, often giving weak positive or negative results. A few drops of hydrogen peroxide added to urine catalyze the formation of acetone, which is detected on urinalysis strips, from β-hydroxybutyrate. Packed cell volume and total protein give quick information about hydration status. If available, venous or arterial blood gases rapidly detect acid–base derangements, and serum osmolality rules HDM in or out.

8. How can acid–base balance and serum osmolality be assessed without access to blood gas analyzers or freezing point osmometers?

Acid–base balance can be evaluated by calculating the anion gap:

$$\text{Anion gap} = (Na + K) - (Cl + TCO_2)$$

where Na = sodium, K = potassium, Cl = chloride, and TCO_2 = total carbon dioxide. Normal values range from 15–25 mEq/L. An increased anion gap is compatible with metabolic acidosis.

Serum osmolality is calculated as follows:

$$\text{Serum osmolality} = 2(Na + K) + glucose/18 + BUN/2.8$$

where N = sodium, K = potassium, and BUN = blood urea nitrogen. Normal values range from 285–310 mOsm.

9. What are the goals in treating DKA?

- To identify and manage the underlying diseases
- To replace body fluids
- To restore electrolyte and acid–base balance
- To reduce blood glucose

10. How are the underlying diseases assessed?

The diseases that most frequently precipitate a DKA crisis include pyelonephritis, pancreatitis, pyometra, hyperadrenocorticism, renal failure, and heart failure. Information gleaned from the physical examination and minimum database should lead the clinician to pursue other diagnostic procedures, including urine culture and sensitivity testing, abdominal and/or thoracic radiographs, serum amylase and lipase concentrations, and adrenocorticotropic hormone stimulation test. Once the condition is identified, therapy must be initiated to treat the diabetic crisis effectively.

11. What is the fluid of choice for treatment of DKA?

The initial fluid of choice is 0.9% saline, which has the highest concentration of sodium among commercially available isotonic crystalloid fluids; thus it is ideal for correcting the hyponatremia in patients with DKA. Hypotonic fluids should be avoided initially because cerebral edema may develop if serum osmolality is decreased too rapidly. Lactated Ringer's solution should be avoided because the hepatic metabolic pathways necessary to generate bicarbonate from lactate are the same pathways necessary to metabolize ketone. Therefore, the ability of the liver to metabolize lactate is often reduced. Poor perfusion may result in retention of lactate and lactic acidosis; in addition, because lactate is negatively charged, more sodium and potassium may be lost by renal excretion to maintain electrical neutrality.

12. How quickly should fluid deficits be replaced?

Fluid requirements should be calculated to restore hydration in 10–12 hours; supply maintenance fluids and replace ongoing losses as they occur. Central venous pressure (CVP) should be monitored along with body weight, packed cell volume, and total protein to prevent volume overload. Serum electrolytes should be reevaluated in 12–24 hours with appropriate adjustments in choice of fluid and rate of delivery.

13. Should potassium be added to fluids?

A normal or elevated serum potassium level does not imply that body potassium stores are normal or increased. Decreased insulin and acidosis result in an extracellular shift of potassium. Once insulin therapy is instituted and metabolic acidosis begins to correct, extracellular potassium moves quickly into the intracellular space and may result in severe hypokalemia. If oliguria and anuria have been ruled out, 20–40 mEq should be added to each liter of fluid. Potassium concentrations should be monitored every 2–4 hours during initial therapy. Because this protocol is not always practical, careful monitoring of the patient for clinical signs of hypokalemia is crucial. Signs include severe muscle weakness, cervical ventroflexion, ileus, and arrhythmias. Electrocardiograms can be evaluated serially for abnormalities associated with hypokalemia including bradycardia, prolonged PR intervals, absence of P-waves, and prolonged QRS and QT intervals.

14. Is bicarbonate therapy necessary for correction of metabolic acidosis?

Once insulin therapy has been initiated, ketoacids are metabolized to bicarbonate, which results in fairly rapid normalization of pH. Administration of exogenous bicarbonate in addition to this newly generated source may lead to iatrogenic metabolic alkalosis. Bicarbonate increases the affinity of oxygen for hemoglobin, decreases oxygen delivery to tissues, and, because it is hyperosmolar, contributes to the hyperosmolar state of DKA. Because of these considerations and the danger of paradoxical central nervous system acidosis, bicarbonate therapy is not recommended unless serum bicarbonate is < 5 mEq/L or pH is < 7.1

15. What type of insulin and insulin delivery methods should I consider?

Regular crystalline insulin is the insulin of choice for critically ill patients with DKA. Subcutaneous (SQ) administration should be avoided in dehydrated patients because poor perfusion leads to unpredictable absorption. Once the animal is rehydrated, a large amount of insulin that was deposited in tissue may be absorbed quickly, leading to profound hypoglycemia.

Insulin can be administered with repeated intramuscular (IM) injections by giving 0.2 U/kg initially, then 0.1 U/kg hourly until the blood glucose concentration is ≤ 250 mg/dl. At this point frequency of injection should be decreased to every 4–6 hours IM, or, if the animal is rehydrated, insulin may be given SQ every 6–8 hours. The dose of insulin may have to be adjusted at this point, depending on serial blood glucose concentrations. The recommended range is 0.1–0.4 U/kg.

Constant-rate intravenous infusion (CRI) of insulin is used routinely in humans and is becoming popular for treatment of DKA in small animals. This technique alleviates the need for hourly injections and allows easy adjustments in insulin dosing as glucose concentrations fall. A 24-hour dose of 2.2 U/kg (dogs) or 1.1 U/kg (cats) is calculated for each patient and added to 0.9% saline. Because insulin binds to plastic IV tubing, the first 50 ml of the solution is allowed to flow through the tubing and discarded. The drip should be administered with an infusion pump. If an infusion pump is used to administer maintenance fluids, the insulin can be "piggy-backed" to the other line. Otherwise, a separate catheter should be placed for insulin infusion. Because periodic adjustments need to be made, the insulin should not be placed in the rehydration/maintenance fluids.

To prevent development of cerebral edema, which occurs with rapid reduction in blood glucose, especially when the reduction in glucose exceeds replacement of lost sodium, blood glucose concentration should be maintained above 250 mg/dl for the first 4–6 hours. When the blood glucose falls below this level, insulin delivery should be adjusted.

Regardless of the route of administration of insulin, blood glucose should be monitored hourly during initial therapy. Once it falls below 250 mg/dl, 2.5% or 5% dextrose should be added to the fluids. Once the animal is eating on its own, a longer-acting insulin, such as NPH or Lente, may be given subcutaneously.

16. Why do ketone levels increase despite insulin therapy?

Most likely, the increase in detectable ketones is due to the metabolism of nondetectable β-hydroxybutyrate to acetoacetate and acetone, which causes an apparent worsening of ketosis.

17. Explain the pathogenesis of hypophosphatemia in patients with DKA.

Hypophosphatemia is not a common complication of DKA but may be life-threatening. Phosphorus is controlled by the body in a similar manner to potassium. Serum phosphorus increases in the absence of insulin and in the presence of acidosis. Because vomiting, anorexia, and osmotic diuresis may cause loss of phosphorus, total body stores may be depleted at the time of presentation, although serum levels may be normal. With therapy, phosphorus is moved into the intracellular space, and hypophosphatemia becomes apparent. Phosphorus is necessary for energy-dependent physiologic processes and cell membrane maintenance. Clinical signs and laboratory abnormalities associated with hypophosphatemia include hemolysis, muscle weakness, and neurologic signs such as seizures, mental dullness, and even coma.

If hypophosphatemia is detected, therapy with potassium phosphate at a dose of 0.03–0.12 mmol/kg/hr should be instituted, and phosphorus should be monitored every 12 hours until the serum level exceeds 2.5 mg/dl. The potassium in this solution should be taken into account in calculating total potassium supplementation.

18. What is the pathogenesis of hyperosmolar diabetes mellitus?

HDM is characterized by extreme hyperglycemia (> 600 mg/dl), hyperosmolality (serum osmolality > 350 mOsm), and neurologic abnormalities. In humans, it generally is associated with nonketotic diabetes mellitus, although it has been described rarely in both ketotic and nonketotic cats. Hyperglycemia causes osmotic diuresis and water and electrolyte disturbances as in DKA. However, compromised renal function results in decreased renal excretion of glucose, which causes a much higher degree of hyperglycemia than in animals with DKA. Severe hyperglycemia leads to an increase in serum osmolality, and the osmotic gradient between extracellular and intracellular compartments causes a shift of water into the extracellular space, resulting in dehydration of tissues. Severe dehydration of neurologic tissues is evidenced by restlessness, ataxia, nystagmus, disorientation, mental dullness, semicoma, and coma.

To prevent excessive shrinkage in brain cells, idiogenic osmoles, which are osmotically active substances, accumulate. If a rapid decrease in serum osmolality occurs because of rapidly declining blood glucose, idiogenic osmoles are dissipated slowly. The resulting osmotic gradient causes a shift of water into the intracellular space and leads to cerebral edema.

19. What are the goals of therapy for HDM?
- To replace the total body water deficit without creating cerebral edema
- To lower blood glucose concentrations slowly
- To correct electrolyte imbalances.

20. How should fluid replacement be addressed?
A balanced electrolyte solution or 0.9% saline is the initial fluid of choice. If the animal has weak, thready pulses, pale mucous membranes, prolonged capillary refill time, and cold extremities, an initial bolus of fluids should be administered. Do not give more than 20–30 ml/kg in 20–30 minutes. After the initial fluid bolus, it is recommended that you replace 80% of the estimated fluid deficit in the next 12–24 hours in addition to maintenance fluids. Another approach to fluid replacement is to calculate total body water deficit from glucose and sodium concentrations and to replace the deficit over the next 24–48 hours along with maintenance fluids and ongoing losses. Electrolyte imbalances can be handled in the same manner as in treatment for DKA.

21. How quickly should blood glucose be lowered?
Rapid decreases in blood glucose concentrations predispose to development of cerebral edema. Therefore, insulin therapy should be delayed until 2–4 hours after initiating fluid therapy, and a decreased dose should be used (1.1 U/kg/24 hr CRI in dogs). Blood glucose concentration should be normalized over 24–48 hours with frequent monitoring. Addition of dextrose to fluids and adjustments in insulin dosage should be handled as for DKA.

22. Describe the clinical signs of insulin overdose.
Lethargy, depression, ataxia, weakness, coma, and seizures may be caused by severe hypoglycemia due to overdose of insulin. Because overdose most often occurs at home, it is important to instruct owners how to look for signs and how to treat. Corn syrup should be applied to oral mucous membranes, and the animal should be brought to the veterinary hospital immediately.

23. How is insulin overdose diagnosed?
The history and clinical signs should increase suspicion. It is important to question the owner closely:
- Has there been any change in the type of insulin?
- How old is the bottle that you are currently using?
- Have you changed the type of insulin syringe that you use?
- Did a new person administer the insulin?
- Has the animal been eating well?
- Has the animal's exercise increased recently? (Increasing exercise decreases insulin requirements.)
- Is the animal being treated for hyperadrenocorticism?
- Has the animal recently finished estrus?

Some cats are transiently diabetic and may no longer need insulin at all. Definitive diagnosis is made fairly easily with a glucose reagent strip or a glucometer.

24. How do I treat insulin overdose?
An IV bolus of 50% dextrose (0.5 mg/kg diluted 1:4 with normal saline) should be given slowly. The animal is placed on a maintenance drip of 5% dextrose and fed as soon as it can eat. Blood glucose should be monitored hourly. Do not reinstitute insulin therapy until the animal is hyperglycemic. This may take several days, depending on severity and duration of hypoglycemia. The insulin dose should be decreased by 25–50%.

BIBLIOGRAPHY

1. Chastain CB, Nichols LS: Low dose intramuscular insulin therapy for diabetic ketoacidosis in dogs. J Am Vet Med Assoc 178:561–564, 1981.
2. Forrester SD, Moreland KJ: Hypophosphatemia: Causes and clinical consequences. J Vet Intern Med 3:149–159, 1989.
3. Macintire DK: Emergency therapy of diabetic crises: Insulin overdose, diabetic ketoacidosis, and hyperosmolar coma. Vet Clin North Am Small Animal Pract 25:639–649, 1995.
4. Macintire DK: Treatment of diabetic ketoacidosis in dogs by continuous low dose intravenous infusion of insulin. J Am Vet Med Assoc 202:1266–1272, 1993.
5. Wheeler SL: Emergency management of the diabetic patient. Semin Vet Med Surg (Small Animal) 3:265–273, 1988.
6. Willard MD, Zerbe CA, Schall WD, et al: Severe hypophosphatemia associated with diabetes mellitus in six dogs and one cat. J Am Vet Med Assoc 190:1007–1010, 1987.

73. HYPOGLYCEMIA

Chris McReynolds, B.A., D.V.M.

1. How is glucose maintained within the normal range in fasting animals?

Most fasting cats and dogs maintain blood glucose above 60 mg/dl. In a fasting state the counterregulatory hormones—glucagon, cortisol, epinephrine, and growth hormone—increase. These hormones stimulate hepatic production of glucose by glycogenolysis and gluconeogenesis. They also decrease peripheral glucose utilization by causing a conversion from carbohydrate metabolism to fatty acid and ketone body utilization by most tissues. Some cells, however, depend on glucose as their primary fuel, including the central nervous system, erythrocytes, and renal medulla.

2. What are the clinical manifestations of hypoglycemia?

Glucose is the primary fuel utilized by the CNS. In acute hypoglycemia the first area to be affected in mammals is the cerebral cortex, which is much more metabolically active than the spinal cord and brainstem. Common clinical signs in neuroglycopenic animals include lethargy, dullness, ataxia, seizures, and bizarre behavior. Hypoglycemia is a potent stimulus for release of counterregulatory hormones that function to increase blood glucose concentrations. With stimulation of the sympathoadrenal axis, muscle tremors, nervousness, restlessness, and hunger may be seen before neurologic signs because of high circulating catecholamine and cortisol blood levels.

3. What is the most common cause of hypoglycemia?

Artifactual reduction in blood glucose of 10 mg/dl/hr may occur when serum is allowed prolonged contact with red blood cells that utilize the glucose for fuel.

4. What are the primary mechanisms of pathologic hypoglycemia (< 65 mg/dl)?

Iatrogenic: inappropriate insulin dose for treatment of diabetes mellitus

Impaired glucose production
Hepatic insufficiency
  Cirrhosis
  Portosystemic shunts
  Necrosis
Fasting in neonates and toy-breed puppies
Hypopituitarism
Adrenocortical insufficiency
Glycogen storage disease
Sepsis

Increased glucose utilization
Insulinoma
Large extrapancreatic tumors
  Hepatoma or hepatocellular carcinoma
  Leiomyoma or leiomyosarcoma
Polycythemia
Sepsis

Decreased intake
Chronic starvation
Malabsorption

5. What diseases cause hypoglycemia due to impaired glucose production?

More than 90% of glucose is produced endogenously by the liver. Thus, hypoglycemia may occur with liver diseases that result in more than 80% loss of hepatic parenchyma. Hypoglycemia also may result from lack of counterregulatory hormones that stimulate hepatic mobilization of glucose, as in hypoadrenocorticism and hypopituitarism. Although most small animals do not become hypoglycemic with 24–48 hour fasting, neonates and toy-breed puppies are at risk for hypoglycemia because of decreased glycogen stores and muscle mass.

6. What diseases cause hypoglycemia due to excessive peripheral glucose utilization?

Insulin-secreting tumors—in particular, pancreatic beta cell tumors—may cause severe hypoglycemia due to inappropriate release of insulin in fasting or exercising animals. Similarly, inappropriate insulin dose for treatment of diabetic animals is a common cause of hypoglycemia. Many other neoplasms have been reported to cause hypoglycemia because of excessive glucose utilization by the tumor and/or inappropriately low hepatic production of glucose. The most common non–insulin-secreting tumors that cause hypoglycemia include hepatocellular carcinoma, hepatoma, leiomyosarcoma, and leiomyoma. Polycythemia (packed cell volume > 65%) may cause hypoglycemia due to increased utilization of glucose by large numbers of red blood cells dependent on glucose for cellular metabolism.

7. Why are septic animals often hypoglycemic?

Sepsis-induced hypoglycemia results from increased utilization of glucose by macrophage-rich tissues, such as the spleen; sepsis-induced enhancement of insulin production; and decreased hepatic production.

8. Describe the acute management of hypoglycemia.

For animals that show signs of agitation or dullness, a small meal usually alleviates clinical signs of hypoglycemia. For animals with hypoglycemic seizures, administer 1–5 ml of 50% dextrose IV slowly over 10 minutes. Once the animal is sternal and alert, feed a small meal. For seizures unresponsive to the dextrose bolus, one should start a 2.5–5% dextrose drip in a stepwise fashion. If seizures continue, add 0.5–1.0 mg/kg of dexamethasone, administered in the IV fluids over 6 hours. Finally, anesthetize the patient for 4–6 hours while continuing the above therapy if there is no response to glucose drip or glucocorticoids. Animals with intractable seizures also should receive treatment for cerebral edema.

9. Why does rebound hypoglycemia occur in animals with insulinomas?

Most animals showing clinical signs of hypoglycemia respond to an IV bolus of 50% dextrose given slowly over 10 minutes. Unfortunately, after the IV bolus of dextrose the beta cell tumor may be excessively stimulated, resulting in insulin release and rebound hypoglycemia. Cycles of hyperglycemia and hypoglycemia can be avoided by administering small amounts slowly; the endpoint should be dictated by control of clinical signs rather than correction of hypoglycemia.

BIBLIOGRAPHY

1. Bagley RS, Levy JK, Malarkey DE: Hypoglycemia associated with intra-abdominal leiomyoma and leiomyosarcoma in six dogs. J Am Vet Med Assoc 208:69–71, 1996.
2. Dyer KR: Hypoglycemia: A common manifestation of cancer. Vet Med 87:42–47, 1992.
3. Feldman EC, Nelson RW: Beta-cell neoplasia: Insulinoma. In Canine and Feline Endocrinology and Reproduction, 2nd ed. Philadelphia, W.B. Saunders, 1996, pp 423–441.
4. Walters PC, Drobatz KL: Hypoglycemia. Comp Cont Educ Pract Vet 14:1150–1158, 1992.

74. ACUTE PANCREATITIS

Chris McReynolds, B.A., D.V.M.

1. Describe the pathophysiology of pancreatitis.

The exocrine pancreas produces a number of digestive enzymes necessary for the degradation of proteins, fats, and polysaccharides. These enzymes are synthesized in inactive proenzyme forms that are activated only after they are secreted into the small intestine. In pancreatitis digestive enzymes are activated in the pancreas rather than the intestine because of damage to the gland or some stimulatory signal that results in pancreatic autodigestion. Systemic complications develop as activated pancreatic enzymes enter the bloodstream.

2. What is the most common cause of acute pancreatitis in people from the island of Trinidad?

The sting from an indigenous scorpion is the most common cause.

3. Why is the ingestion of a meal high in fat implicated as a cause of acute pancreatitis in dogs?

The pancreatic enzyme lipase metabolizes ingested triglycerides to free fatty acids in pancreatic capillaries. These fatty acids are directly injurious to the pancreas. The high incidence of pancreatitis in miniature schnauzers also may be related to the high prevalence of familial hyperlipoproteinemia.

4. Do any drugs cause pancreatitis?

Yes. Drugs implicated in inducing pancreatitis include azathioprine, sulfasalazine, tetracycline, furosemide, cholinesterase-inhibitor insecticides, and corticosteroids.

5. What other conditions may cause pancreatitis in dogs?

Other recognized causes of pancreatitis include hypercalcemia, abdominal trauma, intraoperative manipulation, pancreatic duct obstruction, and hypotension.

6. Are the same causes and mechanisms associated with pancreatitis in both cats and dogs?

Any insult to the feline pancreas, such as hypotension or intraoperative manipulation, may induce pancreatitis. In cats pancreatitis is also associated with concurrent hepatic lipidosis, infection with *Toxoplasma gondii*, and biliary tract inflammation.

7. What are the primary presenting complaints and physical findings in dogs with pancreatitis?

Common clinical findings are vomiting, abdominal pain, dehydration, and fever. In dogs the duration of vomiting may be several days or, in acute hemorrhagic pancreatitis, only a few hours. Uncommon systemic complications include icterus, respiratory distress, and bleeding disorders.

8. Do cats present with the same symptoms as dogs?

Of interest, whereas vomiting is a common historical finding in dogs, most cats present with anorexia and lethargy.

9. What are the radiographic signs of pancreatitis?

The most common radiographic finding is loss of visceral detail (ground-glass appearance) in the right cranial abdomen. Other radiographic signs include displacement of the descending duodenum to the right and of the stomach to the left, presence of a mass medial to the descending duodenum, and a gas-filled duodenum.

10. Are elevations in serum amylase and lipase activities definitive for the diagnosis of pancreatitis?

No. Neither enzyme is pancreas-specific; both are also produced by gastric and intestinal mucosal cells. Furthermore, because both enzymes are eliminated through the urine, a decrease in renal perfusion results in elevations of both enzymes. Finally, the administration of dexamethasone to dogs causes significant elevations in lipase without histologic evidence of pancreatitis.

11. Do normal lipase and amylase values eliminate the possibility of pancreatitis?

Many dogs and even more cats have confirmed pancreatitis with normal levels of both enzymes. Normal enzyme values in animals with pancreatitis may be due to impairment in pancreatic perfusion, depletion of stored enzymes, and/or disruption of the synthesis of new enzymes.

12. How is the diagnosis of pancreatitis confirmed?

Other than by histology, pancreatitis cannot be diagnosed on the basis of one test result. Common laboratory findings include leukocytosis, hyperglycemia, hypocalcemia, and elevations in amylase and lipase. Elevations in trypsinlike immunoreactivity (TLI) correlate well with pancreatitis in both dogs and cats but are also affected by renal perfusion; furthermore, results generally take several days to return. Abdominal fluid analysis—in particular, lipase levels higher than serum lipase values—helps to make a case for pancreatitis. Ultrasound is useful for identifying an enlarged, inflamed pancreas. Diffuse or focal hypoechoic areas in the gland, along with compatible laboratory and physical findings, justify a high index of suspicion of pancreatitis.

13. How can the severity of acute pancreatitis be ascertained?

On admission it may not be easy to predict the severity or probable cause of acute pancreatitis. The clinician should be cognizant of concurrent laboratory abnormalities or clinical signs suggesting systemic complications. Examples include thrombocytopenia or clotting abnormalities, which may suggest disseminated intravascular coagulation (DIC); oliguria, which may indicate acute renal failure; hypotension and tachycardia, which may indicate systemic inflammatory response syndrome; and hypoglycemia, which may suggest sepsis.

14. What are the key components in treatment of pancreatitis?

The most important element of treatment is adequate fluid resuscitation. Decreased pancreatic perfusion due to hypovolemia, which may result from vomiting and third-space losses, may lead to progression of the disease if fluid therapy is inadequate. Recent studies suggest that colloid fluid resuscitation (plasma, hetastarch, and dextran 70) is an important component in the therapy of pancreatitis. In particular, fresh frozen plasma (10–20 ml/kg) is important in treatment of moderate-to-severe cases. Plasma as a colloid provides not only oncotic properties but also clotting factors for management of DIC and protease inhibitors that deactivate pancreatic enzymes in the systemic circulation. Prophylactic antibiotics, pain relief, antiemetics, and antacids are also important components of therapy. Work in cats with experimentally induced acute hemorrhagic pancreatitis has shown that low-dose dopamine (5 µg/kg/min) reduces the severity of pancreatitis by reducing microvascular permeability. Dopamine as an adjunctive treatment awaits clinical evaluation.

15. What is the role of surgery in acute pancreatitis?

In most instances, pancreatitis is treated medically, and surgical intervention is not recommended. In patients that develop septic peritonitis or pancreatic abscess, however, surgery is the treatment of choice to remove necrotic tissue and to lavage the abdomen. Surgery also should be considered in patients who continue to deteriorate even with aggressive medical management.

16. What is done when the patient vomits every time food is offered?

Most patients with mild pancreatitis recover after avoidance of oral ingestion for two days, followed first by gradual introduction of water and then by small meals high in carbohydrates over the next few days. In patients that continue to vomit when offered food, one must first evaluate the case to ensure that no underlying disorder other than pancreatitis explains the persistent vomiting. In cases of smoldering pancreatitis, placement of a jejunostomy tube to provide nutrition with minimal stimulation of the pancreatitis should be strongly considered.

17. What are the long-term complications of pancreatitis?
Recurrent episodes of pancreatitis may result in progressive loss of pancreatic tissue and eventual development of diabetes mellitus and/or exocrine pancreatic insufficiency.

BIBLIOGRAPHY

1. Akol KG, Washabau RJ, Saunders HM, et al: Acute pancreatitis in cats with hepatic lipidosis. J Vet Intern Med 7:205–209, 1993.
2. Cook AK, Breitschwerdt EB, Levine JF, et al: Risk factors associated with acute pancreatitis in dogs: 101 cases (1985–1990). J Am Vet Med Assoc 203:673–679, 1993.
3. Hill RC, Van Winkle TJ: Acute necrotizing pancreatitis and acute suppurative pancreatitis in the cat. J Vet Intern Med 7:25–33, 1993.
4. Karanjia ND, Widdison AL, Lutrin FJ, et al: The antiinflammatory effect of dopamine in alcoholic hemorrhagic pancreatitis in cats. Gastroenterology 101:1635–1641, 1991.
5. Simpson KW: Current concepts of the pathogenesis and pathophysiology of acute pancreatitis in the dog and cat. Comp Cont Educ Pract Vet 15:247–253, 1993.
6. Williams DA: The pancreas. In Strombeck's Veterinary Gastroenterology, 2nd ed. Philadelphia, W.B. Saunders, 1996, pp 381–410.

75. HYPOADRENOCORTICISM

Lynda D. Melendez, D.V.M.

1. Define hypoadrenocorticism.
Hypoadrenocorticism, or Addison's disease, is the lack of production of glucocorticoids and mineralocorticoids by the adrenal glands. It may be due to a pathologic process that affects either the adrenal glands directly (primary hypoadrenocorticism) or the production or release of corticotropin-releasing hormone (CRH) by the hypothalamus or adrenocorticotropic hormone (ACTH) by the pituitary (secondary hypoadrenocorticism). **Typical hypoadrenocorticism** results from combined mineralocorticoid and glucocorticoid deficiency and is characterized by hyponatremia and hyperkalemia.

If only glucocorticoids are deficient, the disease is termed **atypical hypoadrenocorticism**. Because there are no electrolyte imbalances, diagnosis is more difficult than for typical hypoadrenocorticism. All cases of secondary hypoadrenocorticism are deficient only in glucocorticoids (atypical addisonian) because ACTH acts primarily on the adrenal zona fasciculata to stimulate glucocorticoid production and release and has little-to-no effect on mineralocorticoid production. Therefore, affected animals are considered atypical addisonians. Approximately 10% of dogs with primary hypoadrenocorticism are atypical at presentation, but most also develop mineralocorticoid deficiency.

2. What is the common signalment of dogs with hypoadrenocorticism?
Hypoadrenocorticism occurs most frequently in middle-aged females; the median age is 4–5 years. Sexually intact females have a higher risk of developing the disease, and sexually intact males have the lowest risk. Although close to one-third of dogs with hypoadrenocorticism are mixed breed, poodles of any size and flavor, Portuguese water dogs, Leonbergers, and Labrador

retrievers have a familial tendency. Other predisposed breeds include Great Danes, Rottweilers, West Highland white terriers, and German shepherds.

3. What are the most common historical complaints made by owners of dogs with hypoadrenocorticism?

Lethargy, anorexia, vomiting, and weight loss are common historical findings. Less frequent complaints are diarrhea, shaking, polyuria and polydipsia, and weakness. An important feature of hypoadrenocorticism is the waxing and waning nature of clinical signs. In general, the owner comments about marked improvement in the pet after administration of fluids and some "injection."

4. Which abnormalities are most commonly noted on physical examination?

Physical abnormalities include lethargy, weakness, poor body condition, some degree of dehydration, melena, and hypothermia. Approximately 35% of animals present with physical findings consistent with moderate-to-severe shock, including weak pulses, pale mucous membranes, prolonged capillary refill time (CRT), and cold extremities. However, affected animals tend to have bradycardia instead of tachycardia, which is indicative of hyperkalemia.

5. Describe the hematologic abnormalities in patients with hypoadrenocorticism.

Lymphocytosis and eosinophilia (i.e., lack of a stress leukogram in sick animals) occur in approximately 10% and 20% of dogs diagnosed with Addison's disease, respectively. These changes may be the only laboratory clues in the search for the atypical addisonian. A mild normochromic, normocytic nonregenerative anemia is common but often not apparent until dehydration is corrected. However, in patients with melena, anemia may be severe and ultimately regenerative.

6. List the common serum biochemical and electrolyte abnormalities associated with hypoadrenocorticism.

- Moderate-to-severe azotemia (approximately 80% of patients)
- Hyperkalemia (approximately 90–95%)
- Hyponatremia (approximately 80%)
- Hyperphosphatemia (approximately 70%)
- Low total CO_2 (approximately 40%)
- Hypercalcemia (approximately 30%)
- Increased activities of liver enzymes (approximately 30%)
- Hypoglycemia (approximately 17%)

7. Why is the azotemia associated with hypoadrenocorticism generally considered prerenal?

Most addisonians are azotemic at diagnosis and have a urine specific gravity less than 1.030. This finding argues against the assumption that azotemia is due to prerenal causes and supports primary renal failure. However, in most patients, the creatinine levels are typically less elevated than the blood urea nitrogen (BUN) concentrations. In addition, azotemia resolves in most patients with intravenous (IV) fluid administration. The low specific gravity is generally attributed to medullary wash-out from hyponatremia and increased renal excretion of sodium due to the lack of aldosterone, which results in solute diuresis.

8. How does a low sodium:potassium ratio support the diagnosis of hypoadrenocorticism?

A normal sodium:potassium (Na:K) ratio in dogs is 27:1–40:1 with a mean of 30:1. In one study of 225 addisonian dogs, about 95% had a low Na:K ratio; the mean was 19.3:1. However, 20 dogs had a normal Na:K ratio 1–4 weeks previously. Hypoadrenocorticism is placed on the rule-out list of an ill animal with hyponatremia, hyperkalemia, and a Na:K ratio less then 27:1, but hypoadrenocorticism is not the only disease that lowers the Na:K ratio.

9. **List the differential diagnoses for hyperkalemia and hyponatremia.**

Hyperkalemia	Hyponatremia
Anuric or oliguric renal failure	Gastrointestinal disease
Uroabdomen	Nephrotic syndrome
Urinary obstruction	Congestive heart failure
Severe gastrointestinal disease	Hypothyroidism
Metabolic acidosis	Diabetes mellitus
Drugs (potassium-sparing diuretics, nonsteroidal antiinflammatory drugs, angiotensin-converting enzyme inhibitors)	Primary polydipsia Inappropriate secretion of antidiuretic hormone
Pleural effusion	Third spacing
Pseudohyperkalemia of Akitas	Postobstructive diuresis
Thrombocytosis	
Leukocytosis	

10. **What test is used for definitive diagnosis of hypoadrenocorticism?**

Normal dogs may have low resting cortisol levels and so should not be assessed for the diagnosis of hypoadrenocorticism on this basis alone. An ACTH stimulation test is considered the gold standard for diagnosis of hypoadrenocorticism. Dogs with hypoadrenocorticism have low-to-low normal resting serum cortisol levels and show little-to-no response to ACTH administration.

The ACTH stimulation test does not differentiate between primary and secondary hypoadrenocorticism in atypical populations. Dogs with secondary hypoadrenocorticism have only glucocorticoid deficiency and do not develop electrolyte imbalances, whereas dogs with atypical primary hypoadrenocorticism eventually develop mineralocorticoid deficiency. Electrolytes should be monitored periodically in atypical primary patients.

11. **What is an addisonian crisis?**

The term addisonian crisis refers to the development of clinical and biochemical abnormalities associated with acute hypoadrenocorticism and characterized by vascular collapse and shock. Many patients also have EKG abnormalities associated with hyperkalemia. Approximately 35% of all dogs with hypoadrenocorticism are presented to the veterinarian with classic signs of shock, including obtundation, prolonged capillary refill times, pale mucous membranes, hypothermia, and weak, thready pulses. An important clinical feature is the presence of bradycardia in the face of vascular collapse, which suggests hyperkalemia. EKG generally reveals atrial standstill or absence of P-waves, prolonged QRS duration, low R amplitude, and peaked T-waves. A small percentage of dogs exhibit some degree of atrioventricular (AV) block.

12. **What are the goals of management of an acute adrenal crisis?**

Mortality associated with hypoadrenocorticism is usually secondary to shock, hypotension, and hypovolemia rather than hyperkalemia. Therefore, the most important goal of therapy is fluid replacement. Place an IV catheter and collect baseline samples for a complete blood count, chemistry profile, serum cortisol levels, and urinalysis before starting IV fluids. Once the animal is volume-repleted, replacement of glucocorticoid deficits and correction of electrolyte imbalances, hypoglycemia, and acidosis can be addressed.

13. **What is the fluid of choice for hypoadrenocorticism? How should it be administered?**

Normal saline (0.9% NaCl) provides the greatest concentration of sodium and chloride in a physiologic IV fluid preparation. It has the added advantage of being potassium-free. To achieve volume repletion, to correct hypotension and hypovolemia, and to improve tissue perfusion, saline should be administered IV at approximately 40–80 ml/kg in the first hour, with adjustments according to the clinical picture. Fluid administration not only improves vascular parameters but also dilutes extracellular potassium concentrations, decreasing the risk of cardiac arrhythmias. The correction of dehydration with improvement of tissue perfusion may be adequate to correct acidosis. Once heart rate, pulse quality, CRT, and patient attitude improve, the continuing fluid rate is determined by individual requirements (e.g., degree of dehydration, sensible and insensible losses, maintenance needs). If normal saline is not available, a balanced electrolyte solution such as lactated Ringer's, Normosol, or Plasmalyte may be used. Although these preparations contain potassium, concentrations are minimal, and the volume of fluid administered dilutes potassium concentration in the serum.

14. When should hyperkalemia be treated with something other than IV fluid replacement?
Opinions vary; however, it is agreed that if cardiac arrhythmias are present, hyperkalemia should be treated primarily. Others propose that if the potassium concentration is above 7–8 mEq/L, it should be treated with substances that decrease serum potassium concentrations or counteract the cardiac effects of hyperkalemia. Treatment of hyperkalemia is covered in chapter 77.

15. When should an ACTH stimulation test be performed in a crisis setting?
An ACTH stimulation test is a benign procedure and may be performed immediately. The resting cortisol level should be assessed when baseline blood samples are taken, aqueous synthetic ACTH is administered IV, and poststimulation cortisol level is collected in 1 hour for dogs and in 30 and 60 minutes for cats. Because fluid replacement is the most important aspect of therapy, it is generally not detrimental to wait 1 hour before glucocorticoid therapy is instituted. However, if the clinician believes that glucocorticoids should be given immediately, dexamethasone should be used; it is the only commonly used glucocorticoid that is not detected in cortisol assays.

16. When in the course of therapy should glucocorticoids be given?
Because fluid replacement is the most important aspect of therapy, it generally does no harm to delay glucocorticoids until baseline blood samples are taken, the ACTH stimulation test is completed, and the initial shock dose of fluids is administered. Once volume expansion has been accomplished, glucocorticoid replacement should be addressed. Glucocorticoids should not be given until perfusion is improved. If it is not possible to perform an ACTH stimulation test during the initial management of an addisonian crisis, dexamethasone is the drug of choice for glucocorticoid replacement, as explained in the previous question.

17. Which glucocorticoids are recommended for replacement therapy?
1. Hydrocortisone hemisuccinate and hydrocortisone phosphate possess glucocorticoid as well as mineralocorticoid activity and therefore are recommended in an acute crisis. They are given at a dose of 2–4 mg/kg IV every 6–8 hours until shock is corrected, then at a dose of 0.5–1.0 mg/kg every 6–8 hours.
2. Prednisolone sodium succinate also possesses mild mineralocorticoid activity along with its glucocorticoid activity and is given at a dose of 4–20 mg/kg IV every 2–6 hours, depending on the response of the patient.
3. Dexamethasone sodium phosphate has only glucocorticoid activity and may be given initially at a dose of 0.5–2.0 mg/kg. Once the patient is no longer in shock, this dose is decreased to 0.04–0.1 mg/kg twice daily.
4. Once the patient is stable and eating voluntarily, maintenance glucocorticoid replacement is begun. Prednisone or prednisolone is given orally at an initial dose of 0.5–1.0 mg/kg, divided every 12 hours. This dose is decreased by 50% every week and may be discontinued entirely. For animals with atypical hypoadrenocorticism, glucocorticoid therapy is lifelong. Patients that require mineralocorticoid therapy and receive fludrocortisone acetate, which also has some glucocorticoid activity, may not require daily prednisone. If signs of lethargy, anorexia, or depression recur, prednisone should be reinstituted at the physiologic dose of 0.22 mg/kg given daily or divided every 12 hours.
In times of stress animals with hypoadrenocorticism require additional glucocorticoids; thus, owners should keep either prednisone or prednisolone on hand.

18. When should mineralocorticoid replacement be instituted?
In the case of a crisis, saline administration corrects hyponatremia and hypochloremia and improves hyperkalemia while expanding the blood volume. Life-threatening hyperkalemia has already been addressed. Usually, nothing more is needed until the patient is rehydrated and eating

voluntarily. However, in cases that are slow to respond to saline administration, hydrocortisone hemisuccinate or phosphate provides the mineralocorticoid activity needed to improve electrolyte imbalances until a maintenance mineralocorticoid regimen can be instituted.

19. How is maintenance mineralocorticoid replacement assessed?

Maintenance mineralocorticoid replacement may be given in one of two ways:

1. Fludrocortisone acetate, 0.1 mg/10 lb/day orally in divided doses every 12 hours. (This drug has glucocorticoid activity and may not require the addition of prednisone.)

2. Desoxycorticosterone pivalate (DOCP), 1 mg/lb every 25–30 days IM.

Initially, electrolytes should be monitored every 5–7 days until they are stable. Once therapy is adequate, patients receiving fludrocortisone may be monitored every 4–6 months. After the first 1–2 weeks, animals receiving DOCP are monitored on the 25th day of therapy. If electrolytes are normal at that time, the animal may need injection only every 28 or 30 days. Response to DOCP is variable, and dosage and dosing interval must be tailored to each patient.

20. What other problems need to be addressed in dogs with an adrenal crisis?

1. Approximately 17% of patients are hypoglycemic at presentation; some have seizures. Hypoglycemia may be treated by adding dextrose to the saline infusion.

2. Metabolic acidosis is usually mild and may be corrected by volume expansion and improved tissue perfusion. However, if the acidosis is severe, sodium bicarbonate therapy may be required.

3. Renal function should be monitored closely by measuring urine output. If urine production does not meet or exceed 2–4 ml/kg/hr, diuresis with a constant-rate infusion of dopamine, 2–4 μg/kg/min, and furosemide, 2–4 mg/kg IV, may be necessary.

4. Approximately 15% of hypoadrenal dogs present with melena. In some cases, gastrointestinal bleeding may be severe enough to be life-threatening and require blood transfusion. Such animals should be placed on gastric protectants such as sucralfate, H_2 blockers, proton pump inhibitors, and synthetic prostaglandins. Packed cell volumes, platelet counts, and activated clotting times should be monitored closely. As odd as it seems, glucocorticoid therapy should not be withheld. It is postulated that the lack of physiologic glucocorticoids is the cause for loss of gastromucosal integrity and is necessary for healing.

21. What are the principal differences between hypoadrenocorticism in cats and dogs?

• There is no sex predilection in cats with hypoadrenocorticism.
• Diarrhea has not been reported in cats with hypoadrenocorticism.
• EKG abnormalities are uncommon in cats with hyperkalemia but present in 80% of dogs.
• Cats take 3–5 days to respond to therapy as opposed to 1–2 days for dogs.
• Serum cortisol concentrations in cats must be measured at 30 and 60 minutes after administration of aqueous ACTH and at 60 and 120 minutes after IM administration of ACTH gel.

BIBLIOGRAPHY

1. Hardy RM: Hypoadrenal gland disease. In Ettinger SJ, Feldman EC (eds): Textbook of Veterinary Internal Medicine. Philadelphia, W.B. Saunders, 1995, pp 1579–1592.
2. Lynn RC, Feldman EC, Nelson RW, et al: Efficacy of microcrystalline desoxycorticosterone pivalate for treatment of hypoadrenocorticism in dogs. J Am Vet Med Assoc 202:392–396, 1993.
3. Medinger TL, Williams DA, Bruyette DS: Severe gastrointestinal tract hemorrhage in three dogs with hypoadrenocorticism. J Am Vet Med Assoc 202:1869–1872, 1993.
4. Peterson ME, Greco DS, Orth DN: Primary hypoadrenocorticism in ten cats. J Vet Intern Med 3:55–58, 1989.
5. Peterson ME, Kemppainen RJ: Comparison of intravenous and intramuscular routes of administering cosyntropin for corticotropin stimulation testing in cats. Am J Vet Res 53:1392–1395, 1992.
6. Peterson ME, Kintzer PP, Kass PH: Pretreatment clinical and laboratory findings in dogs with hypoadrenocorticism: 225 cases (1979–1993). J Am Vet Med Assoc 208:85–91, 1996.
7. Rogers W, Straus J, Chew D: Atypical hypoadrenocorticism in three dogs. J Am Vet Med Assoc 79:155–158, 1981.
8. Williard MD, Schall WD, McGraw DE, et al: Canine hypoadrenocorticism: Report of 37 cases and review of 39 previously reported cases. J Am Vet Med Assoc 180:59–62, 1982.

76. PERITONITIS

Catriona MacPhail, D.V.M.

1. What are the primary functions of the peritoneum?

The peritoneum is the highly permeable lining of the abdominal wall and viscera, forming an empty cavity. Small amounts of free fluid that act as a lubricant between the abdominal organs are constantly being formed. Water and other soluble products freely diffuse across the membrane. This property allows such life-saving procedures as peritoneal dialysis.

2. What is the normal character and amount of peritoneal fluid?

Normal abdominal fluid is clear with a specific gravity of 1.016, less than 2 gm/dl of protein, and typically 2000–2500 large mononuclear cells/µl. There is usually less than 1 µl/kg body weight of peritoneal fluid.

3. List the types of abnormal fluid, along with the cellular and protein characteristics of each, found in the peritoneal space.

Fluids with different characteristics are classified as transudates, modified transudates, or exudates, according to the following criteria:

Characteristics of Transudates, Modified Transudates, and Exudates

	PROTEIN		
CELLS	< 2.5 gm/dl	2.5–7.5 gm/dl	> 3.0 gm/dl
< 1,500/µl	Transudate		
1,000–7,000 µl		Modified transudate	
> 7,000/µl			Exudate

4. List the most likely differential diagnoses for transudates, modified transudates, and exudates.

Transudates	Modified Transudates	Exudates
Hepatic insufficiency	Cardiovascular disease	Septic peritonitis
Protein-losing enteropathy	Feline infectious peritonitis	Bile peritonitis
Protein-losing nephropathy	Bile peritonitis	Hemoabdomen
Uroperitoneum	Hemoabdomen	Chylous effusion
	Chylous effusion	Uroperitoneum
	Uroperitoneum	Neoplasia
	Neoplasia	

5. What is peritonitis?

The term *peritonitis* describes any inflammatory process involving the peritoneum and peritoneal cavity. Feline infectious peritonitis is the only primary peritoneal disease. More often peritonitis is a sequela of another disease process or an insult associated with disruption of the abdominal viscera or an external wound into the abdominal cavity. Secondary peritonitis usually has an acute or peracute onset with serious systemic symptoms and signs.

6. What is the etiology of feline infectious peritonitis (FIP)?

FIP is a highly contagious, systemic, immune-mediated disease caused by a coronavirus. Chronic effusive peritonitis is the classic manifestation of the wet form of the disease, but the peritoneum is only one of many systems affected. Effusion and inflammation result from perivasculitis and subsequent increase in vascular permeability.

7. Outline the major causes of secondary peritonitis.

Causes of Secondary Peritonitis

BACTERIAL	CHEMICAL	COMBINED/ MISCELLANEOUS
Pyometritis	Uroabdomen	Neoplasia
Gastrointestinal compromise	Pancreatitis (pancreatic enzymes)	Iatrogenic foreign bodies (e.g.,
Surgical wound dehiscence	Gastrointestinal fluid (rupture,	sponges, suture)
Pancreatic abscess	perforation)	Granulomatous (glove powder)
Prostatic abscess	Bile (biliary tract disruption)	Contrast media (barium, iodides)
Penetrating foreign body		Feline infectious peritonitis
Puncture or bite wound		

8. What are the main categories of peritonitis?

Peritonitis is categorized as either **localized** or **diffuse (generalized)**. Presentation, diagnosis, treatment, and prognosis differ dramatically between the two forms. Localized peritonitis may or may not require medical intervention; however, if uncontained, it may rapidly develop into a diffuse or generalized condition that is potentially life-threatening. Because of the nature of the peritoneum, generalized peritonitis may have profoundly damaging effects on other organ systems.

9. What are the typical manifestations of generalized peritonitis?

Animals with generalized peritonitis commonly present with historical and physical abnormalities associated with the primary disease (see question 7). Patients are usually in hypovolemic shock and have marked abdominal pain. The patient may present with obvious abdominal distention, and a fluid wave (succussion) may be elicited on abdominal ballotment. Many animals with peritonitis have a recent history of abdominal surgery.

10. Is peritonitis always painful?

With acute or peracute onset of diffuse peritonitis, the animal exhibits signs of pain on abdominal palpation. Animals with severe abdominal pain often assume a praying position (the forelimbs are bent, and the rear quarters are elevated in the air with extended legs). Peritonitis that develops over an extended period, such as FIP, is usually not painful.

11. How does the peritoneum respond to injury?

The initial response is an increase in vascular permeability with subsequent influx of fluid. Increases in cell population and total protein are due to the presence of blood, albumin, fibrin, and debris. Fibrin is produced in an attempt to wall off the insult; it also allows adhesions to form between structures in the peritoneal cavity.

12. What is the simplest and most rewarding way to diagnose peritonitis?

Abdominocentesis for collection of fluid for cytologic evaluation is the least invasive and quickest way to diagnose peritonitis. If a fluid wave can be balloted, a single midline pericentesis is usually successful. A four-quadrant pericentesis is performed if there are small amounts of fluid, if compartmentalized disease is suspected, or if a midline pericentesis is negative. Usually the animal is standing or in lateral recumbency. The bladder is expressed to avoid unintentional cystocentesis. The abdomen is clipped, antiseptically prepared, and divided into four quadrants, cranial and caudal to the umbilicus and on either side of the ventral midline. A 20-gauge, 1-inch needle is inserted perpendicular to the midline into each of the four quadrants. Fluid should be allowed to drip out the open end of the needle and initially collected into a tube of ethylenediamine tetraacetic acid (EDTA) for cytologic analysis, which should include protein measurement and differential cell count. Other potential tests, as dictated by the suspected primary cause, include culture and sensitivity testing and measurement of packed cell volume, blood urea nitrogen (BUN), creatinine, total bilirubin, amylase, lipase, or triglycerides.

13. What if no fluid is retrieved from the abdominocentesis?

A negative abdominocentesis does *not* rule out peritonitis. The technique described in question 12 commonly yields false-negative results, especially if only a small amount of fluid is present. Alternatives include use of a larger-gauge needle or over-the-needle catheter and placement of a peritoneal dialysis catheter. Diagnostic peritoneal lavage may be performed with an 18- or 20-gauge, 1¼-inch over-the-needle catheter. After the area is prepared, the catheter is inserted into the abdomen and the stylet is removed. Isotonic fluid (22 ml/kg) is then infused into the abdomen through the catheter. After the fluid is allowed to disperse and mix in the abdomen momentarily, it is then aspirated back into the catheter and examined cytologically and biochemically.

14. After a routine, uncomplicated exploratory laparotomy, what type of fluid does postoperative abdominocentesis retrieve?

The fluid should be highly cellular, representing a mild inflammatory reaction due to tissue manipulation. The primary cell population should be nondegenerative neutrophils.

15. When is peritonitis characterized as septic? What are the most common causes of septic peritonitis?

The presence of one bacterium in the abdominal fluid characterizes the fluid as septic. The route of infection is usually from rupture of the gastrointestinal tract secondary to gastric dilatation-volvulus, mechanical obstruction, or breakdown of a previous surgical intestinal resection and anastomosis or enterotomy site. Other possibilities include rupture of localized hepatic, pancreatic, or prostatic abscesses and contamination from a pyometra.

16. What are the most common causes of nonseptic exudate?

Nonseptic exudate is usually associated with inflammation from a chemical irritant such as urine, bile, pancreatic enzymes, or blood. The term *nonseptic* implies the absence of bacteria; however, nonseptic generalized peritonitis may quickly progress to septic peritonitis if not treated. Chemical, nonseptic peritonitis may cause adynamic ileus of the small intestine, resulting in compromise of the lumen and possible induction of septic peritonitis due to bacterial translocation.

17. What are the typical characteristics of an FIP effusion?

The effusion associated with FIP is usually a nonseptic, protein-rich, straw-colored fluid with a relatively low cell count. The fluid is viscous and foamy because of high protein content and often has visible strands or flecks of fibrin. The cell population is typically characterized as pyrogranulomatous because of the predominance of macrophages and nondegenerative neutrophils. If the ratio of albumin to globulin in the effusion is > 0.81, FIP is unlikely.

18. How can suspected uroabdomen be confirmed?

Uroabdomen generally results in a transparent serosanguinous fluid and is initially aseptic unless an underlying urinary tract infection was already established. BUN and creatinine should be measured in the abdominal fluid and serum. The BUN level should be roughly the same in both fluids because BUN rapidly equilibrates over the compromised membrane, whereas the concentration of creatinine is greater in abdominal fluid than in serum. Of interest, BUN is now found to be as accurate as creatinine in identifying acute uroabdomen.

19. Can pancreatitis-associated peritonitis be diagnosed using peritoneal effusions?

Peritoneal effusions associated with pancreatitis are generally classified as nonseptic, suppurative modified transudates or exudates. Comparison of serum and effusion lipase activities generally reveals higher activities in the effusion.

20. How do you differentiate between hemorrhagic effusion and blood pericentesis from a vessel or organ?

The packed cell volume of the fluid should be compared with that from the peripheral blood; if the values are different, hemorrhagic effusion should be suspected. The absence of platelets and the presence of erythrophagocytosis on cytologic examination of the fluid is also consistent with hemorrhagic effusion. If a moderate-to-large amount of fluid is collected, a sample should be evaluated for clotting; if clotting occurs, the fluid is either peripheral blood or peracute abdominal hemorrhage. Traumatic rupture of abdominal organs or vessels, coagulopathies, and neoplasia are common causes of hemoperitoneum.

21. Describe the lethal factors in peritonitis.

The prognosis for a patient with generalized peritonitis depends on the underlying primary cause or preexisting or concurrent disease, duration of the condition, and the patient's physical status. However, certain concurrent conditions increase the likelihood of mortality. If hypovolemic shock develops or a mixed bacterial population or free hemoglobin is found in the effusions, alone or in combination, the prognosis is dramatically worsened. Hemoglobin is believed to enhance the virulence of bacteria by a mechanism not well understood.

22. Do abdominal radiographs have any diagnostic value in patients with confirmed peritonitis?

Fluid in the abdomen causes a ground-glass appearance on radiographs, which obscures serosal detail of abdominal organs. However, abdominal radiographs may delineate free gas in the abdomen, suggestive of gastric or intestinal perforation. This scenario is best appreciated on a standing lateral radiograph, which demarcates a line between fluid and free gas. Plain abdominal radiographs also demonstrate the presence of functional intestinal ileus, which is a common complication of generalized peritonitis. The presence of the urinary bladder or abdominal masses also may be determined from survey films, if fluid volumes are minimal.

23. What other diagnostic tests may help to determine the cause of peritonitis?

Abdominal ultrasound is useful in finding an underlying cause of peritonitis such as pancreatitis. It also may detect pockets of small amounts of fluid, as in a localized peritonitis that may be associated with pancreas or liver abscess. A positive contrast cystourethrogram may help to differentiate between a ruptured bladder and an avulsed ureter. An upper gastrointestinal series is indicated in some cases to confirm mechanical obstruction or perforation of the bowel.

24. What are the significant metabolic alterations and sequelae of generalized peritonitis?

Shock, metabolic acidosis, acute renal failure, hypoglycemia, pancreatitis, sepsis, and disseminated intravascular coagulation are the most common secondary problems in animals with generalized peritonitis.

25. What is a suitable antibiotic choice for a septic abdomen?

Because the bowel is the usual source of bacteria in animals with septic peritonitis, single or combination antibiotics for empirical treatment of gram-negative, gram-positive, and anaerobic bacteria are indicated. In combination therapy, enrofloxacin or aminoglycosides are usually chosen for gram-negative organisms and combined with penicillins, first-generation cephalosporins, or clindamycin, each of which has a broad spectrum of action against gram-positive anaerobic organisms. If a single antibiotic is preferred, second-generation cephalosporins, third-generation cephalosporins, and imipenem are good choices.

26. At what point is surgery indicated? What are the primary goals of surgical intervention?

Every patient with septic peritonitis should be surgically explored to locate and correct the underlying cause and source of contamination. Surgery also allows removal of foreign material, lavage of the peritoneal cavity, and, potentially, placement of peritoneal drains, gastrostomy feeding tubes, or jejunostomy feeding tubes. Irrigation of the abdominal cavity with large volumes of warm isotonic fluid aids removal of necrotic debris, potentially reduces adhesion formulation, and dilutes the bacterial population, thus lessening the potential for abscess formation.

27. What is the role of peritoneal drain systems in the treatment of peritonitis?

Peritoneal drains are useful for providing local drainage of intraabdominal abscesses or other pockets of localized peritonitis. Placement of a closed peritoneal drain for management of generalized peritonitis has been associated with many complications. Because of the peritoneum's ability to respond rapidly to injury, most drainage systems are sealed over within 6 hours by fibrin and adhesion formation. Efficacy of peritoneal drains for continual effusion of abdominal fluid may be enhanced by placement of multiple drains and by intermittent or continuous peritoneal lavage. Cytologic evaluation of the effluent measures the patient's progress and determines when the drains may be removed. The most effective type of abdominal drain is the sump-Penrose system, whereby a sump drain is placed inside a fenestrated Penrose drain. This configuration is thought to protect the abdominal viscera and to provide more efficient drainage than the use of Penrose, tube, or sump drains alone.

28. Describe the complications associated with closed abdomen peritoneal drainage and peritoneal lavage.

Any type of drainage system provides a route for ascending infection. The introduction of foreign material into the peritoneal cavity causes an increase in inflammatory response and formation of adhesions. Drains may be directly damaging to abdominal viscera by erosion of the serosal surface. Problems with peritoneal lavage are associated with the introduction and removal of large amounts of fluid and loss of cells, protein, and electrolytes. The most likely complications are anemia, hypoproteinemia, hypokalemia, hyponatremia, and hypocalcemia. Hypothermia is easily avoided by use of warm lavage fluids. Sterile occlusive dressings around the drain sites may minimize the risk of ascending infection.

29. How beneficial is open drainage of the abdomen? What are its advantages, disadvantages, and complications?

Open abdominal drainage is believed to provide a more rapid and more effective means of drainage of the peritoneal cavity. The obvious risks are infection and sepsis as well as dehiscence and evisceration, but such complications can be avoided by frequent sterile bandage changes and close observation of the patient. At surgery, the abdomen is incompletely closed by loose apposition of the external rectus sheath in a simple continuous pattern. Subcutaneous tissue and skin may be left open or closed, depending on the amount of local contamination. Sterile dressings are placed over the incision and secured to the patient with a circumferential abdominal wrap. The bandage should be changed as often as necessary, typically once or twice daily, and the quantity and appearance of the fluid should be evaluated. A major disadvantage is that this technique requires a second surgical procedure for complete abdominal closure. However, it also provides an opportunity for additional intraoperative lavage. Other complications include significant fluid and protein loss, resulting in hypovolemia, anemia, and hypoproteinemia. These conditions need to be recognized and treated appropriately.

BIBLIOGRAPHY

1. Burrows CF, Bovee KC: Metabolic changes due to experimentally induced rupture of the canine urinary bladder. Am J Vet Res 35:1083–1088, 1974.
2. Cowell RL, Tyler RD, Meinkoth JH: Abdominal and thoracic fluid. In Cowell RL, Tyler RD (eds): Diagnostic Cytology of the Dog and Cat. Goleta, CA, American Veterinary Publications, 1989, pp 151–156.
3. Crowe DT, Bjorling DE: Peritoneum and peritoneal cavity. In Slatter DH (ed): Textbook of Small Animal Surgery. Philadelphia, W.B. Saunders, 1993, pp 407–430.
4. Hosgood G, Salisbury SK: Generalized peritonitis in dogs: 50 cases (1975–1986). J Am Vet Med Assoc 193:1448–1450, 1988.

5. King LG: Postoperative complications and prognostic indicators in dogs and cats with septic peritonitis: 23 cases (1989–1992). J Am Vet Med Assoc 204:407–414, 1994.
6. MacCoy D: Peritonitis. In Bojrab MJ (ed): Pathophysiology in Small Animal Surgery. Philadelphia, Lea & Febiger, 1981, pp 142–147.
7. Rubin MJ, Blahd WH, Stanisic TH, et al: Diagnosis of intraperitoneal extravasation of urine by peritoneal lavage. Ann Emerg Med 14:433–437, 1985.
8. Shaw PM, Kim KH, Ramirez-Schon G, et al: Elevated blood urea nitrogen: An aid to the diagnosis of intraperitoneal rupture of the bladder. J Urol 122:741–743, 1979.
9. Shelly SM, Scarlett-Krantz J, Blue JT: Protein electrophoresis in effusions from cats as a diagnostic test for feline infectious peritonitis. J Am Animal Hosp Assoc 34:495–500, 1988.
10. Sparkes AH, Gruffydd-Jones TJ, Harbour DA: An appraisal of the value of laboratory tests in the diagnosis of feline infectious peritonitis virus infection. J Am Animal Hosp Assoc 30:345–350, 1994.
11. Withrow SJ, Black AP: Generalized peritonitis in small animals. Vet Clin North Am (Small Animal Pract) 9:363–379, 1979.
12. Woolfson JM, Dulisch ML: Open abdominal drainage in the treatment of generalized peritonitis in 25 dogs and cats. Vet Surg 15:27–32, 1986.

77. POTASSIUM ABNORMALITIES

Wayne E. Wingfield, D.V.M., M.S.

1. Where is most of the potassium in the body located?

Potassium concentrations equal approximately 150 mEq/L in the intracellular fluid (ICF) compartment, whereas extracellular fluid (ECF) or plasma concentrations are about 4–5 mEq/L.

2. How is the large chemical gradient between ICF and ECF potassium concentration maintained?

The sodium/potassium (Na+/K+) adenosine triphosphatase pump actively extrudes sodium from the cell and pumps potassium into the cell. This pump is present in all cells of the body. In addition, the cell is electrically negative compared with the exterior, which serves to keep potassium inside the cell.

3. Given the small ECF compared with ICF concentration of potassium, why are some electrical processes so sensitive to changes in ECF potassium concentration?

It is the ratio of ECF to ICF potassium concentration that determines the sensitivity of electrical processes such as cardiac conduction and smooth and skeletal muscle contraction. Because the ECF potassium concentration is small, a slight absolute change in ECF potassium concentration results in a large change in the ratio of ECF to ICF potassium concentration.

4. What common factors influence the movement of potassium between ECF and ICF compartments?

- **Acid–base changes.** Acidemia leads to intracellular buffering of the hydrogen ion, with subsequent movement of potassium to the extracellular compartment, thus increasing the potassium in ECF. In alkalosis, potassium moves from the extracellular to the intracellular space.
- **Hormones.** Insulin, epinephrine, growth hormone, and androgens promote movement of potassium into cells.
- **Cellular metabolism.** Synthesis of protein and glycogen is associated with intracellular binding of potassium.
- **Extracellular potassium concentration.** When ECF potassium levels are high, potassium tends to move into the ICF and vice versa.

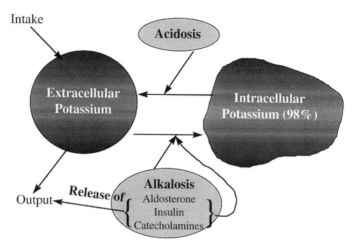

Control of potassium in the body.

5. How is potassium handled by the kidney?

Most potassium is reabsorbed by the proximal tubule, with net secretion or reabsorption by the distal nephron. Most normal animals have a net excess of potassium, requiring its excretion.

6. What is the main regulatory hormone for potassium?

Aldosterone, produced in the adrenal cortex, promotes sodium reabsorption and potassium secretion in the distal nephron, gut, and sweat glands. The main effect is in the kidneys. Release of aldosterone is increased when ECF potassium increases and decreased when ECF potassium decreases.

7. What factors lead to increased renal excretion of potassium?

- Potassium supplementation in intravenous fluids.
- Volume depletion leads to increased aldosterone secretion.
- Alkalosis promotes renal excretion of potassium.
- Increased sodium delivery to the distal nephron promotes sodium reabsorption in exchange for potassium secretion in the distal nephron.
- Decreased chloride concentration in the distal nephron allows sodium to be reabsorbed with a less permeable ion, such as bicarbonate or sulfate, and thus increases the negativity of the tubular lumen in the distal nephron. The increased negativity promotes potassium secretion.
- Drugs, particularly diuretics.

8. What are the other sources of potassium loss?

The gastrointestinal (GI) tract is the other route of potassium loss. Generally, diarrhea increases gut loss of potassium. Vomiting from the upper GI tract causes renal potassium losses from alkalosis, volume depletion (increased aldosterone secretion), or chloride depletion (see question 7).

9. When does serum concentration of potassium falsely estimate total body concentration?

The reciprocal movement of potassium and hydrogen ions across the cell membrane results in a rise in serum potassium of approximately 0.6 mEq/L for every drop in pH of 0.1 units in patients with acidemia. Alkalemia results in a fall in serum potassium of 0.1–04 mEq/L for every rise in pH of 0.1 units. Thus, it is important to consider acid–base status in interpreting serum potassium.

HYPERKALEMIA

10. What concentration of potassium results in a diagnosis of hyperkalemia?
The serum potassium concentration should be > 5.5 mEq/L to diagnose hyperkalemia.

11. What are the most common causes of hyperkalemia in dogs and cats?
  1. **Increased intake**
    • Most commonly due to excessive potassium chloride or inadequate mixing in intravenous fluids
    • Transcellular shifts
      Lack of insulin
      Acute mineral acidosis (HCl, NH_4Cl)
      Acute tumor lysis syndrome
      Massive tissue injury
      Digitalis toxicity
      Reperfusion after thromboembolism
  2. **Decreased renal excretion**
    • Urethral obstruction
    • Anuric or oliguric renal failure (requires significant reduction in glomerular filtration rate and urinary output)
    • Adrenal insufficiency
    • Drugs
      Angiotensin-converting enzyme (ACE) inhibitors
      Potassium-sparing diuretics
      Nonsteroidal antiinflammatory drugs (NSAIDs)
      Heparin

12. What are the clinical manifestations of hyperkalemia?
Weakness and neuromuscular paralysis (without CNS disturbances), suppression of renal ammoniogenesis (which may result in metabolic acidosis), and bradycardia commonly result from hyperkalemia.

13. What are the most common electrocardiographic (EKG) signs of hyperkalemia?
Decreased heart rate, decreased P-wave amplitude, and increased QRS duration are the most sensitive EKG indicators of hyperkalemia. The spiked T-wave, which is classically considered an EKG sign of hyperkalemia, is rarely recognized clinically.

14. What are the goals in treating hyperkalemia?
  • To reverse the toxic effects on the heart.
  • To shift potassium from the ECF compartment into the ICF compartment.
  • To lower total body potassium levels.

15. How is hyperkalemia managed?
  • Discontinue potassium administration (e.g., IV fluids, salt substitutes, potassium chloride, potassium penicillin).
  • Administer calcium gluconate (2–10 ml of 10% solution) (reverses toxic effects on the heart).
  • Consider administering sodium bicarbonate (0.25–1 mEq/kg IV) or 25% dextrose (1 gm/kg IV) with regular insulin (0.5–1.0 U/kg IV) to shift potassium from the ECF into the ICF.
  • Administer bolus potassium-free intravenous crystalloids to dilute ECF potassium.

HYPOKALEMIA

16. What level of serum potassium is necessary to diagnose hypokalemia?

Moderate-to-severe hypokalemia is present when the serum potassium concentration is < 3.0 mEq/L. In hypokalemia, many veterinarians forget that acidosis elevates serum potassium concentrations by shifting potassium from the ICF to the ECF compartment. Thus, in patients with acidosis, the actual total body serum potassium concentration is lower than the measured serum potassium concentration (see question 9).

17. What is the most common electrolyte disorder in critically ill animals?

Since you are reading about hypokalemia, surely you can guess the answer! In fact, about 43.5% of 460 animals in a study by Van Pelt were found to be hypokalemic. When you read the chapter about magnesium, you may find the claim that magnesium imbalance is the most common electrolyte disorder. It makes little difference which ion is abnormal most often; the important point is to expect many dogs and cats with low serum concentrations of both. An association between the two ions is very likely. Often, refractory hypokalemic animals respond rapidly after magnesium supplementation is instituted.

18. What are the common causes of hypokalemia?
1. **Decreased dietary intake**
2. **Transcellular shift**
   - Catecholamines (epinephrine, dobutamine)
   - Alkalosis
   - Metabolic acidosis
   - Insulin- or glucose-containing fluids
   - Hypothermia (?)
   - Hypokalemic periodic paralysis (Burmese cats)
3. **Potassium loss**
   - Renal
     Diuretic therapy
     Vomiting
     Hyperventilation
     Cirrhosis
     Steroid therapy
     Excessive gastric suction losses
     Administration of potassium-free crystalloids or glucose
     Chronic renal failure in cats
     Postobstructive polyuria
     Mineralocorticoid excess (hyperadrenocorticism and primary hyperaldosteronism)
     ACE inhibitor therapy
   - Extrarenal
     Diarrhea
     Vomiting (mostly via renal losses with alkalosis)

19. What are the clinical signs of hypokalemia?

Signs of hypokalemia are associated with cervical ventroflexion (cats) and polyuria/polydipsia from impaired renal concentrating ability. In general, these findings occur with moderate-to-severe potassium depletion. Thus, any reduction in serum potassium concentration is significant, regardless of magnitude.

The most important effect of hypokalemia is on cardiac muscle (arrhythmias). This effect is magnified when the animal is given cardiac glycosides. Hypokalemia also affects striated and smooth muscles. Most animals have signs of muscle weakness or even paralysis and abnormal gastrointestinal function (ileus).

20. How do you estimate the magnitude of total body potassium losses in dogs and cats?
Currently no method is available to estimate total potassium losses; thus, serum potassium concentration is used to govern replacement therapy.

21. What are the guidelines for intravenous supplementation of potassium chloride?

Serum Potassium Concentration (mEq/L)	Amount of Potassium (mEq) Added to 1 Liter of Crystalloid Fluids
< 2.0	80
2.1–2.5	60
2.6–3.0	40
3.1–3.5	30
3.6–5.0	20

22. What are the two main complications of potassium supplementation in animals?
1. When potassium is administered too rapidly, cardiac arrhythmias (often fatal) result.
2. Potassium chloride is an irritant that may induce phlebitis when given parenterally or vomiting during oral supplementation.

BIBLIOGRAPHY

1. Braxmeyer DL, Keyes JL: The pathophysiology of potassium balance. Crit Care Nurs 16(5):59–71, 1996.
2. Dhein CR, Wardrop KJ: Hyperkalemia associated with potassium chloride administration in the cat. J Am Vet Med Assoc 206:1565–1566, 1995.
3. DiBartola SP, de Morais HAS: Disorders of potassium: Hypokalemia and hyperkalemia. In DiBartola SP (ed): Fluid Therapy in Small Animal Practice. Philadelphia, W.B. Saunders, 1992, pp 89–115.
4. Dow SW, Fettman MJ, LeCouter RA, et al: Potassium depletion in cats: Renal and dietary influences. J Am Vet Med Assoc 191:1569–1575, 1987.
5. Nemzek JA, Kruger JM, Walshaw R, et al: Acute onset of hypokalemia and muscular weakness in four hyperthyroid cats. J Am Vet Med Assoc 205:65–68, 1994.
6. Rose BD: Introduction to disorders of potassium balance. In Rose BD (ed): Clinical Physiology of Acid–Base and Electrolyte Disorders, 3rd ed. New York, McGraw-Hill, 1994, pp 702–714.
7. Van Pelt DR, Meyer DJ, Salman MD, et al: Serum electrolyte values in emergency patients: A review of 460 dogs and cats. J Vet Emerg Crit Care 1997 [accepted for publication].
8. Wingfield WE: Potassium and magnesium: The two most important ions in critically ill patients. Vet Prev 3(2):8–13, 1996.

78. MAGNESIUM ABNORMALITIES

Linda G. Martin, D.V.M., M.S.

1. What are the important functions of magnesium?
Magnesium participates in the regulation of vascular smooth muscle tone, signal transduction, adenosine triphosphate (ATP) production, synthesis of nucleic acids, lymphocyte activation, and cytokine production.

2. Which cellular membrane-bound pumps utilize magnesium as a coenzyme?
Sodium-potassium ATPase, calcium ATPase, and proton pumps.

3. How is magnesium distributed within the body?
Magnesium is primarily an intracellular cation. The majority of magnesium is found in bone (60%) and muscle (20%). The remainder is found in other tissues, primarily the heart and

liver. Approximately 1% of total body magnesium is present in the serum and interstitial body fluids.

4. What are the three general causes of hypomagnesemia?
• Decreased intake
• Increased losses
• Alterations in distribution

5. Is short-term anorexia likely to cause significant hypomagnesemia?
No. Decreased dietary intake of magnesium must be sustained for several weeks to cause magnesium depletion.

6. In the clinical setting, how can hypomagnesemia be induced by decreased intake?
Prolonged intravenous fluid therapy, peritoneal dialysis, or total parenteral nutrition without magnesium replacement or supplementation of maintenance levels.

7. What are the primary routes for loss of magnesium from the body?
Gastrointestinal and renal.

8. Which drugs have been known to increase urinary excretion of magnesium?
Digitalis, furosemide, thiazide diuretics, and mannitol.

9. Which drugs may predispose to renal tubular injury and subsequent renal loss of magnesium?
Aminoglycosides, amphotericin, cisplatin, carbenicillin, and cyclosporine.

10. How can redistribution of circulating magnesium result in hypomagnesemia?
Hypomagnesemia can be produced by extracellular to intracellular shifts and chelation or by sequestration of magnesium. Administration of glucose, insulin, or amino acids may cause magnesium to shift intracellularly. Elevation of catecholamines in animals with sepsis or trauma may cause hypomagnesemia by beta-adrenergic stimulation of lipolysis. Free fatty acids are generated and chelate magnesium, thereby producing insoluble salts. Also, when administered in large quantities, citrated blood products avidly chelate magnesium ions. In acute pancreatitis, magnesium may form insoluble soaps, and sequestration of magnesium may occur in areas of fat necrosis.

11. What are the two most commonly affected organ systems in patients with significant hypomagnesemia?
Cardiovascular and neuromuscular systems.

12. Which arrhythmias have been associated with hypomagnesemia?
• Atrial fibrillation
• Supraventricular tachycardia
• Premature ventricular contractions
• Ventricular tachycardia
• Ventricular fibrillation
• Digitalis-induced arrhythmias

13. How does hypomagnesemia predispose patients to digitalis-induced arrhythmias?
Magnesium deficiency not only enhances digitalis uptake by the myocardium but also inhibits the myocardial sodium-potassium ATPase pump, as does digitalis. This inhibition results in disturbances in the resting membrane potential and the repolarization phase of the action potential. In addition, the calcium channel-blocking effect of magnesium appears to be decreased in states of magnesium deficiency and subsequently increases intracellular calcium

content. This increase results in enhanced sensitivity to toxic effects of cardiac glycosides and development of digitalis-mediated arrhythmias.

14. What are the neuromuscular manifestations of hypomagnesemia?
- Weakness
- Ataxia
- Muscle twitching
- Hyperreflexia
- Seizures
- Coma

15. Which other electrolyte abnormalities are commonly associated with hypomagnesemia in critically ill dogs?
Hypokalemia and hyponatremia.

16. Why is the evaluation of magnesium deficiency so difficult?
Because 99% of the total body magnesium is located in the intracellular compartment, serum magnesium levels do not consistently reflect total body stores. Therefore, serum magnesium levels may be normal in the presence of total body magnesium deficiency.

17. Besides measuring serum magnesium concentrations, what are other methods of evaluating magnesium status?
Alternate methods of evaluating magnesium status include determination of ultrafilterable, ionized, and mononuclear blood cell magnesium levels.

18. How may hypomagnesemia cause hypokalemia that is refractory to potassium supplementation?
Because magnesium is a cofactor for the membrane-bound sodium-potassium ATPase pump, magnesium deficiency results in impaired pump function and allows potassium to escape from the cell. Ultimately the potassium is lost in urine. In some instances, total body potassium depletion is profound, and massive supplementation of potassium may fail to correct the hypokalemia until the magnesium deficit is replaced.

19. When is supplementation of magnesium recommended?
Supplementation is recommended if serum magnesium levels are less than 1.2 mg/dl or at higher serum concentrations in the presence of clinical signs (refractory hypokalemia, seizures, cardiac arrhythmias) that can be attributed to hypomagnesemia.

20. What two factors should be assessed before supplementing magnesium?
Renal function and cardiac conduction disturbances. Because magnesium is excreted primarily by the kidneys, the dose of magnesium should be reduced by 50% in azotemic patients and serum levels should be monitored frequently to prevent development of hypermagnesemia. Magnesium also prolongs conduction through the atrioventricular (AV) node. Therefore, any patient with cardiac conduction disturbances should have judicious supplementation of magnesium and frequent EKG monitoring.

21. Which type of magnesium should be administered parenterally when hypocalcemia is present?
Magnesium chloride. Parenteral administration of magnesium sulfate may further aggravate hypocalcemia because of chelation of calcium with sulfate.

22. What are the causes of hypermagnesemia?
- Acute or chronic renal failure
- Hypoadrenocorticism
- Hyperparathyroidism
- Iatrogenic overdose of magnesium, especially in patients with impaired renal function

Because magnesium excretion decreases as the glomerular filtration rate declines, it is not surprising that most cases of hypermagnesemia involve patients with some degree of renal insufficiency. Hypoadrenocorticism and hyperparathyroidism tend to cause only mild elevations in serum magnesium concentrations.

23. What are the cardiovascular manifestations of hypermagnesemia?

Hypermagnesemia produces EKG changes, including prolongation of the PR interval and widening of the QRS complex, due to delayed atrioventricular and interventricular conduction. At severely elevated serum magnesium levels, third-degree AV block and asystole may occur. Hypermagnesemia also has been reported to produce hypotension secondary to relaxation of vascular resistance vessels. Myocardial contractility is probably not affected by hypermagnesemia.

24. What are the neuromuscular manifestations of hypermagnesemia?

The most common clinical signs of hypermagnesemia are weakness and hyporeflexia. Profound magnesium toxicity has been associated with coma and respiratory depression secondary to respiratory muscle paralysis.

25. Describe the treatment for hypermagnesemia.

The first step is to stop all exogenous magnesium administration. Further treatment is based on the degree of hypermagnesemia, clinical signs, and renal function. A patient with mild clinical signs may be treated with supportive care and observation, provided that renal function is normal. More severe cases, which involve unresponsiveness, respiratory depression, and hemodynamic instability, should be treated with saline diuresis and furosemide to accelerate renal magnesium excretion. Intravenous calcium also may be given if arrhythmias or hemodynamic instability is present. Calcium acts as a direct antagonist of magnesium at the neuromuscular junction and may be beneficial in reversing the effects of hypermagnesemia.

BIBLIOGRAPHY

1. Arsenian MA: Magnesium and cardiovascular disease. Prog Cardiovasc Dis 35:271–310, 1993.
2. Cannon LA, Heiselman DE, Dougherty JM, et al: Magnesium levels in cardiac arrest victims: Relationship between magnesium levels and successful resuscitation. Ann Emerg Med 16:1195–1199, 1987.
3. Cobb M, Michell AR: Plasma electrolyte concentrations in dogs receiving diuretic therapy for cardiac failure. J Small Animal Pract 33:526–529, 1992.
4. Dhupa N: Magnesium therapy. In Bonagura JD (ed): Kirk's Current Veterinary Therapy XII. Philadelphia, W.B. Saunders, 1995, pp 132–133.
5. Martin LG, Matteson VL, Wingfield WE, et al: Abnormalities of serum magnesium in critically ill dogs: Incidence and implications. J Vet Emerg Crit Care 4:15–20, 1994.
6. Martin LG, Van Pelt DR, Wingfield WE: Magnesium and the critically ill patient. In Bonagura JD (ed): Kirk's Current Veterinary Therapy XII. Philadelphia, W.B. Saunders, 1995, pp 128–131.
7. Martin LG, Wingfield WE, Van Pelt DR, et al: Magnesium in the 1990's: Implications for veterinary critical care. J Vet Emerg Crit Care 3:105–114, 1993.
8. Olerich MA, Rude RK: Should we supplement magnesium in critically ill patients? New Horizons 2:186–192, 1994.
9. Salem M, Kasinski N, Munoz R, et al: Progressive magnesium deficiency increases mortality from endotoxin challenge: Protective effects of acute magnesium replacement therapy. Crit Care Med 23:108–118, 1995.
10. Salem M, Munoz R, Chernow B: Hypomagnesemia in critical illness: A common and clinically important problem. Crit Care Clin 7:225–252, 1991.

79. HYPOPROTEINEMIA

Michael R. Lappin, D.V.M,. Ph.D.

1. What constitutes hypoproteinemia?

Hypoproteinemia exists if the total serum protein is < 5.4 gm/dl for dogs and < 5.9 gm/dl for cats. Hypoproteinemia usually results from decreased globulins (dogs, < 1.9 gm/dl; cats, < 2.9 gm/dl), decreased albumin (dogs, < 2.7 gm/dl; cats, < 2.3 gm/dl), or decreased globulins and albumin (panhypoproteinemia). Other proteins found in the body include lipoproteins, glycoproteins, mucoproteins, fibrinogen, and clotting factors.

2. What are the primary sources of serum globulins?

Alpha, beta, and gamma globulins make up total serum globulin concentrations. Alpha and beta globulins are produced primarily by the liver. Gamma globulins are produced by B-lymphocytes and plasma cells.

3. What is the primary source of serum albumin?

Albumin is produced by the liver.

4. What are the primary causes of hypoalbuminemia?

The most clinically relevant causes of hypoalbuminemia are losses from the vascular space, decreased hepatic production, or hemodilution with excessive intravenous fluids. The most common sites for albumin loss from the vascular space include the kidneys, gastrointestinal (GI) tract, and third spacing of albumin in tissues or serosal spaces, including the pleural space and peritoneal cavity. Decreased production of albumin from severe hepatic insufficiency is also a common cause of hypoalbuminemia. Rarely, starvation or malnutrition results in hypoalbuminemia.

5. What are the primary causes of hypoglobulinemia?

Hypoglobulinemia results almost exclusively from gastrointestinal loss; albumin is usually lost concurrently, resulting in panhypoproteinemia. Renal diseases and third spacing rarely result in loss of globulins from the vascular space. Hypoglobulinemia rarely results from hepatic insufficiency; although alpha and beta globulins are decreased, gamma globulins are generally increased. This polyclonal gammopathy results from decreased antigen removal by the hepatic reticuloendothelial system; the increased peripheral antigen load stimulates peripheral B-lymphocytes and plasma cells to produce antibodies. Congenital hypoglobulinemias are extremely rare.

6. Why are animals with hypoproteinemia presented for emergency care?

Most animals with hypoalbuminemia are evaluated for respiratory distress, abdominal distention, or peripheral edema. Albumin is the most important protein for maintenance of oncotic pressure; hypoalbuminemia is the most common cause of transudative pleural and peritoneal effusions. Rarely, pericardial effusion and cardiac tamponade result from hypoalbuminemia. Clinical signs referable to the primary cause of hypoproteinemia are often recognized. Occasionally, respiratory distress results in pulmonary thromboembolic disease from antithrombin III (AT III) deficiency; AT III is approximately the same molecular weight as albumin and so is lost with protein-losing enteropathies and protein-losing nephropathies.

7. What are the causes and clinical signs of protein-losing nephropathy?

Polyuria and polydipsia are the most common signs; anorexia and other signs of renal failure occur in some cases. Protein-losing nephropathy is associated with glomerulonephritis and amyloidosis. In dogs and cats, glomerulonephritis is generally an immune complex disease. Systemic lupus erythematosus is the most common primary immune disease. Any chronic antigenic stimulation from bacteria, fungi, parasites, neoplasia, drugs, or vaccines may result in protein-losing nephropathy. *Ehrlichia canis, Brucella canis,* and *Dirofilaria immitis* are infectious examples of glomerulonephritis.

8. What are the causes and clinical signs of protein-losing enteropathy?

Most animals with protein-losing enteropathy have vomiting and small bowel, large bowel, or mixed bowel diarrhea. Approximately 5–10% have no known GI tract signs. Protein-losing enteropathy can result from any diffuse or focal disease of the GI tract; parasites, inflammatory bowel disease, neoplasia, and lymphangiectasia are common causes.

9. What are the causes and clinical signs of hepatic insufficiency?

Hepatic insufficiency generally is due to either congenital portosystemic shunts, which result in hepatic atrophy, or chronic inflammatory hepatic disease, which results in hepatic cirrhosis. Animals with hepatic insufficiency generally present for evaluation of inappetence, ptyalism, vomiting, diarrhea, failure to thrive, hepatic encephalopathy, or lower urinary tract signs from urate calculi formation.

10. What are the causes and clinical signs of third spacing of albumin?

Albumin can be lost from the vascular space into the pleural space, peritoneal cavity, or tissues. Tissue third spacing generally results from vasculitis due to immune-mediated or infectious diseases, such as ehrlichiosis or Rocky Mountain spotted fever. High-protein ascites (modified transudate) results most frequently from right heart disease, vena caval disease, or cardiac tamponade. Neoplasia may result in the loss of albumin and other proteins into the pleural space or peritoneal cavity. Animals with vasculitis generally have depression, fever, and inappetence. Nonspecific clinical signs depend on the tissues with third spacing of fluids. Dyspnea and abdominal distention are common.

11. What is the initial diagnostic plan for animals suspected of hypoproteinemia?

Diagnostic and therapeutic thoracocentesis is indicated in all animals with dyspnea. Abdominal paracentesis is indicated if a fluid wave is balloted on physical examination. Cell counts, protein quantitation, and cytologic analysis should be performed on fluid obtained. Hypoalbuminemia, hypoglobulinemia, or both are confirmed by measurement in serum; a complete blood cell count, serum biochemical panel, and urinalysis are performed in most animals with clinical signs referable to hypoproteinemia. Differential diagnoses can be ranked based on albumin and globulin results.

Differential Diagnoses in Animals with Hypoalbuminemia Based on Globulin Concentrations

SYNDROME	GLOBULIN CONCENTRATION
Protein-losing nephropathy	Normal
Protein-losing enteropathy	Decreased
Hepatic insufficiency	Normal or increased
Third spacing	Normal or increased

12. What specialized diagnostic procedures are used to assess animals with hypoalbuminemia?

- If proteinuria without pyuria or hematuria is detected, a protein:creatinine ratio is performed to assess magnitude of protein loss. Infectious disease serologic tests, antinuclear antibody testing, and thoracic and abdominal radiographs are often performed in the search for an antigen source.
- If panhypoproteinemia is detected, fecal fats, fecal flotation, abdominal radiographs, GI contrast studies, and endoscopy are commonly used to assess potential primary causes.

- If hematologic, serum biochemical, and urinalysis abnormalities consistent with hepatic insufficiency are detected, preprandial and postprandial serum bile acids may be measured to confirm hepatic dysfunction. Ultrasound evaluation and hepatic biopsy are commonly included in the further diagnostic plan for animals with proven hepatic insufficiency.
- If protein-losing enteropathy or nephropathy is present, AT III may be measured to assess risk for developing thromboembolic disease.

13. How do you manage hypoproteinemic animals in the emergency setting?
- Perform diagnostic and therapeutic thoracocentesis if dyspnea is present.
- Remove only enough fluid from the pleural space or peritoneal cavity to relieve dyspnea and to obtain fluid for cytologic evaluation. Until the primary cause is identified and corrected, fluid will reform, potentially further lessening serum protein concentrations.
- Collect blood and urine samples for diagnostic evaluations.
- Administer plasma or synthetic colloids if hypoalbuminemia is life-threatening. The goal of therapy is to increase oncotic pressure enough to lessen transudate formation. It requires large volumes of plasma to normalize albumin concentrations. Hetastarch or low-molecular-weight dextrans are the synthetic colloids used most frequently (see chapter 80).

14. How do I manage hypoproteinemic animals chronically?
The only effective management is to diagnose and treat successfully the underlying cause. Some recommend aspirin administered at 1–5 mg/kg/day orally to lessen risk of thromboembolic disease in animals with hypoalbuminemia (and presumed AT III deficiency) due to protein-losing nephropathy or protein-losing enteropathy.

BIBLIOGRAPHY

1. Forrester SD: Diseases of the kidney and ureter. In Leib MS, Monroe WE (eds): Practical Internal Medicine. Philadelphia, W.B. Saunders, 1997, pp 293–299.
2. Fossum TW: Protein-losing enteropathy. Semin Vet Med Surg 4:219–225, 1989.
3. Leib MS, Matz ME: Diseases of the intestine. In Leib MS, Monroe WE (eds): Practical Internal Medicine. Philadelphia, W.B. Saunders, 1997, pp 698–699.
4. Leib MS: Hepatobiliary diseases. In Leib MS, Monroe WE (eds): Practical Internal Medicine. Philadelphia, W.B. Saunders, 1997, pp 778–796.

80. FLUID AND ELECTROLYTE THERAPY

Wayne E. Wingfield, D.V.M., M.S.

1. What is plasma osmolality?
Plasma osmolality is a function of the ratio of body solute to body water; it is regulated by changes in water balance. Water intake is derived primarily from three sources: ingested water, water contained in food, and water produced from oxidation of carbohydrates, proteins, and fats. Water losses occur in the urine and stool as well as through evaporation from the skin and respiratory tract. Alterations in plasma osmolality of as little as 1–2% are sensed by osmoreceptors in the hypothalamus. These receptors initiate mechanisms that affect water intake (via thirst) and water excretion (via antidiuretic hormone [ADH]) to return plasma osmolality to normal.

2. Define effective circulating volume.
Effective circulating volume is defined as the part of the extracellular fluid (ECF) in the vascular space that effectively perfuses tissues. It varies directly with ECF volume and also with total body sodium, because sodium salts are the primary solutes that hold water in the extracellular

space. Therefore, regulation of sodium balance by changes in renal sodium ion and maintenance of effective circulating volume are closely related.

3. What are the major effectors of effective circulating volume?

Three major effectors alter effective circulating volume: (1) sympathetic nervous system, (2) angiotensin II, and (3) renal sodium excretion. Volume depletion, sensed by arterial baroreceptors as hypotension, causes an increase in peripheral sympathetic tone. Increased sympathetic tone returns volume to normal by initiating specific compensatory changes, including the following:

- Venous constriction, which increases venous return
- Increased myocardial contractility and heart rate, which increases cardiac output
- Arterial vasoconstriction, which increases systemic vascular resistance and blood pressure
- Increased renin secretion, which increases levels of angiotensin II, a potent vasoconstrictor
- Increased renal tubular sodium resorption (due to increased levels of angiotensin II and aldosterone)

Sympathetic tone-induced changes in effective circulating volume are transient and compensatory; appropriate changes in renal sodium excretion are required to restore normal volume.

4. What is the body's main defense against hyperosmolality?

The major defense against hyperosmolality (accumulation of solute in excess of body water) is increased thirst. Although the kidney can minimize water losses via the action of ADH, water deficits can be corrected only by increased dietary intake.

5. When does hypoosmolality result?

Hypoosmolality may result from excessive body water retention with subsequent dilution of body solutes or from solute loss in excess of water loss (e.g., diarrhea). Because the kidney excretes large volumes of water daily, persistent water retention resulting in hypoosmolality occurs only in the presence of decreased renal water excretion. In patients with normal renal function, hypoosmolality must therefore be due to solute loss in excess of body water loss.

6. How does hypovolemia (i.e., dehydration) increase the circulating volume?

Hypovolemia causes an increase in renin secretion. The subsequent increase in angiotensin II causes an increase in blood pressure (as a result of arterial vasoconstriction) as well as renal sodium retention (which is both a direct effect and also the result of increased aldosterone secretion). With sodium retention, water is also retained.

7. How do you determine the degree of dehydration in an animal?

Clinical assessment of dehydration is best accomplished by serial body weight monitoring. Experience has shown that the physical findings often underestimate the degree of dehydration. During the acute phase of volume depletion, only classical physical findings are available. The general guidelines below assume that more serious hypovolemia is present.

Estimated % Dehydration	Physical Findings
< 5	History of fluid loss but no findings on physical examination
5	Dry oral mucous membranes but no panting or pathologic tachycardia
7	Mild-to-moderate degree of decreased skin turgor, dry oral mucous membranes, slight tachycardia, and normal pulse pressure
10	Moderate-to-marked degree of decreased skin turgor, dry oral mucous membranes, tachycardia, and decreased pulse pressure
12	Marked loss of skin turgor, dry oral mucous membranes, and significant signs of shock

8. When and how much fluid can be given via the subcutaneous route?

In mild dehydration, subcutaneous fluids are useful. Isotonic fluids should be used, and no more than 5–10 ml/lb should be given at each injection site. The rate of subcutaneous fluid flow usually is governed by patient comfort. These fluids are aseptically administered, and multiple sites are required to provide adequate fluid volume. In general, all subcutaneous fluids are resorbed within 6–8 hours. If fluids are still noted subcutaneously after this time, the use of intravenous fluids to reestablish peripheral perfusion should be considered.

9. How about using the intraperitoneal route for fluid administration?

The intraperitoneal route is quick and easy, and the fluids generally are resorbed, thus increasing the circulating volume. However, intraperitoneal administration involves the risk of bacterial peritonitis, visceral perforation, and decreased ventilation due to impending diaphragmatic excursion. Experience with peritoneal dialysis in dogs has shown that peritoneal fluids often traverse the diaphragm, enter the thoracic space, and further affect ventilation. Currently, intraperitoneal fluids cannot be recommended.

10. When and how do you administer intravenous fluids?

In general, intravenous fluid administration is indicated in dogs and cats with 7% or greater dehydration. Potential routes for intravenous fluid administration include peripheral veins, jugular veins, and the intraosseous route.

11. When and how do you estimate the volume of fluids to be given?

The amount of fluid needed for replacement depends on the patient's status. Of primary concern is the status of blood volume; later concern is directed to restoration of total body water and electrolytes.

12. What are the three phases of fluid therapy?

• Emergency phase (see chapter 14)
• Replacement phase
• Maintenance phase

13. How much fluid should be given during replacement therapy?

The volume of fluid administered during the dehydration phase is based on assessment of fluid needs for the following:

1. Returning the patient's status to normal (deficit volume)
2. Replacing normal ongoing losses (maintenance volume)
3. Replacing continuing abnormal losses (continuing losses volume)

14. How do you calculate the deficit volume?

The deficit volume is an estimate based on findings from the physical examination or on known changes in body weight. To calculate the deficit volume, the estimated dehydration is multiplied by the body weight. It is difficult to replace all deficits in a 24-hour period. An attempt to do so may result in urinary losses that further dehydration. Thus, it is recommended that only 75–80% of the deficit volume be replaced during the first 24 hours. You must also add daily maintenance volumes to the calculated deficit volume if the animal is not eating or drinking.

Example: A 22-lb (10-kg) dog is assessed to be 7% dehydrated. What volume of fluid deficit should be given during the first 24 hours? Remember that 454 ml = 1 lb of water and that 1000 ml = 1 kg of water.

Total deficit replacement volume = deficit volume + maintenance volume

Deficit replacement volume (ml) = % dehydration × body weight (lb) × 454 × 0.80

Deficit replacement volume (ml) = 0.07 × 22 lb × 454 × 0.80 = 560 ml

or

Deficit replacement volume (ml) = % dehydration × body weight (kg) × 1000 × 0.80

Deficit replacement volume (ml) = 0.07 × 10 × 1000 × 0.80 = 560 ml

15. What are maintenance volumes for fluid therapy?

Maintenance volumes are normal ongoing losses. Ongoing losses are divided into sensible and insensible losses. Sensible losses, or water losses in urine and feces, can be measured. Insensible losses are normal but are not easily quantitated. Insensible water losses occur during panting or sweating. One-third of the maintenance volume is made up of insensible volumes and two-thirds of sensible volumes. For calculation of maintenance volume, see controversies at end of chapter.

16. How do you account for continuing losses during the replacement phase of fluid therapy?

A crude but effective guideline for replacing continuing abnormal losses is to estimate the volume of fluid loss and then double the estimate. The result is surprisingly close to the actual volume of vomitus, diarrhea, and urine.

17. How do you tell when an animal is receiving inadequate fluid volume?

Any acute change in body weight results from losses or gains in water. The animal that loses body weight while receiving crystalloid fluids is probably receiving inadequate volumes of fluid. Body weight may be deceptive in animals with third spacing of fluids (peritonitis, pyometritis, pleural effusions). Such animals may still be dehydrated, but body weight may not have changed. Monitoring of central venous pressure results in a value that is well below 5 cm H_2O. In addition, if renal function is adequate, a dehydrated animal has a urine specific gravity above 1.025.

18. What are the clinical signs of overhydration?

Classically, pulmonary edema is associated with overhydration. Clinically, however, pulmonary edema is the terminal event of overhydration. Before pulmonary edema results, you first note an increased serous nasal discharge, followed by chemosis; finally, pulmonary congestion is auscultated before edema develops.

19. List the common crystalloid fluids and their electrolyte composition, pH, and osmolality.

Solution	Na^+	K^+	Cl^-	Ca^{2+}	Mg^{2+}	Buffer (mEq/L)	Calories (kcal/L)	Osmolality (mOsm/L)
Dextrose 5% in water	—	—	—	—	—	—	170	278
Dextrose 2.5% in 0.45% saline	77	—	77	—	—	—	85	280
Ringer's lactate	130	4	109	3	—	Lactate, 28	9	272
Ringer's	147	4	156	4.5	—	—	—	309
Normosol-R	140	5	109	—	3	Acetate, 27 Gluconate, 23	15	294
Dextrose 5% in Ringer's lactate	130	4	109	3	—	Lactate, 28	179	525
Normal saline (0.9%)	154	—	154	—	—	—	—	308
Dextrose 50%	—	—	—	—	—	—	1700	2525
Dextrose 5% in saline (0.9%)	154	—	154	—	—	—	170	—
Potassium chloride	—	2	2	—	—	—	—	—

20. How do you select the parenteral fluid?

In selecting a fluid, it is important to know which electrolytes are lost and to institute replacement therapy based on knowledge of the pathophysiology of the disease.

Selection of Fluids for Specific Diseases

CONDITION	SERUM					FLUID OF CHOICE
	Na^+	Cl^-	K^+	HCO_3^-	VOLUME	
Diarrhea	D	D	D	D	D	Normosol-R + KCl *or* lactated Ringer's + KCl
Pyloric obstruction	D	D	D	I	D	0.9% saline + KCl
Dehydration	I	I	N	N/D	D	Normosol-R + KCl, lactated Ringer's + KCl, 0.9% saline + KCl, 5% dextrose
Congestive heart failure	N/D	N/D	N	N	I	0.45% saline + 2.5% dextrose + KCl, 5% dextrose
End-stage liver disease	N/I	N/I	D	D	I	0.45% saline + 2.5% dextrose + KCl
Acute renal failure						
Oliguria	I	I	I	D	I	0.9% saline
Polyuria	D	D	N/D	D	D	Normosol-R + KCl, lactated Ringer's + KCl
Chronic renal failure	N/D	N/D	N	D	N/D	Normosol-R, lactated Ringer's, 0.9% saline
Adrenocortical insufficiency	D	D	I	N/D	D	0.9% saline
Diabetic ketoacidosis	D	D	N/D	D	D	0.9% saline (± KCl)

D = decreased, I = increased, N = normal, KCl = potassium chloride.

CONTROVERSIES

21. How much fluid should you give for maintenance volume if the animal is not eating or drinking?

Data about water needs for dogs and cats are few. Water and energy requirements are numerically the same (1 kcal of energy = 1 ml of water). Unfortunately, many authors recommend dramatically different fluid and energy requirements. Estimates of water needs include 66 ml/kg/day (30 ml/lb/day), 132 kcal × $kg^{0.75}$, 156 × $kg^{0.667}$, (30 × kg) + 70, and 70 × $kg^{0.75}$. Studies using indirect calorimetry document that previously recommended formulas overestimate energy (and thus water) needs for dogs and cats.

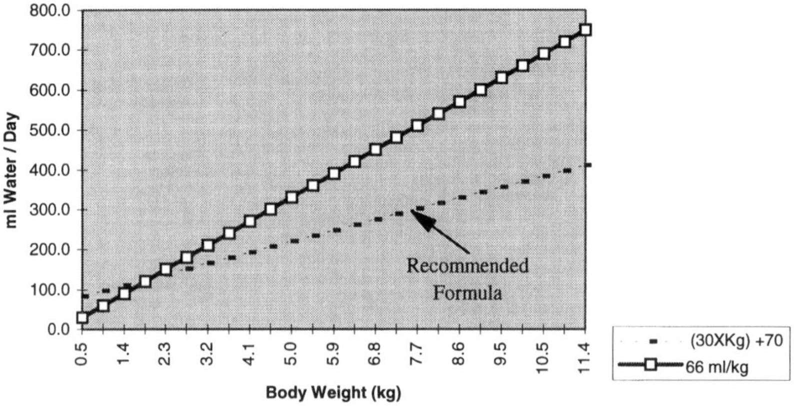

Maintenance fluid volumes for cats. Recommended volumes are calculated from the formula (30 × body weight [kg]) + 70.

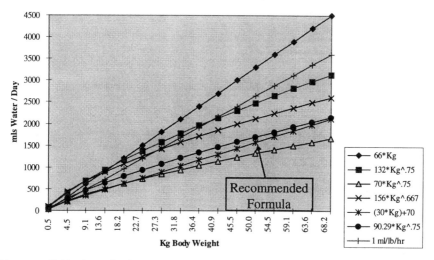

Maintenance fluid volumes for dogs. Recommended volumes are calculated from the formula (30 × body weight [kg]) + 70.

Example: A 22-lb (10-kg) dog is assessed to be 7% dehydrated and has been vomiting. How much fluid should be given during the next 24 hours?

$$\text{Volume (ml of fluid required)} = \text{deficit volume} + \text{maintenance volume}$$
$$= [0.07 \times 22 \text{ lb} \times 454 \times 0.80] + [(10 \times 30) + 70]$$
$$= [560] + [370] = 930 \text{ ml}$$
$$or$$
$$= [0.07 \times 10 \text{ kg} \times 1000 \times 0.80] + [(10 \times 30) + 70]$$
$$= [560] + [370] = 930 \text{ ml}$$

22. Does the above formula satisfy water needs in sick animals?

The question of energy (water) requirements in sick animals continues to elicit controversy. Traditionally, it has been taught that illnesses, injuries, and surgery result in increased need for energy (water). These teachings were extrapolated from human and rodent data. Mounting evidence indicates that increased energy requirements are not common in sick, injured, or surgical dogs. In fact, increasing numbers of publications document lower energy (water) requirements for both normal and sick or traumatized dogs. In addition, from an evolutionary perspective, it seems logical to expect dogs to preserve available energy with illness or injury. The reserves are already minimal, and it makes little sense to increase metabolic requirements in order to survive. It makes more sense to conserve available energy and to reduce metabolic (thus energy and water) requirements. Studies of dogs in a critical care unit have documented significant hypothyroid function. Thus, metabolic requirements are reduced. The decision to change the formulas for calculating water requirements will come only with more objective evidence from normal and sick dogs and cats.

BIBLIOGRAPHY

1. Aberman A: The ins and outs of fluids and electrolytes. Emerg Med 14(7):121–127, 1982.
2. Adams LG, Polzin DJ: Mixed acid–base disorders. Vet Clin North Am Small Animal Pract 19:307–326, 1989.
3. Bonner CW, Stidham GL, Westenkirchner DF, Tolley EA: Hypermagnesemia and hypocalcemia as predictors of high mortality in critically ill pediatric patients. Crit Care Med 18:921–928, 1990.
4. Concannon KT: Colloid oncotic pressure and the clinical use of colloidal solutions. J Vet Emerg Crit Care 3:49–62, 1993.

5. Dubick MA, Wade CE: A review of the efficacy and safety of 7.5% NaCl/6% dextran-70 in experimental animals and in humans. J Trauma 36:323–330, 1994.
6. Duval D: Use of hypovolemic saline solutions in hypovolemic shock. Comp Cont Educ Pract Vet 17:1128–1231, 1995.
7. Garvey MS: Fluid and electrolyte balance in critical patients. Vet Clin North Am Small Animal Pract 19:1021–1057, 1989.
8. Haskins SC: A simple fluid therapy planning guide. Semin Vet Med Surg 3:227–236, 1988.
9. Kronfeld DS: Protein and energy estimates for hospitalized dogs and cats. Proceedings of the Purina International Nutrition Symposium, January 15, 1991, Orlando, FL, pp 5–11.
10. Ogilvie GK, Salman MD, Kesel ML, et al: Effect of anesthesia and surgery on energy expenditure determined by indirect calorimetry in dogs with malignant and nonmalignant conditions. Am J Vet Res 57:1321–1326, 1996.
11. Ogilvie GK, Walters LM, Salman MD, et al: Resting energy expenditure in dogs with nonhematopoietic malignancies before and after excision of tumors. Am J Vet Res 57:1463–1467, 1996.
12. Schaer M: General principles of fluid therapy in small animal medicine. Vet Clin North Am Small Animal Pract 19:203–213, 1989.
13. Schertel ER, Allen DA, Muir WW, et al: Evaluation of a hypertonic saline-dextran solution for treatment of dogs with shock induced by gastric dilatation-volvulus. J Am Vet Med Assoc 210:226–230, 1997.
14. Thatcher CD: Nutritional needs of critically ill patients. Comp Cont Educ Pract Vet 18:1303–1337, 1996.
15. Walters LM, Ogilvie GK, Salman MD, et al: Repeatability of energy expenditure measurements in clinically normal dogs by use of indirect calorimetry. Am J Vet Res 54:1881–1885, 1993.
16. Walton RS, Wingfield WE, Ogilvie GK, et al: Energy expenditure in 104 postoperative and traumatically injured dogs with indirect calorimetry. J Vet Emerg Crit Care 6(2):71–75, 1996.

81. ACID–BASE DISORDERS

Wayne E. Wingfield, D.V.M., M.S., and Suzanne G. Wingfield, R.V.T., V.T.S.

1. List the five common acid–base disorders and give an example of each.

Acid–base disorder	Common example
Metabolic acidosis	Cardiopulmonary arrest
Metabolic alkalosis	Vomiting from pyloric obstruction
Respiratory acidosis	Chronic obstructive pulmonary disease
Respiratory alkalosis	Hyperventilation
Mixed acid–base disorder	Gastric dilatation-volvulus

2. How do you diagnose the four primary acid–base disorders? How does the body compensate for each disturbance?

Acid-base disorder	Primary disturbance	Compensation
Metabolic acidosis	$\downarrow HCO_3^-$	$\downarrow PaCO_2$
Metabolic alkalosis	$\uparrow HCO_3^-$	$\uparrow PaCO_2$
Respiratory acidosis	$\uparrow PaCO_2$	$\uparrow HCO_3^-$
Respiratory alkalosis	$\downarrow PaCO_2$	$\downarrow HCO_3^-$

3. The integrated actions of which three organs are involved in acid–base homeostasis?
- Liver: hepatic metabolism of organic acids (lactate)
- Lungs: excretion of carbon dioxide
- Kidneys: reclaim filtered bicarbonate and excrete accumulated acid

4. List the common causes of metabolic acidosis.
- Renal failure
- Diarrhea
- Chronic vomiting
- Severe shock
- Diabetes mellitus
- Hypoadrenocorticism

5. List the common causes of metabolic alkalosis.
- Acute profuse vomiting
- Pyloric outflow obstruction
- Excessive use of diuretics
- Bicarbonate therapy

6. List the common causes of respiratory acidosis.
- Anesthesia
- Respiratory depressant drugs
- Obesity
- Chronic obstructive lung disease
- Brain injuries

7. List the common causes of respiratory alkalosis.
- Fever
- Left-to-right shunts
- Shock
- Hypoxemia

8. What is meant by the anion gap?

The anion gap represents the difference between the routinely measured cations and anions in a plasma or serum sample. It is usually calculated as follows:

$$([Na^+] + [K^+]) - ([Cl^-] + [HCO_3^-])$$

where Na = sodium, K = potassium, Cl = chloride, and HCO_3^- = bicarbonate. Because potassium makes such a small contribution to the anion gap, it is often not used in the above formula. The normal values at our hospital for anion gap are 10–27 in cats and 8–25 in dogs. The negative charges on plasma proteins account for most of the missing anions, because the charges of the other cations (calcium [Ca^{2+}] and magnesium [Mg^{2+}]) and anions (phosphate, sulfate, and organic anions) tend to balance out. Determining the anion gap is useful in the differential diagnosis of metabolic acidosis because the causes of the disorder may be divided into those that elevate the anion gap and those that do not.

As acid accumulates in the body, there is rapid extracellular buffering by bicarbonate. If the acid is hydrochloric acid (HCl), the following formula applies:

$$HCl + NaHCO_3 \rightarrow NaCl + H_2CO_3 \rightarrow H_2O + CO_2$$

The net effect is an mEq-for-mEq replacement of extracellular bicarbonate by chloride ion. Because the sum of Cl^- and HCO_3^- concentrations remains constant, the anion gap is unchanged. Because of the increase in the plasma chloride ion concentration, this state is often referred to as hyperchloremic acidosis. Conversely, if H^+ accumulates with any anion other than Cl^-, extracellular HCO_3^- is replaced by an unmeasured anion. The results are a decrease in the sum of the chloride and bicarbonate concentrations and an increase in the anion gap.

9. List the common causes of an increased anion gap metabolic acidosis.
- Ethylene glycol ingestion
- Ketoacidosis
- Uremia
- Lactic acidosis
- Salicylate toxicity
- Severe starvation

10. List the common causes of a decreased anion gap.
- Increased unmeasured cations (K^+, Mg^{2+}, Ca^{2+})
- Addition of abnormal cations (lithium)
- Increase in cationic immunoglobulins (plasma cell dyscrasias)
- Loss of unmeasured anions such as albumin (hypoalbuminemia)
- Severe acidosis resulting in loss of effective negative charge on albumin

11. What is a strong ion?

Strong ions are salts that are completely dissociated in water (e.g., Na^+, K^+, and Cl^-).

12. What is the strong ion difference (SID)?

The SID is the difference in all positive and negative strong ions (normally Na^+, K^+, and Cl^-). When SID increases, it is usually due to metabolic alkalosis; decreases in SID usually result from metabolic acidosis.

13. What is the base excess (BE)?

Base excess is the amount of base (substances that can accept a hydrogen ion) above or below the normal buffer base. BE is expressed in mEq/L. Positive BE values reflect an excess of base (or a deficit of acid), whereas negative BE values reflect a deficit in base (or an excess of acid).

14. What four factors influence BE?
- Free water (Na^+)
- Chloride concentration
- Protein concentration
- Unidentified anions (lactic acid)

15. What is lactic acidosis? List the common causes.

Lactic acidosis is due to the accumulation of lactic acid, the end-product of glycolysis. This accumulation leads to depletion of the body's buffers and drop in pH. Common causes of lactic acidosis include the following:
- Cellular hypoxia
- Decreased hepatic utilization of lactic acid
- Cyanide poisoning
- Neoplasms with large tumor burden
- Diabetic ketoacidosis
- Carbon monoxide poisoning
- Sodium nitroprusside infusions

16. How do you determine the efficiency of oxygenation in patients?

Oxygenation is determined by calculating the alveolar–arterial oxygen gradient (A–a gradient). The formula used for this calculation when the animal is breathing room air (e.g.,. 21% oxygen) is as follows:

$$A = \text{calculated alveolar oxygen} = (\text{barometric pressure} - 47)(0.21) - PaCO_2/0.8$$

$$a = \text{measured } PaO_2$$

$$\text{A–a gradient} = A - a$$

In this equation you need the barometric pressure, water vapor pressure (47), concentration of oxygen in room air (21% or 0.21), measured $PaCO_2$, respiratory quotient (0.8), and measured PaO_2.

17. What are the normal values for the A–a gradient when an animal is breathing room air?
- Normal = 0–10
- Normal (?) = 11–20
- Acute respiratory distress syndrome (?) = 21–30
- Acute respiratory distress syndrome ≥ 30

18. How do you assess oxygenation if the animal is breathing supplemental oxygen?

If the animal is breathing supplemental oxygen, you cannot use the equation in question 16; you must use the following equation:

$$\text{A–a gradient (supplemental oxygen)} = PaO_2/FIO_2$$

In this case an arterial PO_2 is required along with the concentration of inspired oxygen (FIO_2). When breathing via a face mask or nasal insufflation cannula, the FIO_2 is approximately 40% ($FIO_2 = 0.40$). If an endotracheal tube is in place and the cuff is inflated, the concentration is 100% ($FIO_2 = 1.0$). If the result of the above equation is ≥ 200 mmHg, the animal is oxygenating adequately.

19. What are the common causes of alveolar hypoxia? What are their effects on the A–a gradient?

Cause	Effect on PaO_2	Effect on A–a gradient
Diffusion abnormality	Decreased	Increased
Ventilation–perfusion mismatch	Decreased	Increased
Right-to-left shunt	Decreased	Increased

20. How do you assess the animal's ability to ventilate?

Examine the $PaCO_2$ in an arterial blood sample. If the animal is hypoventilating, the $PaCO_2$ is increased. With hyperventilation the animal's $PaCO_2$ is decreased.

21. What are the normal values for an arterial blood gas (ABG) sample?

Parameter	Normal value	Range
pH	7.40	7.35–7.45
$PaCO_2$	38	35–45
HCO_3^-	24	22–27
PaO_2	92	80–110

22. Does the environmental altitude affect normal values?

Yes. Living in a state such as Colorado results in an increase in red blood cells in response to the hypoxia (normal PaO_2 = 78–92) of altitude. In addition, animals at altitude breathe more rapidly, resulting in decreased $PaCO_2$ (normal = 28–32) and bicarbonate (normal = 18–22).

23. Describe the sequence of steps in assessing an ABG sample.

1. The first question that you must answer is whether the sample is arterial or venous blood. The distinction is commonly based on oxygen saturation (> 90%) and PaO_2 (> 75 mmHg).
2. Next, determine the pH. Is the animal acidotic (pH < 7.35) or alkalotic (pH > 7.45)?
3. Assess $PaCO_2$:
   - Respiratory acidosis: $PaCO_2$ > 45 mmHg
   - Respiratory alkalosis: $PaCO_2$ < 32 mmHg
4. Assess HCO_3^-:
   - Metabolic acidosis: HCO_3^- < 20 mEq/L and BE < –5 mEq/L
   - Metabolic alkalosis: HCO_3^- > 27 mEq/L and BE > +5 mEq/L
5. Determine whether there is compensation in response to the primary metabolic or respiratory disorder.
6. Examine BE for evidence of a mixed acid–base disorder.
7. Assess oxygenation by calculating the A–a gradient.
8. Calculate the anion gap.

24. What do ABGs and tic-tac-toe have in common?

Simplifying the interpretation of ABGs to diagnose an acid–base imbalance involves asking three questions:

1. Does the pH indicate acidosis or alkalosis?
2. Is the cause of the pH imbalance respiratory or metabolic?
3. Is there compensation for the acid–base imbalance?

To answer these questions, set up a tic-tac-toe grid and write the words *acid, normal,* and *alkaline* in the boxes across the top row:

Acid	Normal	Alkaline

Comparing the patient's ABG results with normal values, write *pH, PaCO₂,* and *HCO₃⁻* under the appropriate column head. Once three items—including the head—are in a vertical column, you are ready to diagnose the patient's condition.

For example, let us consider the case of Sage, a 3-year-old, yellow Labrador retriever with diabetes mellitus. The following ABG results are reported: pH = 7.26, $PaCO_2$ = 42, and HCO_3^- = 17. Plug these values into the grid as follows:

Acid	Normal	Alkaline
pH	$PaCO_2$	
HCO_3^-		

The column in which the pH is located tells you whether the patient has acidosis or alkalosis. The relative positions of pH, $PaCO_2$, and HCO_3^- reveal the origin of any acid–base imbalance. If the pH and $PaCO_2$ fall in the same column (other than normal), the problem is respiratory. If the pH and HCO_3^- fall in the same column, the problem is metabolic. Thus, Sage's diagnosis is metabolic acidosis.

25. Which electrolyte is most commonly affected by a change in acid–base balance?

Serum potassium. Animals with severe metabolic acidosis tend to have elevated serum potassium concentrations, whereas animals with severe alkalosis tend to have low serum potassium concentrations. A change in pH of 0.1 is consistent with a corresponding change in serum potassium of about 0.6 (0.3–0.8) mEq/L. If the pH is elevated by 0.1, the serum potassium falls by about 0.6 mEq/L; if the pH is diminished by 0.1, the serum potassium rises by about 0.6 mEq/L. This concept is extremely important in treating diabetic ketoacidotic patients. Although total body potassium may be severely depleted, initial serum potassium concentrations may actually be elevated in severely acidotic animals. As the patient is treated with intravenous crystalloids and insulin, the acidosis resolves and the serum concentrations of potassium fall precipitously, requiring potassium supplementation.

26. How does the core body temperature of an animal affect ABGs?

With hypothermia, uncorrected ABGs yield falsely elevated pH as well as falsely decreased PaO_2 and $PaCO_2$. For every 1° C (1.8° F) decrease in body temperature, the pH increases by 0.015, $PaCO_2$ (mmHg) decreases by 4.4%, and PaO_2 decreases by 7.2% (37° C reference). Hyperthermia decreases the pH and increases the $PaCO_2$ and PaO_2 by an equivalent amount. All samples should be corrected for temperature before interpretation of ABG results.

27. What does pulse oximetry contribute to the understanding of acid–base status?

Nothing. Pulse oximetry measures oxygen saturation and does not provide a measurement of acid–base or ventilatory status. ABG analysis is necessary to determine acid–base status.

28. Can venous blood gases be used to assess acid–base balance?

Yes. There is good statistical correlation between arterial vs. venous pH, PCO_2, and HCO_3^-. Unfortunately, you must insert venous blood gas values into regression equations, as follows:

(1) Arterial pH $= 0.329 + (0.961 \times$ venous pH)
(2) Arterial $PCO_2 = 7.735 + (0.572 \times$ venous $PCO_2)$
(3) Arterial $HCO_3^- = 0.538 + (0.845 \times$ venous $HCO_3^-)$

29. In circulatory failure, which is less severe than cardiopulmonary arrest, why should you assess both arterial and central venous samples?

In patients with severe hemodynamic compromise, ABGs provide useful information about pulmonary gas exchange. However, in the presence of severe hypoperfusion, hypercapnia and acidemia at the tissue level are better detected in central venous blood.

30. What is a mixed acid–base disorder?

Thus far, we have assumed that only one primary disorder is present. Real patients, however, often have more than one disorder (mixed acid–base disorder). These disturbances can be identified by determining the expected compensatory response to a given change in the primary abnormality and assuming that any value that falls outside this range represents an additional primary disorder. Numerous nomograms and mathematical formulas are available. Unfortunately, mathematical equations, especially ones that are different for acute and chronic disorders, are difficult to memorize. Nomograms are relatively simple but further mystify acid–base analysis by providing answers without necessarily requiring an understanding of the relevant pathophysiology. A simpler alternative is first to identify the most clinically important disorders as outlined by the rules below:

Rule 1. *Look at the pH.* On whichever side of 7.40 the pH falls, the process that caused it to shift is the primary abnormality. *Principle:* The body does not fully compensate for primary acid–base disorders.

Rule 2. *Calculate the anion gap.* If the anion gap is ≥ 20 mEq/L, the patient has a primary metabolic acidosis, regardless of the pH or bicarbonate concentration. *Principle:* The body does not generate a large anion gap to compensate for a primary disorder.

Rule 3. *Calculate the excess anion gap* (the total anion gap minus the normal anion gap) and add this value to the measured bicarbonate concentration. If the sum is greater than normal serum bicarbonate, there is an underlying metabolic alkalosis; if the sum is less than normal serum bicarbonate, there is an underlying nonanion gap metabolic acidosis. *Principle:* 1 mEq of unmeasured acid titrates 1 mEq of bicarbonate ($+ \Delta$ anion gap $= - \Delta$ [HCO_3^-]).

CONTROVERSY

31. When do you use sodium bicarbonate to treat metabolic acidosis?

Most acid–base disorders correct themselves if adequate fluid volume is provided to normalize tissue perfusion. The difficult question is whether to administer sodium bicarbonate to severely acidotic animals (pH < 7.10; bicarbonate < 8). In this case sodium bicarbonate should be administered, but do not try to replace the entire base deficit with bicarbonate because you will usually induce metabolic alkalosis. The bicarbonate replacement formula that we use is as follows:

$$\text{Amount of bicarbonate} = 0.4 \times \text{body weight (kg)} \times (12 - \text{patient's bicarbonate})$$

In most cases, one-third of this volume is administered in a slow intravenous bolus, and the remainder is given over the next 8 hours. Ideally, sodium bicarbonate is given only if blood gases can be monitored. If empirical doses are used, no more than 0.25 mEq/kg should be given.

BIBLIOGRAPHY

1. Adrogué HJ, Nashad N, Gorin AB, et al: Assessing acid–base status in circulatory failure: Differences between arterial and central venous blood. N Engl J Med 320:1312–1316, 1989.
2. Cornelius LM, Rawlings CA: Arterial blood gas and acid–base values in dogs with various diseases and signs of disease. J Am Vet Med Assoc 178:992–995, 1981.
3. Haber RJ: A practical approach to acid–base disorders. West J Med 155:146–151, 1991.
4. Kollef MH, Schuster DP: The acute respiratory distress syndrome. N Engl J Med 332:27–37, 1995.
5. Mays D: Turn ABGs into child's play. RN Jan:36–40, 1995.
6. Van Pelt DR, Wingfield WE, Wheeler SL, et al: Oxygen-tension based indices as predictors of survival in critically ill dogs. J Vet Emerg Crit Care 1:19–25, 1991.
7. Wingfield WE, Van Pelt DR, Hackett T, et al: Usefulness of venous blood in estimating acid–base status of the seriously ill dog. J Vet Emerg Crit Care 4:23–27, 1994.

82. PORTOSYSTEMIC SHUNTS

Derek P. Burney, D.V.M.

1. What is a portosystemic shunt?

A portosystemic shunt is an abnormal vessel that connects the portal vein to a systemic vein. The most common locations for portosystemic shunts are a patent ductus venosus or a connection between the portal vein and caudal vena cava or azygous vein.

2. What is the difference between congenital and acquired portosystemic shunts?

Most acquired shunts are multiple and extrahepatic. Acquired shunts develop because of sustained portal hypertension from chronic liver disease and cirrhosis. Congenital portosystemic shunts are usually single and may be intra- or extrahepatic. The most common intrahepatic portosystemic shunt is a patent ductus venosus.

3. Are certain breeds associated with portosystemic shunts?

Congenital portosystemic shunts may occur in any breed of dog but are common in minia-ture schnauzers, miniature poodles, Yorkshire terriers, dachshunds, Doberman pinschers, golden retrievers, Labrador retrievers, and Irish setters. Acquired portosystemic shunts are secondary to chronic hepatic disease and so may occur in any breed.

4. Why do patients with portosystemic shunts have decreased liver function?

Portal venous blood is important because it brings hepatotropic growth factors and insulin to the liver. If insulin bypasses the liver in a shunt, significant quantities are utilized by other organs and the liver receives less benefit. Portal venous blood flow is important for normal liver devel-opment as well as glycogen storage, hypertrophy, hyperplasia, and regeneration. Congenital por-tosystemic shunts are often associated with hepatic atrophy, hypoplasia, and dysfunction.

5. What are the most common clinical signs of portosystemic shunts?

Failure to thrive and failure to gain weight are appropriately common. Most clinical signs are referable to hepatic encephalopathy, which is defined as clinical signs of neurologic dysfunction secondary to hepatic disease. Signs include ataxia, stupor, lethargy, unusual behavior, disorienta-tion, blindness, and seizures. Some animals display anorexia, vomiting, and diarrhea. Polyuria and polydipsia may be present. Some animals have ammonium urate urolithiasis, which may result in pollakiuria, hematuria, stranguria, or obstruction. Increased production of saliva (ptyal-ism) and abdominal distention due to ascites occur in some animals.

6. What causes hepatic encephalopathy associated with portosystemic shunts?

Products of bacterial metabolism in the intestine, such as ammonia, short-chain fatty acids (SCFAs), mercaptans, and gamma-aminobutyric acid (GABA), have been suggested as mediators of hepatic encephalopathy. In addition, the ratio of aromatic amino acids to branched-chain amino acids is often increased in patients with portosystemic shunts. The aromatic amino acids may act as false neurotransmitters. Phenylalanine and tyrosine may act as weak neurotransmit-ters in the presynaptic neurons of the CNS. Tryptophan causes increased production of serotonin, which is a potent inhibitory neurotransmitter. The GABA receptor has binding sites for barbitu-rates, benzodiazepines, and substances with similar chemical structure to benzodiazepines. These agents may be responsible for depression of the CNS in hepatic encephalopathy.

7. What factors may precipitate an hepatic encephalopathy crisis? By what mechanism?

Factor	Mechanism Inducing Hepatic Encephalopathy
High protein meals	Increased synthesis of ammonia by enteric bacteria
Constipation	Increased synthesis of ammonia by enteric bacteria
Transfusion with stored blood	Ammonia increases in stored blood with length of storage
Infection	May increase systemic ammonia levels
Alkalosis	Shifts ammonium ion to ammonia, allowing it to penetrate the CNS and become trapped as ammonia
Vomiting	Fluid, electrolyte, acid–base disturbances
Hypovolemia with prerenal azotemia	Increased blood urea nitrogen (BUN), which may increase ammonia production
Hypokalemia	Increases trapping of ammonia within cells
Hypoglycemia, ammonia, SCFAs	Synergistic in increasing chances of seizures

8. How is hepatic encephalopathy treated?

The animal should be evaluated for hypoglycemia immediately and treated appropriately if it is present. Appropriate fluid therapy based on acid–base and electrolyte status (see chapter 80) should be initiated to correct abnormalities. Ammonia concentration and production should be decreased by administering lactulose and neomycin (10–20 mg/kg orally every 6 hr) if a swallow response is present. Oral metronidazole may be used at a dose of 10 mg/kg every 8 hr in place of neomycin. If the animal is comatose, 20–30 ml/kg of lactulose diluted 1:2 with water or a 1:10 dilution of povidone-iodine solution may be given as an enema. Seizures may be treated initially with diazepam at a dose of 0.2 mg/kg IV. However, some animals with hepatic encephalopathy have difficulty metabolizing benzodiazepines such as diazepam. If diazepam is ineffective, flumazenil, a benzodiazepine antagonist, has been suggested as a possible treatment because in some patients benzodiazepinelike substances in the circulation may contribute to the encephalopathic state. If these drugs do not control seizures, intravenous phenobarbital may be titrated slowly to effect. Patients often have decreased clearance of barbiturates.

9. What routine blood work and urinalysis abnormalities suggest portosystemic shunts?

Microcytosis is a consistent abnormality of complete blood cell count in animals with portosystemic shunts. Some animals manifest acid–base, electrolyte, and glucose disturbances (hypoglycemia). Because of vomiting and dehydration, prerenal azotemia may be present. There is no consistent finding with regard to alanine aminotransferase (ALT), aspartate aminotransferase (AST), and serum alkaline phosphatase (ALP); activities of these enzymes may be elevated, decreased, or normal in patients with portosystemic shunts. Hypoalbuminemia is common, as are coagulopathies. Some animals have isothenuric urine due to medullary wash-out; ammonium biurate crystals may be identified on microscopic examination of urine sediment.

10. What are the best ways to diagnose a portosystemic shunt?

Elevated serum pre- and postprandial bile acids in a young animal with signs of hepatic encephalopathy and stunted growth are consistent with but not diagnostic for portosystemic shunts. A nuclear medicine scan using transcolonic sodium pertechnetate Tc99m demonstrates radioactivity in the heart before the liver in an animal with portosystemic shunt. Nuclear medicine is rapid, noninvasive, and safe to the animal. The disadvantages are that the animal is radioactive for 24 hours, studies can be performed only by specially trained personnel, exact location of the shunt cannot be determined, and cases of hepatic microvascular dysplasia, which have shunting within the liver (as in Cairn terriers), may give false-negative results. When nuclear medicine facilities are unavailable, positive contrast portography may demonstrate the anomalous vessel. Portography, however, is technically demanding and invasive. Furthermore, a second surgical procedure is required to repair the shunt because of an otherwise dangerously long period of anesthesia. The major advantage of positive contrast portography is that it definitively locates the shunt.

11. What is the best way to manage a patient with portosystemic shunt?

Although medical management may be beneficial, surgical ligation of the shunt is optimal. In one study, animals that receive total ligation, even if it had to be done in two or more surgeries, showed more clinical improvement than patients with incomplete shunt ligation.

12. Describe the preoperative management of a patient with portosystemic shunt.

In animals displaying hepatic encephalopathy, it is important to correct acid–base and electrolyte disturbances before surgery. Measures to control hepatic encephalopathy also should be performed before surgery, including a low protein diet, oral lactulose, and neomycin or metronidazole. Some have recommended supplementation with vitamins A, B, C, E, and K. Medical stabilization for 1–2 weeks before surgery is recommended for all patients with portosystemic shunts. A preoperative coagulation screen should be performed, and crossmatched fresh whole blood should be available. Fresh frozen plasma transfusions may be necessary for hypoalbuminemic patients. Most surgeons administer a broad-spectrum antibiotic (e.g., first-generation cephalosporin) intravenously before and during surgery.

13. What considerations must be given to drug therapy and anesthetic use in patients with portosystemic shunts?

Because liver function decreases in patients with portosystemic shunts, drugs that are potentially hepatotoxic should be avoided. In addition, hepatic clearance of drugs and anesthetic agents may be delayed.

14. What parameters should be monitored postoperatively in patients with portosystemic shunts?

After surgery, many patients with portosystemic shunts are hypoglycemic, hypothermic, and hypoalbuminemic. A postoperative database should include body weight, temperature, packed cell volume, total solids, and glucose. Additional useful information is provided by electrolytes and albumin. Maintaining hydration status and perfusion with a balanced electrolyte solution is important. Mucous membrane color, capillary refill time, pulse rate and quality, and temperature should be assessed, and the patient should be monitored for seizures. In addition, serial measurement of abdominal circumference is helpful because a number of patients develop portal hypertension and ascites postoperatively.

15. What are common postsurgical complications?

Sepsis, seizures, and portal hypertension are the most critical complications that may develop postoperatively, although pancreatitis and intussusceptions have been reported. Animals with seizures should be treated with appropriate measures to normalize acid–base and electrolyte balance. Diazepam and phenobarbital may be required to control seizures. Sepsis should be treated aggressively.

16. What are common signs of postoperative portal hypertension?

Portal hypertension most commonly results in abdominal distention secondary to ascites. In some cases, portal hypertension is subclinical and ascites resolves in several days. Some patients develop abdominal distention, pain, and hypovolemia; others have abdominal distention with severe pain, hypovolemia, cardiovascular collapse, hemorrhagic diarrhea, and septic or endotoxic shock.

17. How should postoperative portal hypertension be treated?

If the animal develops abdominal distention with no clinical signs of pain or discomfort, continued medical therapy is indicated. Most animals with pain and abdominal distention stabilize with colloid fluid therapy. Patients with severe pain, abdominal distention, bloody diarrhea, and cardiovascular shock should be treated for shock with fluids, stabilized as much as possible, and taken for exploratory surgery to remove the ligature or thrombus that has probably developed in a partially attenuated portosystemic shunt.

18. Why may a patient with portosystemic shunt become septic postoperatively?

A patient with portosystemic shunt may develop septic peritonitis postoperatively because of bacteremia in the portal vein. The monocyte-phagocyte system in the liver may not be fully functional. Sepsis may develop as a result of inadequate filtering of portal blood by the liver before the blood reaches the systemic circulation.

BIBLIOGRAPHY

1. Birchard SJ, Sherding RG: Feline portosystemic shunts. Vet Med 14:1295–1300, 1992.
2. Holt D: Critical care management of the portosystemic shunt patient. Comp Cont Educ Pract Vet 16:879–892, 1994.
3. Hottinger HA, Walshaw R, Hauptman JG: Long-term results of complete and partial ligation of congenital portosystemic shunts in dogs. Vet Surg 24:331–336, 1995.
4. Johnson SE: Disease of the liver. In Ettinger ST, Feldman EC: Textbook of Veterinary Internal Medicine, 4th ed. Philadelphia, W.B. Saunders, 1995, pp 1341–1347.

5. Koblik PD, Hornoff WJ: Transcolonic sodium pertechnetate Tc 99m scintigraphy for diagnosis of macrovascular portosystemic shunts in dogs, cats, and potbellied pigs: 176 cases (1988–1992). J Am Vet Med Assoc 207:729–733, 1995.
6. Lawrence D, Bellah JR, Diaz R: Results of surgical management of portosystemic shunts in dogs: 20 cases (1985–1990). J Am Vet Med Assoc 201:1750–1753, 1992.
7. Matushek KJ, Bjorling D, Mathews K: Generalized motor seizures after portosystemic shunt ligation in dogs: Five cases (1981–1988). J Am Vet Med Assoc 196:2014–2017, 1990.

83. HEPATIC LIPIDOSIS AND ACUTE HEPATITIS

Cynthia Stubbs, D.V.M.

1. What is hepatic lipidosis?

Hepatic lipidosis is a common disease of cats in which excessive fat accumulates in hepatocytes and may lead to severe intrahepatic cholestasis and progressive liver failure. Most cases in cats are idiopathic. Diabetes mellitus, pancreatitis, cholangiohepatitis, hyperthyroidism, hypertrophic cardiomyopathy, renal disease, chronic cystitis, chronic upper respiratory infections, hyperadrenocorticism, and neoplasia also have been detected in some cats with hepatic lipidosis. Most dogs with hepatic lipidosis have another underlying disease process.

2. What is acute hepatitis?

Acute hepatitis refers to any condition that causes inflammation and swelling of the liver. Injury may be precipitated by drugs, trauma, toxins, and infectious agents. In addition, immune-mediated diseases, inborn errors of metabolism (copper toxicity in Bedlington terriers is an example), and neoplastic diseases may result in acute hepatitis. Acute hepatitis also accompanies acute pancreatitis in both dogs and cats.

3. What historical questions should be asked of clients with animals with suspected acute hepatitis?

Drug administration, trauma, and toxin exposure should be ruled out by history. Many drugs, including potentiated sulfonamides and anthelmintics such as metronidazole, have been associated with acute hepatitis or acute hepatic necrosis. It should be determined whether the animal has ingested moldy food; aflatoxins produced by some fungi are potent hepatotoxins. Travel and vaccination histories are important; leptospirosis may result in acute hepatitis in dogs and is a direct zoonosis.

4. What population of cats typically develops idiopathic hepatic lipidosis?

Middle-aged cats are primarily affected, but cats of any age may develop hepatic lipidosis. There does not appear to be a breed or sex predisposition. A large percentage of affected cats are obese before onset of clinical signs.

5. What historical complaints are commonly associated with acute hepatitis or lipidosis?

Anorexia occurs in most animals. In cats with idiopathic lipidosis, a stressful episode such as surgery, boarding, moving, or a new member in the household may precede appetite loss. Lethargy, depression, icterus, ptyalism, and vomiting are also commonly reported with acute hepatic diseases. Diarrhea is uncommon with idiopathic lipidosis but occurs in some animals with acute hepatitis. Hepatic encephalopathy (HE), characterized by head pressing, stupor, and coma, occurs in some animals with acute hepatic diseases.

6. What physical abnormalities are commonly detected in animals with acute hepatitis or lipidosis?

Depression, icterus, and dehydration are common. At presentation, most cats with idiopathic hepatic lipidosis have lost as much as 25–50% of their previous body weight. Most animals with acute hepatitis have clinical signs of shock, including elevated heart rate, pale mucous membranes, increased capillary refill time, and weak pulse. Liver size may be normal, increased, or decreased, depending on the primary cause and duration of the disease process before acute presentation. Animals with chronic hepatic disease that present with an acute exacerbation may have abdominal distention due to sustained portal hypertension or hypoalbuminemia-associated transudative ascites.

7. What diagnostic tests should be considered for animals with suspected acute hepatitis or lipidosis?

Complete blood count, platelet count, serum biochemistry panel, activated clotting time, and urinalysis should be assessed on admission. Packed cell volume, total protein, blood glucose, electrolytes, and coagulation should be assessed as soon as possible and emergency treatment initiated as indicated. Coagulation should be assessed because hepatic aspiration or biopsy is often indicated and disseminated intravascular coagulation is common, particularly in animals with acute hepatitis.

8. What routine laboratory abnormalities are most consistent with acute hepatitis or lipidosis?

Although no pathognomonic changes in complete blood count are associated with hepatic lipidosis, mild nonregenerative anemia, neutrophilia, or neutropenia may be noted. Increases in liver enzyme activities are common; any combination of increased activity of alanine transferase (ALT), aspartate aminotransferase (AST), alkaline phosphatase (ALP), or gamma-glutanyl transferase (GGT) may occur. In most cats, increases in ALP and GGT activities are greater than increases in ALT and AST activities. Lack of increased liver enzyme activities does not exclude the diagnosis of idiopathic hepatic lipidosis. Hyperbilirubinemia and bilirubinuria occur in most cats with idiopathic hepatic lipidosis. Findings are similar with acute hepatitis, but increases in ALT and AST activities are usually greater than increases in ALP and GGT activities.

9. What ancillary diagnostic tests help to determine the cause of liver disease in animals with suspected acute hepatitis or lipidosis?

Fasting and postprandial serum bile acids are usually markedly increased but do not need to be measured if hyperbilirubinemia is present. Fasting serum ammonia concentrations may be elevated and can be used for indirect assessment of the presence of hepatic encephalopathy. Abdominal radiographs, hepatic ultrasound, and pancreatic ultrasound may be used to narrow the differential list in animals with acute hepatic disease.

10. Do I need to perform a hepatic biopsy for all animals with suspected acute hepatitis or lipidosis?

A presumptive diagnosis of idiopathic hepatic lipidosis in cats may be made by the combination of appropriate history, laboratory abnormalities, and vacuolated hepatocytes on cytologic evaluation of a fine aspirate of the liver. If the cause of hepatitis is determined by history (trauma, drugs, toxins) or other findings (pancreatitis), biopsy may not be needed. However, the reference test for hepatic diseases is hepatic histologic evaluation. If hepatic aspiration or biopsy is performed, samples should be cultured for aerobic and anaerobic bacteria.

11. What immediate supportive care should be provided to animals with suspected acute hepatitis or lipidosis?

Fluid, electrolyte, acid–base, coagulation, and glucose abnormalities should be corrected as discussed in other chapters. Depending on acid–base and electrolyte status, 0.45% NaCl and

2.5% dextrose or Normosol-R are appropriate fluid choices. Potassium supplementation is required for most cases. Antibiotics should be administered to all animals with suspected acute hepatitis because bacterial translocation from the intestines into the liver is common. Penicillin derivatives or first-generation cephalosporins administered parenterally are adequate if clinical findings of sepsis are not present. Enrofloxacin should be considered in animals with suspected gram-negative sepsis. Vitamin K should be given subcutaneously to animals with increased activated clotting time. Supplementation with B vitamins is suggested for most cases. Hepatic encephalopathy, if present, is managed as described for portosystemic shunts (see chapter 82). Appetite stimulants, including cyproheptadine and benzodiazepams, generally are not successful alone. Benzodiazepams may lead to severe sedation if hepatic dysfunction is severe.

Whether enteral feeding is indicated depends on the cause of the disease. Early, aggressive nutritional therapy is the key to successful treatment of idiopathic hepatic lipidosis in cats. Initial short-term nutritional support may be provided by a nasoesophageal tube. However, because nutritional support is required for at least 3–6 weeks in most cases, a gastrostomy tube is strongly recommended. Multiple small meals should be fed to cats to provide a total of 60–80 kcal/kg/day. Most full-grown cats can handle 50–80 ml of food per feeding when the volume of food at each meal is gradually increased over several days. Protein should not be restricted unless signs of hepatic encephalopathy are present. Food should always be offered by mouth; the tube can be pulled after eating begins.

12. What is the prognosis for recovery from idiopathic hepatic lipidosis?
The prognosis is guarded to fair, depending on how early the disease is recognized. The conditions can be reversed with aggressive nutritional therapy. Owners must be counseled that recovery may require up to 20 weeks before spontaneous eating occurs. Without treatment, hepatic lipidosis is usually fatal, leading to progressive liver failure.

BIBLIOGRAPHY

1. Bunch SE: Hepatotoxicity associated with pharmacologic agents in dogs and cats. Vet Clin North Am 23:659, 1993.
2. Center SA: Hepatobiliary infections. In Greene CE (ed): Infectious Diseases of the Dog and Cat, 2nd ed. Philadelphia, W.B. Saunders, 1990, pp 146–156.
3. Dimski DS, Taboada J: Feline idiopathic hepatic lipidosis. Vet Clin North Am 25:357–373, 1995.
4. Marks SL, Rogers QR, Strombeck DR: Nutritional support in hepatic disease. Part II: Dietary management of common liver disorders in dogs and cats. Comp Cont Educ Pract Vet 10:1287–1295, 1994.
5. Sherding RG: Acute hepatic failure. Vet Clin North Am 15:119, 1985.

X. Digestive Emergencies

Section Editor: Wayne E. Wingfield, D.V.M., M.S.

84. FOREIGN BODIES IN THE DIGESTIVE SYSTEM

Howard B. Seim, III, D.V.M.

ESOPHAGEAL OBSTRUCTION

1. What is the most common cause of esophageal obstruction? Where are most obstructions located?

Foreign bodies (e.g., bones, cartilage, fish hook) are the most common cause of esophageal obstruction. Esophageal stricture and neoplasia also may cause signs of obstruction. The most common locations are the heart base and lower esophageal sphincter. Foreign bodies occasionally lodge in the cervical esophagus and thoracic inlet. Esophageal strictures are generally located in the cranial thoracic esophagus, whereas neoplasms occur at the lower esophageal sphincter.

2. Describe the most common clinical signs and physical findings in patients with esophageal obstruction.

Patients with esophageal obstruction present with various signs, depending on the duration of obstruction. Initially, regurgitation, hypersalivation, gagging, and retching are common signs. Some patients may exhibit dysphagia, distress, or slow continual swallowing. Later, these signs may disappear and become less specific (e.g,. depression, anorexia, weight loss). Physical findings are generally nonspecific. Occasionally, cervical or thoracic inlet foreign bodies are palpable.

3. What tests are most likely to confirm the diagnosis of esophageal obstruction?

Approximately 50% of esophageal foreign bodies are radiopaque; in such cases, survey radiographs are diagnostic. Radiographic findings suggestive of a nonradiopaque foreign body include gas in the esophagus and mediastinitis or pleuritis, which suggest a perforated esophagus. Contrast radiography should be performed if the diagnosis is in reasonable doubt. If suspicion of perforation is high, an organic iodide contrast media should be used instead of barium. Contrast radiographs also diagnose esophageal stricture and neoplasia. Rigid or flexible fiberoptic esophagoscopy is the definitive diagnostic procedure.

4. List the most common methods of removing esophageal foreign bodies.

Ninety percent of esophageal foreign bodies can be removed without surgical intervention by one of the following methods:

1. **Rigid esophagoscopy.** Advantages include dilation of the esophagus proximal to the obstruction, removal of the foreign body within the scope without trauma to the proximal esophagus, advancement of the foreign body into the stomach, relatively low cost of equipment, and low risk of pneumothorax if an esophageal perforation is present. Disadvantages include lack of clear visualization and difficulty in evaluating the esophageal wall after removal.

2. **Flexible fiberoptic endoscopy.** Advantages include precise view of the foreign body, ability to grasp the foreign body, advancement of the foreign body into the stomach, and accurate evaluation of the esophagus after removal. Disadvantages include high risk of tension pneumothorax if an esophageal perforation is present, high cost of equipment, and inability to protect the orad esophagus during removal.

5. What is the first step after removal of the foreign body?

The first step is to evaluate the esophageal mucosa for evidence of erosion, ulceration, or perforation. If perforation is present, consider surgery to repair the defect. If ulceration and erosion are present, treat for esophagitis.

6. List the components of treatment after removal of a foreign body and explain the reason for each.

1. An **H₂ receptor blocker** decreases acid content of the stomach, thus decreasing the risk of reflux of acid-rich gastric juice into the esophagus.

2. **Dietary restriction** eliminates mechanical trauma to eroded or ulcerated esophageal mucosa. Either the patient is given nothing orally for several days, or a gastrostomy feeding tube is placed.

3. **Corticosteroids** decrease the incidence of esophageal stricture formation. The esophagus is unique among bodily organs in its lack of an organized dermis; a stratified squamous epithelium lies directly on loose submucosal connective tissue. Healing, therefore, may be more simple and rapid than in complex organs such as skin, and early retardation of collagen synthesis with corticosteroids seems to make a significant difference in the quality and quantity of the final scar.

4. **Antibiotics** protect the patient against bacterial infection and possible abscess, particularly in the presence of small, undetectable perforations.

5. **Prokinetic agents** increase normograde gastric motility and pressure at the lower esophageal sphincter; both actions decrease reflux of gastric contents into the esophagus.

7. Should all patients with esophageal perforation be treated surgically?

In patients suspected of esophageal perforation after removal of a foreign body, an organic iodide esophagram should be done. Small perforations (1–3 mm) should be treated conservatively (see question 6). Placement of a gastrostomy feeding tube should be considered. Large perforations (> 3 mm) should be surgically explored, debrided, and sutured.

SMALL INTESTINAL OBSTRUCTION

8. How are small intestinal obstructions classified?

1. **Strangulating vs. nonstrangulating (simple) obstruction.** Strangulation implies that the blood supply to the segment of obstructed bowel is compromised to some degree. Nonstrangulating obstructions do not cause vascular compromise to the affected intestinal segment. Strangulating obstruction is generally more life-threatening than nonstrangulating obstruction.

2. **Complete vs. partial obstruction.** A complete obstruction implies that gas and fluid located above the obstruction cannot pass below the obstruction. A partial obstruction implies that some gas and fluid can pass beyond the obstruction. Complete obstructions are generally more life-threatening than partial obstructions.

3. **High vs. low obstruction.** High obstructions generally imply pyloric, duodenal, and mid-jejunal involvement. Low obstructions generally imply distal jejunum and ileal involvement. In general, the closer the obstruction to the pyloric region and the more complete the obstruction, the greater the severity of signs.

9. **What are the causes of small intestinal obstruction? Give common examples of each.**
   1. Luminal foreign bodies (e.g., bones, rocks, rags, socks, string)
   2. Mural lesions (e.g., adenocarcinoma, leiomyoma, leiomyosarcoma, lymphosarcoma)
   3. Extraluminal (e.g., intussusception, volvulus, hernia, torsion)

10. **What are the most common presenting signs?**
   Clinical signs of small bowel obstruction include vomiting, abdominal pain, restlessness, abdominal distention, dehydration, hyporexia, and anorexia. Severity and duration of signs depend on location and completeness of the obstruction and whether vascular occlusion (i.e., strangulation) is present.

11. **Describe the most common physical findings in patients with small bowel obstruction.**
   Abdominal tenderness or pain, palpation of an abdominal mass, low-grade fever, and dehydration are common physical findings. Patients with complete, high obstruction or strangulating obstruction of long duration (i.e., several days to weeks) may be severely moribund, with low body temperature, muddy mucous membranes, capillary refill time greater than 2 seconds, elevated heart rate, and variable breathing patterns, depending on acid–base status.

12. **What is the single best test to establish a definitive diagnosis?**
   Survey and contrast abdominal radiographs are the best diagnostic tests. Characteristic findings of survey radiographs include: (1) multiple loops of gas-dilated small intestine of various diameters, (2) gas–fluid interfaces in dilated loops of small intestine on standing lateral projections, (3) visualization of a radiopaque foreign body, (4) ground-glass appearance if peritoneal fluid is present, and (5) free gas in the peritoneal cavity if intestinal perforation has occurred. Contrast radiographic examination may confirm the diagnosis by outlining the intraluminal mass with contrast, or the contrast may be compressed by a mural or extraluminal lesion.

13. **What laboratory abnormalities are generally present?**
   Patients suspected of small bowel obstruction should have a complete blood count, biochemical profile, and urinalysis. Changes in blood parameters are influenced by location and degree of intestinal obstruction as well as presence or absence of strangulation. In general, patients have a normal or slightly elevated white blood cell count, hyponatremia, hypochloremia, hypokalemia, metabolic alkalosis, prerenal azotemia, and increased urine specific gravity. A shift to metabolic acidosis occurs as continued vomiting and dehydration cause further losses of fluid and electrolytes, resulting in hypovolemic shock. Severe fluid loss may be due to (1) vomiting, (2) intraluminal pooling, and (3) bowel wall edema.

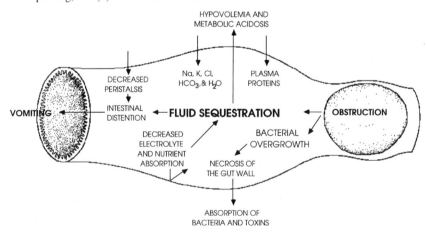

Pathophysiology of intestinal obstruction.

14. List the steps in the initial medical management of small bowel obstruction.

1. Intravenous fluid resuscitation to correct dehydration, replace electrolyte losses, correct acid–base abnormalities, and treat hypovolemic shock.

2. Consider corticosteroid or flunixin meglumine in patients suspected of strangulating obstruction or sepsis.

3. Consider antimicrobial therapy in (1) old, debilitated patients, (2) patients with sepsis, (3) patients suspected of strangulating obstruction, and (4) patients in whom perforation is associated with the obstruction (e.g., linear foreign body, necrotic tumor). In addition, antimicrobial therapy should be considered if the surgical procedure will take longer than 90 minutes.

4. Consider adding glucose to the intravenous fluids in septic patients, especially if the serum biochemistry profile reveals a low glucose level or your index of suspicion is high.

15. What is the differential diagnosis for small bowel obstruction?

1. **Paralytic ileus.** Most patients have a history of dietary indiscretion. Physical examination reveals no palpable abdominal mass, and the abdomen is not as tender. Survey radiographs reveal generalized rather than segmental ileus.

2. **Mesenteric volvulus.** Most patients have a history of sudden, severe abdominal pain and hematochezia. Physical examination reveals severe abdominal distention and abdominal pain out of proportion with other physical findings. Survey radiographs reveal generalized ileus with abdominal distention.

16. When does the patient with small intestinal obstruction become a "stable" surgical candidate?

- *Never let the sun set on a small bowel obstruction.*
- *When a patient is unable to pass feces or flatus per rectum, he is sick and will surely die, unless surgically relieved.*

Both axioms apply to veterinary patients with signs of small intestinal obstruction. The nearer the obstruction to the pylorus, the greater the surgical urgency. Stabilization before surgical intervention is defined as the time necessary to deliver a shock dose of fluids, to ensure cardiovascular stability, to begin resolving electrolyte and acid–base abnormalities, and to institute additional shock therapy as needed (i.e., antibiotics, corticosteroids, glucose, flunixin meglumine).

17. List the surgical options at the time of laparotomy. Give examples of settings in which each option is appropriate.

1. Enterotomy (e.g., luminal foreign body, intestinal wall mass, intestinal biopsy)

2. Enterotomy with transverse closure (e.g., resection of intestinal wall mass in which linear closure will result in unacceptable lumen compromise)

3. Anastomosis (e.g., mural lesion, nonviable bowel segment, multiple mesenteric wounds)

4. Enteroplication (e.g,. after intussusception reduction or resection and anastomosis)

5. Enterostomy feeding tube (e.g,. bypass of surgical site for immediate postoperative enteral feeding)

18. What are the most reliable criteria for assessing small bowel wall viability at surgery?

The most reliable criteria include color, peristalsis, arterial pulsations, intravenous fluorescein dye injection, and a second look. Intravenous fluorescein is the method of choice in dogs and cats.

Fluorescein dye is injected via any peripheral vein. Sixty to 90 seconds after injection the lights in the operating room are dimmed and ultraviolet illumination (e.g., Wood's lamp) is provided. The affected segment of bowel is evaluated according to established criteria.

Second look refers to laparotomy 24–36 hours after the original laparotomy to reexamine the bowel in question. Less accurate methods include Doppler studies, surface oximetry, and serosal bleeding of a cut surface.

19. What is the most common postoperative complication of intestinal surgery?

Breakdown of the enterotomy or anastomosis and subsequent leakage of intestinal contents into the peritoneal cavity is the most common postoperative complication of intestinal surgery. The causes may include (1) less than 3-mm bite in the submucosa, (2) sutures spaced more than 3 mm apart, (3) traumatic handling of the cut edge of intestine, (4) improper knotting of suture material, and (5) suturing of nonviable bowel.

20. What is the most accurate test for diagnosis of postoperative intestinal leak?

Peritoneal tap and evaluation of peritoneal fluid cytology is the most sensitive diagnostic test for peritonitis secondary to anastomotic leak. Presumptive diagnosis is based on elevated body temperature, vomiting, abdominal tenderness, drainage from the incision, inflammatory leukogram, and low glucose. Survey abdominal radiographs are generally not helpful; they are difficult to assess critically because of the presence of postoperative air and fluid. Barium should not be used because it may cause peritoneal irritation. Aqueous contrast agents are not sensitive enough to pick up small perforations. If the presence of a leak is in doubt, remember the axiom, "It is better to have a negative exploratory laparotomy than a positive postmortem."

CONTROVERSY

21. Should anastomosis of small intestine be performed with 8–10 sutures?

For: Several authors have suggested that intestinal anastomosis can be successfully performed with minimal sutures (i.e., 8–10). This technique is less time-consuming and causes less trauma to intestinal tissue and blood supply.

Against: Patients with intestinal obstruction frequently have associated bowel pathology (e.g., inflammation, edema, vascular compromise). Eight to 10 sutures are likely to leave gaps of significant size that encourage leak. Sutures should be placed no further apart than 3 mm; a typical anastomosis requires 20–25 sutures.

BIBLIOGRAPHY

1. Lantz GC: The pathophysiology of acute mechanical small bowel obstruction. Comp Cont Educ 3:910–918, 1981.
2. Nemzek JA, Walshaw R, Hauptman JG: Mesenteric volvulus in the dog: A retrospective study. J Am Animal Hosp Assoc 29:357–362, 1993.

85. CANINE HEMORRHAGIC GASTROENTERITIS

Wayne E. Wingfield, D.V.M., M.S.

1. What is canine hemorrhagic gastroenteritis (HGE)?

Canine HGE is a syndrome characterized by the acute onset of profuse vomiting and bloody diarrhea with significant hemoconcentration.

2. What is the cause of HGE?

The cause is unknown. Although the term HGE implies an inflammatory condition, the disease is more likely due to altered intestinal mucosal permeability and perhaps mucosal hypersecretion. Cultures of GI contents from HGE-affected dogs have yielded large numbers of *Clostridium perfringens*, leading to speculation that this organism or its exotoxins are the cause.

3. Which dogs are most likely to be affected with HGE?

Toy and miniature breeds seem particularly prone to HGE, especially toy and miniature poodles and schnauzers, but the syndrome may affect any breed.

4. What are the clinical signs of HGE?

- Acute onset of vomiting
- Severe depression
- Profuse, bloody, fetid diarrhea
- Shock

5. How is the diagnosis of HGE made?

- Extreme hemoconcentration (packed cell volume > 50–60%)
- Bloody, fetid diarrhea
- No leukopenia
- Fecal cytology with increased numbers of clostridial organisms

6. Describe the treatment for HGE.

- Intensive fluid therapy until the packed cell volume is in the normal range and then continued intravenous crystalloid fluids (Normosol-R + potassium chloride) until vomiting is controlled.
- Antibiotics to control *C. perfringens* (ampicillin or amoxicillin)
- Restriction of food and water
- Antiemetic drugs (metoclopramide)

7. What is the prognosis of HGE?

- Early, aggressive fluid therapy consistently results in significant improvement within 24 hours.
- If vomiting and diarrhea are not resolved in 48 hours, a search for other causes mimicking HGE should be conducted (parvovirus, coronavirus, GI foreign bodies, intussusception, intestinal volvulus, clostridial enteritis, lymphocytic–plasmocytic enteritis).

BIBLIOGRAPHY

1. Sherding RG, Johnson SE: Diseases of the intestines. In Birchard SJ, Sherding RG (eds): Saunders Manual of Small Animal Practice. Philadelphia, W.B. Saunders, 1994, p 704.
2. Twedt DC: *Clostridium perfringens*-associated enterotoxicosis in dogs. In Kirk RW, Bonagura JD (eds): Current Veterinary Therapy XI (Small Animal Practice). Philadelphia, W.B. Saunders, 1992, pp 602–604.

86. ESOPHAGEAL DISORDERS

Wayne E. Wingfield, D.V.M., M.S.

1. What is the most common clinical sign of an esophageal disorder?

Regurgitation.

2. What is the difference between regurgitation and reflux?

Regurgitation refers to passive, retrograde movement of ingested material to a level proximal to the upper esophageal sphincter; usually this material has not reached the stomach. In most cases, regurgitation results from abnormal esophageal peristalsis, esophageal obstruction, or asynchronous function of the gastroesophageal junction.

Reflux refers to the movement of gastric and duodenal contents into the esophagus without associated eructation or vomiting.

3. List the causes of regurgitation.

1. Megaesophagus
   - Idiopathic
   - Secondary
     - Myasthenia gravis
     - Polyneuropathy
     - Systemic lupus erythematosus
     - Polymyositis
     - Toxicosis (lead, thallium)
     - Hypothyroidism
     - Hypoadrenocorticism
2. Esophageal foreign body
3. Esophageal stricture
   - Intraluminal stricture
   - Extraluminal stricture due to compression
     - Abscess
     - Cranial mediastinal mass
     - Thoracic hilar lymphadenopathy
4. Vascular ring anomaly
5. Neoplasia (primary or metastatic)
6. Granuloma (e.g., *Spirocerca lupi*)
7. Hiatal hernia
8. Esophageal diverticula

4. What is megaesophagus?

Megaesophagus refers to a specific syndrome characterized by a dilated hypoperistaltic esophagus.

5. What is the most common complication of megaesophagus?

Aspiration pneumonitis.

6. Does esophageal dilatation on thoracic radiographs confirm an esophageal disorder?

No. The following conditions often produce transient dilatation of the esophagus:

- Aerophagia
- Anxiety
- Respiratory distress (dyspnea)
- Anesthesia
- Vomiting

7. How is esophageal motility evaluated?

Thoracic radiography initially evaluates for evidence of an esophageal foreign body, esophageal dilatation, or thoracic mass. Ideally a barium esophagram with fluoroscopy should be performed. It is best to mix food with the barium to observe for decreased contractility.

8. Why is abnormal esophageal motility not demonstrated by a liquid barium esophagram?

Often the liquid barium esophagram shows *decreased* motility in the esophagus, but mostly it is useful for confirming esophageal motility. Abnormal motility is best demonstrated by mixing barium with food. The esophagus with abnormal motility is unable to propel the mixture of barium and food in the normal aboral direction.

9. What is myasthenia gravis?

Myasthenia gravis is an immune-mediated disorder, either acquired or congenital (familial), resulting from the action of autoantibodies against nicotinic acetylcholine receptors at the neuromuscular junctions.

10. What are the most common clinical signs of myasthenia gravis?

- Premature fatigue with exercise
- Spastic pelvic limb gait
- Tetraparesis
- Collapse
- Tachypnea
- Respiratory distress
- Sialosis
- Regurgitation
- Dysphagia
- Weakness of facial muscles
- Decreased palpebral reflex

11. What is the test of choice for myasthenia gravis?

Acetylcholine receptor antibody titers.

12. Describe the typical profile of a dog with myasthenia gravis.
• Breeds most commonly affected: golden retriever, German shepherd
• Bimodal age of onset: 2–4 years and 9–13 years

13. How is myasthenia gravis treated?
1. Anticholinesterase drugs—neostigmine
    • Injectable (Prostigmin [Roche]): 0.02 mg/lb IM every 6 hr
    • Oral (Mestinon [Roche]): 0.25–0.45 mg/lb every 8–12 hr
2. Corticosteroids

14. Describe the principles for management of megaesophagus.
1. Remove the cause if possible.
2. Minimize chances for aspiration of esophageal contents. (Feed the animal in an upright position so that the upper body is elevated to at least 45° above the lower body. Maintain this position for at least 10 minutes after eating and before bedtime.)
3. Maximize nutrient intake to the GI tract (if possible, feed 2–4 times/day).

15. What is an alternative means of feeding dogs with megaesophagus?
Gastrostomy tube.

16. What is the prognosis for a dog with megaesophagus?
Guarded to poor.

17. List causes of esophageal stricture in dogs.
• Esophagitis
• Reflux of gastric acid during general anesthesia (on a tilted operating table)
• Ingestion of a strong acid or alkali material
• Esophageal foreign bodies
• Thermal burns
• Hairballs (cats)

18. How is esophageal stricture diagnosed?
Esophageal stricture is diagnosed by barium esophagram and esophageal endoscopy.

19. List the treatment options for esophageal stricture and the success rate for each.
• Surgery (esophagotomy, patch grafting, resection and anastomosis): < 50% success
• Esophageal bougienage: 50–70% success
• Balloon catheter dilatation: > 50–70% success (treatment of choice, ideally done under fluoroscopy)

20. What are the most common areas of the esophagus in which foreign bodies lodge?
• Thoracic inlet
• Base of the heart
• Hiatus of the diaphragm

21. How do you manage dogs with an esophageal foreign body?
Esophageal foreign bodies are considered an emergency. The following steps are recommended:
1. Endoscopic removal of the foreign body is usually successful. Either extract the foreign body or carefully push it into the stomach. If the foreign body is a bone, it is often best to push it into the stomach. Gastrostomy is not usually required for removal of the bone, but serial radiography should be done to ensure digestion or passage of the bone.
2. If esophagoscopy is unsuccessful, surgical removal is required.

3. Assess the esophageal mucosa for hemorrhage, erosions, lacerations, or perforations.

4. Withhold food and water for 24–48 hours, and give crystalloid fluids and parenteral antibiotics.

22. What treatments are available for esophageal reflux?

- **Metoclopramide** (Reglan) increases gastroesophageal sphincter tone and decreases gastric reflux into the stomach.
- **H₂ receptor-blocking agents** (e.g., cimetidine or ranitidine) reduce the acidity of refluxed gastric contents.
- **Sucralfate suspension** is an aluminum salt that selectively binds to injured gastro-esophageal mucosa and acts as an effective barrier against the damaging actions of gastric acid, pepsin, and bile acids associated with reflux esophagitis.

BIBLIOGRAPHY

1. Johnson SE, Sherding RG: Diseases of the esophagus and disorders of swallowing. In Birchard SJ, Sherding RG (eds): Saunders Manual of Small Animal Practice. Philadelphia, W.B. Saunders, 1994, pp 630–654.
2. Shelton GD: Disorders of neuromuscular transmission. Semin Vet Med Surg (Small Animals) 4:126, 1989.
3. Shelton GD, Willard WD, Cardinet GH III, et al: Acquired myasthenia gravis: Selective involvement of esophageal, pharyngeal, and facial muscles. J Vet Intern Med 4:281, 1990.
4. Tams TR: Esophagoscopy. In Tams TR (ed): Small Animal Endoscopy. St. Louis, Mosby, 1990, pp 47–88.
5. Zawie DA: Esophageal strictures. In Kirk RW (ed): Current Veterinary Therapy X. Philadelphia, W.B. Saunders, 1989, pp 904–906.

87. CANINE PARVOVIRUS

Wayne E. Wingfield, D.V.M., M.S., and Dennis W. Macy, D.V.M., M.S.

1. What are the common clinical signs in dogs with canine parvovirus (CPV)?

- Lethargy
- Inappetence
- Acute-onset diarrhea
- Vomiting
- Fever
- Profound neutropenia (white blood cells < 1000/mm³)

Puppies between the ages of 6 weeks to 6 months are most commonly affected. In a Canadian study, sexually intact dogs had a 4-fold greater risk than spayed or neutered dogs, and the months of July, August, and September had a 3-fold increase in cases of CPV.

2. What systems other than the GI tract are involved with CPV?

In a study of dogs with the GI form of CPV, arrhythmia was diagnosed in 21 of 148 cases, including supraventricular arrhythmias and conduction disturbances. Some dogs developed significant enlargement of the cardiac silhouette and other radiographic cardiac abnormalities. CPV can replicate in bone marrow, heart, and endothelial cells; replication in endothelial cells of the brain produces neurologic disease.

3. What other infectious diseases may be mistaken for CPV infection?

Infection with *Salmonella* sp., *Campylobacter* sp., or *Escherichia coli* may mimic CPV symptoms and also cause the shift in white blood cells. CPV infection also may be confused with hemorrhagic gastroenteritis (HGE), although HGE is seen most commonly in smaller breeds and usually resolves in 24 hours. Coronavirus often presents with GI signs, but neutropenia tends to resolve more rapidly than with CPV infection. Clinical signs of infection with coronavirus are usually seen only in dogs also infected with parvovirus.

4. What is the primary mode of transmission of CPV?

The number of viral particles in the feces is quite high; the fecal-oral route is the most likely means of transmission. No studies of vomitus have been done, but it probably contains viral particles.

5. How does CPV infect the intestines?

Viral replication occurs in the oropharynx during the first 2 days of infection, spreading to other organ systems via the blood. By the third to fifth day a marked viremia develops. The virus reaches the intestinal mucosa from the blood rather than from the intestinal lumen. Clinical signs are seen 4–5 days after exposure, and the incubation period ranges from 3–8 days, with shedding of the virus on day 3.

6. Where does CPV replicate in the body?

The virus replicates in rapidly dividing cells, which include lymph nodes, spleen, bone marrow, and intestines. In the intestines, viral replication kills the germinal epithelium of the intestinal crypts, leading to epithelial loss, shortening of the intestinal villi, vomiting, and diarrhea. Lymphoid necrosis and destruction of myeloproliferative cells result in lymphopenia and, in severe cases, panleukopenia. Only about one-third of CPV cases have defined neutropenia or lymphopenia.

7. How has the clinical presentation of CPV infection changed since the 1970s?

There are several strains of CPV, including the original strain, CPV-1; the minute virus; and the most severe strain, CPV-2 (with subtypes 2a and 2b). CPV-2b is now the most common strain in the United States. CPV-1, which dominated in the 1970s, caused a milder disease associated with fever and a larger window for treatment. CPV-2b causes a more explosive acute syndrome that affects young dogs 6–12 weeks of age, making the window between the first signs of GI upset and treatment much narrower and more critical. There have been no major changes in presentation in the past 6 years; lethargy, listlessness, and bloody diarrhea are the most common presenting signs. Partially vaccinated dogs respond much faster to treatment; fully vaccinated dogs, usually over 1 year old, that present with CPV have a history of immunosuppression involving corticosteroids or other diseases. Other diseases associated with or mistaken for CPV are canine distemper virus, coccidial or giardial infection, hookworms, roundworms, or a combination of these.

8. When and how does one diagnose CPV?

CPV is most easily diagnosed with a fecal enzyme-linked immunosorbent assay (ELISA). If the test is negative but CPV is still suspected, isolate the animal and run the test again in 48 hours. The virus is not usually shed until day 3, and conscientious clients may bring the animal to the hospital at the first sign of illness. The period during which CPV is shed in the feces is brief, and the virus is not usually detectable until day 10–12 after infection. Usually the acute phase of illness has passed by this time. Modified live CPV vaccines shed in the feces may give a false-positive ELISA result 4–10 days after vaccination.

One also may use a combination of ELISA, complete blood count, and radiographs to diagnose CPV. Radiographs may help to rule out the possibility of an intestinal foreign body, and detection of generalized ileus with fluid-filled loops of intestines supports the diagnosis of CPV. Be sure to have enough antigen in the fecal sample when running the ELISA; watery stools may dilute the antigen and give a false-negative result.

Conclusive proof of CPV infection is made with electron microscope identification of the virus.

9. What are the recommendations for inpatient care of dogs with CPV?

1. **Aggressive fluid therapy.** Correct dehydration and provide intravenous maintenance fluid volumes of a balanced crystalloid solution. Make every attempt to replace continuing

losses (vomitus and diarrhea) with equal volumes of crystalloid fluids. The easiest method is simply to estimate the volume lost and *double* your estimate. Continuing losses need to be replaced at the time that they occur. Use Normosol with at least 20 mEq/L of potassium chloride supplementation. Monitor glucose level. If necessary, add 2.5–5% dextrose to intravenous fluids. A 5% dextrose solution creates an osmotic diuresis, but it also allows assessment of progress in dealing with a septic case (glucose increases when the animal receives 5% dextrose if the sepsis is resolving). Low levels of magnesium chloride may be added to fluids to help correct unresponsive hypokalemia.

2. **Antibiotic therapy.** Broad-spectrum parenteral antibiotics are recommended because of disruption of the mucosal barrier and potential sepsis. A combination of ampicillin and gentamicin every 8 hours is recommended, but one should be cautious about using an aminoglycoside because of renal toxicity. Most veterinarians use only a first-generation cephalosporin in dogs without neutropenia or fever and reserve ampicillin and gentamicin or amikacin for dogs with signs of sepsis.

3. **Endotoxin-neutralizing products.** Endotoxin-neutralizing products may be administered along with antibiotic therapy. The rationale for their use is based on the large population of gram-negative bacteria; by killing the bacteria, antibiotic therapy may shower the body with endotoxin, thus exacerbating the CPV condition. Studies have shown that endotoxin-neutralizing products decrease the incidence of septic shock. They may be diluted (4 ml/kg) with an equal volume of saline and administered intravenously over 30–60 minutes.

4. **Antiemetics.** Metoclopramide is the drug of choice. Phenothiazine derivatives should be used with caution and only after adequate volume replacement is initiated to avoid severe hypotension. Antiemetics are especially useful when continued vomiting makes it difficult to maintain hydration or electrolyte balance.

5. **Motility modifiers.** The use of motility modifiers is controversial. Anticholinergic antidiarrheal medications may suppress segmental contractions and actually hasten transit time. Narcotic analgesics and synthetic opiates are better choices but should be reserved for severe or prolonged cases because slowing the flow through the intestine may increase toxin absorption.

6. **Nothing per os (NPO).** Begin a slow return to water 24 hours after the animal stops vomiting, and slowly progress to gruel made from a bland diet.

10. What is granulocyte colony-stimulating factor (GCSF)? What role does it have in treating dogs with CPV?

GCSF selectively stimulates release of granulocytes form the bone marrow. Preliminary studies have shown that it reduces morbidity and mortality due to CPV. Unfortunately, it is available only as a human drug and is expensive, but when the positive benefits are considered, its use is justified.

11. How is a dog with CPV monitored?

Monitor respiration and central venous pressure (CVP) to prevent overhydration. With osmotic diarrhea the animal loses protein. If abdominal or extremity swelling is observed or if the total solids drop by 50% from admission values or go below 2.0 gm/dl, the animal should be supplemented with either 6% hetastarch or plasma to maintain colloid oncotic pressures. Blood glucose should be monitored at least 4 times/day on the first two days. Glucose level may drop precipitously and suddenly. Most importantly, weigh the dog at least twice each day. If adequate crystalloid replacement is provided, body weight does not decrease from initial values. Ideally body weight should increase at a rate comparable to the degree of dehydration originally assessed.

Dogs that can hold down water for 12 hours may be offered a gruel made from bland foods. Most dogs force-fed by hand will vomit. This response may be physical or psychological (association of food with vomiting). Nasogastric tubes seem to help this problem. Metoclopramide speeds gastric emptying, acts as an antiemetic, and decreases gastric distention when added to the liquid diet. Dogs that are not vomiting should be offered food even if the diarrhea has not totally stopped. A low-fat, high-fiber diet is a good choice to stimulate intestinal motility.

12. How do you know when to send a dog home?

The dog should stay in the hospital for 12 hours after it has ingested solid food with no vomiting. Clients should report immediately any vomiting in the next 7 days or refusal to eat for 24 hours. A high-fiber diet is recommended for reducing diarrhea. A recheck appointment in 1 week with a stool sample helps the clinician to assess progress.

13. What recommendations do you offer to clients who have had a CPV-infected animal in their household and now want a new pet?

Prevention involves a proper vaccination regimen, limited exposure to other animals (especially in puppies less than 12 weeks of age), cleaning contaminated areas with bleach (allowing prolonged contact time), and vacuuming all surfaces with which the previous pet came into contact (rugs, carpet, walls, furniture). Wait at least 1 month before bringing the new pet into the home. It is doubtful that the environment (especially outdoors) will ever be completely free of the virus. CPV is a hardy and ubiquitous organism.

14. How long can a dog with CPV be expected to retain immunity?

A dog that has recovered from CPV can maintain immunity for 20 months or longer.

15. What is the recommended vaccination schedule for dogs? Is it the same for every breed?

Some breeds are more susceptible to CPV than others. Rottweilers, American pitbull terriers, Doberman pinschers, and German shepherds are the most susceptible, whereas toy poodles and Cocker spaniels are less susceptible. The new higher-titer vaccines have a higher antigen level and a more virulent vaccine strain that can overcome maternal antibodies, unlike the older lower-titer vaccines. These vaccines narrow the window of infection, especially for susceptible breeds. The vaccination protocol for the new high-titer vaccines is 6, 9, and 12 weeks. Susceptible breeds should be vaccinated only with the high-titer CPV vaccine and then with a combination vaccine at 6–8, 12, and 16 weeks. For less susceptible breeds, the combination vaccines at 6–8, 12, and 16 weeks should be adequate.

16. How do you manage a sick puppy when the client is unwilling to pursue hospital treatment for CPV?

CPV can be treated on an outpatient basis. A combination of dietary restriction, subcutaneous fluids, and, in some cases, GI medications may be used with a follow-up appointment in 1–3 days. Outpatient recommendations include the following:
- Small, frequent amounts of fluid
- Bland food
- Oral antibiotics
- Strong recommendation to have the pet reexamined and admitted for therapy if vomiting returns or anorexia persists

Nine of ten clients bring the dog back for inpatient care shortly after taking it home. Before treating an outpatient, remember that mildly depressed dogs may have a rectal temperature of 106° F and a blood glucose of 30 mg/dl in 12 hours or less.

CONTROVERSIES

17. Should a dog with suspected CPV be hospitalized and placed in isolation?

Undoubtedly hospitalization provides the best chance for survival. Isolation is more controversial. In most veterinary hospitals, isolation means that the animal is housed in a section of the hospital that is not staffed at all times. The adage "out of sight, out of mind" has led to the demise of many CPV-infected dogs. Experience with housing dogs with CPV in the critical care unit at the Veterinary Teaching Hospital of Colorado State University has shown that nosocomial infections can be avoided with a common-sense approach to patient management. The animal is placed in the least traveled area and has its own cleaning supplies; gowns and gloves are worn each time the animal is handled; and the animal's cage is kept as clean as humanly possible. These procedures are no different from those in an isolation area. By being housed in an area where constant attention can be given, the animal receives adequate fluid replacement therapy and is monitored for changes, which occur rapidly.

18. How is nutrition provided for vomiting dogs?

Tough question! Dogs that have not eaten for 3–5 days are probably in a negative nitrogen balance, and certainly intestinal villi have undergone atrophy if not already destroyed by the CPV. The sooner patients begin receiving oral nutrition, the more rapidly they will recover. In addition, micronutrient therapy for the intestinal mucosa is required for maintenance of the mucosal barrier. Without this barrier, sepsis and bacteremia are more likely. Unfortunately, the only means to provide micronutrients is the oral route.

Glucose therapy does not provide nutritional support. It is best to think of dextrose as simply a source of water. One liter of 5% dextrose solution contains a mere 170 kcal. Increasing dextrose concentrations beyond 5% usually results in glycosuria and osmotic diuresis.

Patients that have not eaten for several days are primed for fat metabolism; thus, Intralipid (20%) may be added to fluids. It should be administered through a central IV catheter and requires strict aseptic management, which may be difficult if the patient is in an isolation area of the hospital.

For dogs that retain water without vomiting, glutamine may be added directly to the water bowl. Often placing electrolyte solutions in the water bowl is a good way to start the animal drinking. Placing dextrose in these fluids or even using commercial solutions such as Ensure-Plus in the bowl helps to provide intestinal nutrients.

19. Should parvovirus antibody levels be measured to check the immune status of the puppy?

Although antibodies to parvovirus can be measured, a negative titer does not necessarily mean that the dog is susceptible to CPV. Repeated revaccination of antibody-negative dogs usually does not result in significant titers.

BIBLIOGRAPHY

1. Dunn T, Abood SK, Polley D, et al: Clinical management of canine parvovirus. Part I. Canine Pract 20(5):10–14, 1995.
2. Dunn T, Abood SK, Polley D, et al: Clinical management of canine parvovirus. Part II. Canine Pract 20(6):11–16, 1995.
3. Dunn T, Abood SK, Polley D, et al: Clinical management of canine parvovirus. Part III. Canine Pract 21(1):21–26, 1995.
4. Houston DM, Ribble CS, Head LL: Risk factors associated with parvovirus enteritis in dogs: 283 cases (1982–1991). J Am Vet Med Assoc 208:542–546, 1996.
5. Pollock RVH, Coyne MJ: Canine parvovirus. Vet Clin North Am (Small Animals) 23:555–568, 1993.

88. INTUSSUSCEPTION

Howard B. Seim, III, D.V.M.

1. What is intussusception?

Intussusception is produced by a vigorous intestinal wall contraction that forces a segment of intestine into the lumen of the adjacent relaxed segment. The invaginated segment is called the intussusceptum, and the enveloping segment is called the intussuscipiens.

2. What causes intussusception?

The cause of intussusception is unknown. It is considered a sign, not a primary disorder, and is commonly associated with various causes of gastrointestinal upset such as parvovirus infection, severe parasitic infestation, or intestinal obstruction (e.g., foreign body, neoplasia).

3. At what age is intussusception most commonly diagnosed? What segment of bowel is most often affected?

Intussusception generally occurs in animals less than 1 year of age at the ileocecolic junction. Intussusception in older animals is most often due to an intestinal foreign body or mural neoplasm and may occur in any segment of the intestine.

4. List the cardinal clinical signs and physical findings in patients with intussusception.

1. **Vomiting.** Severity of vomiting often depends on location of the intussusception, degree of luminal compromise, and associated disorders (e.g, parvovirus, parasites). In general, the closer the obstruction to the pylorus and the greater the degree of luminal compromise, the more severe the vomiting.

2. **Abdominal pain.** Intussusception is a strangulating obstruction. In general, as the degree of strangulation and duration of obstruction increase, so does the severity of abdominal pain.

3. **Melena or hematochezia.** When the wall of the intussusceptum is strangulated enough to alter its normal mucosal barrier, hemorrhage may occur in the bowel lumen. Upper intestinal intussusception (i.e., jejunal) may cause melena; lower intestinal intussusception (i.e., ileocecolic) may cause hematochezia.

4. **Palpable abdominal mass.** Intussusception produces an abdominal mass that is easily palpable, sausage-shaped, movable, and mildly painful (depending on degree of strangulation). Young animals have a relatively underdeveloped abdominal musculature, which allows unrestrained abdominal palpation.

5. What about patients with characteristic clinical signs and physical findings that seem to come and go?

Occasionally, animals present with clinical signs and physical findings that are consistent with intussusception but seem to come and go. This pattern may occur in patients with a sliding intussusception. The intussusception intermittently reduces itself, then reinvaginates, allowing clinical signs and physical findings to come and go. Sliding intussusception generally occurs in young animals with associated gastrointestinal disorders (e.g, parvovirus, parasites).

6. How do you definitively diagnose intussusception?

Definitive diagnosis is based on cardinal clinical signs and physical findings along with survey and contrast radiography and ultrasonography. Survey radiographs may reveal gas- and fluid-filled loops of small intestine proximal to the intussusception and a fluid-dense abdominal mass. Contrast radiographs (i.e., upper GI or barium enema) reveal compression of the contrast column at the intussuscepted segment of bowel. Ultrasonography produces a pathognomonic image of the intussuscepted bowel.

7. Barium enemas are often the definitive treatment for intussusception in humans. Are they successful in dogs and cats?
No. Barium enemas may be used for diagnostic purposes but are rarely beneficial as a definitive treatment.

8. What is the presurgical treatment for patients with intussusception?
Preoperative treatments are generally based on presenting clinical signs, physical findings, and results of laboratory data:
• Patients with severe abdominal pain, profuse vomiting, and bloody mucoid stools (i.e., complete, strangulating obstruction) are generally treated with intravenous fluids (i.e., shock dose), glucose, corticosteroids or flunixin meglumine, and antibiotics; they are taken to surgery as soon as fluid and medications have been given and the cardiovascular system is stable.
• Patients with mild presenting signs are volume-expanded and taken to surgery as soon as an operating room becomes available.

9. How do you reduce an intussusception?
Reduction is attempted by grasping the intussuscipiens and squeezing out the intussusceptum as if you were squeezing a sausage from its casing. Care is taken to place minimal, if any, traction on the intussusceptum because traction forces are transmitted along the invaginated mesenteric blood supply of the intussusceptum.

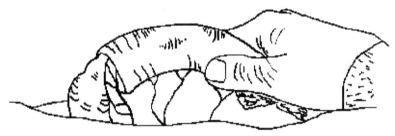

Reducing an intussusception at surgery.

10. If the intussusception does not reduce without causing seromuscular tears, what is the proper course of action?
Consider intestinal resection and anastomosis. Forced reduction of adhered, strangulated bowel may release sequestered endotoxins into the peritoneal cavity and systemic circulation. In addition, forced reduction may cause intestinal perforation and peritoneal leakage of intestinal contents.

11. If the intussusception is successfully reduced, viable bowel is present, and no cause is identified, what is the proper course of action?
Consider enteroplication. The recurrence rate of intussusception is reported to be as high as 27%. Enteroplication is performed by suturing the seromuscular layers of duodenum, jejunum, and ileum in an organized, plicated fashion (see figure at top of next page). Enteroplication effectively prevents recurrence of intussusception.

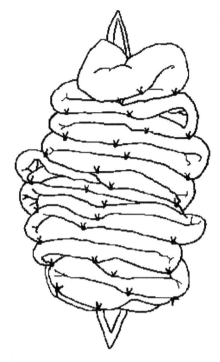

Enteroplication to prevent recurrence of
intussusception.

12. If the intussusception is successfully reduced and bowel wall viability is questionable, what is the proper course of action?

The most reliable criteria for surgical assessment of small intestinal viability include color, peristalsis, arterial pulsations, and intravenous fluorescein dye injection. Intravenous fluorescein dye has been shown to be > 95% accurate for predicting bowel wall viability vs. nonviability. If the bowel wall is viable, replace the affected intestine and close routinely. If the bowel wall is nonviable, perform intestinal resection and anastomosis.

13. If the intussusception is successfully reduced and a foreign body or neoplasm is found, what is the proper course of action?

Perform an enterotomy (for a foreign body, small mural neoplasm, or intestinal biopsy) or anastomosis (for a foreign body causing strangulation or larger mural neoplasm) to remove the cause of the intussusception and perform enteroplication of the remaining bowel to prevent recurrence.

14. The ileocecocolic junction is the most common location for intussusception in young dogs. What is the consequence of removing the ileocecocolic valve?

If bowel resection results in removal of the ileocecocolic valve, malabsorption syndrome and chronic diarrhea may result. The valve functions to control bacterial numbers in the small and large bowel. The small bowel has a relatively low bacterial count, whereas the large bowel has a high bacterial count. If the valve is removed, reflux of bacteria from the colon into the ileum may occur. Overgrowth of bacteria in the small intestine results in increased deconjugation of bile acids and hydroxylation of dietary fatty acids as well as production of bacterial metabolites toxic to epithelial cells. The absorptive capacity of the epithelial cells is then decreased, resulting in malabsorption. The toxic effect on villi results in inflammation and edema, causing fluid secretion into the lumen and further malabsorption that results in chronic diarrhea. Treatment with intestinal antibiotics may help to control the overgrown bacterial population in the small bowel.

15. What suture patterns are considered acceptable for performing intestinal anastomosis in dogs and cats?

1. Simple continuous appositional sutures
2. Simple interrupted apposing sutures
3. Simple interrupted crushing sutures

16. What suture material and needles are recommended for intestinal surgery?

- Suture material: synthetic monofilament absorbable, monofilament nonabsorbable, and synthetic multifilament absorbable
- Suture size for dogs: 3–0 to 4–0; for cats: 4–0 to 5–0
- Needle: swaged-on taper point, taper-cut, or reverse cutting

CONTROVERSY

17. Is it necessary to perform enteroplication in patients that have a surgically treatable cause of the intussusception (i.e., foreign body, neoplasm)?

For: Because recurrence of intussusception is relatively high (i.e., 27%) and a second exploratory procedure is needed to reduce or repair the recurring intussusception, it seems justified to perform a prophylactic enteroplication. In addition, enteroplication does not cause abnormal side effects such as diarrhea, vomiting, weight loss, anorexia, or hyporexia.

Against: The inciting cause of the intussusception has been identified and treated. It seems unwise to perform a second procedure that is necessary in only 27% of patients. In addition, enteroplication increases total operating time and potentially jeopardizes an already debilitated patient.

BIBLIOGRAPHY

1. Lewis DD, Ellison GW: Intussusception in dogs and cats. Comp Cont Educ 9:523–532, 1987.
2. Oakes MG, Lewis DD, Hosgood G, Beale BS: Enteroplication for prevention of intussusception recurrence in dogs: 31 cases (1978–1992). J Am Vet Med Assoc 205:72–75, 1994.
3. Wilson GP, Burt JK: Intussusception in the dog and cat: A review of 45 cases. J Am Vet Med Assoc 164:515–518, 1974.

89. COLITIS

Wayne E. Wingfield, D.V.M., M.S.

1. What is the typical signalment for acute colitis?

- German shepherds and golden retrievers are the most commonly affected breeds.
- 1–4 years old is the most common age.
- Males are more commonly affected than females (3:2).

2. What are the common clinical signs of acute colitis?

- Diarrhea or soft stool (watery, mucus, fresh blood, frequent small amounts)
- Tenesmus
- Normal appetite with little or no weight loss
- Vomiting (30%)
- Abdominal pain

3. What is the typical scenario for a nosocomial clostridial infection?

Acute, bloody diarrhea beginning 1–3 days after exposure to a veterinary hospital.

4. What are the possible causes of acute colitis?

The cause of acute colitis is usually unknown, but the following possibilities should be considered:

1. Mucosal injury by a foreign body or trauma
2. Infection
   - Parasitic (whipworms [*Trichuris* sp.])
   - Bacterial (*Salmonella, Campylobacter, Clostridium* spp.)
   - Fungal (histoplasmosis)
3. Systemic disease (especially uremia)

5. What differential diagnoses should be considered in patients suspected of acute colitis?

1. Other gastrointestinal problems
   - Chronic colitis
   - Neoplasia (adenocarcinoma, lymphoma, leiomyosarcoma, polyp)
   - Ileocolic intussusception
   - Cecal inversion
   - Irritable colon (diagnosis by exclusion)
   - Rectal stricture
   - Perianal fistula
   - Uremic ulcers
2. Painful abdomen
   - Hemorrhagic gatroenteritis (HGE)
   - Viral enteritis
   - GI foreign bodies
   - Bowel ischemia due to thrombi
   - Intestinal volvulus
   - Pancreatitis
   - Hepatobiliary problems
   - Urologic disorder (renal calculi, pyelonephritis, urinary tract infection)
   - Peritonitis (ruptured abdominal organ, sepsis)
   - Splenic torsion
   - Genital problems (uterine torsion or rupture, testicular torsion, prostatic abscess)
3. Thoracolumbar pain

6. Which diagnoses are most commonly confused with acute colitis?

- Neoplasia (adenocarcinoma, lymphoma, leiomyosarcoma, polyps)
- Rectal stricture

7. What are the most common physical findings?

1. Physical examination is usually normal.
2. Deep palpation may or may not produce abdominal pain.
3. Rectal examination may be painful and show fresh blood and mucus.

8. How do you approach the diagnosis of acute colitis?

- Rectal examination
- Fecal flotation for ova or parasites
- Direct and stained fecal smears
- Fecal culture
- Routine laboratory evaluation (complete blood count, biochemical profile, urinalysis)
- Abdominal radiographs and barium enema
- Colonoscopy
- Mucosal biopsy via colonoscopy

9. Describe the appropriate symptomatic treatment.

1. Withhold food for 24–48 hours or until diarrhea resolves. If lymphocytic-plasmocytic enteritis is suspected, withholding food will not resolve the problem.

2. Give crystalloid fluids with potassium chloride.

3. Give medication to decrease fecal water and increase colonic motility (loperamide).

10. What cause-specific treatments may be used for acute colitis?

- Correction of underlying cause if known (e.g., foreign body removal)
- Reduction of clostridial overgrowth (tylosin preferred; also metronidazole)
- Treatment of inflammatory bowel disease (i.e., chronic colitis) with tylosin, mesalazine, sulfasalazine (oral, enema, or foam), or prednisone (antiinflammatory doses)
- High-fiber diet (often supplemented with Metamucil)

BIBLIOGRAPHY

1. Burrows C: Canine colitis. Comp Vet Cont Educ 14:1347–1354, 1992.
2. Bush B: Colitis in the dog. In Practice 17:410–415, 1995.
3. Gilford WG: New ideas for the dietary management of gastrointestinal tract disease. Small Animal Pract 35(12):620–624, 1994.
4. Macintire DK: The acute abdomen—Differential diagnosis and management. Semin Vet Med Surg 3:302–310, 1988.
5. Willard MD: Selected bacterial problems of the alimentary tract. Vet Ann 35:96–106, 1995.

XI. Reproductive Emergencies

Section Editor: Lori A. Wise, D.V.M., M.S.

90. PYOMETRITIS

Donald A. Ostwald, Jr., D.V.M.

1. What is pyometritis?

Pyometritis is the accumulation of pus within the lumen of the uterus. It is one of the few life-threatening conditions of the female reproductive tract. The resulting extragenital effects may include shock, septicemia, toxemia, glomerulonephritis that leads to renal dysfunction, and uterine rupture with secondary peritonitis. Pyometras are loosely defined as open-cervix or closed-cervix based on the amount of vaginal discharge, which depends in part on the degree of cervical patency. Many animals presenting with slight-to-no vaginal discharge (closed pyometras) are in a more advanced state of disease and often in more serious clinical condition. Pyometritis has been reported in many species, including dogs, cats, rabbits, ferrets, and guinea pigs.

2. How are progesterone and estrogen involved in the pathogenesis of pyometritis?

Cystic endometrial hyperplasia results from an inappropriate response of the endometrium to progesterone. Pyometritis develops when opportunistic bacteria from the vagina (most commonly *Escherichia coli*) ascend into a uterus affected by cystic endometrial hyperplasia. Progesterone also suppresses the local immune system, stimulates the endometrial glands to provide secretions favoring bacterial growth, decreases myometrial contractility, and closes the cervix, preventing drainage of the ensuing uterine exudate. The endometrial hyperplasia caused by progesterone occurs with or without estrogen. Estrogen, however, profoundly increases the severity by increasing the number of progesterone receptors in the endometrium. Thus pyometritis develops in 25% of bitches given estradiol as an abortifacient (mismate shot) during diestrus. The incidence of pyometritis is lower in queens than in bitches because queens are induced ovulators and therefore progesterone usually is secreted only after mating.

3. Describe the presenting signs and symptoms of pyometritis.

Pyometritis is more common in middle-aged to older females that have had an estrus within 2 months before the onset of clinical signs. Presenting complaints include vulvar discharge, lethargy, anorexia, vomiting, polydipsia/polyuria, and weight loss. The most common physical findings include vulvar discharge, abdominal distention, enlargement of the uterus, and dehydration. A fever is present in less than one-third of the cases. Vulvar discharge may be less obvious in cats because of their fastidious grooming habits.

4. Explain why polyuria with polydipsia is a common symptom.

Approximately 50% of dogs with pyometritis present with polyuria/polydipsia. These renal manifestations are poorly understood but may result from prerenal azotemia secondary to dehydration and/or shock; antigen–antibody complex glomerulopathy; endotoxin interference with renal tubular function (renal diabetes insipidus); or a combination of the above. Although many dogs with pyometritis develop renal dysfunction, few have lesions severe enough to produce renal failure.

5. List the differential diagnoses for pyometritis.

- Pregnancy
- Fetal abortion
- Postpartum endometritis
- Normal estrus
- Vaginitis
- Vaginal neoplasia
- Renal failure
- Diabetes mellitus
- Hepatic failure
- Hypoadrenocorticism

6. How is pyometritis diagnosed?

Diagnosis is strongly suggested by a history of recent estrus and a clinical presentation of vaginal discharge. Laboratory findings include leukocytosis with a left shift and mild-to-moderate normocytic, normochromic anemia. Some patients may be consuming white blood cells and present with a leukopenia. Serum alkaline phosphatase levels are elevated in 50–75% of the bitches. Azotemia is seen in fewer than one-third of the cases. Most bitches with pyometritis present with concurrent urinary tract infections.

7. What is the role of ultrasound in diagnosing pyometritis?

Although abdominal radiographs may reveal an enlarged uterus, they cannot distinguish between pyometritis and a gravid uterus in the first two trimesters (before fetal calcification is detectable). Ultrasonography is the best tool to demonstrate uterine enlargement and to visualize uterine contents.

8. How do you treat a patient with pyometritis?

Treatment of pyometritis should be prompt and aggressive. Intravenous fluid therapy should be administered first to correct dehydration, improve renal function, and maintain adequate tissue perfusion. Intravenous, broad-spectrum, bactericidal antibiotics should be administered until culture and sensitivity results are known. Surgical ovariohysterectomy is the recommended treatment for pyometritis unless the owner strongly desires to breed the animal.

9. When should you perform surgery?

According to an old adage, don't let the sun set on a pyometra. Surgical removal of the uterus should be performed within 6–12 hours or even sooner if the uterus is thought to have ruptured. Patients should be stabilized before surgery. Dehydration, azotemia, hypotension, shock, acid-base imbalance, and electrolyte abnormalities should be corrected before anesthesia.

10. Is there a medical alternative to surgery?

Yes. Open-cervix pyometras have been successfully treated with prostaglandin F_2-alpha (PGF_2-alpha) and long-term, broad-spectrum antibiotics. Medical treatment of pyometritis with PGF_2-alpha should be reserved for clinically stable bitches who will be bred in the next heat cycle. A closed-cervix pyometra should be treated cautiously with PGF_2-alpha because of the greater risk of rupturing the uterus. Natural PGF_2-alpha (Lutalyse) is given at a dose of 0.05–0.25 mg/kg subcutaneously once or twice daily for 3–5 days. Synthetic PGF_2-alpha (Fluprostenol, Cloprostenol) is more potent than natural PGF_2-alpha and should not be used. PGF_2-alpha is not labeled for use in small animals in the United States, and informed consent should be obtained before it is used.

11. Describe the methods of action of PGF_2-alpha.

PGF_2-alpha stimulates uterine motility, forcing the excretion of uterine contents through the cervix. Its relaxing effects on the cervix are inconsistent; therefore, its use is restricted to treatment of open-cervix pyometras. Because PGF_2-alpha is luteolytic, it reduces progesterone levels in both bitches and queens. In bitches, however, the luteolytic effect may not be a factor in treatment because it occurs late in diestrus. The response to PGF_2-alpha likely depends on underlying uterine pathology rather than dosage. The lower dose should be used first and increased only if there is no initial response.

12. What are the side effects of PGF₂-alpha?

Side effects of PGF$_2$-alpha include panting, salivation, vomiting, defecation, and micturition. These effects are transient and disappear within the first hour after treatment. Subsequent injections result in progressively less severe side effects.

13. What is the prognosis for pyometritis?

The prognosis for surgical treatment of pyometritis is good for patients surviving the perioperative period. Medical management of open-cervix pyometras with prostaglandins resolves clinical signs and illness in over 90% of bitches and queens. Breeding during the next estrus after treatment should be recommended strongly. More than 70% of bitches successfully treated with PGF$_2$-alpha redevelop pyometritis within 2 years. Fewer than 30% of patients with closed-cervix pyometras recover when treated with prostaglandins.

BIBLIOGRAPHY

1. Davidson AP, Feldman EC, Nelson RW: Treatment of pyometra in cats, using prostaglandin F$_2$-alpha— 21 cases (1982–1990). J Am Vet Med Assoc 200:825–828, 1992.
2. Gilbert RO: Diagnosis and treatment of pyometra in bitches and queens. Compend Contin Educ Pract Vet 14:777–785, 1992.
3. Grieve GR: Pyometra in cats. Vet Rec 129:516, 1991.
4. Johnson JH, Wolf AM: Ovarian abscesses and pyometra in a domestic rabbit. J Am Vet Med Assoc 203:667–669, 1993.
5. MacIntire DK: Emergencies of the female reproductive tract. Vet Clin North Am Small Animal Pract 24:1173–1188, 1994.
6. Memon MA, Mickelsen WD: Diagnosis and treatment of closed-cervix pyometra in a bitch. J Am Vet Med Assoc 203:509–512, 1993.
7. Okkens AC, Bevers MM, Dieleman SJ, et al: Fertility problems in the bitch. Animal Reprod Sci 28:379, 1992.
8. Potter K, Hancock DH, Gallina AM: Clinical and pathological features of endometrial hyperplasia, pyometra, and endometritis in cats—79 cases (1980–1985). J Am Vet Med Assoc 198:1427–1431, 1991.
9. Threlfall WR: Diagnosis and medical management of pyometra. Semin Vet Med Surg Small Animal 10:21, 1995.
10. Tobias KMS, Wheaton LG: Surgical management of pyometra in dogs and cats. Semin Vet Med Surg Small Animal 10:30–34, 1995.
11. Wheaton LG, Barbee DD: Comparison of 2 dosages of prostaglandin-F$_2$-alpha on canine uterine motility. Therio 40:111, 1993.

91. PARAPHIMOSIS

Adam J. Reiss, D.V.M.

1. What is paraphimosis?

Paraphimosis is the inability of a male animal to retract the penis into normal position within the prepuce.

2. What is the difference between phimosis and paraphimosis?

Phimosis is the inability to extrude the penis from the prepuce, whereas in paraphimosis the penis is extruded and cannot be replaced within the prepuce.

3. What are the clinical signs of paraphimosis?

Engorged penis protruding from the prepuce	Drying or necrosis of the exposed penis
Excessive licking of the exposed penis	Stranguria, hematuria, and anuria

4. What factors predispose to paraphimosis?

The following factors, in conjunction with sexual excitement, often precede the development of paraphimosis:

- Reduced size of the preputial opening secondary to congenital malformation or trauma
- Penile strangulation caused by preputial hair or foreign bodies (e.g., string or hair)
- Penile swelling secondary to trauma, infection, neoplasia, or priapism
- Chronic balanoposthitis

5. Describe the pathophysiology of paraphimosis.

The pathophysiology of paraphimosis is related to the blood flow dynamics of the penis. Paraphimosis results from a decrease or blockage of venous drainage of the engorged penis that prevents shrinkage and retraction into the prepuce. Prolonged exposure eventually causes desiccation, trauma, and necrosis, which increase existing swelling, tighten constrictive forces, and further inhibit venous drainage and retraction.

6. What other conditions may appear similar to paraphimosis?

- Chronic priapism
- Paralysis of the retractor penis muscles
- Malformation or fracture of the os penis
- Abnormally large preputial opening
- Congenital shortening of the prepuce

7. How is paraphimosis differentiated from similar-appearing conditions?

Differentiation is often made by a good history. Paraphimosis is acute in onset and associated with coitus, whereas similar-appearing conditions are often chronic.

8. What advice can you give to owners over the telephone to prevent further damage before presentation?

- Do not let the dog lick or bite his penis.
- Lubricate the penis with jelly or ointment.
- Keep the dog calm and quiet.

9. How do you treat paraphimosis?

Dogs that present with paraphimosis are in pain, agitated, and potentially in shock. Cardiovascular status must be evaluated and addressed first. Sedation or general anesthesia is required for replacement of the penis. Before manipulation, the exposed penis should be cleansed, freed of hair and foreign material, debrided if necessary, and generously lubricated. Gentle manipulation is often all that is required to replace the penis in its proper position. Cold packs and hyperosmotic solutions help to reduce swelling and ease replacement. A preputial incision may be required to replace the penis. If penile viability is in question, a Doppler examination may be used to search for active blood flow.

10. What are the potential sequelae of paraphimosis? How can they be prevented or treated?

- Penile necrosis and urethral obstruction are the most serious sequelae. Penile resection and urethrotomy are required in cases of necrosis and urethral obstruction.
- Preputial adhesions to the penis also may occur. Adhesions are best prevented by daily extrusion of the penis and infusion of steroid/antibiotic ointments into the prepuce.

11. How can recurrence of paraphimosis be prevented?

- Correct congenital malformations
- Address underlying musculoskeletal or neurologic problems
- Preputial hygiene and regular trimming of preputial hair
- Castration

BIBLIOGRAPHY

1. Bjorling DE: Reproductive emergencies—Surgical treatment. In Proceedings of the Fourth IVECCS, San Antonio, TX, 1994, pp 246–248.
2. Boothe HW: Penis, prepuce and scrotum. In Slatter D (ed): Textbook of Small Animal Surgery. Philadelphia, W.B. Saunders, 1993, pp 1344–1345.
3. Feldman EC, Nelson RW: Canine and Feline Endocrinology and Reproduction. Philadelphia, W.B. Saunders, 1996, pp 692–693.
4. Hall MA, Swenberg LN: Genital emergencies. In Kirk RW (ed): Current Veterinary Therapy VI—Small Animal Practice. Philadelphia, W.B. Saunders, 1977, pp 1216–1217.
5. Held JP, Prater PE: Diseases of the external genitalia. In Morgan RV (ed): Handbook of Small Animal Practice. New York, Churchill Livingstone, 1992, pp 670–671.
6. Hobson HP: Surgical procedures of the penis. In Bojrab MJ (ed): Current Techniques in Small Animal Surgery. Philadelphia, Lea & Febiger, 1990, pp 428–430.
7. Holst PA: Canine Reproduction: A Breeder's Guide. Loveland, CO, Alpine Publications, 1985, pp 203–204.

92. ECLAMPSIA

Teresa Dye, D.V.M.

1. What is eclampsia?

Eclampsia is a hypocalcemic tetany associated with pregnancy in bitches or queens.

2. What other terms are used for eclampsia?

- Puerperal tetany
- Lactation tetany
- Periparturient hypocalcemia

3. Are certain animals predisposed to eclampsia?

Eclampsia is seen most commonly in small-breed dogs and is uncommon in cats and large-breed dogs. Bitches with a previous history of eclampsia may have recurrence with subsequent litters.

4. What are the common causes of the hypocalcemia associated with eclampsia?

Calcium is lost to fetuses during gestation and through milk during lactation. Improper perinatal nutrition may result in limited calcium intake. The stress of lactation may result in a decreased appetite and poor intake of calcium even when an adequate diet is provided. Excessive supplementation of calcium during gestation may lead to atrophy of the parathyroid gland and inhibit release of parathyroid hormone, thus interfering with mobilization of calcium stores and utilization of dietary calcium after parturition. Metabolic factors, such as alkalosis, that promote increased protein binding of calcium and therefore decreased levels of ionized calcium also may contribute to development of eclampsia.

5. What are the clinical signs of eclampsia?

Initial signs of eclampsia are restlessness, anxiety, irritability, and panting. These signs may progress within minutes to hours to early signs of tetany, including hypersalivation, stiffness of gait, and ataxia. Severe tetany is characterized by tonic-clonic muscle spasms, which may be provoked by auditory or tactile stimuli, recumbency, and seizures. Such signs are generally accompanied by tachycardia, miosis, and pyrexia. Death may result from severe respiratory depression, hyperthermia, and cerebral edema.

6. What is the pathophysiology of eclampsia?

Hypocalcemia alters cell membrane potentials, allowing spontaneous discharge of nerve fibers and induction of tonic contractions of the skeletal muscles. Both degree of hypocalcemia and rate of decline in calcium level determine the onset and degree of clinical signs.

7. When does eclampsia occur?

Eclampsia is typically seen within the first 2 weeks postpartum but also may occur in late pregnancy or during parturition when hypocalcemia may be a contributing factor to uterine inertia.

8. How is eclampsia diagnosed?

Diagnosis is typically based on history, clinical signs, and response to treatment. Pretreatment calcium level should be assessed, but treatment should not be delayed for laboratory confirmation. Serum calcium levels are usually less than 7 mg/dl. Serum glucose levels also should be evaluated for concurrent hypoglycemia.

9. What is the initial treatment for eclampsic patients?

Treatment consists of slow (over 15–30 minutes) intravenous infusion of 10% calcium gluconate to effect. A total dose of 1–20 ml may be required. Heart rate and electrocardiogram should be monitored during infusion. If bradycardia or arrhythmias develop, the infusion is discontinued until the heart rate and rhythm normalize and is then resumed at one-half of the initial infusion rate. Once the animal is stable, the initial required dose of calcium gluconate is diluted with an equal volume of saline and injected subcutaneously 3 times daily to prevent recurrence of clinical signs. Concurrent hypoglycemia, hyperthermia, and cerebral edema should be treated if present. Corticosteroids should be avoided because they lower serum calcium levels through promotion of calciuria, decreased intestinal absorption of calcium, and inhibition of osteoclasis.

10. What if the patient does not respond to calcium infusion?

If clinical signs do not resolve despite calcium infusion, diazepam or phenobarbital may be used to control seizures. Other causes for seizure activity should be considered, including concurrent hypoglycemia, cerebral edema, toxicosis, or primary neurologic disorder.

11. What instructions are given for the patient at the time of discharge from the hospital?

The patient should be placed on oral supplementation with calcium gluconate, calcium lactate, or calcium carbonate tablets. Various dosages have been recommended. Suggested doses are 10–30 mg/kg of calcium carbonate 3 times/day or 150–250 mg/kg of calcium gluconate 3 times/day. Over-the-counter antacid products may be used to provide calcium carbonate. A well-balanced growth formula diet should be fed.

Puppies older than 3 weeks should be weaned. If puppies are younger, they may be allowed to nurse but should be supplemented with hand-feeding to reduce lactational demands on the bitch. If a relapse occurs, puppies should be weaned, regardless of age, and hand-fed.

12. What steps can be taken to prevent development of eclampsia in pregnant bitches?

A balanced growth formula diet should be fed during the second half of gestation and through lactation. Calcium should *not* be supplemented during gestation but may be desirable during lactation in bitches with a previous history of eclampsia. Calcium carbonate may be used at a dosage of 10–30 mg/kg 3 times/day.

BIBLIOGRAPHY

1. Feldman EC, Nelson RW: Canine and Feline Endocrinology and Reproduction. Philadelphia, W.B. Saunders, 1987, pp 444–445.
2. Davidson AP: Postpartum disorders. In Morgan RV (ed): Handbook of Small Animal Practice, 2nd ed. New York, Churchill Livingstone, 1992, pp 670–699.

3. Jones DE, Joshua JO: Reproductive Clinical Problems in the Dog. Boston, Wright, 1982, pp 108–109.
4. Wallace MS, Davidson AP: Abnormalities in pregnancy, parturition, and the periparturient period. In Ettinger SJ, Feldman EC (eds): Textbook of Veterinary Internal Medicine, 4th ed. Philadelphia, W.B. Saunders, 1995, p 1620.

93. DYSTOCIA

Adam J. Reiss, D.V.M.

1. What is dystocia?
A dystotic animal is unable to expel fetuses from the uterus.

2. To recognize dystocia one must know the normal stages and signs of eutocia (normal parturition). What are the stages and signs of eutocia?
Stage 1. Stage 1 consists primarily of behavioral changes. The commonly seen signs are restlessness, nesting, panting, and shivering. Such signs may occur up to 48 hours before parturition but are not reliable indicators of parturition.

Stage 2. The second stage of labor consists of strong, externally visible contractions that result in expulsion of the fetus through the birth canal. This stage may last up to 24 hours in large canine litters and up to 36 hours in cats.

Stage 3. The passage of the placenta is the hallmark of the third stage of labor. Stages 2 and 3 may occur alternatively. Stage 3 may not be observed if the bitch or queen is allowed to ingest the placenta. This stage is completed with uterine involution.

3. What common signs may help pet owners and veterinarians to recognize a dystotic animal?
• Prolonged gestation (concern should be raised in dogs and cats after the 68th day of gestation, as determined by the last breeding date)
• No active stage 2 labor within 24 hours of temperature drop below 100°F
• Visible abdominal contractions for 30 minutes or more without passage of a fetus
• Visible fetal membranes for 15 minutes or longer
• Weak, nonproductive abdominal contractions for 4 hours after onset of stage 2 labor
• More than 3 hours between puppies without signs of labor
• Abnormal vulvar discharge (foul-smelling, purulent, green, without production of a puppy or kitten)
• Crying or biting of flanks or vulvar area, with repeated attempts to urinate
• Depressed or obtunded bitch or queen
• Failure to deliver all puppies in 24 hours or all kittens in 36 hours

4. What is the most reliable and available indicator of impending parturition?
The most reliable and available indicator of impending parturition is a drop in body temperature below 100°F (97–99°F). This drop usually occurs within 24 hours of parturition. Owners should monitor temperature twice daily for the last 7–10 days of the predicted date. Temperature drop in the queen is not as reliable an indicator as in the bitch.

5. What steps should be taken to diagnose a dystotic animal?
1. Obtain a complete history. Important question to ask:
   • When is the predicted date of parturition?
   • What was the last breeding date?

- Was vaginal cytology done?
- What was the first day of diestrus?
- What signs of labor have you seen?
- How long ago were they observed, and how long did they last?
- When was the last puppy delivered?
- Has the bitch or queen had dystocia previously? If so, how was she treated?
- Did you record a temperature drop?

2. Perform a complete physical exam. Address dehydration, shock, and toxemia quickly. Perform a sterile vaginal exam and relieve obstructions, if possible.

3. Take abdominal radiographs (two views). Abdominal radiographs may be helpful and do not harm the fetuses. Gestational length (fetal calcification at 45 days), number in litter, orientation, size of the fetus vs size of the birth canal, and fetal viability can be assessed. Radiographic evidence of fetal death includes gas in the uterus, overlapping of skull and spinal bones, fetal bone resorption, and abnormal positions.

6. How is fetal viability best determined?

Fetal viability is best determined by ultrasonographic identification of a heartbeat.

7. Once the animal has been diagnosed as dystotic, how is the type of dystocia classified?

Dystocia can be broadly divided into maternal (60–75%) and fetal causes (25–40%). Dystocia of maternal origin may be divided into anatomic, physiologic (primary uterine inertia), or combined (secondary uterine inertia) anatomic and physiologic etiologies.

Uterine inertia (failure of the uterine musculature to expel the fetus with an open birth canal) is the physiologic cause of dystocia. Primary uterine inertia also may be divided into two groups, complete and partial. Animals suffering from complete primary uterine inertia do not reach the second stage of labor. Animals experiencing partial primary uterine inertia reach the second stage of labor, but attempts to expel the fetus are weak and unsuccessful.

Anatomic causes imply obstruction of the birth canal. Birth canal obstructions may be due to narrowing of the pelvis (congenital or acquired), uterine malposition, mass lesions, vaginal stricture or bands, and vulvar hypoplasia and mucosal hyperplasia.

Secondary uterine inertia is a combination of anatomic and physiologic causes. Persistent uterine contractions against a closed or obstructed birth canal result in exhaustion of the uterine musculature and secondary inertia.

Fetal causes of dystocia include oversized fetus (single pup litters), developmental abnormalities (monsters, ascites, hydrocephalus, and hydropic conditions), faulty orientation, deficiency of fetal fluids, and fetal death.

8. Why is it important to know the underlying cause of dystocia?

It is essential to know the underlying cause to determine the best course of therapy. Ecbolic drugs, such as oxytocin, administered to animals with obstructive causes of dystocia may lead to uterine rupture and placental separation, resulting in fetal death.

9. What types of dystocia are most likely to respond to medical therapy? What is the best course of medical treatment?

All nonobstructive causes or obstructive dystocias that respond to manual manipulation or episiotomy can be addressed medically. It has been reported that 60–70% of medically managed dystocias require surgical intervention. Animals that are toxic should not receive medical management for dystocia but should be stabilized first.

Most authors recommend the use of oxytocin, 10% calcium gluconate, and dextrose in various combinations and dosages. No single combination is necessarily right or wrong. Oxytocin should be administered initially at a dose of 1.1–2.2 U/kg IM, with the dosage not to exceed 20 U. This dosage may be repeated at 30-minute intervals as long as it is working. Oxytocin also may be administered intravenously (10 U of oxytocin per liter of fluids). The initial fluid rate of oxytocin should be slow, $\frac{1}{8}$–$\frac{1}{4}$ maintenance. The rate of administration should be adjusted every 15–30 minutes until effective abdominal contractions are visualized.

If no response is seen after 2–3 repeated dosages of oxytocin, 10% calcium gluconate and/or dextrose should be administered intravenously. Ten percent calcium gluconate may be administered at a dosage of 1cc/3–5 kg of body weight. Calcium should be given slowly, and the animal's heart rate and rhythm should be monitored during administration. Dextrose also may be added to the treatment regimen. The recommended dosage of 50% dextrose is 0.5 ml/kg, which should be diluted minimally (1:1) with sterile saline before administration. If oxytocin is given intravenously, it may be added to a liter of 5% dextrose.

If productive abdominal contractions are not stimulated by the above protocols surgical intervention should be pursued.

10. Can oxytocin be overdosed?

Yes. If the IM dose of oxytocin is too large or if the rate of IV administration is too fast, tetanic uterine contractions result. Such contractions do not contribute to expulsion of the fetus and may lead to uterine tears and placental separation. Tetanic uterine contractions appear as extremely strong, intense contractions persisting for several minutes or longer. Oxytocin dosages must be decreased by at least 50% before normal contractions will return.

11. What other ecbolic drug is available? What are its advantages and disadvantages?

Ergonovine maleate is the other available ecbolic drug. The recommended dose is 0.125–0.5 mg/15 kg IM or PO. Advantages include longer duration of action, stronger uterine contractions, and less cervical contraction than oxytocin. The advantages also may be disadvantages; overdose is more likely as well as uterine rupture.

12. What are the indications for Cesarean section?

- Uterine inertia not responsive to medical management
- Pelvic or vaginal obstruction nonamenable to manipulation
- Fetal oversize
- Fetal death
- Planned surgery
- Malpresentations not amenable to correction
- Fetal monstrosities
- Deficiency or excess of fetal fluids

13. What preanesthetic protocols may be instituted to ensure maternal and fetal survival?

The goal should be to minimize the time from anesthetic induction to removal of the fetuses. The following suggestions may help:

- Prepare surgical site prior to induction.
- Preoxygenate to prevent maternal and fetal hypoxia. Because of the physical and physiologic changes of pregnancy, maternal lung volumes, diaphragmatic function, and oxygen-carrying capability may be decreased, whereas oxygen consumption is increased.
- Fluid therapy. Dehydration and shock should be corrected before anesthesia. Removal of the uterus from the peritoneal cavity during surgery results in a large increase in vascular space and potential secondary hypovolemia.
- Drug dosages. Pregnant animals are prone to overdosage because they have decreased requirements based on weight. Anesthetics should be administered in titrated doses until the desired effect is achieved. Most drugs cross the placenta to the fetus, which has immature organ systems; thus, drug excretion is prolonged.

14. The most controversial issue related to dystocia is the anesthetic protocol used during Cesarean section. Which anesthetic drugs are right, and which are wrong?

Many anesthetic protocols are available for pregnant animals; no single protocol is right or wrong. Each method has advantages and disadvantages. Factors in deciding which protocol to use include condition of the animal, expertise and familiarity of the practitioner, and availability of certain drugs. The three basic approaches are as follows:

1. Administration of a tranquilizer and subsequent local block
2. Use of epidural regional anesthesia with or without sedation
3. Use of general anesthesia

Although local and epidural blocks have minimal effects on the fetus, many animals require sedation or tranquilization to ensure their cooperation and to provide some degree of visceral anesthesia. All sedatives and tranquilizers cross the placental barrier, but narcotics depress the central nervous system and respiratory function of the fetuses. A combination of narcotic and tranquilizing agents to produce neuroleptanalgesia may be a useful supplement to regional techniques as well as appropriate premedication for general anesthesia.

15. What anesthetic combinations are commonly used?

- Acepromazine (0.05–0.1 mg/kg) with morphine (0.1–0.2 mg/kg) or oxymorphone (0.025–0.05 mg/kg) IV
- Butorphanol (0.45 mg/kg) with diazepam (0.45 mg/kg) IM

For both combinations reversal agents are available, such as naloxone for opioids and flumazenil for benzodiazepines. Because both combinations may result in severe hypotension, animals should receive intravenous fluids simultaneously. Other drugs, such as propofol and etomidate, are useful but should be used only by practitioners with experience in their administration.

Lidocaine used for local anesthesia in doses that exceed 5 mg/kg may result in systemic toxicity. Bupivacaine (1 ml/3.5 kg) and/or morphine (0.1 mg/kg) may be administered epidurally to provide regional anesthesia.

Halothane and isoflourane may be delivered with or without preanesthetics. Inhalant anesthetics are generally considered the safest for bitches or queens, and fetal exposure to sedatives, tranquilizers, and narcotics may be avoided. Although these anesthetic agents are fairly safe, standard protocols should be followed—i.e., premedication with anticholinergics and intravenous fluids.

16. What are the advantages and disadvantages of each of the above anesthetic protocols?

The advantage of a local block is its minimal effect on the fetus. The disadvantages are the need for concurrent tranquilization, possible systemic effects of the drug, and lack of visceral anesthesia. Epidural anesthesia does not affect the fetus and provides better visceral analgesia and immobilization of the hind end than local blocks. The disadvantages of epidural anesthesia include difficulty of technique, regional vasodilatation, and subsequent hypotension and need for tranquilization. The main advantages of general anesthesia include ease of administration, avoidance of fetal exposure to narcotics and tranquilizers, rapid recovery, and complete analgesia and immobilization. Disadvantages include depression of the fetus and dam, restraint during induction, and possible catecholamine release during the excitement stage.

17. What breed or type of pregnancy has increased susceptibility to dystocia?

Dystocia has been reported in almost all breeds of dog. The most common include miniature and small breeds and dogs with large heads and wide shoulders. The breeds at increased risk include chihuahuas, dachshunds, pekinese, Yorkshire terriers, miniature poodles, pomeranians, bulldogs, pugs, Boston terriers, and Scottish terriers. Persians have been reported to have an increased incidence of dystocia. In addition, primigravid, single pup litters have been reported to have a higher incidence of dystocia. Single fetal litters are suspected to contribute to dystocia by allowing increased fetal size and inadequate fetal hormonal stimulation to initiate parturition.

BIBLIOGRAPHY

1. Ekstrand C, Forsberg CL: Dystocia in the cat: A retrospective study of 155 cases. J Small Animal Pract 35:459–464, 1994.
2. Darvelid AW, Forsberg CL: Dystocia in the bitch: A retrospective study of 182 cases. J Small Animal Pract 35:402–407, 1994.

3. Davidson AP: Dystocia. In Morgan RV (ed): Handbook of Small Animal Practice. New York, Churchill Livingstone, 1992, pp 697–699, 709.
4. Feldman EC, Nelson RW: Canine and Feline Endocrinology and Reproduction. Philadelphia, W.B. Saunders, 1987, pp 432–438.
5. Gaudet DA, Kitchell BE: Canine dystocia. Compend Contin Educ 7:406–416, 1985.
6. Gaudet DA: Retrospective study of 128 cases of canine dystocia. J Am Animal Hosp Assoc 21:813–818, 1985.
7. Johnson CA: Disorders of pregnancy. Vet Clin North Am Small Animal Pract 16:477–494, 1986.
8. Jones DE, Joshua JO: Reproductive Clinical Problems in the Dog. London, Wright PSG, 1982, pp 61–101.
9. Macintire DK: Emergencies of the female reproductive tract. Vet Clin North Am Small Animal Pract 24:1173–1188, 1994.
10. Robbins MA, Mullen HS: En bloc ovarihysterectomy as a treatment for dystocia in dogs and cats. Vet Surg 23:48–52, 1994.
11. Root MV, et al: Vaginal septa in dogs: 15 cases (1983–1992). J Am Vet Med Assoc 206:56–58, 1995.
12. Sharpe DE, et al: Detrusor atony of the urinary bladder following prolonged dystocia in a dog. J Am Animal Hosp Assoc 29:299–302, 1993.
13. Wallace MS: Management of parturition and problems of the periparturient period of dogs and cats. Semin Vet Med Surg Small Animal 9:28–37, 1994.
14. Wykes PM, Olson PN: Normal and abnormal parturition. In Slatter D (ed): Textbook of Small Animal Surgery. Philadelphia, W.B. Saunders, 1993, pp 1316–1325.

94. ABORTION

Lori A. Wise, D.V.M., M.S.

1. How common are abortions in dogs and cats?

The true incidence of abortion is unknown because early fetal resorption may occur in animals not known to be pregnant. In addition, cats and dogs may consume aborted fetuses before they are noticed by the owner.

2. What are the common causes of abortion?

Causes can be divided into three main categories:

1. Fetal problems: abnormalities of development or chromosomal defects.

2. Maternal problems: systemic diseases such as uterine disease (infection, neoplasia, cystic endometrial hyperplasia), hypoluteoidism, or failure to maintain progesterone levels above 2.0 ng/ml, hypothyroidism in bitches, nutritional deficiencies, or exposure to certain drugs or compounds.

3. Infectious agents: *Brucella canis, Escherichia coli*, streptococci, canine herpesvirus, canine parvovirus, canine distemper virus, *Mycoplasma* sp., *Ureaplasma* sp., *Campylobacter* sp., *Toxoplasma gondii, Neospora caninum* in bitches; panleukopenia, feline leukemia virus infection, rhinotracheitis, toxoplasmosis, and various bacteria in queens.

3. What medications may cause abortion in dogs or cats?

Corticosteroids have been incriminated in bitches as well as doxorubicin, methotrexate, xylazine, and misoprostol. In general, try to avoid giving any medications or vaccinations during pregnancy.

4. What signs may indicate impending abortion?

The animal may vomit; become anorectic, listless, or febrile; show abdominal pain; or have abdominal contractions. A vaginal discharge that is purulent, bloody, black, dark green, or fetid is abnormal and may signify abortion. A portion of a litter may be aborted, with viable fetuses remaining.

5. Should anything be done to manage an animal that may be aborting?

The animal should be evaluated, and a thorough reproductive history should be taken. Include breeding dates, results of previous pregnancies, vaccination history, results of *Brucella* sp. testing, and information about diet, husbandry, and medications. Complete laboratory evaluation should include a complete blood count, biochemical profile, urinalysis, thyroid hormone level, and serologic tests for *Brucella canis*, *Toxoplasma gondii*, and canine herpesvirus. Plasma may be collected for a progesterone level. The progesterone level will drop once abortion has occurred but should not be low at the time of abortion. Exercise should be limited, and antibiotic treatment should be given if infection is suspected.

6. What if the animal presents after abortion has occurred?

Using physical examination (palpation), radiography, and possibly ultrasound, the animal should be evaluated for pyometra, retained fetuses, and retained placenta. If uterine infection is suspected, antibiotic therapy plus prostaglandin treatment may be necessary. An ovariohysterectomy should be considered if there are no future breeding plans. In bitches, a *Brucella* titer should be obtained. If possible, the owner should collect aborted fetuses and placentas and keep them refrigerated until they can be examined.

7. What specific tests help to diagnose the cause of abortion?

Fetal lung and liver should be cultured for *Brucella* sp. and herpesvirus. Fetal stomach contents should be cultured for other bacterial species. *Campylobacter* sp. requires specific culture techniques. Fetal and placental tissues should be submitted for histopathologic examination. Collect vaginal samples from bitches for cytologic examination and culture. In addition to routine bacterial culture, samples should be placed in Aimes media for *Mycoplasma* sp. and *Ureaplasma* sp. culture. Results of vaginal cultures should be interpreted with caution because various organisms may be isolated from healthy animals. Serum should be collected from bitches to test for *Brucella canis*, canine herpesvirus, and *Toxoplasma gondii*.

8. If abortion is recurrent, what should be done?

First, document the pregnancy with ultrasound (as early as 16 days) or radiography (at 42–45 days). Collect a *Brucella* titer of the bitch, dog, and previous mates. Perform a physical examination, vaginal examination, vaginal culture, and cytology. Perform titers for various infectious diseases. A progesterone assay should be done during pregnancy. Finally, uterine biopsy and culture may be indicated.

9. Hypoluteoidism is a common cause of early abortion in humans. Is this condition common in dogs and cats?

Hypoluteoidism, or inadequate secretion of progesterone for maintenance of pregnancy, has not been confirmed in dogs and cats. The diagnosis is made by confirming pregnancy in conjunction with an abnormally low (< 1.0 ng/ml) level of circulating progesterone.

BIBLIOGRAPHY

1. Feldman EC, Nelson RW: Canine and Feline Endocrinology and Reproduction. Philadelphia, W.B. Saunders, 1996, pp 574–578, 757–759.
2. Floss JL, Hardin DK: Diagnosing, treating, and preventing canine abortion. Vet Med 91:846–849, 1996.
3. Purswell BJ: Differential diagnosis of canine abortion. In Kirk RW, Bonagura JD (eds): Current Veterinary Therapy XI. Philadelphia, W.B. Saunders, 1992, p 925.
4. Zone M, et al: Termination of pregnancy in dogs by oral administration of dexamethasone. Therio 43:487, 1995.

XII. Urologic Emergencies

Section Editor: India F. Lane, D.V.M., M.S.

95. ACUTE BACTERIAL PROSTATITIS AND PROSTATIC ABSCESS

Cary L. Matwichuk, D.V.M., M.V.Sc., and India F. Lane, D.V.M., M.S.

1. What organisms are commonly implicated in prostatic infections in dogs?

Organisms commonly implicated in prostatic infections in dogs are the common pathogens of the urinary tract. *Escherichia coli* is the most frequently isolated organism. Other commonly identified organisms include staphylococci, streptococci, and *Proteus, Klebsiella,* and *Pseudomonas* spp. Anaerobic infections are uncommon but may occur with prostatic abscesses.

2. What historical and clinical findings are suggestive of acute bacterial prostatic infection?

Historical and clinical signs reflect systemic illness; examples include lethargy, anorexia, and vomiting. Affected dogs may walk with a stiff rear limb gait. Physical findings include fever; caudal abdominal pain, which may be localized to the prostate gland on digital rectal examination; and hemorrhagic or purulent urethral discharge. Some dogs with severe depression do not react dramatically to palpation, however. Vague abdominal pain or "splinting" of the abdomen may be detected instead. Bacterial prostatitis should be considered a primary differential diagnosis in intact male dogs presented for vomiting, lethargy, back pain, or fever.

3. How do signs of prostatic abscess differ from signs of acute bacterial prostatitis?

Clinical findings in dogs with prostatic abscess include those associated with acute bacterial prostatitis as well as signs of generalized peritonitis and septic shock. The prostate gland may be enlarged and asymmetric. Dogs may exhibit stranguria or tenesmus due to pressure placed on the urethra or colon by the enlarged prostate gland. With prostatic abscess caused by *E. coli*, polyuria and polydipsia may be included in the preliminary complaints. Just as in female dogs with pyometra, *E. coli* endotoxin may interfere with responsiveness to antidiuretic hormone and urine concentrating ability.

4. Formulate a plan to confirm the diagnosis of acute bacterial prostatic disease.

A presumptive diagnosis of acute bacterial prostatitis is usually made on the basis of history, physical examination, complete blood count, urinalysis, and urine culture. Dogs presenting with historical signs suggestive of acute bacterial prostatic disease should have a complete physical examination, including digital rectal examination. Leukocytosis, with or without a left shift, may be observed in a complete blood count. Hematuria, pyuria, and bacteriuria may be observed in urine sediment examination. A urine sample, preferably collected by cystocentesis, should be submitted for culture and sensitivity testing. In the case of suspected prostatic abscess, abdominal radiographs and ultrasound are indicated. An enlarged asymmetrical prostate gland may be visible on radiographs; hypoechoic or anechoic areas within the prostate may be observed sonographically.

5. Should prostatic fluid samples be obtained from dogs with suspected acute bacterial prostatitis?

All intact male dogs with a urinary tract infection should be considered to have prostatic involvement. Analysis of prostatic fluid probably provides no additional information in a dog with an inflammatory urine sediment, positive urine culture, and clinical and physical signs compatible with acute bacterial prostatitis. Dogs are usually in too much pain to produce an ejaculate. Urethral brushings or prostatic massage should not be performed because of the possibility of producing bacteremia.

6. Should prostatic cysts or abscesses be aspirated for cytologic evaluation and culture?

Ultrasound may be used to guide collection of fluid by fine-needle aspiration. Complications include seeding of bacteria along the needle tract and peritonitis. Fine-needle aspiration is probably contraindicated in dogs with fever or leukocytosis. With guided technique and a 22-gauge needle, the benefit of obtaining cyst fluid for cytologic evaluation, culture, and confirmation of diagnosis may outweigh the risk associated with aspiration. Fine-needle aspirates can be obtained sequentially to assess therapy. If an abscess is inadvertently aspirated, antibiotic therapy should be instituted.

7. What considerations are important in selecting an antimicrobial agent for acute bacterial prostatitis? For long-term antimicrobial therapy?

Identification of the causative organism, its antimicrobial sensitivity pattern, the ability of the antimicrobial to reach effective concentration within the prostate gland, and the animal's clinical condition should be considered in choosing an antimicrobial treatment for acute bacterial prostatitis. The choice should be based on the results of urine culture and sensitivity testing. While awaiting culture results, the clinician should initiate therapy with a broad-spectrum antibiotic with good activity against gram-negative bacteria. Gram stain results may be helpful for guiding initial therapy. During acute inflammation the blood–prostate barrier is not intact, and most antimicrobials penetrate the prostate gland. In a severely ill dog, antibiotics should be administered intravenously.

For chronic therapy, it is essential to choose an antibiotic that crosses the blood–prostate barrier. A highly lipid-soluble antibiotic that is weakly basic with a high pK_a is desired. Recommended antimicrobials for treatment of gram-negative infections include trimethoprim-sulfadiazine, enrofloxacin, and chloramphenicol. Trimethoprim-sulfadiazine, chloramphenicol, erythromycin, and clindamycin are good choices for gram-positive infections. Commonly used antibiotics such as penicillins, cephalosporins, and aminoglycosides penetrate the prostate poorly and are not recommended.

8. Formulate a treatment plan for acute bacterial prostatitis.

Supportive care, including intravenous fluids, should be initiated in ill patients. Choice of initial antibiotic before culture and sensitivity results are available should be based on Gram stain results. If the dog is very ill, parenteral antibiotic therapy is indicated initially. Antimicrobial choices for the acute phase of disease include trimethoprim-sulfadiazine, ampicillin, cephalosporins, chloramphenicol, and enrofloxacin. The dog then may be switched to oral therapy with an antimicrobial chosen on the basis of culture and sensitivity results and predicted prostatic penetrance. Antibiotic therapy should be continued for 21–28 days.

9. After resolution of the acute episode, how should the patient with acute bacterial prostatitis be monitored?

A follow-up evaluation should be performed 5–7 days after completion of antimicrobial therapy. The evaluation should include a complete physical examination, urinalysis and urine culture, and cytologic evaluation and culture of prostatic fluid. Urethral brushings or fine-needle aspirates of intraprostatic cysts are useful methods for obtaining prostatic samples. An assumption that the infection has been eliminated should not be based solely on resolution of clinical signs. Castration may be considered after resolution of acute disease to facilitate clearance of bacteria and to prevent recurrence of prostatic disease.

10. What surgical options are available for management of prostatic abscesses?
Surgical drainage of prostatic abscesses may be accomplished by needle aspiration, placement of drains over the prostate gland, marsupialization of the abscess, or subtotal prostatectomy. Complications of needle aspiration include septic shock and absorption of bacterial toxins. Complete drainage and resolution of the abscess are difficult with this method alone, although clinical signs can be minimized with intermittent drainage and antimicrobial treatment. Complications of prostatic drains include fistula formation, ascending infection, and recurrence of the abscess. Marsupialization creates a draining stoma to the exterior. If the stoma closes too early, the abscess may recur. On the other hand, a chronic draining tract may develop. More extensive prostatic surgery is associated with a high incidence of postoperative urinary incontinence. Complete excisional prostatectomy is not recommended because of high morbidity, but subtotal prostatectomy may be required in severely abscessed glands. Because of the numerous potential complications of medical or surgical treatment, prostatic abscess carries a guarded prognosis.

BIBLIOGRAPHY

1. Dorfman M, Barsanti J: Diseases of the canine prostate gland. Comp Cont Educ Pract Vet 18:791–806, 1995.
2. Dorfman M, Barsanti J: CVT update: Treatment of canine bacterial prostatitis. In Bonagura JD (ed): Kirk's Current Veterinary Therapy XII. Philadelphia, W.B. Saunders, 1995, pp 1103–1108.
3. Hardie EM, Barsanti JA, Rawlings CA: Complications of prostatic surgery. J Am Animal Hosp Assoc 20:50–56, 1984.
4. Klausner JS, Johnston SD, Bell FW: Canine prostatic disorders. In Bonagura JD (ed): Kirk's Current Veterinary Therapy XII. Philadelphia, W.B. Saunders, 1995, pp 1029–1032.
5. Kraweic DR, Heflin D: Study of prostatic disease in dogs: 177 cases (1981–1986). J Am Vet Med Assoc 200:1119–1122, 1992.

96. URINARY TRACT INFECTION AND ACUTE PYELONEPHRITIS

Cary L. Matwichuk, D.V.M., M.V.Sc., and India F. Lane, D.V.M., M.S.

1. What are the differential diagnoses for acute pollakiuria, hematuria, and dysuria?
The clinical signs of pollakiuria (frequent urination), hematuria (blood in the urine), and dysuria (difficult urination) indicate lower urinary tract inflammation but are not specific for a particular disorder. Differential diagnoses for an animal exhibiting lower urinary tract signs include bacterial urinary infection, urolithiasis, neoplasia, trauma, feline lower urinary tract disease, and prostatic disorders.

2. What clinical signs suggest involvement of the upper urinary tract (kidneys, renal pelves, ureters)?
Determining the extent of infection along the urinary tract is important because more aggressive treatment is indicated with involvement of the upper urinary tract. Localization of infection may be difficult. However, animals with disorders confined to the lower urinary tract do not exhibit systemic signs of illness. Fever, lethargy, anorexia, vomiting, polyuria and polydipsia, and lumbar pain are suggestive of upper urinary tract infection, neoplasia, or injury. If pyelonephritis

is secondary to ascending infection from the lower urinary tract, concurrent lower urinary tract signs may be observed.

3. How can the origin of hematuria be localized?

Hemorrhage from the kidney, ureters, urinary bladder, urethra, or external genitalia leads to microscopic or macroscopic hematuria. Clinical signs, physical examination (including digital rectal and vaginal examination), timing of hematuria during urination, comparison of a voided urine sample with a sample collected by cystocentesis, and identification of urinary tract pathology on radiographs or ultrasound help to localize the source of the hematuria.

Blood observed at the beginning of urination suggests bleeding from the bladder neck, urethra, or genital tract (uterus, vagina, prostate, prepuce). Blood observed throughout urination is most consistent with diffuse bladder disease or upper urinary tract hemorrhage (kidneys, ureters); hemorrhage due to coagulopathy also may lead to this pattern of hematuria. With focal (especially ventral or cranioventral) lesions of the urinary bladder or large dependent cystouroliths, blood may enter urine primarily at the end of voiding. Bleeding or discharge from the genital tract may occur independently of urination and may be detected only in voided samples. Hematuria in the absence of other lower urinary tract symptoms (pollakiuria, dysuria, stranguria) may indicate upper urinary tract disease, genital hemorrhage, or coagulopathy.

4. List differential diagnoses for acute changes in urinary volume (polyuria or oliguria).

Urine concentration and volume vary in response to water and solute intake in normal animals. Changes in urine output may simply represent homeostatic mechanisms of body water balance; however, dramatic changes in urine output may signify pathologic states. Acute polyuria may be associated with increased sodium or water intake, hypoadrenocorticism, pyometra, nonoliguric acute renal failure, pyelonephritis, urinary tract or prostate infection with *Escherichia coli,* or diabetes mellitus. Most of these disorders can be differentiated by physical evaluation and minimal database. An abrupt decline in urine output may indicate physiologic urine concentration (dehydration), acute oliguric renal failure, urine retention, or urinary tract rupture or obstruction.

5. When is cystocentesis contraindicated for the diagnosis of urinary tract infection (UTI)?

Cystocentesis is the preferred method for urine collection. Urine collected by free flow or catheter may be contaminated by cells or normal bacterial flora residing in the distal urethra and genital tract, whereas urine obtained by cystocentesis should be sterile. Performed correctly, cystocentesis is a safe procedure. Contraindications to cystocentesis include thrombocytopenia or other coagulopathies, suspected or confirmed pyometra, major abdominal trauma, or severe skin infection at the needle entry site. A relative contraindication is a distended urinary bladder secondary to urethral obstruction because of the possibility of a compromised bladder wall.

6. What urinalysis findings are suggestive of acute UTI?

Urinalysis findings suggestive of UTI include hematuria, pyuria, and bacteriuria. Hematuria and proteinuria may be noted on urine dipstick examination. Urine dipstick leukocyte assays are generally unreliable and should not replace urine sediment examination for detection of inflammatory cells. Urine pH may be increased with infection by urease-producing bacteria (staphylococci, *Proteus* sp.). However, alkaline urine in the absence of compatible clinical signs or urine sediment findings does not necessarily suggest a diagnosis of UTI.

7. What is the significance of crystals in patients with acute pollakiuria, polyuria, hematuria, or dysuria?

Crystals are formed when urine is oversaturated with mineral and other substrates. In normal dogs and cats, crystals often are insignificant findings and are readily shed in urine without causing clinical signs. Magnesium ammonium phosphate (struvite) crystals may be a component of idiopathic lower urinary tract disease or urolithiasis in cats. Other crystals are more suggestive of metabolic (cystine, urate) or pathologic (calcium oxalate monohydrate) disorders. Identification of crystals in urine, however, may aid in the detection, classification, and management of urolithiasis in dogs and cats.

8. What is the significance of casts in patients with acute polyuria or oliguria?

Casts are cylindrical structures formed in the tubular lumen and shed into urine. They are molds of cells and Tamm-Horsfall protein, which is secreted by tubular epithelial cells in the loops of Henle, distal tubules, and collecting ducts. Casts may contain epithelial cells, bacteria, inflammatory cells, bilirubin, or fat globules. A few hyaline or granular casts may be observed in the urine of normal animals. In significant numbers, casts indicate an active pathologic process with renal tubular involvement, usually acute tubular injury. Cellular casts indicate hemorrhage or inflammation within renal tubules. Casts are shed into urine intermittently; the absence of casts does not rule out acute renal injury.

9. Why should urine cultures be completed in patients with suspected UTI?

The findings of hematuria and pyuria indicate only urinary tract inflammation, for which there are many differential diagnoses. Urine culture should be completed to distinguish between infectious and noninfectious causes of inflammation. With a negative urine culture, investigation for other causes of lower urinary tract disease may be initiated earlier in the course of evaluation. In many patients with UTI, overt bacteriuria may not be observed in the urine sediment, and culture is used to confirm infection. Bacterial culture and sensitivity testing are the only methods to identify antibiotic sensitivity patterns of individual organisms and to ensure that appropriate antimicrobial therapy is instituted.

Urine culture in especially important in animals with recurrent UTIs to distinguish between relapse (infection with the same organism) and reinfection (infection with a different organism or different susceptibility pattern). This distinction is important because patient evaluation and follow-up differ. In patients with relapse, a persistent nidus of infection is likely or antimicrobial treatment was ineffective, whereas reinfection is more likely due to an abnormality of the urinary tract predisposing to infection.

10. How are urine samples best handled for urinalysis? For urine culture?

To ensure reliable results, urinalysis should be performed immediately after collection. Allowing urine to sit at room temperature may result in lysis of red and white blood cells and changes in crystal composition. Urine may be refrigerated but should be analyzed within 12 hours. Urine culture is best initiated within 30 minutes after collection, because at room temperature bacterial counts may double rapidly. If culture cannot be done immediately, urine may be refrigerated for up to 6 hours. Urinalysis and urine culture should be performed before administration of antimicrobials or radiographic contrast agents.

11. How can in-house urine cultures be initiated?

If a laboratory is not readily available, urine cultures can be performed easily in the practice setting. Calibrated loops or mechanical pipettes may be used to apply a known quantity of urine to blood agar and MacConkey plates and incubated at 37° C for 18–30 hours. Plates demonstrating significant bacterial growth may be sent to a commercial laboratory for identification of the organism and antimicrobial sensitivity testing.

12. What clinicopathologic findings support a diagnosis of upper UTI?

Bacteria are inconsistently observed in urine of patients with upper UTI. Additional urinalysis findings that suggest upper UTI include isosthenuric or suboptimally concentrated urine (urine specific gravity of 1.008–1.029 in dogs, 1.008–1.034 in cats), inflammatory urine sediment (pyuria and hematuria), and casts (especially white blood cell casts). An inflammatory leukogram may be detected in acute pyelonephritis, and azotemia may be evident with severe bilateral pyelonephritis. The absence of these findings does not preclude a diagnosis of pyelonephritis, however; chronic pyelonephritis may be associated with minimal hematologic and biochemical abnormalities.

13. How can a tentative diagnosis of upper UTI be confirmed?

Supportive evidence for pyelonephritis may be obtained by imaging the kidneys with intravenous urography or ultrasound. Findings consistent with pyelonephritis include dilation, blunting or asymmetry of the renal pelves, and dilation of the ureters. A definitive diagnosis of pyelonephritis requires isolation of bacteria from the kidneys via pyelocentesis or renal biopsy. Because these diagnostic tests are moderately invasive, a tentative diagnosis of upper UTI is usually based on identifying urinary tract infection in the presence of clinical, laboratory, and radiographic signs consistent with upper urinary tract involvement.

14. What are reasonable first-line antimicrobial agents for suspected lower UTI?

Antimicrobial selection is best based on results of antimicrobial sensitivity testing. Ideally, minimal inhibitory concentrations (MICs) are determined; an antimicrobial that reaches urine concentrations of at least 4 times the MIC is likely to be effective in vivo. Before culture and sensitivity results are available, initial therapy may be based on Gram stain of urine and knowledge of best choices for the urinary tract. In general, ampicillin or amoxicillin is a good choice for gram-positive infection, and trimethoprim-sulfonamide combination is usually effective for gram-negative infections. Cephalosporins are appropriate choices for treatment of *Klebsiella* sp.; tetracyclines or fluoroquinolones are effective against *Pseudomonas* sp.

15. What are reasonable first-line antimicrobial agents for suspected upper UTI?

An antimicrobial that concentrates well in serum and renal tissue is desired for treatment of upper UTIs. Good initial choices include trimethoprim-sulfonamide or chloramphenicol. Aminoglycosides also may be used, although in renal patients they should be used only with extreme caution and appropriate monitoring. With the advent of fluoroquinolones, aminoglycosides are now rarely indicated for upper UTIs.

16. What supportive treatment is indicated in patients with suspected upper UTI?

Patients with acute pyelonephritis may be severely ill. Appropriate supportive care includes intravenous fluid therapy, parenteral antibiotic therapy, pain management, and nutritional support if needed. Fluids should be administered to replace volume deficits quickly (over 6–8 hours) and to maintain moderate diuresis. With effective antimicrobial treatment, most patients improve clinically and can support hydration requirements orally within a few days.

17. When should surgical therapy be considered in patients with pyelonephritis?

If long-term therapy with an appropriate antimicrobial fails to eliminate renal infection or if a nidus of continued infection remains (e.g., nephroliths), surgical intervention may be necessary. Nephroliths may be removed by nephrotomy. Nephrectomy is indicated if the infection appears to be unilateral, if the kidney becomes abscessed, and if the remaining kidney is able to maintain adequate function. Nuclear scintigraphy may be used to measure glomerular filtration rate in individual kidneys and is therefore a useful tool for documenting function in the remaining kidney.

18. What follow-up recommendations should be made for small animals with simple lower UTI?

A simple or uncomplicated UTI is defined as a single or rare infection in an animal in which no underlying cause can be identified. Such animals usually respond quickly to an appropriate course of antimicrobial therapy. Appropriate therapy includes treatment for 10–14 days with an antimicrobial to which the identified organism is susceptible. Ideally urinalysis or urine culture is performed 3–5 days after completion of therapy to ensure that the infection has been eliminated.

19. What conditions suggest that an animal with UTI should be followed more aggressively?

An animal in which an underlying condition predisposing to UTI has been identified requires more careful follow-up to ensure successful eradication of the infection. Every effort should be made to identify and remove reversible complicating factors. Factors that compromise host defenses include conformational or anatomic abnormalities, urine retention or voiding dysfunction, changes in urine composition, urolithiasis or neoplasia, and immunocompromising diseases or treatments. Animals with an identifiable compromise in host defenses are said to have a complicated infection and should be treated with an appropriate antimicrobial for no less than 4 weeks. A negative urine culture 3–5 days after initiation of therapy indicates that the chosen antibiotic is efficacious. A urine culture should be performed 3–5 days before discontinuing therapy and 5–7 days after completion of therapy to ensure that the infection has been eliminated. Urinalysis with or without urine culture is indicated 30 and 60 days after completion of antimicrobial therapy. Upper UTIs, UTIs in intact male dogs, and UTIs in cats should be considered complicated and treated as such.

20. What emergency patients may be at increased risk for development of UTI?

Any factor that impairs normal host defenses predisposes an animal to development of nosocomial (hospital-acquired) infections. Common predisposing factors include prolonged hospitalization, immunosuppression, indwelling urinary catheter placement, intravenous catheters, chronic debilitating disease, previous antibiotic therapy, and burns or skin wounds. In veterinary medicine, urethral catheterization (obstructed cats, urethral surgery), dysfunctional voiding (neurogenic disorder, bladder atony), and immunosuppression (diabetes mellitus, glucocorticoid or chemotherapy administration) are the most common scenarios in which nosocomial infections occur.

21. How can nosocomial infections be prevented?

Because nosocomial infections are often caused by bacteria exhibiting multidrug resistance, every effort should be made to prevent their development. Guidelines for minimizing the risk of nosocomial infections include awareness of factors predisposing to infection, minimizing the duration of hospitalization, placement of indwelling urinary catheters only when necessary, strict attention to cleanliness when handling intravenous or urinary catheters, frequent hand washing, disinfection of equipment, maintaining environmental cleanliness, and judicious use of antimicrobials.

22. How common are catheter-induced UTIs?

Catheterization of the urinary tract predisposes animals to UTIs both by providing a direct route of entry for bacteria into the bladder and by allowing bacteria to bypass many normal host defense mechanisms. Catheter-induced infections are common, with the reported incidence ranging from 20–75% in small animals. The risk of infection increases with duration of catheterization, open indwelling catheters, concurrent administration of glucocorticoids, and immunocompromising disease. Because of the potential for UTI, careful consideration should be given to the necessity of urinary catheterization; catheterization should be avoided in patients particularly susceptible to infection. Intermittent urinary catheterization is preferred over indwelling catheters whenever possible; however, the risks of repeated catheterization (trauma, introduction of infection) must be weighed against the potential benefit in individual patients.

23. When should antimicrobial treatment be given to catheterized patients?

Antimicrobial therapy is initiated in patients with an indwelling urinary catheter only after the catheter has been removed and infection has been documented. Prophylactic antimicrobial treatment while the catheter remains in place does not prevent infection and increases the likelihood of development of resistant infection. To minimize the possibility of catheter-induced UTI, indwelling urinary catheters should be kept in place for as short a duration as possible. Urine culture or culture of the catheter tip should be performed at the time of catheter removal to identify the current causative organisms and antimicrobial sensitivity pattern.

Antimicrobial therapy is indicated while an indwelling catheter is in place in the presence of clinical signs of systemic illness suggestive of upper UTI. If antibiotic therapy is instituted in a patient with an indwelling catheter, urine culture and sensitivity testing should be performed when the catheter is removed to identify resistant infections that may have developed during therapy.

BIBLIOGRAPHY

1. Barsanti JA: Urinary tract infections. In Greene CE (ed): Infectious Diseases of the Dog and Cat. Philadelphia, W.B. Saunders, 1990, pp 158–170.
2. Barsanti JA: Effect of therapy on susceptibility to urinary tract infection in male cats with indwelling urethral catheters. J Vet Intern med 6:64–70, 1992.
3. Jones RL: Control of nosocomial infections. In Kirk RW (ed): Current Veterinary Therapy IX. Philadelphia, W.B. Saunders, 1986, pp 19–24.
4. Lees GE: Diagnosis and localization of urinary tract infection. In Kirk RW (ed): Current Veterinary Therapy IX. Philadelphia, W.B. Saunders, 1986, pp 1118–1123.
5. Lees GE: Bacterial urinary tract infections. Vet Clin North Am (Small Animal Pract) 26:297–304, 1996.
6. Lees GE: Use and misuse of indwelling urethral catheters. Vet Clin North Am (Small Animal Pract) 26:499–505, 1996.
7. Osborne CA: Three steps to effective management of bacterial urinary tract infections: Diagnosis, diagnosis, and diagnosis. Comp Cont Educ Pract Vet 17:1233–1248, 1995.
8. Polzin DJ: Management of recurrent bacterial urinary tract infections. Comp Cont Educ Pract Vet 16:1565, 1994.
9. Senior DF: The use of enrofloxacin in the management of urinary tract infections in dogs and cats. Suppl Comp Cont Educ Pract Vet 18:89–95, 1996.

97. ACUTE RENAL FAILURE

India F. Lane, D.V.M., M.S.

1. What pathophysiologic events lead to the abrupt decline in glomerular infiltration rate characteristic of acute renal failure (ARF)?

Glomerular filtration rate (GFR) and nephron function are maintained by the balance of afferent and efferent blood flow, glomerular capillary pressure, and intratubular pressure. Disruption of vascular flow, glomerular capillary function, or intratubular dynamics causes reductions in GFR.

2. What are the major mechanisms that initiate or perpetuate ARF?

• Failure of afferent arteriolar blood flow, usually afferent arteriolar vasoconstriction
• Reduced functional glomerular capillary surface area
• Efferent arteriolar vasodilation leading to a drop in glomerular capillary pressure
• Tubular epithelial damage leading to backleak of filtrate into peritubular capillaries
• Tubular obstruction with cellular debris, cellular edema, casts, or crystals

3. What are the most common causes of ARF in small animals?

The most common causes of ARF are nephrotoxic and ischemic injury. Nephrotoxicity, especially ethylene glycol intoxication, is much more common than ischemic injury in small animals. Hospital-acquired ARF also may be due to nephrotoxic therapeutic agents or iatrogenic ischemic injury. Toxicant-induced ARF may be precipitated by amphotericin B, aminoglycosides, chemotherapeutic agents, or nonsteroidal antiinflammatory agents. Ischemic injury is associated with hypovolemia and hypotension, which lead to diminished renal blood flow. Trauma, cardiopulmonary failure, and hyperthermia may lead to ischemic renal injury. Iatrogenic causes include hypotension associated with surgery or anesthesia and vasodilatory therapy (especially angiotensin-converting enzyme inhibitors).

A third category of patients with ARF includes dogs and cats with acute-on-chronic renal failure, in which an acute exacerbation of azotemia develops in an animal with established renal insufficiency or failure. Acute renal dysfunction also may result from renal neoplasia, hypercalcemia, acute pyelonephritis, or leptospirosis.

4. What patients are at highest risk for acquired ARF?

Patients with preexisting renal disease, major trauma, or major systemic disease such as pancreatitis, diabetes mellitus, cardiovascular disease, and hepatic disease are at increased risk for development of acquired ARF. In addition, clinical conditions such as volume depletion, electrolyte disturbances, hypotension or hypertension, fever, and sepsis are contributing risk factors. For patients at risk, administration of nephrotoxic drugs, anesthesia, surgery, or administration of radiographic contrast media may precipitate ARF.

5. How can at-risk patients be protected from development of ARF?

Volume deficits, electrolyte disturbances, and major medical problems should be addressed before the use of anesthetics, radiographic contrast media, or potentially nephrotoxic agents. During required procedures, anesthesia, or surgery, systemic blood pressure should be monitored and maintained above 60 mmHg by fluid support or pharmacologic means. Potentially nephrotoxic agents should be discontinued, avoided, or used only with appropriate therapeutic drug monitoring. Pretreatment with saline diuresis or mannitol infusion may be protective.

High-risk patients should be monitored for early deterioration of renal function by frequent monitoring of hydration status, body weight, blood urea nitrogen, serum creatinine, and serum electrolyte concentrations. Urine output should be estimated or measured, and urine should be monitored for blood, casts, protein, or cellular debris. Urinary enzymes may be useful parameters for monitoring aminoglycoside and chemotherapeutic treatments.

6. Describe the historical and physical clues that suggest ARF.

ARF is defined as an abrupt decline in GFR, leading to rapid development of azotemia and clinical signs of uremia. Anorexia, depression, vomiting, diarrhea, and sudden changes in urine output (either polyuria or oliguria) may be clinical indicators of ARF. Patients with acute nephrotoxic injury without preceding illness are usually in good condition and active, with minimal preliminary signs. Ethylene glycol intoxication is characterized by an early stage of ataxia, vomiting, and polyuria and polydipsia, followed first by a transient period of apparent recovery, then by established renal failure. At this stage, minimal outward signs of intoxication or ARF may be observed.

On physical examination, uremic breath odor may be detected. Oral ulcerations develop in some cases and may lead to severe stomatitis or tongue-tip necrosis. Pallor, weakness, and dehydration are common findings. Subnormal body temperature often is detected. Kidneys may become enlarged or painful if intracapsular swelling occurs.

7. Describe the clinicopathologic abnormalities that suggest a diagnosis of ARF.

Rapid development of azotemia is the hallmark of ARF. Increases in urea and creatinine are usually parallel. Hyperphosphatemia and metabolic acidosis accompany azotemia. Hyperkalemia is most common in oliguric patients, patients with postrenal azotemia, and patients with severe metabolic acidosis. Anemia develops relatively rapidly over the course of established ARF but is usually not evident at diagnosis. Urine specific gravity often is isosthenuric but varies and may be normal with acute glomerular injury. Proteinuria, glucosuria, and urinary casts or cellular debris may be observed in urinalysis samples.

8. With acute azotemia, how is renal azotemia distinguished from prerenal causes?

In prerenal azotemia associated with volume depletion or hypotension, urine concentrating ability should reflect body water conservation, with urine specific gravity measurements > 1.030 (dogs) or > 1.035 (cats). Many nonrenal disorders influence urine concentrating ability, however, and distinction of prerenal azotemia may be complicated in the face of hypoadrenocorticism, hyperadrenocorticism, diabetes mellitus, or diuretic or steroid therapy. Other findings suggestive of prerenal azotemia include urinary sodium concentration < 20 mEq/L, fractional excretion of sodium < 1.0%, urine osmolality:plasma osmolality ration > 5, and urine creatinine:plasma creatinine ratio > 20. Without the availability of these quantitative measurements, response to fluid therapy may be used to distinguish the prerenal component of azotemia. Prerenal azotemia should resolve rapidly with correction of volume deficits and restoration of renal perfusion.

9. What other methods can be used to characterize renal function?

In some referral hospitals and veterinary teaching hospitals, nuclear scintigraphy is used for rapid quantification of renal function. Individual kidney filtration and excretory function can be assessed. Serial assays provide an assessment of disease severity, progression, and response to therapy. If scintigraphy is not available, excretory urography may be used for a subjective assessment of individual kidney function and to rule out postrenal obstruction; however, the large dose of contrast agent required for adequate renal opacification increases the risk of further renal damage. In patients with urine collection systems in place, timed measurements of endogenous creatinine clearance may be completed to monitor GFR objectively.

10. What is oliguric ARF? How does it differ from polyuric ARF?

Oliguria has been defined as urine production < 0.27 ml/hr/kg, but urine production < 0.5–1.0 ml/hr/kg should be considered inappropriate in rehydrated patients with ARF. Oliguria or anuria signifies severe renal dysfunction or bilateral postrenal obstruction. In oliguric renal failure, management becomes more difficult because fluid administration may be dramatically attenuated, making it difficult to resolve azotemia and hyperkalemia. Oliguric ARF also involves a greater potential for overhydration and volume overload. The degree of azotemia and hyperkalemia tends to be blunted in nonoliguric ARF, and the potential for overhydration is reduced.

11. What extrarenal complications may develop with ARF?

Nausea, anorexia, diarrhea, and oral ulcerations are common gastrointestinal signs that accompany ARF. A caustic effect of ammonia produced locally by bacterial ureases may lead to oral ulceration. Gastritis and enteritis are attributed to local ammonia production, impairment of the gastric mucosal barrier, and reduced renal clearance of gastrin. Nausea and vomiting also may be centrally mediated, because uremic toxins affect the chemoreceptor trigger zone. Malnutrition develops quickly from the combination of metabolic demands and lack of food intake.

Impaired leukocyte function and cellular immunity increase the risk of concurrent infection or sepsis. A bleeding tendency characterized by platelet dysfunction is occasionally observed with severe uremia. Uremic encephalopathy, manifested as altered mentation, bizarre behavior, tremors, head bobbing, or seizures, is observed with severe renal dysfunction. Rare complications of ARF include uremic pneumonitis, pulmonary edema, and cardiac arrhythmias.

12. What are the major objectives in the treatment of ARF?

Specific treatment of underlying disease (obstruction, hypercalcemia, lymphoma, leptospirosis) should be undertaken when possible. Supportive treatments should be formulated to correct fluid, electrolyte, and acid–base disorders, initiate diuresis, and manage systemic complications. Drugs commonly used in the management of ARF, along with their specific actions, recommended dosages, adverse effects, and contraindications, are listed in the table on the next page.

Drugs Used in the Management of Acute Renal Failure

AGENT	ACTIONS	DOSAGE	ADVERSE EFFECTS	CONTRA-INDICATIONS
Agents to enhance urine production				
Furosemide	Loop diuretic ↑ RBF	2–3 mg/kg IV q 6–8 hr 2–6 mg/kg IV q 30–60 min 1 mg/kg/hr IV CRI	Volume depletion Hypokalemia	Gentamicin Nephrotoxicity
Dopamine	↑ RBF, ↑ GFR ↑ Natriuresis	1–5 µg/kg/min IV CRI	Arrhythmias Hypertension Vomiting	
Mannitol	Osmotic diuresis ↓ Cellular edema Free radical scavenger	0.5–1.0 gm/kg IV slow bolus (as a 10–20% solution)	Pulmonary edema GI upset	Overhydration Cardiac disease
Dextrose (10–20%)	Osmotic diuresis Caloric support	25–50 ml/kg IV slow infusion q 8–12 hr	Volume expansion Hyperglycemia Hyperosmolality	
Agents to treat hyperkalemia				
Calcium gluconate (10% solution)	Cardioprotection	0.5–1.0 ml/kg IV slow bolus	Arrhythmias	
Sodium bicarbonate	Alkalinization of ECF	0.5–2 mEq/kg IV slow bolus	Hypernatremia ↓ Ionized calcium Hypokalemia	Hypocalcemia
Dextrose	↑ Insulin	0.1–0.5 gm/kg IV (1–2 ml/kg 25% solution)	Hyperglycemia Hyperosmolality	
Insulin/dextrose	Intracellular movement of potassium	0.25–0.5 U/kg insulin with 1–2 gm dextrose per unit insulin	Hypoglycemia	
Agents to treat metabolic acidosis				
Sodium bicarbonate	Alkalinization	See text for dosage	Hypernatremia Hypokalemia ↓ Ionized calcium	
Agents to treat nausea and vomiting				
Cimetidine	H₂ antagonist	2.5–5.0 mg/kg IV q 8–12 hr	Altered drug metabolism	Severe renal or hepatic failure
Ranitidine	H₂ antagonist	2 mg/kg IV q 8–12 hr		Severe renal or hepatic failure
Metoclopramide	Dopamine antagonist	0.2–0.4 mg/kg IM, IV or 1–2 mg/kg/24 hr IV CRI	CNS signs Interference with dopamine Constipation	GI obstruction Seizures
Misoprostol	Prostaglandin analog	1–5 µg/kg PO q 6–12 hr	GI upset Uterine contraction	Pregnancy Hypertension ? Seizures ?

RBF = renal blood flow, GFR = glomerular filtration rate, CRI = constant-rate infusion, ECF = extracellular fluid, CNS = central nervous system, GI = gastrointestinal.

13. What fluid composition is appropriate in the initial treatment of ARF?

In polyuric ARF, sodium and chloride are usually lost in concert with water losses. Sodium and extracellular fluid losses are exacerbated by gastrointestinal losses. Potassium may be retained because of poor excretion or lost by renal or gastrointestinal routes. In most patients with ARF, normal (0.9%) saline is an appropriate initial fluid choice because it is isotonic to plasma and contains no potassium. Normosol-R and lactated Ringer's solution are other isotonic replacement fluids that contain minimal potassium and are suitable alternative fluids. In patients with cardiopulmonary disease, half-strength (0.45%) saline in 2.5% dextrose or half-strength lactated Ringer's solution is preferable. In hypernatremic patients, isotonic fluids are used for volume replacement, followed by judicious administration of low sodium fluids (0.45% sodium chloride or 5% dextrose in water) to drop serum sodium concentrations slowly.

14. How is the initial fluid rate calculated for patients with suspected ARF?

Volume deficits are estimated (estimated percentage hydration × body weight in kg = liters required) and replaced within 4–6 hours. Fluids for maintenance requirements (40–60 ml/kg/day) and ongoing losses associated with polyuria, vomiting, and diarrhea should be added to the daily total and replaced over 24 hours. Ongoing losses can be estimated at 10–20 ml/kg/day; alternatively, 1.5–2 times maintenance requirements can be added to fluids calculated for volume replacement. Ideally, fluids are administered via a jugular catheter while urine output and serial central venous pressures are measured.

15. When is specific correction of hyperkalemia or metabolic acidosis indicated?

Correction of fluid deficits and initiation of diuresis are usually sufficient to reverse mild-to-moderate hyperkalemia and metabolic acidosis. Occasionally specific treatment may be required to prevent or counteract cardiotoxic effects of hyperkalemia (see chapter 77). Effects of pharmacologic treatment are short-lived, however, and urinary excretion must be restored or dialytic therapy considered. Bicarbonate therapy is indicated in patients with severe metabolic acidosis (blood pH < 7.2, bicarbonate or total CO_2 < 12–15 mmol/L). Partial correction of bicarbonate deficits over a period of 12–24 hours is advised (see chapter 81).

16. When is pharmacologic manipulation indicated to enhance urine output?

Urine production should be measured with an indwelling urinary catheter and closed collection system, metabolic cage, or serial weighing of litter pans or absorbent padding. After replacement of the estimated volume deficit, urine production should exceed 1 ml/kg/hr. If urine production is inadequate, mild volume expansion may be considered (administer an additional 3% body weight in fluid) and urine production reassessed. If urine production remains inadequate, pharmacologic treatment with furosemide and dopamine or mannitol is warranted.

17. What pharmacologic agents are available for enhancing urine output?

Diuretics and vasodilatory agents have been used to enhance urine output in ARF. Furosemide, mannitol, and hypertonic dextrose are used as diuretics. Dopamine at subpressor doses leads to renal vasodilation. For the most part, little change in GFR or clinical outcome is documented despite improvement in urine flow.

18. How can furosemide be useful in the treatment of ARF?

Furosemide is readily available and easy to administer as an intermittent IV bolus (2–3 mg/kg IV every 6–8 hr) or constant-rate infusion (1 mg/kg/hr). As a loop diuretic, furosemide helps to increase tubular flow and to improve renal blood flow but does not significantly affect GFR. Furosemide also may protect tubular epithelial cells in the thick ascending loop of Henle by reducing active transport at this site. The effectiveness of furosemide is enhanced by concurrent administration of dopamine. Furosemide may lead to excessive potassium losses, and it is contraindicated in the treatment of gentamicin nephrotoxicity.

19. What are the potential advantages of dopamine in the treatment of ARF?

Dopamine is a norepinephrine precursor that at low doses (1–5 mg/kg/min) causes dilation of splanchnic and renal arterial beds and acts at specific renal receptors to enhance sodium excretion. In cats, dopamine appears to stimulate alpha-adrenergic receptors, leading to increased blood pressure and natriuresis. Effects on urine production may be significant, but effects on GFR are modest.

20. What are the potential advantages of mannitol in the treatment of ARF?

Mannitol is a safe and effective osmotic diuretic when used in rehydrated, normovolemic patients with ARF and normal cardiopulmonary function. As an osmotic diuretic, mannitol creates volume expansion and increases tubular flow and urine production. A renal vasodilatory effect is also observed, perhaps mediated by enhanced prostaglandin activity or release of atrial natriuretic peptide. By virtue of volume expansion and vasodilatory effects, mannitol results in mild improvements in renal blood flow and GFR. Mannitol also may exert a cytoprotective action in ARF because the osmotic agent helps to minimize swelling of injured or hypoxic cells. Weak free radical scavenging activity also may help to minimize ischemic and reperfusion injury.

21. When is maintenance fluid therapy initiated?

Once volume deficits have been restored, electrolyte concentrations are stabilized, and diuresis has been established, fluid therapy should be tailored to match urine volume and other sensible and insensible losses. Insensible losses (e.g., water lose due to respiration) are estimated at 13–20 ml/kg/day. Urine output (the most variable sensible loss) is quantitated during 6- or 8-hour intervals; the amount lost is replaced during an equivalent period, along with measured or estimated gastrointestinal losses.

Fluid composition during maintenance therapy should be tailored to the individual patient. Polyionic replacement solutions that provide buffering activity and electrolyte replacement may be administered during the first few days of treatment, especially if gastrointestinal or electrolyte losses are great. For longer-term therapy, lower sodium solutions designed to meet maintenance fluid needs are preferred.

22. How are fluid requirements managed in ARF with oliguria or anuria?

Fluid requirements in oliguric patients must be based on urine output. As with typical maintenance fluid therapy, insensible losses are calculated at 13–20 ml/kg/day and urinary losses are measured and replaced. The fluid rate is adjusted frequently as hydration status is assessed. Serial measurements of central venous pressure are valuable for detecting early fluid overload.

23. When is dialytic therapy indicated in ARF?

Dialytic therapy should be considered in patients with ARF caused by dialyzable nephrotoxicants; patients with life-threatening fluid overload, hyperkalemia, or metabolic acidosis; oliguric or anuric patients that do not respond to pharmacologic manipulation; and patients that do not respond to medical management within 24–48 hours.

24. How are patients with ARF monitored?

Body weight, hydration status, blood pressure, food and fluid intake, and urine output should be monitored frequently. Clinicopathologic monitoring should include records of packed cell volume, total protein measurements, and concentrations of blood urea nitrogen, serum creatinine, sodium, potassium, and phosphorus as well as acid–base status. Frequency of monitoring is based on the severity and phase of illness; once- to twice-daily monitoring is ideal in critical patients.

25. How can progress and recovery be monitored in ARF?

Stabilization of azotemia, resolution of electrolyte and acid–base disturbances, and maintenance of polyuria are favorable signs in the management of ARF. Slow improvement of azotemia may be expected during fluid support in the maintenance phase if recovery is likely. Recovery of renal function and histologic renal repair may require several weeks before the animal is able to be weaned from fluid or dialytic support. Serial percutaneous kidney biopsies (at initiation of therapy and 3–4 weeks later) are most helpful in establishing accurate prognosis and monitoring recovery.

26. What factors affect prognosis and survival in patients with ARF?

Established ARF carries a guarded-to-grave prognosis unless an underlying disease process can be rapidly reversed (e.g., treatment of leptospirosis, removal of a nephrolith). Prognosis of acute intrinsic renal failure is affected by severity of dysfunction, extent of histologic damage, and response to therapy. Nonoliguric ARF generally has a more favorable prognosis than oliguric ARF, and patients with complete anuria are unlikely to survive. Nephrotoxicant-induced ARF (except ethylene glycol toxicosis) may have a better prognosis than ischemia-induced ARF because tubular basement membranes frequently remain intact. Preexisting cardiac disease, renal disease, neoplasia, pancreatitis, and major trauma as well as development of oliguria, respiratory failure, coma, or sepsis are poor prognostic indicators in human patients with ARF.

Early use of diuretics or renal vasodilators and early application of dialytic support may ultimately improve the outcome in ARF in veterinary medicine. Dialysis provides extended time for renal repair but is fraught with complications. In animals that survive or are maintained by dialysis, partial renal recovery is expected in 3–6 weeks (up to 12 weeks in patients that are initially oliguric).

BIBLIOGRAPHY

1. Behrend EN, Grauer GF, Mani I, et al: Hospital-acquired acute renal failure in dogs: 29 cases (1983–1992). J Am Vet Med Assoc 208:537–541, 1993.
2. Chew DJ: Fluid therapy during intrinsic renal failure. In Dibartola SP (ed): Fluid Therapy in Small Animal Practice. Philadelphia, W.B. Saunders, 1992, pp 554–572.
3. Forrester SD, Brandt KS: The diagnostic approach to the patient with acute renal failure. Vet Med 212:214–218, 1994.
4. Lane IF, Grauer GF, Fettman MR: Acute renal failure. Part I: Risk factors, prevention, and strategies for protection. Comp Cont Educ Pract Vet 16:15–29, 1994.
5. Lane IF, Grauer GF, Fettman MR: Acute renal failure. Part II: Diagnosis, management and prognosis. Comp Cont Educ Pract Vet 16:625–645, 1994.
6. Rubin SI: Management of fluid and electrolyte disorders in uremia. In Bonagura JD (ed): Kirk's Current Veterinary Therapy XII—Small Animal Practice. Philadelphia, W.B. Saunders, 1995, pp 951–955.

98. OBSTRUCTIVE FELINE LOWER URINARY TRACT DISEASE

Kristi L. Graham, D.V.M., and India F. Lane, D.V.M., M.S.

1. What are the most common causes of urethral obstruction in cats?

The two most common causes of urethral obstruction include mucoproteinaceous plugs and urethroliths. Urethral plugs are composed of minerals embedded in a proteinaceous matrix. The mineral composition within urethral plugs varies but often includes magnesium ammonium phosphate (struvite), calcium oxalate, calcium phosphate, or a mixture of these crystals. The matrix is a proteinaceous substance suspected to consist primarily of Tamm-Horsfall mucoprotein. Uroliths are a less common cause of urethral obstruction but are found in 15–22% of cats with clinical signs of hematuria, pollakiuria, and dysuria. The composition of feline uroliths most frequently consists of magnesium ammonium phosphate or calcium oxalate. Other, less frequent causes of urethral obstruction include bladder neck or urethral neoplasia, luminal strictures, extraluminal compression, and functional urethral obstruction or detrusor-urethral dyssynergia.

2. Obstructive uropathy is most frequently associated with what metabolic abnormalities?

Metabolic derangements associated with postrenal azotemia include volume depletion, hyperkalemia, and metabolic acidosis. Volume depletion may be a result of adipsia, anorexia, and vomiting; it is often underestimated by physical examination. The urethral blockage impairs excretion of potassium and hydrogen ions, leading to hyperkalemia and metabolic acidosis. With time, increased pressure within the bladder and ureters impairs glomerular filtration, renal blood flow, and tubular function, leading to postrenal azotemia.

3. What is the typical clinical course of complete urethral obstruction over 24–72 hours?

A urethral plug or urolith initially leads to dysuria, stranguria, and pollakiuria. Distention of the bladder and inflammation of the bladder and urethra contribute to hematuria and pain. Cats may become irritable, vocalize, or groom the perineum incessantly. Within 12–48 hours, the cat becomes anorectic, lethargic, and depressed. Postrenal uremia usually develops within 24 hours of complete obstruction. Vomiting and weakness are observed as uremia progresses. With prolonged obstruction, cats may become recumbent, shocky, or comatose. Without treatment, death usually occurs within 3–6 days of complete urethral obstruction.

4. What are the primary goals of medical therapy when complete urethral obstruction is suspected?

The immediate therapeutic goals are relief of the obstruction and reversal of concurrent metabolic abnormalities. The status of the patient directs priorities in management. Relieving the obstruction is required for ultimate resolution of azotemia and hyperkalemia. However, hypovolemia and hyperkalemia may be life-threatening in more compromised cats; thus, fluid support and cardioprotective treatments become top priorities. In more severely affected cats, intravenous fluid treatment is initiated while preparations are made for urethral catheterization. In alert and stable cats, urethral catheterization may be completed first.

5. What is the appropriate fluid therapy for obstructive lower urinary tract disease (LUTD)?

Goals of fluid therapy are to replace volume needs, to reduce hyperkalemia and uremia, and to minimize acid–base imbalance. Normal saline (0.9% sodium chloride) is a safe and efficacious initial choice. As a potassium-free solution, saline corrects volume deficits and promotes diuresis of retained potassium, urea, and hydrogen ions. Alkalinizing solutions such as Normosol-R or lactated Ringer's solution may be preferable for reversing acidemia and hyperkalemia, although these fluids contain minimal amounts of potassium. Improvements in tissue perfusion, acidosis, and potassium excretion often outweigh the risk of a small added potassium load. As urinary excretion of potassium is restored and diuresis ensues, hypokalemia is likely to develop, depending on duration of therapy and composition of the fluid. Fluids then need to be supplemented with potassium.

6. How should cats be restrained for urethral catheterization?

Urethral obstruction is an extremely painful condition, and patients often need chemical restraint to facilitate urethral catheterization. However, risks associated with anesthetic or analgesic administration in compromised cats must be considered. The choice of sedative agents is dictated by the clinical condition of the cat. Severely depressed and obstructed cats often require no anesthesia. In other cats, ketamine and diazepam are the most common agents chosen. Ketamine alone often provides adequate depth and duration for most catheterization. However, it is unlikely to provide analgesia. Ketamine must be used judiciously because it is excreted by the kidneys. Repeated doses are not advised. Additional muscle relaxation may be gained with the addition of diazepam. If cardiac stability is a concern or if urethral catheterization was unsuccessful with injectable agents, masking the cat with isoflurane may be a safer choice for restraint. Isoflurane provides adequate depth and duration for the procedure, and its effects can be removed quickly by discontinuing inhalation.

Approximate Doses of Pharmacologic Agents Used in Obstructed Cats

DRUG	APPLICATION	DOSE	COMMENTS
Ketamine	Chemical restraint	3–5 mg/kg	No analgesia No muscle relaxation
Ketamine with diazepam	Chemical restraint	K: 3–5 mg/kg D: 0.25–0.5 mg/kg	
Calcium gluconate	Cardioprotective in hyperkalemia	2–10 ml in 10% solution IV	Give slowly, monitor EKG
Sodium bicarbonate	Hyperkalemia	1–2 mEq/kg	
Glucose	Hyperkalemia	5–10% dextrose in water or 1–2 ml/kg 50% dextrose bolus (diluted to 25% with saline)	
Glucose with insulin	Hyperkalemia	I: 0.5–1 U/kg G: 2 gm dextrose per unit insulin	Monitor serum glucose levels
Bethanechol	Detrusor contraction	1.25–7.5 mg/cat orally every 8 hr	
Prazosin	Urethral smooth muscle relaxant	0.03 mg/kg IV	Hypotension
Phenoxybenzamine	Urethral smooth muscle relaxant	2.5–7.5 mg/cat orally every 12–24 hr	Hypotension
Diazepam	Urethral striated muscle relaxant	1–5 mg/cat orally every 8 hr or 1 mg/kg IV	Sedation possible

7. What methods are available for relieving difficult urethral obstruction?

The urethra may be catheterized with a sterile, open- or closed-tip, 3.5-French "tomcat" catheter (Sherwood Medical, St. Louis). Minnesota olive-tipped catheters (Ejay International, Glendora, CA) also are available in several different lengths and diameters; they are composed of steel and designed to be minimally traumatic to the urethra. If the obstruction is not easily dislodged, flushing the catheter with sterile saline occasionally forces the plug back into the bladder or breaks up the obstructive material sufficiently to allow passage of the urinary catheter into the bladder. If simple reverse flushing is ineffective, retropulsion with a closed urethral orifice may dilate the urethra around the plug and release it. If bladder size and intra-luminal pressure are excessive, hindering retropulsion and passage of the catheter, a decompressive cystocentesis may be cautiously performed (see controversies). Occasionally, a small amount of lidocaine (solution or gel) instilled through the catheter helps to decrease urethral spasm and facilitates catheter placement. Large quantities of anesthetic solutions should be avoided because they may be readily absorbed through inflamed urinary bladder mucosa. Injection of pharmacologic agents that may decrease urethral pressure (alpha antagonists, skeletal muscle relaxants) has been investigated as a means of facilitating urethral catheterization. The magnitude of change in urethral pressure with these drugs, however, is unlikely to enhance catheter passage dramatically.

8. Does flushing the bladder help to minimize dysuria or reobstruction?

After the obstruction is relieved, flushing the bladder with a sterile saline solution has been recommended. Justification for this practice is based on the assumption that removal of crystals, "sand," or mucoid precipitate remaining in the bladder decreases the chance of reobstruction. Saline hydrodistention and flushing also may promote release and excretion of inflammatory mediators that contribute to feline LUTD. Hydrodistention provides temporary relief in some women with interstitial cystitis, probably by exhausting sensory nerve firing, promoting release of inflammatory mediators, and creating epithelial trauma, which heals over time. However, patients usually have more pain for several weeks after the procedure before improvement is appreciated. In cats, the effects of aggressive bladder flushing are not established, but the technique is unlikely to cause harm as long as care is taken not to overdistend the bladder.

9. What are the main criteria for maintaining an indwelling urinary catheter?

The decision to leave an indwelling catheter is based on the condition of the patient and postobstructive bladder and urethral function. With severe azotemia or metabolic acidosis, the catheter is often maintained to assess urine output during postobstructive diuresis. An indwelling catheter also averts immediate reobstruction, which compromises recovery in critically ill cats. Indwelling catheters also may be maintained to minimize reobstruction in cats after difficult, traumatic catheterization or early reobstruction or in cats with heavy crystalluria, hematuria, or urine debris. Finally, temporary indwelling catheters are indicated when detrusor atony or functional urethral obstruction is likely to interfere with voiding. Ideally, the polypropylene catheter is removed, and urine stream is assessed by gentle bladder expression. The catheter may then be replaced, if necessary, with a soft flexible alternative. With difficult catheterization, the original catheter is usually left in place for short-term use (12–24 hours) to avoid additional trauma and to allow urethral inflammation and spasm to subside.

10. How are indwelling catheters maintained?

Soft polyvinyl ("red-rubber") catheters are preferred to minimize iatrogenic urethral and bladder irritation during longer-term urethral catheterization. A 5-French catheter is usually needed to maintain good urine flow. Alternatives include infant feeding tubes (Argyle feeding tube, Sherwood Medical, St. Louis) and recently available silicone or Teflon-based products (Slippery Sam catheter, Cook Veterinary Products, Bloomington, IN). Soft catheters can be stiffened in the freezer to facilitate placement. The tip of the catheter is ideally situated within the bladder neck so that drainage is effective but excessive catheter material does not remain in the bladder. The catheter is then secured by tape, which is attached to the catheter and sutured to the prepuce. Tension is avoided by taping the catheter or drainage tubing to the cat's tail.

Indwelling urinary catheters may be maintained as an open system or a closed collection system. Open systems ensure that the urethra remains open but allow easy bacterial colonization of the urinary bladder and do not allow quantification of urine output. A closed urinary catheter system can be created by using a fluid infusion line to connect the catheter to an empty, sterile collection bag (usually a recently emptied fluid bag). Commercial urine collection systems also are available. A closed system initially minimizes bacterial colonization. With increased time, however, ascending infection becomes more likely as bacteria gain access by migrating along the outside of the urinary catheter.

11. Why does postobstructive diuresis occur?

The dramatic diuretic effect after relief of urinary obstruction probably results from appropriate physiologic responses and residual tubular concentrating defects. The homeostatic response to retained loads of urea, sodium, potassium, phosphate, and hydrogen ions is an increase in excretion. An accumulation of atrial natriuretic factor during obstruction also may promote natriuresis and diuresis. Intrarenally, residual tubular defects may impair concentrating ability. The medullary gradient and tubular responsiveness to antidiuretic hormone also may be ineffective after periods of obstruction.

12. How can measured urine production help to direct fluid therapy?

Urinary losses during the postobstructive phase may be great. Because maintenance fluid requirements include both sensible (primarily urinary) and insensible losses, urine output may be used to prepare fluid therapy in previously obstructed cats. Insensible losses are estimated at 13–20 ml/kg/day. Urinary losses are measured over 6- or 8-hour intervals and replaced over intervals of similar duration. With this "ins-and-outs" method, fluid replacement more equally matches true requirements. Over 24–72 hours, fluids may be tapered to prevent ongoing diuresis.

13. When is removal of the indwelling catheter indicated?

Because of the risk of urinary tract infection and iatrogenic trauma, urinary catheters should be removed as soon as the cat is clinically and metabolically stable and likely to urinate voluntarily. Postobstruction voiding function is difficult to predict but is more likely when hematuria is resolving and when the bladder is small and tonically contracted around the catheter tip. A decision to remove the catheter is usually made within 24–48 hours of placement.

14. Are antimicrobials necessary? If so, when are they indicated?

Primary bacterial infections are rarely documented in obstructive or nonobstructive LUTD in cats. However, iatrogenic introduction of bacteria into the urinary tract is possible during the placement and maintenance of urinary catheters. Prophylactic antimicrobial administration is not recommended while an indwelling urinary catheter is in place unless symptomatic infection or urosepsis develops (excessive straining, lethargy, fever). Prophylactic antimicrobial treatment often leads to development of complicated infections with a resistant species of bacteria. Ascending infections of the upper urinary tract are also possible. Urinary tract colonization increases over time; use of sterile technique and a closed collection system may delay the development of urinary tract infection. Ideally, antibiotic therapy is based on urine culture obtained after removal of the urinary catheter.

15. List possible reasons for persistent voiding dysfunction in previously obstructed cats.

In the early postobstructive period, inability to void is usually attributable to physical reobstruction, functional outlet obstruction, or detrusor atony. Outlet resistance and bladder function can be assessed by attempting manual expression of a moderately full bladder. If a good urine stream can be produced with gentle sustained compression, detrusor atony is the most likely cause of urine retention. If voiding is not stimulated and an appropriate urine stream cannot be generated, physical or functional outlet obstruction is likely. Physical reobstruction is common as a result of persistent mucocrystalline debris, small uroliths, or urethral edema. Resistance to urethral catheterization may be used to distinguish physical from functional obstruction; however, small uroliths can be easily bypassed or pushed back into the urinary bladder. Development of dysuria several weeks to months after obstruction may indicate urethral stricture, an uncommon complication of urethral trauma, by either the plug, urolith, or catheter.

16. How can functional urethral obstruction be detected?

Excessive urethral outlet resistance is commonly observed after urethral obstruction in cats. Cats usually strain to void, producing minimal amounts of urine. Expression of the bladder is difficult or impossible, whereas urethral catheterization is usually easy. Some cats demonstrate detectable perineal contractions while straining to void. Extensive urethral spasm makes withdrawal of a urinary catheter difficult.

17. What treatments are effective for voiding dysfunction attributed to functional outlet obstruction?

Smooth and striated muscle of the urethra can be manipulated pharmacologically. Alpha-adrenergic antagonists (prazosin, phenoxybenzamine) are useful in modulating smooth muscle of the urethra in dogs and have been effective experimentally in reducing urethral pressures in cats. However, in cats striated muscle relaxants may be more effective in reducing outlet resistance in the distal urethra, which is the usual site of injury in recently obstructed cats. Diazepam and dantrolene have been investigated for this purpose. In clinical usage, diazepam appears to facilitate bladder expression and may be most helpful when initiated early after relief of obstruction.

In most cases, however, patience and tincture of time are the only effective treatments for restoring normal voiding function.

18. When is surgical intervention indicated?

Perineal urethrostomy has been used to avert urethral obstruction. Emergency perineal urethrostomy may be necessary when repeated attempts to catheterize the urethra fail, although decompressive cystocentesis may be used to provide additional time for medical attempts to succeed in dislodging the obstruction. Urethrostomies are most commonly performed in cats with frequent reobstruction. Because of the short clinical course typically associated with feline LUTD, surgery should be performed only when all attempts at medical control fail. Surgery helps to prevent future urethral obstruction, but owners should be advised that signs of idiopathic inflammation (hematuria, pollakiuria, dysuria) are still likely to occur.

CONTROVERSIES

19. Should corticosteroids be used in obstructive feline LUTD?

The decision to use glucocorticoids in obstructive feline LUTD should be given careful consideration. Certainly inflammation plays a role in the development of dysuria, pollakiuria, and hematuria associated with urethral obstruction. The antiinflammatory properties of glucocorticoids help to minimize clinical signs and reduce the possibility of reobstruction. However, the immunosuppressive and catabolic effects of glucocorticoids may be detrimental in obstructed cats with postrenal azotemia and associated metabolic abnormalities. Furthermore, the efficacy of glucocorticoids in nonobstructive disease remains unproved. Glucocorticoids are contraindicated in cats with indwelling urinary catheters or bacterial urinary tract infection.

20. Should decompressive cystocentesis be used in urethral obstruction?

Decompressive cystocentesis may be indicated when the urethral obstruction cannot be immediately removed. Advantages of a carefully performed cystocentesis include rapid decompression of an overly distended bladder, relief from pain, temporary attenuation of renal compromise, and facilitation of reverse flushing and retropulsion of urethral plugs. Samples obtained via cystocentesis are suitable for initial urinalysis and culture. However, cystocentesis may be dangerous, especially if the bladder wall is compromised. Urine may extravasate around the needle, or the bladder wall may be further injured, occasionally leading to rupture. Thus, the decision to perform decompressive cystocentesis is based on immediacy of need for decompression and assessment of likely bladder wall integrity.

BIBLIOGRAPHY

1. Barsanti JA, Shotts EB, Crowell WA, et al: Effect of therapy on susceptibility to urinary tract infection in male cats with indwelling urethral catheters. J Vet Intern Med 6:64–70, 1992.
2. Osborne CA, Kruger JM, Lulich J, et al: Medical management of feline urethral obstruction. Vet Clin North Am 26:483–498, 1996.
3. Polzin DJ, Osborne CA, Bartges JW: Management of postrenal azotemia. Vet Clin North Am 26:507–513, 1996.
4. Ross LA: The protocol for treating cats with urethral obstruction. Vet Med 85:1206–1214, 1990.
5. Straeter-Knowlen IM, Marks SL, Rishniw M, et al: Urethral pressure response to smooth and skeletal muscle relaxants in anesthetized, adult male cats with naturally acquired urethral obstruction. Am J Vet Res 56:919, 1995.

99. PERITONEAL DIALYSIS AND HEMODIALYSIS

India F. Lane, D.V.M., M.S., and Leslie Carter, M.S., C.V.T., V.T.S.

1. How does dialysis work?

All forms of dialysis are based on the interaction of plasma water with a solution across a semipermeable membrane that allows movement of selected substances from plasma into removable dialysate or vice versa. Movement of water and solute is directed by principles of **diffusion** (the movement of molecules from areas of high concentration or activity to areas of low concentration or activity), **osmosis** (the movement of water toward increasing solute concentration), and **solute drag** (the movement of substances en masse in response to diffusion or osmotic forces). In peritoneal dialysis, the peritoneum serves as the membrane for transfer of solute or water, and movement is driven predominantly by osmotic gradients. In hemodialysis, an artificial membrane within the dialyzer allows transfer, which is driven by artificially generated hydrostatic forces as well as diffusion gradients. The ultimate goal of dialysis in renal failure is transfer of undesirable solutes and excessive fluids from blood of the uremic patient to the dialysate.

2. What are the indications for dialytic therapy in veterinary medicine?

Dialysis is most commonly used in veterinary medicine for the management of refractory acute intrinsic renal failure. Dialysis is indicated when clinical signs, azotemia, acidosis, or hyperkalemia is unresponsive to appropriate medical management (see chapter 97). Guidelines for severity of azotemia that warrants dialysis include blood urea nitrogen > 100 mg/dl or serum creatinine > 10 mg/dl. Dialysis is chosen early in treatment of acute renal failure if life-threatening hyperkalemia or fluid overload cannot be medically reversed or if oliguria is persistent. Ideally, dialysis is initiated for reversible acute renal disease but may be useful in chronic renal disease, perioperatively for renal transplantation, or temporarily while awaiting renal biopsy results. In chronic renal failure, intermittent dialysis may be undertaken for selected patients to minimize signs of uremia and to improve overall quality of life. Although azotemia worsens between dialysis periods, maximal urea concentrations and time-averaged urea concentration are reduced. Other indications for dialysis include acute intoxicoses or refractory fluid overload due to nonrenal causes.

PERITONEAL DIALYSIS

3. What factors affect peritoneal clearance of a solute?

Although the peritoneal surface area is large, the capillary surface area for fluid movement is relatively small. Transport may be intercellular, transcytoplasmic, or via vesicle formation. Movement of solute depends not only on diffusion gradients but also on molecular size and weight, charge, and protein binding. Interstitial and vascular hydrostatic pressures, peritoneal permeability, and dwell time also influence transfer. Use of warmed dialysate, increased dwell time, or hypertonic dialysate solutions may enhance diffusion and solute drag.

4. How does peritoneal dialysis compare with hemodialysis?

Peritoneal dialysis is effective for removal of most retained uremic toxins, acids, and potassium. Peritoneal dialysis may be more effective than hemodialysis in the removal of larger-molecular-weight substances (middle molecules of uremia) because of larger pore size, but hemodialysis is generally more efficient than peritoneal dialysis. In its simplest form, peritoneal dialysis is practical for any veterinary practice; however, dialysis is labor-intensive and fraught with complications. Hemodialysis requires additional technical equipment, reliable vascular access, and specially trained personnel. In the dedicated laboratory, intermittent hemodialysis requires less time and labor than continuous peritoneal exchanges.

5. How do you perform a peritoneal dialysis exchange?

After surgical placement of the dialysis catheter, the tail of the catheter tubing is aseptically connected to a transfer tubing set that previously has been attached to and primed with a pre-warmed bag of dialysate. With a single-spike system, exchanges are made as follows:

1. After a fresh bag of dialysate is prepared, the collapsed empty dialysate bag is unrolled and placed below the level of the animal for drainage.

2. The roller clamp on the transfer tubing is opened to allow slow drainage of fluid from the peritoneal cavity.

3. The fresh dialysate bag is connected to the transfer set spike, and dialysate is infused by gravity flow.

4. Dialysate remains in the peritoneal cavity for 1–6 hours (depending on the intensity of dialysis required), and the process is repeated.

With a Y-set system, the Y-set is attached to the catheter tubing or transfer set, with a fresh dialysate bag and collection container attached to either segment of the Y. For exchanges, a small amount of fresh dialysate is first flushed into the drainage bag so that any contaminants introduced during the connections procedures are flushed into the drainage bag and not into the peritoneal cavity. The peritoneal cavity is then drained, and fresh dialysate is infused for the next dialysis cycle. If desired, the Y-set can be disconnected between exchanges and the caps protected with disinfectant. Details of dialysis procedures are reviewed in works listed in the bibliography.

6. How is dialysate prepared for peritoneal dialysis?

Dialysate solutions are buffered, slightly hyperosmolar crystalloid solutions designed to pull fluid, potassium, urea, and phosphate from the plasma into dialysate while providing diffusible buffer and other needed compounds such as magnesium and calcium. Potassium-free commercial dialysate solutions are available with dextrose concentrations of 1.5%, 2.5%, or 4.25% and lactate as the primary buffer. Potassium supplementation may be required during long-term dialysis of normokalemic or hypokalemic patients. Similar solutions can be prepared by adding dextrose to lactated Ringer's solution; however, magnesium supplementation may be necessary. Acetate-based solutions may damage the peritoneum and are not recommended.

7. Why are hypertonic solutions used for peritoneal dialysis?

Hypertonic dextrose-containing solutions are effective for minimizing edema in over-hydrated patients and for enhancing ultrafiltration (removal of water) in all patients. Hypertonic dextrose appears to favor capillary vasodilation and increased pore size in the peritoneum and enhances solute drag. Dialysate containing 1.5% dextrose is used in dehydrated or normovolemic patients, whereas 2.5% and 4.25% solutions are used in mildly to severely overhydrated patients. Intermittent use of 4.25% dextrose solution may increase the efficiency of dialysis in all patients.

8. What is the recommended volume for dialysis exchange?

The recommended infusion volume for small animals is 30–40 ml/kg per exchange. For the first 12–24 hours after catheter placement, exchange volumes should be one-half of the calculated ideal volume to assess the degree of abdominal distention, effect on respiratory function, and potential for dialysate leakage.

9. How can small exchanges be facilitated in cats or small dogs?

Multiple exchanges can be completed with a single bag of dialysate. The exchange volume is calculated and administered by weighing the bag during infusion (1 liter of fluid equals 1 kg). Dialysate can be drained into a separate collection container using a Y-infusion set or directly back into the infusion bag. Dilution of drained effluent with fresh dialysate still allows infusion of effective dialysate for several exchanges.

10. What catheters are available for peritoneal dialysis?

Peritoneal dialysis catheters are available in straight, curled, and column-disk designs. The column-disk design is preferred for veterinary patients, because it appears to be less easily obstructed than other designs. However, commercial availability has been sporadic. Curled catheters may be adaptable to small animals for long-term dialysis. Straight catheters designed for human use are readily available and satisfactory for acute dialysis in dogs and cats. Without immediate access to specially designed peritoneal catheters, thoracostomy tubes and other sterile fenestrated tubing may be used temporarily while preparations are made for long-term dialysis.

11. How can catheter occlusion be prevented?

A full or partial omentectomy at the time of catheter placement may minimize physical occlusion of catheter pores. Heparin (100 U/L initially, tapered to 250 U/L) is added to dialysate solution during the first few days of dialysis to minimize fibrin formation and obstruction by blood clots.

12. What measures should be taken if the effluent is not draining effectively?

Less fluid may be recovered from the abdomen than was delivered for the first few exchanges. As dialysis proceeds, outflow should approximate or exceed inflow. If drainage persistently lags behind infusion, excessive fluid is being resorbed by the patient, fluid is leaking around the catheter, or catheter outflow is obstructed. If the patient appears to be resorbing most of the dialysate fluid, a higher dextrose concentration may be chosen for a few exchanges. Leakage into bandage material or subcutaneous leakage can be detected by examination of the catheter site. Significant leakage impedes effective dialysis. Dwell volume may be decreased temporarily. Corrective sutures may be necessary to resolve persistent leakage. If dialysate is retained in the peritoneal cavity (progressive abdominal distention and discomfort), the integrity of the catheter system must be evaluated.

13. What measures should be taken if effluent exceeds dialysate input?

Fluid losses from the patient into the dialysate may be excessive. On the other hand, this scenario may be desirable if the patient is fluid over-loaded or receiving large volumes of parenteral fluid supplementation. Deviations from ideal exchange efficiency can be monitored to demonstrate inappropriate fluid loss or gain. If effluent production is inappropriately excessive, the osmolality of the dialysate solution should be reduced to minimize osmotic pull. Intravenous fluid supplementation is adjusted to prevent dehydration or fluid overload.

14. What findings suggest the development of peritonitis?

Bacterial peritonitis is a serious complication of peritoneal dialysis and usually results from touch contamination of catheter tubing or bag spikes. Clinical findings or effluent characteristics may be the first indicator of peritonitis. Abdominal pain, vomiting, depression, and fever may indicate peritonitis; however, most of these signs may be difficult to differentiate from signs of uremia. Cloudy or bloody effluent may suggest peritonitis; periodic cytologic evaluation of effluent is recommended regardless of gross appearance. Peritonitis is diagnosed if two of the following three criteria are met: (1) cloudy dialysate fluid with neutrophilic inflammatory cells (> 100 µl); (2) detection of organisms in effluent by Gram stain or culture; and (3) clinical signs of peritonitis.

15. How is peritonitis managed in peritoneal dialysis?

When peritonitis is suspected, effluent is cultured for aerobic and anaerobic organisms. Broad-spectrum antimicrobial treatment (e.g., parenteral cephalosporin) is initiated pending culture and antimicrobial susceptibility results. Antimicrobial agents are often added to dialysate in human patients but are probably best administered systemically in veterinary patients, especially when dosing becomes difficult because multiple or partial exchanges will be made from a single dialysate bag.

16. What are other complications of peritoneal dialysis?

Complications of peritoneal dialysis include catheter complications, metabolic complications, and other miscellaneous problems. Catheter occlusion, exit site and subcutaneous tunnel infections, and leakage of dialysate are the most common catheter complications. Metabolic complications include blood and protein losses, hyponatremia, hypokalemia, and hyperglycemia. Dialysis dysequilibrium is an uncommon complication of early dialysis. Rapid removal of urea and other osmotic products from the plasma creates an osmotic gradient with subsequent movement of water into cells and the potential for cerebral edema. Symptoms include restlessness, vomiting, dementia, seizures, or death.

17. When should peritoneal dialysis be terminated?

Ideally, dialytic support is continued until renal function recovers sufficiently to maintain a clinically acceptable level of azotemia with infrequent or no dialysate exchanges. In reversible acute renal failure, this phase may require several weeks. For acute toxicoses or corrected postrenal azotemia, dialysis may be required for a much shorter period. In other patients, dialytic support and remaining renal function are insufficient to support a reasonable quality of life. The decision to terminate treatment is usually made when clinical signs of uremia are not managed by dialysis, biochemical abnormalities are not corrected, or refractory peritonitis is encountered.

HEMODIALYSIS

18. How does hemodialysis work?

In hemodialysis, blood is removed from the body, circulated through an artificial kidney that simulates the excretory and regulatory functions of the kidney, and returned to the body. Undesirable uremic toxins are removed by transfer across a membrane into the dialysate. Water removal (ultrafiltration) is regulated by manipulating hydrostatic pressures generated in the extracorporeal circuit.

19. How does hemodialysis compare with peritoneal dialysis?

Hemodialysis is 10–20 times more efficient than peritoneal dialysis for management of acute and chronic azotemia. Although the equipment and personnel costs for hemodialysis exceed those for peritoneal dialysis, the procedure can be completed efficiently and conveniently in specialized centers. With experience and dedicated personnel, hemodialysis is a practical option for aggressive management of renal failure and intoxications.

20. What are the characteristics of a suitable hemodialyzer?

The ideal artificial kidney must be able to remove small- and medium-molecular-weight waste products while preventing loss of blood proteins, cells, and needed solutes. The system must be able to independently regulate ultrafiltration (water removal) and must be biocompatible.

21. Describe the typical construction of a hemodialyzer.

Hemodialyzers are classified based on construction design and composition of the limiting membrane. The most common type of dialyzer in current use is the hollow-fiber design. The dialyzer is constructed of bundles of small-diameter capillary fibers with multiple tiny pores for diffusion. Blood flows through the hollow fibers in one direction while dialysate is distributed around the fiber bundle in a countercurrent direction. This design provides a large surface are for exchange and minimizes resistance to blood flow while retaining compact size. Membranes are comprised of disposable natural cellulosic material or more expensive but durable synthetic plastic polymers.

22. What are the other components of the hemodialyzer unit?

In addition to the dialyzer, reliable vascular access and an adjustable delivery system are required for hemodialysis. Dialysis delivery can be prepared and completed manually, but automated systems have simplified this laborious process and minimized the supervision required during dialysis. The delivery system controls dialysate and blood flow, delivers anticoagulant, and creates the appropriate dialysate composition and pressure. Alarms are incorporated into the system to alert operators to blood and air leaks, disconnections, and pressure or temperature changes in the circuit. Infant and pediatric systems have advanced sufficiently to be readily adaptable to dogs and cats.

23. How is vascular access maintained for hemodialysis?

Arteriovenous shunts created by cannulating the femoral artery and vein or carotid artery and jugular vein have been traditionally used for vascular access. During dialysis, blood is shunted from the arterial limb into the dialyzer and returned to the vasculature via the venous limb. Between dialysis periods, the limbs of the shunt are connected, leaving a permanent, flowing arteriovenous shunt. Unfortunately, shunts require surgical placement, easily become clotted, and are difficult to maintain in active veterinary patients. Double-lumen transcutaneous vascular catheters have replaced shunts for short- and long-term dialysis in dogs and cats. The catheter tip is placed in the right atrium via the jugular vein, and blood is removed from and returned to this compartment using the two lumens of the same catheter.

24. What is a typical hemodialysis plan for a patient with acute renal failure?
Patients with acute renal failure are usually prepared for dialysis and dialyzed once daily, with dialysis designed to drop the predialysis urea concentration by 40–50%. Once the predialysis blood urea nitrogen concentration is below 90 mg/dl, treatments can be extended to 48–72-hour intervals. Intensity of dialysis may be increased by increasing dialysis time, blood flow rate through the dialyzer, and/or ultrafiltration pressure.

25. What is a typical hemodialysis plan for a patient with chronic renal failure?
Dialysis times and prescriptions are modified in patients with chronic renal failure to provide an acceptable interdialysis quality of life with minimal treatments. In moderately azotemic dogs and cats (serum creatinine: 6–8 mg/dl), weekly dialysis may be sufficient. In more severely affected animals (serum creatinine > 8 mg/dl), dialysis may be required every 4–5 days. Dialysis sessions for animals with advanced chronic renal failure are designed to achieve an acute drop in urea concentrations by 85–90% of the predialysis value and to maintain a time-averaged urea concentration of 60 mg/dl or less.

26. What are the common complications of hemodialysis?
During dialysis, transient hypotension, vomiting, seizures, cramping, clotting in the extracorporeal circuit, and blood loss are the most common complications. These complications can be minimized by alterations in dialysis delivery and fine-tuning of anticoagulant delivery. Dialysis dysequilibrium may occur with the rapid osmotic shifts of early dialysis and can be avoided by appropriately graded sodium delivery and by starting therapy with conservative prescriptions. After dialysis, common complications include clotting, failure or infection of the vascular access, venous thrombosis attributed to the vascular access, sepsis, and bleeding associated with heparinization.

BIBLIOGRAPHY

1. Birchard SJ, Chew DJ, Crisp MS, Fossum TW: Modified technique for placement of a column disc dialysis catheter. J Am Animal Hosp Assoc 24:663–666, 1988.
2. Carter LJ, Wingfield WE, Allen TA: Clinical experience with peritoneal dialysis in small animals. Comp Cont Educ Pract Vet 11:1335–1343, 1989. (Updated in The Compendium Collection: Renal Disease in Small Animal Practice. Trenton, NJ, Veterinary Learning Systems, 1994, pp 125–132.)
3. Chew DJ, Dibartola SP, Crisp MS: Peritoneal dialysis. In Dibartola SP (ed): Fluid Therapy in Small Animal Practice. Philadelphia, W.B. Saunders, 1992, pp 573–597.
4. Cowgill LD: Application of peritoneal dialysis and hemodialysis in the management of renal failure. In Osborne CA, Finco DR (eds): Canine and Feline Nephrology and Urology. Baltimore, Williams & Wilkins, 1995, pp 573–596.
5. Cowgill LD, Maretzki CH: Veterinary applications of hemodialysis: An update. In Bonagura JD (ed): Kirk's Current Veterinary Therapy XII. Philadelphia, W.B. Saunders, 1995, pp 975–977.
6. Crisp MS, Chew DJ, Dibartola SP, Birchard SJ: Peritoneal dialysis in dogs and cats: 27 cases (1976–1987). J Am Vet Med Assoc 195:1262–1266, 1989.
7. Lane IF, Carter LJ, Lappin MR: Peritoneal dialysis: An update on methods and usefulness. In Kirk RW, Bonagura JD (eds): Current Veterinary Therapy XI. Philadelphia, W.B. Saunders, 1992, pp 865–870.
8. Parker HR: Peritoneal dialysis and hemofiltration. In Bovee KC (ed): Canine Nephrology. Media, PA, Harwal Publishing, 1984, pp 723–753.
9. Thornhill JA: Peritonitis associated with peritoneal dialysis: Diagnosis and treatment. J Am Vet Med Assoc 182:721–724, 1983.
10. Thornhill JA: Hemodialysis. In Bovee KC (ed): Canine Nephrology. Media, PA, Harwal Publishing, 1984, pp 755–802.

XIII. Toxicology

Section Editor: J. Michael McFarland, D.V.M.

---

100. GENERAL TOXICOLOGY AND APPROACHES

Tam Garland, D.V.M., Ph.D.

---

1. What is toxicology?

Toxicology is the knowledge of poisons, including their chemical properties, identification, biologic effects, and treatment.

2. How is poison defined?

A poison is any substance in any state, whether solid, liquid, gas, ionic, or nonionic radiation, that when placed into or applied to the body interferes with the life processes of the cells by its own inherent qualities without mechanical action and with regard to temperature.

3. Are there natural toxicants?

Yes. Many herbs, plants, mycotoxins, and microbial agents are toxic, although they are natural. Biotoxins from snakes and spiders are natural but are also toxic. The fact that a substance is "all natural" does not mean that it is safe.

4. How is acute toxicity defined?

Acute toxicity refers to the effects of a single dose or multiple doses during a 24-hour period. The toxic effects may become obvious over several days or weeks.

5. What is a chronic toxicity?

Chronic toxicity refers to the effects produced by prolonged exposure of 90 days or longer.

6. What factors should be considered in evaluating potential toxicity?

The physiologic factors, such as breed, species, age, sex, pregnancy, and lactation, are considerations. Also consider the environmental factors such as season, temperature, humidity, and air circulation. Other environmental factors may include the quality and quantity of water, diet, caging size and material used in the cage, and presence of other animals.

7. Is duration of exposure important?

Yes. The duration greatly affects the toxicity. The animal may survive a single exposure but multiple exposures over time may prove lethal. Likewise, multiple exposures may produce a type of tolerance, as with rodents and rodenticides. Both duration of exposure and dose are important.

8. Is the route of exposure important?

Yes. Most common are dermal, oral, and inhalation routes. However, toxicities also occur through intravenous, intraperitoneal, and subcutaneous routes.

9. How much of a substance does it take to poison an animal?

The amount depends on the substance, size of the animal, and even species.

10. What clinical signs may a poisoned animal exhibit?

Poisoned animals exhibit a full range of clinical signs, including vomiting, diarrhea, trembling, shaking, convulsing, coma, problems with the heart, difficulty with breathing, clotting problems, muscle weakness, and muscle stiffness. Poisonings may mimic a number of diseases and can affect all body systems.

11. Are species and breed important in dealing with toxicities?

Yes. Physiologic factors are always a concern. Some species are more sensitive than others. For example, cats may be more sensitive to some insecticides than dogs. Likewise, some breeds may be more sensitive than others. For example, collie and collie-cross dogs may be more sensitive to some heartworm products.

12. Is it possible for more than one animal to be involved?

Yes. Always ask the owners if other pets could have been exposed.

13. Is it important to know immediately if an animal was poisoned?

Sometimes. Some toxic substances, such as cyanide or strychnine, require immediate attention. Other situations are not as critical, and stabilizing the animal may be more important.

14. What is the first thing to do once it is known that an animal has been poisoned?

Make sure that the animal is in stable condition. Treat with appropriate antidote, if available. Treat the clinical signs, and do not harm.

15. Does the length of time between the incident and the time the animal is seen by a veterinarian make a difference?

Yes. The sooner an animal is seen by a veterinarian, the better the prognosis, in most cases.

16. What substances are best to induce emesis?

Apomorphine is the most reliable and most effective. However, it may cause protracted emesis. Apomorphine may be controlled by appropriate narcotic antagonists administered intravenously. It was at one time withdrawn from the market but is now available from pharmacies with the capability to compound substances.

17. Do other products besides apomorphine induce emesis?

Syrup of ipecac is available but it is only 50% effective in dogs. It can be repeated only once within 20 minutes. If emesis does not occur after the second dosage, the syrup of ipecac must be removed by gastric lavage. Syrup of ipecac may be toxic. Copper sulfate is occasionally effective, but it is dangerous. Table salt is dangerous but has been known to cause emesis. Hydrogen peroxide is not highly effective in companion animals, although it does occasionally work. Rompun (xylazine) also has been used as an emetic and is usually effective.

18. When is emesis contraindicated?

Emesis is contraindicated if the animal is unconscious or shows signs of central nervous system (CNS) depression. Respiratory depression may be an indication of CNS depression. If the animal has been intoxicated with a petroleum distillate, emesis is contraindicated. If more than 4 hours have passed since ingestion, emesis is contraindicated. At more than 4 hours after ingestion, probably no toxic substance remains in the stomach, and to cause emesis is to put undue stress on the animal. If you suspect that the animal has ingested an acid or an alkali, the stomach wall may be weakened. Retching may rupture the stomach and allow the substance to reinjure the esophagus and oral cavity.

19. When has it been too long after consumption to consider inducing emesis?

The general rule is that when it is longer than 4–5 hours since ingestion, emesis will probably not benefit the animal.

20. What is the mechanism of activated charcoal?

Charcoal is activated by increasing the surface area of the charcoal and heating it. It provides a surface onto which the substance is absorbed.

21. How much activated charcoal should be given?

Make a slurry with water and activated charcoal. Use 1 gm charcoal/5–10 ml of water, and calculate the dose at 2–8 gm of charcoal/kg of body weight. Administer through an orogastric tube using a funnel or large syringe. Administer a saline cathartic 30 minutes after the charcoal. For best results, the activated charcoal should be readministered 4 times/day for several days after intoxication.

22. What type of activated charcoal is best?

Use an activated charcoal of vegetable or petroleum origin. Do not use activated charcoal of animal origin.

23. Why is syrup of ipecac not recommended if charcoal is used?

Syrup of ipecac renders the charcoal inactive and incapable of adsorbing toxic particles. Likewise, the charcoal binds the syrup of ipecac and renders it unable to produce vomition.

24. What is a saline cathartic?

A cathartic is a substance causing evacuation of the bowels. Sometimes evacuation results from increasing bulk, sometimes from stimulating peristaltic action. A saline cathartic increases fluidity of the intestinal contents by retention of water by osmotic forces and indirectly increases motor activity. Sodium sulfate is a salt, and saline refers to a salt.

25. How is a saline cathartic made? How is it administered?

A saline cathartic is made by mixing either sodium sulfate or magnesium sulfate with enough water to form a thin paste, similar to the consistency of Milk of Magnesia or slightly thinner. The mixture should be administered orally or through a gavage tube or esophageal tube, if the animal is anesthetized. Sodium sulfate is generally preferred and should be administered at approximately 1 gm/kg of body weight. Magnesium sulfate is an alternative to sodium sulfate.

26. Why is a cathartic, especially a saline cathartic, recommended after treatment with activated charcoal?

Activated charcoals are adsorbents. Substances adsorbed to the charcoal also may desorb; hence, the use of a cathartic hastens elimination of the substance while it is still adsorbed to the surface of the charcoal. The mechanism of a saline cathartic is to increase fluid in the bowel osmotically and cause emptying. It does not interfere with other physiologic processes within the body that result from treatment or poisoning.

27. Why is pentobarbital better for a seizing animal than phenobarbital when the seizure is not epileptic?

Pentobarbital allows much faster control of the seizing animal. In cases such as strychnine poisoning, it is important to give the patient relief as quickly as possible because the respiratory muscles are paralyzed. Phenobarbital has a latent period between administration and action. This latent period may be as long as 20 minutes, in which time a seizing patient can die. Therefore, it is appropriate to use an agent that relieves the seizure activity quickly.

28. If I suspect that my patient has eaten a toxic plant, can the diagnosis be confirmed before the patient dies?

Yes, sometimes. History and access to vomitus are the most useful tools. The easiest method is a complete history. Some animals shred a plant without actually consuming it. If portions of the plant can be brought to the clinic, they should be carefully examined to ascertain whether the plant was shredded or eaten. The vomitus can be inspected in a laboratory, usually by a toxicologist competent with microscopic plant particles, to determine what plant was consumed. If the stomach is gavaged, then resulting fluid may be examined.

29. What is the best way to treat an animal suspected of having a poisonous plant intoxication?

If the plant is identified and specific treatment is available, that is the best treatment. If the plant does not have a specific treatment or the plant is unknown, symptomatic treatment is best. Emesis may be indicated to remove as much of the plant from the animal's system as possible.

30. What is the best approach when an animal is believed to have been poisoned?

The first step is to stabilize the animal. If it is seizing, control the seizures; otherwise it is important to follow the ABC rule. That is, establish an airway that is not blocked by some structure; make sure the animal is breathing; and make sure that cardiac output is sufficient to sustain life. Treat the signs exhibited by the animal. Often an owner is convinced that the animal was poisoned by some other substance that may not be consistent with the clinical picture.

31. What information should be recorded in case of litigation in relation to a poisoned animal?

With any case, it is important to keep accurate and detailed records. Records should indicate what procedures were performed and the results. If you are suspicious that the case may involve a legal issue, notify the laboratory. You can always save some samples of vomitus or other tissues in a refrigerator—not a freezer. Your records are legal documents and can be subpoenaed.

32. How can I really find out if the animal has been poisoned?

A thorough history is important. It is probably the best start to solving the mystery. However, at times a toxic diagnosis is the only thing left. Many cases of toxicosis mimic other diseases and situations and may be difficult to definitively diagnose. Others are highly specific, and there is no question. Submitting the proper samples to a diagnostic laboratory can be helpful in determining whether the animal has been poisoned.

33. Why are some substances classified as more toxic than other substances?

Classification is based primarily on how much of the substance is required to induce an intoxication. Perhaps it is best explained by the chart below:

Toxicity Rating Chart

CLASS	TOXICITY
Extremely toxic	< 1 mg/kg
Highly toxic	1–50 mg/kg
Very toxic	50–500 mg/kg
Moderately toxic	0.5–5 gm/kg
Slightly toxic	5–15 gm/kg
Practically nontoxic	> 15 gm/kg

34. What is a dose-response relationship?

For every dose of a substance there is a response, even if the response is death. The dose-response relationship is defined as the level of exposure vs. the magnitude of the biologic reaction. It is possible for a veterinarian to induce toxicity by administering an improper dose of a pharmacologic agent or for an inappropriate amount of time. Pharmacologic agents can cause toxicities, and veterinarians may be responsible for toxicities if proper procedures are violated.

35. Is there a difference between tolerance and action level?

Tolerance level is the maximal quantity of chemical or drug that can legally appear in food for human consumption or in animal feeds. This level is legally set by regulatory agencies and is published in the Code of Federal Regulation or Federal Register. An action level is similar, but it is a guideline and is not legally established. However, regulatory agencies use it in a similar manner as a tolerance.

36. Is there a difference in first-order and zero-order toxicokinetics?

In zero-order kinetics a fixed quantity is excreted during a given time, e.g., 10/mg/kg/day. First-order kinetics is a constant fraction or percentage of a chemical excreted per unit time. First-order kinetics is most common.

37. Why is it important to know if a substance is first-order or zero-order kinetics?

This information allows an estimate of how long the animal may have a potentially dangerous amount of a substance in the body, particularly pharmaceutical products that pets occasionally consume, usually in an accidental setting.

38. When I take a history of an animal, what factors may help to determine whether the animal has been poisoned?

A thorough history is informative and helpful. Histories of particular interest include prior consumption of nonfood items. Sometimes a plant is shredded without consumption. Clues to toxicities are often found in the vomitus or urine. A toxicologic or diagnostic laboratory study is most useful. How attentive the owner is to the animal and its surroundings may give clues to the health status of the animal. Animals that are prone to investigate garbage are more likely to experience toxicities of various natures. Indications from the owner concerning new additions to the surroundings are important. For example, new rugs, new plants, or recent insect treatment to the yard or home are important clues.

39. What are the goals of therapy in treating a poisoned animal?

Goals of therapy always involve emergency intervention and prevention of further exposure. Delay further absorption, whether by bathing or emesis. Application of specific antidotes and remedial measures is important. If possible, hasten the elimination of the absorbed toxicant. Be sure to institute appropriate supportive therapy. If possible, determine the source of the toxicant, and educate the client.

40. Describe the procedure of gastric lavage.

Gastric lavage may be an important way to remove a substance from an animal's stomach. The animal should be unconscious or under light anesthesia with a cuffed endotracheal tube that extends beyond the teeth. Measure the orogastric tube from muzzle to xiphoid cartilage, and mark the tube. The orogastric tube should be the same size as the endotracheal tube. Slightly lower the head and thorax of the animal. Use 5–10 ml/kg of lavage solution for infusion. Aspirate the solution from the stomach using a large aspirator bulb or 50–60-ml syringe. Repeat the cycle 10–15 times. Activated charcoal increases efficiency. It is important to use low pressures and not to force the fluid. Reduce the volume if there are signs or suspicion of a weakened stomach. Do not rupture the esophageal or gastric walls.

41. Is it important to rid the body quickly of a toxin?

Yes. The more quickly a toxicant is removed, the less damage is likely to be done.

42. How can I hasten the elimination of a toxic substance from the body?

Activated charcoal followed by a cathartic, especially a saline cathartic, is one of the best methods to hasten elimination. Always follow activated charcoal with a cathartic. If the substance is water-soluble and can be excreted in the urine, fluid diuresis and ion trapping may be helpful.

43. What methods of eliminating a toxicant from the body are important to consider?

Animals eliminate waste by defecating and urinating. Vomiting may on occasion be a method of elimination as well as gastric lavage. Exhalation and lactation are also routes of elimination. Lactation may intoxicate nursing animals also. If a substance is not water-soluble and is not absorbed by the body, it is likely to be passed in the feces or enter the enterohepatic circulation, which may prolong exposure to a toxic substance. If the substance is water-soluble, it may be excreted in the urine. Fluid diuresis and ion trapping may be helpful.

44. Describe the mechanism of ion trapping. Where in the body can it be used?
The pH of urine may be manipulated so that the substance in question is not reabsorbed. By alkalinizing the urine, products that are acidic are trapped and not reabsorbed; therefore, they are excreted. Likewise, basic substances may be trapped in the bladder by acidifying the urine. This phenomenon is known as ion trapping. Ion trapping may also occur within the stomach.

45. What is the best way to submit stomach contents to a veterinary diagnostic laboratory?
Stomach contents should be submitted in a clean glass jar or clean plastic bag. Stomach contents should be refrigerated, not frozen. If you must ship them to a laboratory, be sure to include adequate ice to keep the sample cool.

46. What is the best tissue to test for organophosphate? How should the tissue be submitted to a veterinary diagnostic laboratory?
The best tissue to test for organophosphates is the brain. Testing the brain for organophosphates is a bit of a misnomer. The brain is actually tested for depressed acetylcholine activity, which indicates probable exposure to organophosphates. If the brain is autolyzed, acetylcholine activity is depressed also. Be sure to keep the brain well chilled, but not frozen.

47. How do you treat a cat that presents with aspirin or acetaminophen intoxication?
Methylene blue has been controversial. It has been maintained for years that it is toxic to cats. However, current work suggests that it may be acceptable, if given with care. The standard treatment has been acetylcysteine (Mucomyst) in a sterile 1–20% solution given at 140 mg/kg orally every 8 hours. Ascorbic acid also may be given at the rate of 200 mg orally 3 times/day.

BIBLIOGRAPHY

1. Osweiler GD, Carson TL, Buck WB, Van Gelder GA: Clinical and Diagnostic Veterinary Toxicology, 3rd ed. Dubuque, IA, Kendall/Hunt, 1976.
2. Osweiler GD: Toxicology. Baltimore, Williams & Wilkins, 1996.
3. Timbrell JA: Introduction to Toxicology, 2nd ed. London, Taylor & Francis, 1995.

101. ETHYLENE GLYCOL INTOXICATION

J. Michael McFarland, D.V.M.

1. What is the lethal dose of ethylene glycol?
In dogs the minimal lethal dose is approximately 4.4–6.6 ml/kg or less than $1/2$ cup for a 10-kg dog. Cats are considerably more sensitive, requiring only 1.4 ml/kg of the full strength solution or $1 1/2$ tsp for a 5-kg cat.

2. What is the pathophysiology of ethylene glycol intoxication?
The effects of ethylene glycol are dose-dependent. When a large volume is ingested, the patient may progress to coma and death within a few hours, primarily because of the direct effect of ethylene glycol on the central nervous system (CNS). If the patient survives this initial phase, liver metabolism via alcohol dehydrogenase leads to the production of several substances capable

of causing severe metabolic acidosis and renal damage. The ethylene glycol metabolites include glycoaldehyde, glycolic acid, glyoxalic acid, and oxalic acid. CNS depression from the effects of glycoaldehyde is accentuated by metabolic acidosis and a high osmolal gap. The other metabolites, particularly glycolate, can cause severe damage to the renal tubular epithelium. Oxalic acid (oxalate) combines with calcium and eventually crystallizes in the renal tubules. The damage caused by the presence of calcium oxalate crystals is thought to be relatively minor. If left untreated, anuric renal failure may develop within 1–4 days.

3. Describe the clinical signs and symptoms associated with ethylene glycol intoxication.
The initial symptoms are similar to those of alcohol intoxication, including depression, stupor, ataxia, knuckling, and vomiting. Unfortunately, these symptoms occur within a few hours of ingestion and frequently go unnoticed by the owner. If the quantity ingested is sufficient, polyuria, polydipsia, and dehydration develop within 12 hours. Thereafter symptoms are primarily associated with oliguric renal failure. Ethylene glycol-intoxicated cats develop renal failure in 12–24 hours. Dogs usually experience renal failure within 48–72 hours. Nonspecific signs include oral ulceration, hypersalivation, vomiting, oliguria with isosthenuria, and eventually (within 4 days) anuria.

4. How can serum osmolality be used in diagnosis?
Ethylene glycol is an effective antifreeze due to its low-molecular-weight osmotic activity. After ingestion, ethylene glycol significantly raises serum osmolality within 1 hour. Hyperosmolality usually peaks within 6 hours and remains elevated for up to 24 hours. Normal serum osmolality in the dog and cat is 280–310 mOsm/kg. The normal osmolal gap is less than 10 mOsm/kg. Osmolal gap is the difference between measured serum osmolality and calculated osmolality. A formula for calculating serum osmolality (in mOsm/kg) is as follows:

$$1.86 (Na + K) + glucose/18 + BUN/2.8 + 9$$

where N = sodium, K = potassium, and BUN = blood urea nitrogen. Ingestion of ethylene glycol can cause characteristically high osmolar gaps (> 30 in cats and > 50 in dogs). Discovering a high osmolar gap in an acutely depressed or vomiting animal may be an effective way of diagnosing ethylene glycol intoxication. However, because of the potential delay in presentation, a low serum osmolality does not rule out ethylene glycol exposure.

5. What other common laboratory findings are associated with ethylene glycol intoxication?
The metabolites of ethylene glycol are potent organic acids. Therefore, severe metabolic acidemia develops within a few hours of ingestion. The presence of these organic acids increases anion gap (AG) significantly. Anion gap (normal: 10–15 mEq/L) is calculated as follows:

$$AG = (Na + K) - (HCO_3 + Cl)$$

Urinalysis is important in the diagnosis of ethylene glycol intoxication. Calcium oxalate crystalluria is a consistent finding. These crystals occur in several forms. The most common associated with ethylene glycol ingestion is the monohydrate (6-sided prism) crystal. In addition, urine specific gravity decreases by 3 hours after ingestion to the isosthenuric range (1.012–1.014). Another consistent finding is a low urine pH. Hematuria, proteinuria, and glucosuria are less common findings. With the onset of renal failure, azotemia and hyperphosphatemia develop. As renal failure progresses, hyperkalemia occurs. Consumption of calcium by chelation with oxalic acid leads to hypocalcemia.

6. Are any other reliable diagnostic tests available?
In-house ethylene glycol test kits are readily available, but they are not reliable 18 hours after ingestion. False-positive results may occur if substances containing propylene glycol (e.g., some forms of activated charcoal) are administered before testing. However, a positive result in conjunction with appropriate history and clinical signs is a strong indication for treatment.

7. Describe the goals of treatment in ethylene glycol intoxication.

As with most other types of intoxication, the first goal of treatment is to prevent absorption. Vomiting should be induced if ingestion has occurred within 2 hours. Gastric lavage and administration of activated charcoal are also indicated.

The metabolites of ethylene glycol are primarily responsible for the life-threatening damage. Nearly all of the ethylene glycol ingested is excreted or metabolized within 48 hours. Therefore, it is extremely important to interfere with the action of alcohol dehydrogenase (ADH) on ethylene glycol as soon after exposure as possible. Ideally, therapy with an ADH inhibitor should be started within 3 hours of ingestion in cats and within 8 hours of ingestion in dogs.

Supportive care and close monitoring are crucial. Fluid therapy is necessary to correct electrolyte and acid-base imbalance, restore hydration, increase tissue perfusion, and promote diuresis. Fluid rates should start at 3 times daily fluid maintenance and be adjusted as needed. Use the following formula to calculate daily fluid maintenance requirements:

$$\text{Daily fluid maintenance requirement (ml)} = (30 \times \text{kg body weight}) + 70$$

A conservative approach to bicarbonate supplementation is recommended, taking into account the positive effect of fluid therapy on acid-base disorders. The following formula may be used to determine sodium bicarbonate requirements:

$$\text{mEq of sodium bicarbonate needed} = (\text{body weight [kg]} \times 0.3 \times (12-HCO_3))/3$$

8. What methods can be used to inhibit ethylene glycol metabolism by alcohol dehydrogenase?

The classical method of preventing ethylene glycol metabolism is infusion of 20% ethanol. Ethanol has a higher affinity for ADH than ethylene glycol. In dogs, the suggested dose is 5.5 ml/kg given intravenously every 4 hours for 5 treatments, then every 6 hours for 4 treatments. In cats, the suggested dose is 5 ml/kg IV every 6 hours for 5 treatments, then every 8 hours for 4 treatments. Bolus injections are not recommended. The ethanol should be administered slowly over 1 hour or delivered by constant-rate infusion.

The disadvantages of ethanol infusion include increased severity of CNS depression, acidemia, hyperosmolarity, and hypothermia. An ideal ADH inhibitor in dogs, with no side effects, is 4-methylpyrazole (4-MP). 4-MP is not currently recommended for use in cats. The suggested protocol for 4-MP treatment is as follows:

INITIAL LOADING DOSE	12 AND 24 HOURS AFTER INITIAL DOSE	36 HOURS AFTER INITIAL DOSE
20 mg/kg	15 mg/kg	5 mg/kg

Although 4-MP is an excellent option for treatment of dogs with ethylene glycol intoxication, it has been very difficult for the practitioner to obtain. In early 1997, 4-MP will be commercially available as Antizol-Vet (Orphan Medical, Minnetonka, MN).

BIBLIOGRAPHY

1. Beasley VR, Buck WB: Acute ethylene glycol toxicosis: A review. Vet Hum Toxicol 22(4):255–263, 1980.
2. Connally HE, Thrall MA, Forney SD, et al: Safety and efficacy of 4-methylpyrazole for treatment of suspected or confirmed ethylene glycol intoxication in dogs: 107 cases (1983–1995). J Am Vet Med Assoc 209:1880–1888, 1996.
3. Dial SM, Thrall MA, Hamar DW: The use of 4-methyl pyrazole as treatment for ethylene glycol intoxication in the dog. J Am Vet Med Assoc 195:73–76, 1989.
4. Dial SM, Hull-Thrall MA, Hamar DW: Efficacy of 4-methylpyrazole for treatment of ethylene glycol intoxication in dogs. Am J Vet Res 55:1762–1770, 1994.
5. Dial SM, Hull-Thrall MA, Hamar DW: Comparison of ethanol and 4-methylpyrazole as treatments for ethylene glycol intoxication in cats. Am J Vet Res 55:1771–1782, 1994.
6. Frederick C: Utility of the serum osmol gap in the diagnosis of methanol or ethylene glycol ingestion. Ann Emerg Med 27:343–346, 1996.
7. Grauer GF, Thrall MA, Henre BA, et al: Early clinicopathologic findings in dogs ingesting ethylene glycol. Am J Vet Res 45:2299–2303, 1984.

8. Grauer GF, Thrall MA, Henre BA, Hjelle JJ: Comparison of the effects of ethanol and 4-methylpyrazole on the pharmacokinetics and toxicity of ethylene glycol in the dog. Toxicol Let 35:307–314, 1987.
9. Thrall MA, Grauer GF, Mero KN: Clinicopathologic findings in dogs and cats with ethylene glycol intoxication. J Am Vet Med Assoc 184:37–41, 1984.

102. LEAD POISONING

Colleen Murray, D.V.M.

1. What are the most common sources of lead exposure for companion animals?

The most common route of entry of lead is through the gastrointestinal tract. Lead sources include flaking paint from buildings painted prior to 1950, ashes from lumber painted prior to 1950, curtain weights, fishing sinkers, old lead toys, storage batteries, paint flakes and dust from bridges and water towers, artist's paints, solder, lead shot, lead glazed pottery, linoleum, putty, industrial pipe dope compounds, gasoline, motor oil, tar paper, golf balls, roofing materials, insulations, lead emissions that settle on soil or vegetation, and some inks and dyes.

2. What are the clinical signs of lead intoxication?

The primary signs are gastroenteritis and neurologic problems. As a rule, the neurologic signs predominate in acute, high level exposure to lead, whereas gastrointestinal signs result from lower, long-term exposures. The most common neurologic signs are convulsions, hysteria (barking, crying, running, indiscriminate biting), ataxia, tremors, blindness, clamping of jaws, grinding of teeth, and other behavioral changes. Such clinical signs may be mistaken for canine distemper and rabies. The most common gastrointestinal signs are vomiting, abdominal pain, tense abdomen, and anorexia.

3. What are the most common laboratory and radiographic findings?

Of prime importance is the finding of large numbers of nucleated erythrocytes (5–40+/100 white blood cells) without anemia. Other common findings include neutrophilic leukocytosis, basophilic stippling, and other abnormalities of red blood cell morphology.

The most helpful radiographic finding is the presence of radiopaque material in the gastrointestinal tract. However, it is impossible to differentiate these radiographic densities from substances such as bone and gravel. Lead shot is a common radiographic finding in hunting dogs; it is typically not a problem in mammals but may be in birds. A small number of young, rapidly growing dogs may develop lead lines on the metaphyses of long bones. Lead lines are difficult to distinguish and are best seen proximal to the open epiphysis of the distal radius, ulna, and metacarpal bones.

4. What diagnostic tests are available?

Chemical detection of lead intoxication is best confirmed by abnormally high levels of lead using heparinized whole blood (check with the local laboratory for other blood-testing options). Blood levels > 0.4 ppm associated with clinical signs are diagnostic (normal: 0.05–0.25 ppm). Feces, liver, and kidney can also be tested. Lead levels greater than 35 ppm indicate exposure to lead in the feces. Lead levels greater than 5 ppm in the liver and 10 ppm in the kidney are significant.

5. What is the treatment?

Therapy for lead poisoning involves removal of lead from the gastrointestinal tract, blood, and body tissues; alleviation of neurologic signs; and prevention of reexposure. Lead should be removed from the gastrointestinal tract with enemas, emetics, and possibly surgery for large items in the stomach and intestines. Chelating agents have been used historically to bind to the absorbed lead, forming nontoxic, water-soluble complexes that can be excreted via the urine or bile. In the past, $CaNa_2EDTA$ has been the drug used for treatment. The dosage ranged from 75–110 mg/kg daily for 2–5 days. The daily dose is divided into 4 equal parts and given subcutaneously after dilution to a concentration of about 10 mg $CaNa_2EDTA$/ml in a 5% dextrose solution (high concentrations of $CaNa_2EDTA$ can be painful). $CaNa_2EDTA$ may be given by slow intravenous push in critically ill animals. Multiple treatments can be used in combinations of 5 days on, 5 days off. $CaNa_2EDTA$ is not without side effects. It may produce a reversible, acute necrotizing nephrosis, gastroenteritis, and depression. It should never be given to an animal in the absence of adequate hydration or urine flow. Rapid mobilization of lead from bone can aggravate signs of lead poisoning or even kill dogs with high body burdens of lead. $CaNa_2EDTA$ can also deplete other vital metals by nonspecific binding with zinc, copper, and iron.

The oral chelating agent D-penicillamine can be used in animals that are not acutely ill. It also may be used as a follow-up treatment to $CaNa_2EDTA$. Dosages range from 35–110 mg/kg divided into 3 or 4 daily doses for 1 week on, 1 week off. Multiple treatments may be needed for total recovery. D-penicillamine also may have adverse side effects. It is contraindicated in animals with penicillin allergies and may cause renal damage.

The drug of choice for lead intoxication is meso-2,3 dimercaptosuccinic acid (DMSA) (Chemet, McNeil Consumer Products Co., Fort Washington, PA). DMSA is a more specific chelator than $CaNa_2EDTA$, binding to the highest degree with lead, mercury, and arsenic. It does not deplete other body metals. Chelated metals are excreted in urine. Unlike $CaNa_2EDTA$, DMSA is not associated with chelation-induced absorption of lead from the gut or mobilization of lead into the body during therapy. In the original study by Ramsey, dogs treated with DMSA suffered no side effects except reports of halitosis and malodorous feces, characterized by an unpleasant sulphur smell. Dogs are treated with gelatin capsules at a dosage of 10 mg/kg every 8 hrs orally for 10 days.

6. What is the public health significance of lead intoxication?

The veterinarian should consider companion animals a sentinel for lead. The pet owner should be fully informed of the risk that lead presents for humans, especially children. If the situation indicates potential exposure, everyone in the home should be referred to the family physician for lead testing. Every effort should be made to identify the source of lead intoxication and to eliminate it from the environment. If identifying the source proves impossible, the pet should be tested for reexposure at selected intervals.

BIBLIOGRAPHY

1. Bratton GR, Kowalczyk DF: Lead Poisoning. Current Veterinary Therapy X. Philadelphia, W.B. Saunders, 1989, pp 152–159.
2. Ettinger SJ, Feldman EC: Toxicology. Textbook of Veterinary Internal Medicine. Philadelphia, W.B. Saunders, 1995, p 318.
3. Morgan RV: Lead Poisoning in Small Animals: Recent Trends. Proceedings of the 12th ACVIM Forum. 1994, pp 262–263.
4. Ramsey DT, et al: Use of orally administered succimer (meso-2,3 dimercaptosuccinic acid) for treatment of lead poisoning in dogs. J Am Vet Med Assoc 208:371–375, 1996.

103. ORGANOPHOSPHATE AND CARBAMATE TOXICITY

J. Michael Walters, D.V.M.

1. What are the two classes of cholinergic pesticides? Why do they cause toxicity?

The most common types of cholinergic pesticides formulated for use in cats and dogs are the organophosphates (OP) and carbamates. They are widely used in the control of fleas and ticks. Toxicoses can occur from accidental exposure, intentional misuse, and rarely, from idiosyncratic or allergic hypersensitivity reactions in cats and dogs. These two classes of pesticides differ in chemical structure and site of action on the acetylcholinesterase enzyme. Organophosphates are acetylcholinesterase inhibitors that disable the enzyme by an irreversible binding process known as "aging," whereas carbamates are reversible cholinesterase inhibitors. The signs of poisoning are similar.

2. What nervous pathways are affected by cholinergic pesticides?

Clinical signs are usually correlated with an overriding of the parasympathetic pathways but also may result from sympathetic stimulation. Acetylcholine stimulates nicotinic receptors of the somatic nervous system, parasympathetic preganglionic nicotinic and muscarinic postganglionic receptors, and sympathetic preganglionic nicotinic receptors. The effector organ of the somatic nervous system is skeletal muscle. Effector organs of the parasympathetic nervous system are the iris, cardiac muscle, blood vessels, smooth muscle of the lungs, smooth muscle of the gastrointestinal (GI) system, and exocrine glands. Effector organs of the sympathetic nervous system can be stimulated through preganglionic cholinergic neuron stimulation of the postganglionic adrenergic neurons in the adrenal gland, cardiac muscle, iris, blood vessels, smooth muscle of the lungs, smooth muscle of the GI system, and exocrine glands. The degree to which the parasympathetic or sympathetic nervous pathways is stimulated depends on many factors and explains the mix of clinical signs.

3. Where and how do cholinergic pesticides effect their toxicity?

Under normal conditions there is rapid hydrolysis of acetylcholine by acetylcholinesterase after neurochemical transmission at autonomic and neuromuscular synapses. In OP poisoning, phosphate radicals covalently bind to an active site on the enzyme, rendering it inactive. This process of producing an inactive enzyme is known as "aging," which is believed to fix an extra charge to the protein, altering the active site and thereby preventing regeneration. This inhibition of the acetylcholinesterase activity allows accumulation of acetylcholine at the synapses, resulting in overstimulation and later disruption of transmission in the CNS, parasympathetic nerve endings, some sympathetic nerve endings, somatic nerve, and autonomic ganglia. Carbamates lead to carbamylation of acetylcholinesterase; this bond is broken down within 48 hours with regeneration of acetylcholinesterase to the active form of the enzyme.

4. Where are the compounds absorbed? How are they metabolized?

Most of the compounds are absorbed from the conjunctiva, skin, lungs, and GI tract. Once absorbed, they undergo extensive hepatic biotransformation, the route and rate are highly species-specific.

5. What are the clinical signs of toxicity due to cholinergic pesticides?

Toxicoses from OP or carbamate insecticides may occur in dogs or cats when yard or agricultural formulations are ingested or misused, when dips are incorrectly diluted, when cholinesterase-inhibiting compounds are used in conjunction with other topical or systemic OPs, when products labeled for use in dogs are used on cats, or when unusually sensitive pets are exposed. Chlor-pyrifos formulation is an example of a common pesticide that is misused on cats and may result in either acute or chronic toxicoses. Clinical signs of OP or carbamate toxicoses most commonly result from parasympathetic stimulation. Clinical signs include vomiting, depression, hypersali-vation, muscle tremors, diarrhea, ataxia, anorexia, hyperthermia, dyspnea, seizure, weakness, and death. Classic signs of toxicosis include miosis and bradycardia. Postmortem lesions associated with OP and carbamate toxicoses are nonspecific. Chronic anorexia, muscle weakness, and twitching may occur in cats with or without episodes of acute toxicoses. Occasionally signs of sympathetic nervous system stimulation can occur, such as tachycardia, and should not be con-sidered inconsistent. Carbamate-containing pesticides, such as carbofuran, can produce rapid onset of seizure and respiratory failure and require aggressive therapy.

6. What OP and carbamate pesticides are commonly available?

Organophosphate compounds commonly available include chlorpyrifos, cythioate, diazinon, dichlorvos, fenthion, phosmet, tetrachlorvinphos, and safrotin. Carbamate insecticides include carbaryl, propoxur, methomyl, and bendiocarb. Individual toxicity varies and depends on the route of exposure.

7. How is the diagnosis made?

History of exposure associated with clinical signs of parasympathetic and skeletal muscle stimulation warrants a tentative diagnosis of poisoning. Chemical analyses are generally unre-warding because rapid metabolism results in low tissue levels. Recent evidence has shown that metabolites of these pesticides may be detected in the urine and may aid in the diagnosis. Finding insecticide in the stomach contents can be quite valuable in establishing the diagnosis. An important part of confirming a diagnosis is to assess the degree of inhibition of acetyl-cholinesterase activity in whole blood, serum, or tissue of the affected animal. A reduction in whole blood/serum acetylcholinesterase activity to less than 25% of normal is indicative of ex-cessive exposure. Depending on the insecticide used, the acetylcholinesterase activity in dogs may remain depressed for several days to several weeks after exposure. Some acetyl-cholinesterase activity depression is to be expected after routine use of insecticides. Therefore, whole blood/serum acetylcholinesterase activity should be viewed only as an indication of the status of the acetylcholinesterase enzymes in the body. Acetylcholinesterase activity can be measured in the brain and generally is less than 10% of normal activity in affected animals. For best laboratory results, whole blood/serum and brain tissue samples should be well chilled or frozen before submission. A sagittal half of the brain should be submitted, because laboratories vary in the portion of the brain used for determination of acetylcholinesterase activity. Samples of stomach contents as well as any suspected material should be frozen and submitted to the laboratory for chemical analysis. Other biochemical analysis can be performed such as com-plete blood count, serum chemistry panel, liver function tests, electrocardiogram, and chest radiographs.

8. What is the emergency management?

Effective supportive care is paramount, as is the use of specific antidotes. The ABCs of emergency case management should be followed. Establish an airway, and provide oxygen as necessary. Respiratory distress may be due to excessive secretions, bronchospasm, pulmonary edema, chemical pneumonitis, aspiration, adult respiratory distress syndrome, muscle weakness, or paralysis. Intravenous access should be established in severe cases, and specific therapy should be instituted. A detailed history of pesticide exposure and use, active ingredients, clinical signs, onset and duration of clinical signs, and exposure dose are important. If the patient has ingested an OP or carbamate product within the past 2 hours of presentation and is asymptomatic, an emetic such as 3% hydrogen peroxide (2 ml/kg orally; maximal dose: 45 ml) should be used after feeding a moistened meal. Emesis with hydrogen peroxide is reliable if adequate ingesta are in the stomach. Alternatively, apomorphine may be used to induce emesis. Induction of emesis after ingestion of a liquid OP should be avoided because of potential aspiration and pulmonary injury from petroleum distillate solvents. Induction of emesis after ingestion of carbamates should be avoided or attempted with caution because of the potential for rapid onset of seizures. Activated charcoal after oral ingestion (2.0 ml/kg orally or via stomach tube) mixed with a cathartic such as 70% sorbitol (3.0 ml/kg) diluted with water should be used to absorb any residual pesticide. Patients who are symptomatic after recently ingesting significant quantities of an insecticide product should be anesthetized and intubated with a cuffed endotracheal tube; gastric lavage should be performed using a large-bore orogastric tube. Gastric lavage should be performed until no more ingesta are evident, followed by a final wash of activated charcoal/sorbitol slurry. If some time has passed since the ingestion of the toxin, activated charcoal/sorbitol without emesis or lavage may have greater efficacy.

If the pet presents with seizures, phenobarbital (6 mg/kg, to effect) and atropine (0.2 mg/kg, ¼ intravenously, the remainder subcutaneously or intramuscularly) should be used to control the seizure and combat the parasympathetic signs. Diazepam has been shown to potentiate OP toxicosis; the exact mechanism is unknown but is thought to result from activation of muscarinic signs by CNS sedation or by competitive release of bound insecticide. Because of the potential of worsening clinical signs, diazepam should not be used in cases of suspected OP toxicosis. Atropine is administered as needed to control life-threatening clinical signs such as respiratory depression, bronchoconstriction, and bradycardia. Atropine should not be used unless clinical signs are present and should be titrated to effect. Oxygen and ventilator support may be necessary until respiratory function returns to normal.

Clinical signs such as muscle fasciculation, resulting from the nicotinic receptor stimulation by OP, can be reduced by using pralidoxime chloride (2-PAM, Protopam) administered at 10–15 mg/kg intramuscularly or subcutaneously every 8–12 hours. Pralidoxime chloride is most effective when administered within the first 24 hours of exposure. Pralidoxime chloride should be continued for approximately 36 hours before cessation due to lack of improvement. Unused pralidoxime chloride may be refrigerated for up to 2 weeks if wrapped in foil.

Once the animal is stabilized, a mild detergent bath should be performed to remove adherent chemical in cases of dermal exposure and to help reduce further cutaneous absorption or ingestion while grooming. Activated charcoal may benefit even cases of dermal exposure because of biliary excretion and intestinal reabsorption of some OP compounds or metabolites. Dosages of 1 gm/kg every 6–8 hours should be repeated until improvement is evident.

Intravenous fluids, nutritional support, and maintenance of normal body temperature are important. The owner needs to be aware that nursing care and nutritional support may be needed for 1–4 weeks.

9. Are cats any more or less susceptible to OP or carbamates?

Cats can be extremely sensitive to OP and carbamates, especially chlorpyrifos. Chronic OP toxicosis may develop from the purposeful systemic or topical application of insecticidal agents or from a prolonged exposure to a contaminated environment. Cats appear to be more sensitive to chronic OP toxicosis than dogs.

10. What are the signs of chronic OP toxicosis in cats?

Chronic OP toxicosis in cats causes signs of CNS disturbance, including ataxia, lethargy, or anorexia and nicotinic signs of neuromuscular dysfunction, without the classic SLUD (salivation, lacrimation, urination, defecation) signs of the muscarinic syndrome of acute OP toxicosis. Chronic OP toxicosis is more difficult to diagnose because the signs have a much slower rate of onset (days to weeks), are less specific, and mimic signs caused by other systemic, infectious, nutritional, metabolic, and neuromuscular diseases.

11. What is considered a toxic amount of chlorpyrifos in cats?

The oral minimal lethal dose in cats is 10–40 mg/kg. The acute LD_{50} of chlorpyrifos is 118–245 mg/kg in rats, 504 mg/kg in guinea pigs, and approximately 2000 mg/kg in rabbits.

12. How is chronic chlorpyrifos toxicosis diagnosed in cats?

The diagnosis is similar to that of any other OP toxicosis. History of exposure to a sufficient amount coupled with clinical signs is adequate to make a tentative diagnosis of OP toxicosis. Additional supportive information from blood/serum or tissue acetylcholinesterase activity helps to confirm the diagnosis.

13. How is chronic chlorpyrifos toxicosis treated in cats?

Treatment in cats can be demanding and time-consuming. Most cats are not presented until 2–5 days after exposure. Redistribution of the compound to adipose tissue, particularly subcutaneous fat after dermal exposure, may create a depot effect that slowly releases the pesticide, resulting in continued exposure. Treatment, therefore, may have to be continued for weeks, even if it is initiated within a few hours of exposure.

Atropine (0.2 mg/kg, $^{1}/_{4}$ intravenously, the remainder subcutaneously or intramuscularly) as needed and 2-PAM (10–15 mg/kg intramuscularly or subcutaneously, every 12 hr) should be started before bathing or feeding to help reduce the stress of treatments. Stress can trigger a respiratory crisis. Atropine and 2-PAM may be less than effective in cases of chronic OP exposure because of aging of the enzyme-insecticide complex. Diphenhydramine has been shown to help block the effects of nicotinic receptor overstimulation and to improve muscle strength in some animals with OP toxicosis. Other treatment methods, such as bathing, activated charcoal, and supportive care, are also important.

BIBLIOGRAPHY

1. Aiuto LA, Pavlakis SG, Boxer RA: Life-threatening organophosphate-induced delayed polyneuropathy in a child after accidental chlorpyrifos ingestion. J Pediatr 122(4):658–660, 1993.
2. Fikes JD: Toxicology of selected pesticides, drugs and chemicals. Organophosphate and carbamate insecticides. Vet Clin North Am Small Anim Pract 20(2):353–367, 1990.
3. Hooser SB, Beasley VR, Sundberg JP, Harlin K: Toxicologic evaluations of chlorpyrifos in cats. Am J Vet Res 49:1371–1375, 1988.
4. Levy JK: Chronic chlorpyrifos toxicosis in a cat. J Am Vet Med Assoc 203:1682–1684, 1684–1686, 1993.
5. Nafe L: Selected neurotoxins. Vet Clin North Am Small Anim Pract 18(3):593–604, 1988.
6. Wagner SL, Orwick DL: Chronic organophosphate exposure associated with transient hypertonia in an infant. Pediatrics 94(1):94–97, 1994.

104. ANTICOAGULANT RODENTICIDE TOXICITY

J. Michael Walters, D.V.M.

1. How were the anticoagulant rodenticides developed?

The anticoagulant rodenticides were developed after investigations of moldy sweetclover poisoning in cattle. A naturally occurring coumarin is converted to dicumarol, the toxic agent. Warfarin was synthesized from this toxic agent while its mode of action was under study. Warfarin has subsequently been widely used as a rodenticide. With continued use, warfarin-based anticoagulant rodenticides began to develop resistance in target animals. Subsequently, more potent rodenticides were developed, which had led to some difficulties in treating the nontarget host. Warfarin and other anticoagulant rodenticides (indandione derivatives) that are not effective against warfarin-resistant rodents are considered first-generation rodenticides whereas those effective against the more resistant rodents are second-generation rodenticides.

2. Describe their mechanism of action.

The essential toxic mechanism is depletion of vitamin K_1. Clotting factors II, VII, IX, and X must bind calcium to be active in clot formation. Dicarboxylic acid groups on the clotting factor form the active site that binds calcium. These factors require vitamin K_1 to form the dicarboxylic acid groups. Vitamin K epoxide reductase is the enzymatic lesion of biologic importance; without this enzyme, vitamin K cannot be recycled. This leads to rapid depletion of vitamin K stores, and synthesis of new clotting factors is impaired. Clotting factors II, VII, IX, and X have the shortest half-lives (41, 6.2, 13.9, and 16.5 hours, respectively) in dogs; therefore, they can be rapidly depleted if not replenished. This leads to the "lag-time" that follows ingestion of the bait and onset of clinical signs.

3. How toxic are anticoagulant rodenticides?

Eight different anticoagulant rodenticides are sold over the counter and through exterminators in the United States. Generally, the pest must ingest a first-generation rodenticide for some time before it receives a lethal dose. This led to the development of second-generation rodenticides, which are more lethal with a single dose. Single-dose lethality was achieved by maximizing the potency, biologic duration of action, or both. Therefore, second-generation anticoagulant rodenticides are more potent, last longer, or both compared with first-generation anticoagulant rodenticides.

Toxicity of Rodenticides in Dogs and Cats

CHEMICAL	BAIT CONCENTRATION (PPM)	COMPOUND (MG/KG) DOG	COMPOUND (MG/KG) CAT	BAIT (OZ/LB) DOG
Warfarin	250	20–300	3–30	1.3
Fumarin	250	?	?	?
Pindone	250	5–75	?	?
Valone	250	?	?	?
Diphacinone	50	0.9–8	15	0.3
Chlorphacinone	50	?	?	?
Brodifacoum	50	0.2–4	~ 25	0.06
Bromadiolone	50	11–15	> 25	3.5

4. What are the common clinical signs?

Typically, the initial clinical signs include depression, weakness, and dyspnea. External signs of hemorrhage include melena, epistaxis, hematemesis, hematuria, gingival bleeding, excessive hemorrhage from a wound, or bruising; these signs may or may not be immediately evident. Internal hemorrhage into the pleural and/or peritoneal cavities is also common.

5. How is the diagnosis made?

Differential considerations include disseminated intravascular coagulation, congenital factor deficiencies, von Willebrand's disease, hyperviscosity syndromes, platelet deficiencies, thrombocytopathies, and canine ehrlichiosis. Laboratory tests such as a clotting profile (one-stage prothrombin time [OSPT], activated partial thromboplastin time [APTT], fibrin degradation products, platelet count), factor testing, buccal mucosal bleeding times, activated clotting time (ACT), and serology should be considered whenever possible. A thorough history and exposure potential are by far the most important. A positive response to a 24-hour therapeutic trial of vitamin K_1 is also strongly suggestive. Prolongation of coagulation parameters—ACT (> 120–150 sec), OSPT, and APTT—are common. Platelet counts can be normal or decreased. Conclusive laboratory testing is analytical detection of the rodenticide.

6. Does the type of toxin have any influence on the length of the treatment course?

Yes. Once the diagnosis is made, the type of anticoagulant rodenticide has a major influence on the length of treatment. Because no tests distinguish between first- and second-generation anticoagulant rodenticides, proper identification may rely on recovering a package or portion of the agent to determine how long to treat. If the package is unavailable, the owner should be instructed to return to the store where it was purchased so that the active ingredients can be identified. Most first-generation anticoagulant rodenticides require a much shorter length of therapy (7–10 days), whereas second-generation anticoagulant rodenticides may require as long as 4–6 weeks. Below is a list of the common anticoagulant rodenticides and recommended length of treatment:

Chemical Name	Length of Treatment
Warfarin (first generation)	4–6 days
Diphacinone (second generation)	3–4 weeks
Chlorphacinone (second generation)	3–4 weeks
Brodifacoum (second generation)	3–4 weeks
Bromadiolone (second generation)	3–4 weeks

7. What therapeutic methods are used to treat anticoagulant rodenticides?

Vitamin K_1 is the preferred form of vitamin K. Both parenteral and oral forms are available. The intravenous route should not be used because of the high risk of anaphylaxis. The dosage of vitamin K_1 depends on the type (first- vs. second-generation anticoagulant rodenticide). Second-generation anticoagulant rodenticides require dosages 5–25 times higher than first-generation rodenticides. The most common routes of administration are oral and subcutaneous. Oral absorption of vitamin K may be improved by a fatty meal. A can of food with vitamin K improves absorption 4–5-fold compared with vitamin K administered alone. An initial intramuscular dose of vitamin K_1 may result in a life-threatening intramuscular hemorrhage; therefore, this route should be discouraged for initial therapy. Hypovolemic animals may have poor uptake of the drug from subcutaneous injection, although it is preferred to intravenous injection. With warfarin-based rodenticides, a loading dose of 0.25 to 2.5 mg/kg subcutaneously can be used, followed by oral medications for 4–6 days. Loading doses as high as the oral dose are often used. For second-generation rodenticides the dosage range is 2.5–5 mg/kg subcutaneously and then orally for 4–6 weeks. Higher dose ranges and longer treatment times are imperative. Most treatment failures with second-generation anticoagulant rodenticides are due to use of the lower warfarin-based treatment regimen for an inadequate time. Because vitamin K has no effect on the metabolism or elimination of the rodenticide, therapy must be maintained until toxic amounts of the material are no longer present within the animal.

When prompt control of hemorrhage is needed, an infusion of fresh or fresh frozen plasma provides concentrations of factors II, VII, IX, and X. This infusion can be repeated every 6 hours if needed. The amount of plasma should be approximately 5–10% of the patient's total blood volume, assuming a blood volume of 90 ml/kg for dogs and 70 ml/kg for cats. When anemia is coexistent, fresh whole blood or packed red blood cells and fresh frozen plasma can be used.

8. Can vitamin K_3 be used to treat anticoagulant rodenticide intoxications?

No. Although vitamin K_3 has been used as a feed additive, it is completely ineffective in the treatment of warfarin or dicumarol toxicity. The production and marketing of injectable vitamin K_3 was suspended in 1985 by the Center for Veterinary Medicine of the Food and Drug Administration because it was found to induce Heinz-body anemia, methemoglobinuria, urobilinuria, and hepatic damage at dosages of 25 mg/kg.

9. How do you decide when to stop treatment?

Current recommendations are to measure prothrombin times 2–3 days after cessation of an adequate course of vitamin K_1 for the type of anticoagulant rodenticide. Others feel that prothrombin times are inadequate for mild-to-moderate reductions in factor VII activity (the factor with the shortest half-life) and that more sensitive tests should be used. Proteins induced by vitamin K absence or antagonism (PIVKA) are perhaps unfamiliar to most veterinarians, but once this test is understood, it is quite useful in the diagnosis and treatment of anticoagulant rodenticides. The PIVKA test (Thrombotest, Nycomed Pharma AS, Oslo, Norway) is a sensitive test for coagulation factors II, VII, and X as well as the PIVKA proteins and was developed for the specific control of anticoagulant therapy. If PIVKA remains normal 48 hours after suspected exposure to a rodenticide or 48 hours after cessation of vitamin K_1 therapy, there is no need for continued treatment. In dogs with active hemorrhage due to intoxication with one of the long-acting rodenticides, it is safest to continue treatment for 4–6 weeks. The same may be said for animals exposed to an unknown quantity and type of rodenticide. It is advisable to treat them for an extended time rather than to stop treatment prematurely. Theoretically, there is a possibility of greater sensitivity upon reexposure; therefore, owners may want to change the type of rodenticide that they use.

BIBLIOGRAPHY

1. Bellah JR, Weigel JP: Hemarthrosis secondary to suspected warfarin toxicosis in a dog. J Am Vet Med Assoc 182:1126–1127, 1983.
2. Mount ME: Proteins induced by vitamin K absence or antagonists (PIVKA). In Kirk RW (ed): Current Veterinary Therapy IX. Philadelphia, W.B. Saunders, 1986, pp 513–515.
3. Mount ME, Feldman BF: Mechanism of diphacinone rodenticide toxicosis in the dog and its therapeutic implications. Am J Vet Res 44:2009–2017, 1983.
4. Mount ME, Feldman BF, Buffington T: Vitamin K and its therapeutic importance. J Am Vet Med Assoc 180:1354–1356, 1982.
5. Peterson J, Streeter V: Laryngeal obstruction secondary to brodifacoum toxicosis in a dog [clinical conference]. J Am Vet Med Assoc 208:352–354, 354–355, 1996.
6. Schaer M, Henderson C: Suspected warfarin toxicosis in a dog. J Am Vet Med Assoc 176:535–536, 1980.

105. CHOLECALCIFEROL TOXICITY

J. Michael Walters, D.V.M.

1. Besides warfarin, what other rodenticides are in common use?

Rodenticides that contain vitamin D_3 (cholecalciferol) as the active components have recently been introduced, with the claim that they are less toxic to dogs and human beings than to rats. This claim has been challenged by a recent study concluding that these products pose a significant risk to dogs.

2. How long does it take for cholecalciferol rodenticides to work?

In the nontarget host a few days may be all that is required before clinical signs of toxicosis appear. Vitamin D was reported at one time to be a cumulative toxin, requiring 1–2 weeks before its maximal effects on the mineral metabolism occur, but the time probably depends on the amount of rodenticide ingested.

3. What are the typical clinical signs of cholecalciferol toxicosis?

Signs of toxicosis are relatively nonspecific, such as lethargy, anorexia, vomiting, weakness, ataxia, hematemesis, and shock. A history of polyuria and polydipsia also may be noted. Most commonly the potential for exposure to a cholecalciferol rodenticide is reported. The clinical effects of vitamin D toxicosis result from increases in osteoclastic activity in bone and increased intestinal absorption of calcium, resulting in hypercalcemia and hyperphosphatemia. Death is attributable to the sustained effects of hypercalcemia.

4. What are the common biochemical findings?

Biochemical analysis typically indicates hypercalcemia with concurrent hyperphosphatemia, although normophosphatemia and transient normocalcemia have been reported. Varying degrees of azotemia can be found, coupled with inadequately concentrated urine (isosthenuria). Glucosuria and proteinuria also may be present. Complete blood counts generally yield nonspecific findings; a normal or stress leukogram is common.

5. Do any special laboratory or diagnostic analyses confirm the diagnosis?

High-performance liquid chromatography has been used to determine serum levels of 25-hydroxycholecalciferol. It may be difficult to locate a laboratory that performs this analysis, and normal values vary from laboratory to laboratory. If used, it probably is wise to submit samples from similar-aged animals, if possible, to provide a basis for normal. Abdominal ultrasonography of the kidneys can be performed as well. Increased echogenicity of the renal cortex that is indicative of glomerulonephritis, nephrocalcinosis, or tubular necrosis is a common finding in cholecalciferol rodenticide toxicosis and can be used as supportive data of metastatic calcification.

6. What does a differential list include?

Hypercalcemia of malignancy (pseudohyperparathyroidism), primary hyperparathyroidism, hypoadrenocorticism, primary renal failure, nutritional oversupplementation, and certain plants such as *Cestrum* sp. (day-blooming jessamine, day Cestrum, wild jasmine). Of interest, cod liver oil was at one time used as a source of vitamin A and D and was thought to be a source of toxicosis.

7. Describe the pathophysiologic changes.

Increased bone resorption coupled with increased gastrointestinal absorption of calcium and phosphorus is responsible for pathophysiologic abnormalities. The result is extensive soft tissue mineralization of the endocardium, blood vessels, tendons, kidneys, and lungs. A calcium and phosphorus product greater than 60 mg/dl (growing puppies may have a higher Ca × P product, perhaps in excess of 100 mg/dl) is considered an indication for metastatic calcification and is associated with microscopic mineralization of tissues.

8. What are the common pathologic and histologic findings in animals poisoned with cholecalciferol?

Severe gastric and intestinal mucosal hemorrhage has been reported, along with patchy mineralization of the cortical renal tubular basement membrane. Multifocal necrosis involves crypt cells in the small intestine as well as the pulmonary alveolar basement membrane.

9. How is it treated?

Treatment of cholecalciferol rodenticides should be aggressive, especially with the potential risk of metastatic calcification. Normal (0.9%) saline should be started to promote diuresis. Dehydration should first be corrected, then a minimum of 2–3 times maintenance provided. Furosemide (1.0–2.0 mg/kg, every 12 hours, subcutaneously or intramuscularly) helps in the diuresis once the animal is well hydrated; prednisolone (1–2 mg/kg, every 12 hours, subcutaneously or intramuscularly) helps to diminish calcium uptake in the gut; and salmon calitonin (Calicimar, USV Laboratories, Tarrytown, NY), (4.0–8.0 U/kg, every 6–8 hours subcutaneously) helps to diminish the resorption of calcium from bone. No well-defined dosage ranges have been established for salmon calitonin, although a wide range is reported. Its use for treating cholecalciferol rodenticide toxicosis has also not been well defined, but the principle is sound. The major biologic effect of calcitonin is inhibition of bone resorption by the suppression of osteoclastic activity and suppression of the recruitment of new osteoclasts from precursor cells. Frequent serum calcium determinations are important, and the dose and frequency of the drug may have to be titrated in order to achieve the desired effect. In humans, relatively mild, infrequent transitory side effects are reported. The signs include dermatologic reactions, urticaria, abdominal cramps, diarrhea, pruritus, and pollakiuria. In animals, anorexia and vomiting have been reported; these signs stopped soon after calcitonin was discontinued.

10. What are the long-term treatment goals?

Once the animal is stable and no longer requires intravenous fluid support, it may be possible to discharge. Frequent rechecks of the serum calcium levels should be considered. Oral furosemide, calcitonin, and prednisolone may be continued at home. A calcium-free diet should be suggested. Long-term prognosis is good.

BIBLIOGRAPHY

1. Dorman DC: Toxicology of selected pesticides, drugs, and chemicals. Anticoagulant, cholecalciferol, and bromethalin-based rodenticides [Review]. Vet Clin North Am Small Anim Pract 20:339–352, 1990.
2. Dougherty SA, Center SA, Dzanis DA: Salmon calcitonin as adjunct treatment for vitamin D toxicosis in a dog. J Am Vet Med Assoc 196:1269–1272, 1990.
3. Fooshee SK, Forrester SD: Hypercalcemia secondary to cholecalciferol rodenticide toxicosis in two dogs. J Am Vet Med Assoc 196:1265–1268, 1990.
4. Gunther R, Felice LJ, Nelson, Franson AM: Toxicity of a vitamin D_3 rodenticide to dogs. J Am Vet Med Assoc 193:211–214, 1988.

106. TOXIN-INDUCED SEIZURES

J. Michael McFarland, D.V.M.

1. What are the common causes of seizures induced by toxic products?

- Organophosphates and carbamates
- Chlorinated hydrocarbons
- Pyrethrins
- Strychnine
- Metaldehyde
- Lead
- Caffeine
- Pseudoephedrine
- Ethylene glycol
- Drugs of abuse

2. How important is a good history in diagnosing toxin induced seizures?

History is the most important part of the evaluation, especially when intoxication is suspected. In addition to routine questions about signalment, medical history, systems (e.g., cardiovascular, respiratory, gastrointestinal, renal), and diet, several points should be covered while interviewing the owner:

- Was exposure to a toxin actually observed?
- If so, how was the animal exposed (oral, dermal, inspired)?
- What was the amount and/or duration of exposure?
- Describe the pet's environment and level of confinement.
- When was the pet last seen normal?
- Describe the seizure itself (character, onset, duration).
- Was the seizure triggered by external stimuli (noise, touch, bright light)?
- Describe the pet's behavior and health before the seizure.
- Is anyone in the family taking medications of any kind?
- Is there any possibility for exposure to drugs of abuse? (A little discretion is in order here.)
- Have the neighbors made any threats toward you or your pets?
- Have any baits or insecticides been applied to your yard or your neighbor's yard?

Of course, time is of the essence, especially if the patient presents in status epilepticus. A preprepared questionnaire for the owner may help while you and your staff attend to the immediate medical crisis.

3. What is the minimal database required for toxin-induced seizures?

A complete blood count and chemistry panel with electrolytes should be run immediately. Urine is collected for urinalysis and toxicology screening. Stomach contents may be submitted for toxicology screening. Blood gas analysis is important, because prolonged seizures, apnea, tachypnea, or the toxin itself may have profound effects on acid-base balance. Cardiovascular monitoring (electrocardiogram and blood pressure) detects cardiac arrhythmias, hypotension, or hypertension. Thoracic and abdominal radiographs help to rule out aspiration, pulmonary edema, and foreign body ingestion.

4. What is the most common cause of toxin-induced seizures?

Insecticides. Organophosphates, carbamates and pyrethrins are found in various shampoos, sprays, and dips that are readily available to pet owners. Accidental exposure and overdose are extremely common. Insecticide toxicity is discussed in more detail in the next chapter.

5. How can metaldehyde intoxication be differentiated from strychnine intoxication?

History alone is usually sufficient; on presentation the two intoxications may look exactly alike. Both can lead to tetanic seizures and status epilepticus. Some metaldehyde baits include carbamate and may cause cholinergic signs (hypersalivating, vomiting) as well. Strychnine is a competitive inhibitor of the inhibitory neurotransmitter glycine. The seizures that result from strychnine intoxication are frequently triggered by external stimuli, such as loud noise or bright lights. Metaldehyde is hydrolyzed by stomach acid to acetaldehyde. The muscle tremors and seizures that result from metaldehyde ingestion are not triggered by external stimuli. In addition, acetaldehyde leads to profound metabolic acidosis, with little or no respiratory compensation in patients with seizures. Examination of stomach contents can be helpful. Most strychnine baits contain a green or pink die marker that may be visible in the ingesta. Metaldehyde may cause the odor of the stomach contents to resemble that of formaldehyde.

6. What are the specific treatment considerations in dealing with strychnine or metaldehyde intoxication?

It may take as long as 24–48 hours before strychnine is completely eliminated in the urine; thus, long-term sedation is needed. Repeated doses of pentobarbital (15–30 mg/kg) or inhalation anesthesia are used for seizure control. Higher doses than normal are often required to achieve complete relaxation. Methocarbamol (150 mg/kg intravenously or orally) may improve muscle relaxation. Diuretics and urinary acidifiers such as ammonium chloride enhance urinary excretion. Urinary acidification is contraindicated if the patient has acidosis or myoglobinuria. Close monitoring is extremely important, because respiratory depression and hypothermia are common sequelae of long-term barbiturate sedation. The patient should be kept in a warm, dry, dimly lit location.

Seizure control for metaldehyde intoxication is similar to that for strychnine intoxication. In addition, profound acidosis may require attention. Intravenous fluid administration with lactated Ringers' provides enough buffering to control acidosis in most cases. When possible, blood gases should be evaluated. If serum bicarbonate levels are less than 12 mmol/L, sodium bicarbonate supplementation is recommended. Continued supportive care and monitoring may be necessary for as long as 4 days. In some patients, death occurs 3–4 days later as a result of hepatic failure.

7. What common items found around the house can lead to seizures after ingestion?

Methylxanthines, such as chocolate and caffeine, are the most common. The approximate LD_{50} for methylxanthines is 100–500 mg/kg. Most caffeine-based stimulants contain 100 mg of caffeine. One ounce of milk chocolate contains approximately 5–10 mg of caffeine and 35–50 mg of theobromine. Dark or baker's chocolates are up to 10 times more toxic than milk chocolates. In addition, over-the-counter cold and sinus preparations that contain pseudoephedrine may be a problem.

8. Is seizure prevention the only concern with methylxanthine and pseudoephedrine intoxication?

No. Methylxanthine and pseudoephedrine may lead to significant gastrointestinal (GI) and cardiovascular difficulties as well. After seizure control and detoxification procedures, attention should be focused on cardiovascular monitoring. Tachyarrhythmias and hypertension are significant problems and may lead to sudden death. Propranolol (0.04–0.06 mg/kg by slow intravenous push every 8 hours) is recommended to control most cardiovascular complications. Supraventricular tachycardia and ventricular premature contractions may require lidocaine (2 mg/kg by slow intravenous push or 50–75 µg/kg/min CRI) for control. Rarely, bradycardia develops and can be controlled with atropine (0.02–0.04 mg/kg intravenously, subcutaneously, intramuscularly).

GI irritation may be severe, and hemorrhagic gastroenteritis is common. Supportive care with intravenous fluids is important to maintain hydration and to promote diuresis. In addition, urinary catheterization keeps the bladder empty and prevents reabsorption of toxins. The long half-life of methylxanthines may require treatment for up to 72 hours.

BIBLIOGRAPHY

1. Chrisman CL: Seizures. In Ettinger SJ, Feldman EC (eds): Textbook of Veterinary Internal Medicine. Philadelphia, W.B. Saunders, 1995, pp 152–156.
2. Dorman DC: Toxins that induce seizures in small animals. Proceedings of the 8th ACVIM Forum. 1990, pp 361–364.
3. Drobatz KJ: Clinical approach to toxicities. Vet Clin North Am Small Anim Pract 24:1123–1138, 1994.
4. Hooser SB, Beasley VR: Methylxanthine poisoning (chocolate and caffeine) toxicosis. In Kirk RW (ed): Current Veterinary Therapy IX. Philadelphia, W.B. Saunders, 1986, p 191.
5. Nicholson SS: Toxicology. In Ettinger SJ, Feldman EC (eds): Textbook of Veterinary Internal Medicine. Philadelphia, W.B. Saunders, 1995, pp 312–326.
6. Udall ND: The toxicity of the molluscicides metaldehyde and methiocarb to dogs. Vet Rec 93(15):420–422, 1973.
7. Webster CJ, Webster JM: Anaesthetic control for metaldehyde poisoning [letter]. Vet Rec 119(20):511–512, 1986.

107. BITES AND STINGS

Terri E. Bonenberger, D.V.M.

1. Where do most stings occur on cats and dogs?

Most stings occur on the head and paws, probably because of animals' natural nosy nature.

2. What groups of insects commonly cause the most severe reactions to pets?

The families within the order *Hymenoptera* that cause the most problems and side effects are *Apidae* (bees), *Vespidae* (wasps, hornets, and yellow jackets), and *Formicidae* (ants).

3. How do the stings of bees, wasps, and ants differ?

Apis (the honeybee) has a unique stinging apparatus. The stinger is eviscerated from the bee (killing the bee), and the stinger and venom sac are retained within the victim. The visual presence of the venom sac allows positive identification of *Apis* as the source of the sting. *Vespa* (wasps and hornets) leave no stinger in the victim; therefore, they are free to attack and may sting a victim repeatedly. However, they generally only attack when they are hunting or provoked. The sting of fire ants is unique because it is a two-part process. First the ant bites its victim's skin with two powerful pinching jaws; the ant then stings the victim with its modified ovipositor apparatus.

This process produces a circular pattern of stings with two centralized punctate holes. A sterile pustule forms after the bite.

4. What are the active components responsible for the toxic effects of the venom?

Bee and wasp/hornet venom are similar. They are composed primarily of protein, with phospholipase A1 and A2, hyaluronidase, acid phosphatase, antigen-5, melittin, and apamin. Wasp and hornet venom also contains wasp and hornet kinins, respectively. These specific kinins appear to act similarly to bradykinin and may be important in the pathogenesis of stings. Fire ant stings are again unique within *Hymenoptera*. Their venom is only approximately 5% protein and 95% alkaloid; however, the proteins are similar to those in other *Hymenoptera*.

5. How should a bee stinger be removed from the patient?

Because the stinger can pulsate venom into the animal for up to 2–3 minutes after being separated from the bee, it should be removed as soon as possible. The stinger should be scraped out (a scalpel blade can be used); it should not be squeezed out with fingers or tweezers because the venom sac may rupture, further exposing the animal to its contents.

6. How do the Africanized (killer) bees differ from honey bees?

Apis mellifera scutellata (Africanized or killer bees) resulted from breeding the docile European honeybee with the more aggressive African bee. The Africanized honeybees have retained the aggressive nature and are more militant in regard to colony defense. Although Africanized bees actually release less venom per sting, their aggressive stinging behavior makes them potentially more dangerous because of the possibility of multiple stings and, therefore, systemic toxic reactions.

7. What are the different classifications for insect stings?

Insect stings can be grouped according to the type of reaction that they cause:
Group 1: Small, local (toxic in origin)   Group 3: Systemic, allergic (anaphylaxis)
Group 2: Large, local (allergic in origin) Group 4: Systemic, toxic (massive envenomation)

8. What is the recommended medical treatment for mild reactions?

Group 1 reactions rarely require veterinary attention. The lesions result from local irritation by the venom, which can cause redness, pain, and swelling. Ice compresses and topical lidocaine help to ease the symptoms. Group 2 reactions are allergic in origin and may cause facial or limb edema. Management should include treatment recommended for group 1 as well as antihistamines (diphenhydramine 2–4 mg/kg every 2 hours) and cortisone if swelling is severe (prednisolone, 1 mg/kg every 12 hours, tapered over 5 days). The patient should be monitored for the next 2–3 hours to assess for a positive response to therapy. Unfortunately, antihistamine and corticosteroids have not been shown to be beneficial in preventing or resolving the pustules associated with fire ant bites.

9. What are the clinical signs of anaphylaxis (group 3)?

Anaphylaxis is a rarely reported complication of insect stings. Affected animals generally begin to show symptoms within 15 minutes of the bite. Clinical signs include swelling, vomiting, urination, defecation, muscle weakness, and seizures. Symptoms in cats include pruritus, dyspnea, salivation, ataxia, and collapse.

10. What is the recommended medical treatment for anaphylaxis?

Treatment should be directed at impending vascular collapse. Crystalloid and colloidal fluids are imperative and should be administered at shock volumes. Antihistamine (diphenhydramine hydrochloride, 2 mg/kg by slow intravenous push and intravenous glucocorticoids (prednisolone sodium succinate, 10 mg/kg) may be helpful if given early. The use of epinephrine is questionable and may be helpful only early in the onset of shock.

11. What clinical signs are associated with massive envenomation (group 4)?

Large numbers of stings can cause a toxic reaction due to the large amount of venom. This reaction is toxic and not allergic; therefore, patients may not present with edema or urticaria. Neurotoxic, hepatotoxic, nephrorotoxic, and cytotoxic signs have been seen in cats and dogs. These clinical signs may not be present initially but may develop several days after the attack. The patient is generally febrile and depressed. Neurologic signs include ataxia, facial paralysis, and seizures. Vomiting, red-to-brown urine, brown vomitus, and bloody stool also may be seen.

12. What abnormalities are associated with massive envenomation?

Laboratory results include elevations in total bilirubin, alanine aminotransferase, blood urea nitrogen, and creatinine. The hemogram often reflects leukocytosis with a degenerative left shift or regenerative left shift. Anemia can be present secondary to intravascular hemolysis. More serious cases show increases in clotting times (increased activated partial thromboplastin time, OSPT, fibrin degradation products) and thrombocytopenia. A high index of suspicion for the development of disseminated intravascular coagulation (DIC) is required (treatment is more successful when started before the animal develops the classic signs of DIC). Evidence of renal tubular damage (granular casts in urinalysis) and acute renal failure are possible.

13. What is the recommended treatment for systemic toxicosis from insect stings?

Patients suffering from multiple hymenopteran stings should be hospitalized and observed for immediate or delayed toxic reactions. Systemic inflammatory response syndrome (SIRS) may be a complication; thus, the most important goal of treatment is correction of hypovolemia and vascular stasis. Fluid therapy, supportive care, prophylactic antibiotics, and monitoring of hemodynamic function are the cornerstones of treatment. Intravenous glucocorticoids may be helpful if neurologic or intravascular hemolysis is seen. Antihistamines are helpful only early in the disease process and only if there is an allergic component.

14. Do fire ants pose a serious threat to cats and dogs?

Not usually. Severe and fatal attacks by fire ants are extremely rare. Patients that suffer a massive attack from fire ants usually are debilitated in some way and are unable to move out of the swarm's path. The stings can result in scars or secondary infection.

15. What are the clinical signs of *Lactrodectus* envenomation (black widow spider bite)?

The initial bite is usually not painful, and local tissue changes are generally absent. The bite appears as small puncture wounds with a blanched area surrounded by erythema, which are often difficult to visualize because of the dense hair coat and pigmented skin. Severe cramping of large muscle masses is common; abdominal cramping sometimes interferes with respiration. Abdominal rigidity without pain is considered a hallmark sign. The severe muscle cramping may cause anxiety, spasms, and seizures. The cat is extremely sensitive to the bite; clinical signs include severe pain, restlessness, excessive salivation, and paralysis.

16. What is the treatment for the muscle cramping and other signs caused by *Lactrodectus* envenomation?

The slow intravenous injection of 10% calcium gluconate, 10–30 ml (dogs) and 5–15 ml (cats). The patient's cardiac rate and rhythm should be monitored during administration. Repeated dosing in 4–6 hours may be necessary. If seizures occur, diazepam is recommended. The prognosis may be guarded (especially in cats); therefore, close monitoring over the next 2–3 days is recommended.

17. What are the characteristic signs of *Loxosceles* bite (brown recluse or fiddleback spider)?

The bite is not painful initially, but within 2–6 hours an area of pain and erythema develops, followed by a blister (12 hours) and then classic bulls-eye lesion (a necrotic center surrounded by a white ring of ischemia against an area of erythema). The lesion then progresses to focal ulceration and necrosis. Other symptoms include fever, arthralgia, lethargy, vomiting, and seizures. The wound is slow to heal, and aggressive open wound management with debridement is often necessary.

18. What are the signs of scorpion envenomation?
The sting of a scorpion is acutely painful and generally only pain management of the sting is required (ice compresses and aspirin), however, systemic signs may develop. Some species of scorpions possess neurotoxins which can cause an excitatory neurotoxicity. Clinical signs include salivation, urination, defecation, lacrimation and mydriasis which can easily be confused with organophosphate or carbamate toxicity. Death can result from respiratory collapse, hypertension and cardiac arrhythmias. Treatment is supportive; antihistamines, corticosteroids and atropine are not helpful. Intravenous fluids should be administered with caution due to the possibility of pulmonary edema.

CONTROVERSY

19. Can desensitization therapy help animals who have suffered serious allergic attacks from the stings of *Hymenoptera*?
In humans, immunotherapy decreases the severity of the systemic response to Hymenopteran stings. Therapy is more effective if it is directed at the specific insect; however, cross-sensitivities to various venom are common and multivalent venom is available for desensitization therapy. Because anaphylaxis is a rare complication of stings in animals, relatively few patients present for this therapy. Unless an *Apis* stinger is identified, it is often difficult to determine which insect caused the reaction. However, if the patient is successfully treated for anaphylaxis secondary to Hymenopteran sting, the possibility of desensitization therapy should be discussed with the owner and a veterinary dermatologist.

BIBLIOGRAPHY

1. Cowell AK, Cowell RL: Management of bee and other Hymenoptera stings. In Kirk RW (ed): Current Veterinary Therapy XII—Small Animal Practice. Philadelphia, W.B. Saunders, 1995, pp 226–228.
2. Cowell AK, Cowell RL, Tyler RD, Nieves MA: Severe systemic reactions to Hymenoptera stings in three dogs. J Am Vet Med Assoc 198:1014–1016, 1991.
3. Dart RC, Lindsey D, Schulman A: Snakes and shocks. Ann Emerg Med 17:1262, 1988.
4. Elgart GW: Ant, bee, and wasp stings. Dermatol Clin 8:229–236, 1990.
5. Peterson ME, Meerdink GL: Bites and stings of venomous animals. In Kirk RW (ed): Current Veterinary Therapy—Small Animal Practice. Philadelphia, W.B. Saunders 1989, pp 177–186.
6. Reedy LM, Miller WH Jr: Allergic Skin Diseases of Dogs and Cats. Philadelphia, W.B. Saunders, 1989, p 28.
7. Synder CC, Knowles RP: Snakebites: Guidelines for practical management. Postgrad Med 83(6):52–75, 1988.

108. OVER-THE-COUNTER NONSTEROIDAL ANTIINFLAMMATORY INTOXICATION

J. Bruce Nixon, D.V.M.

1. What dosage of nonsteroidal antiinflammatory drugs (NSAIDs) can cause toxic symptoms in dogs and cats?
Aspirin in dogs can be toxic at 15 mg/kg every 8 hours (1 regular strength tablet/50 lbs 3 times/day). Because of the much longer half-life in cats, 25 mg/kg/day of aspirin ½ regular strength tablet daily) may be toxic.

Acetaminophen toxicosis in dogs occurs at a dose of 150 mg/kg (2 regular strength tablets per 10 lbs). Cats are extraordinarily poor conjugators of the active metabolite of acetaminophen and become intoxicated at a dose of 50 mg/kg (as little as $^1/_2$ tablet).

Ibuprofen has been reported to produce toxicity at a dose of 50 mg/kg (1 regular strength tablet per 10 lbs).

2. What is the pathophysiology of NSAID intoxication?

Gastric irritation, leading to ulceration, is the hallmark of aspirin toxicosis. Aspirin inhibits prostaglandin production and alters prostaglandin's protective abilities. This combination of events results in damaged gastric mucosa. In addition, aspirin can gain direct entry into mucosal cells by virtue of its lipid solubility and cause cellular damage. An acid-base disturbance develops—respiratory alkalosis followed by metabolic acidosis. Cats are prone to develop Heinz-body anemia and bone marrow hypoplasia. Toxic hepatitis also may develop, especially with chronic administration.

Acetaminophen overdosage results in toxic levels of an active metabolite that is normally conjugated by glutathione. A limited glutathione supply, coupled with a diminished ability to biotransform and eliminate the drug, may rapidly lead to toxicosis, especially in cats. The cat's hemoglobin molecule is particularly prone to methemoglobinemia in such circumstances. Hemolysis and Heinz-body anemia also may occur. As with aspirin, hepatic necrosis may develop, particularly with chronic administration.

3. What are the symptoms of NSAID toxicity?

For aspirin, watch for vomiting (with or without blood) and abdominal pain. Early respiratory alkalosis results in tachypnea. Elevated body temperature and depression are common. Untreated, signs may progress to coma and death. Icterus may develop over time.

In acetaminophen toxicosis, the major symptoms in dogs are usually related to hepatotoxicosis, whereas in cats the greatest clinical symptoms are related to methemoglobinemia. The development of methemoglobinemia causes tachypnea and cyanosis. Cats particularly may void dark brown urine (from hematuria and hemoglobinuria). Edema may develop in the face and distal extremities. As with aspirin toxicosis, vomiting and abdominal pain may be seen, especially early after ingestion. Depression develops progressively. Icterus from toxic hepatitis also may be seen, especially in dogs. Cats show more severe signs and more rapid progression in NSAID overdosage.

4. What laboratory findings are useful?

Aspirin	*Acetaminophen*
Heinz-body anemia (especially in cats)	Methemoglobinemia
Elevated bilirubin, alanine aminotransferase (especially in chronic dosing)	Elevated bilirubin, alanine aminotransferase, alkaline phosphatase (dogs)
Acid/base disturbances Respiratory alkalosis followed by metabolic acidosis	Heinz-body anemia (cats) Hematuria/hemoglobinuria
Hypokalemia	
Hyponatremia	

5. What is appropriate treatment for aspirin toxicosis?

Induce vomiting and/or perform gastric lavage, even as long as 12 hours after ingestion, because aspirin tends to remain in the stomach as an insoluble mass. Vomiting and lavage should be followed by 2 gm/kg of activated charcoal. Fluids and electrolytes should be replaced, particularly in depressed patients. Consider using sodium bicarbonate at 1 mEq/kg intravenously to alkalinize urine. This treatment increases excretion of salicylate.

Gastric ulceration may be addressed in various ways; the most common is administration of cimetidine, 5 mg/kg subcutaneously, intravenously, or orally 4 times/day. Ranitidine (Zantac) is an H_2 blocker that is reportedly more potent than cimetidine and has the advantage of twice daily dosing at 2 mg/kg intravenously, subcutaneously, or orally. Also consider using sucralfate (Carafate) if you are fairly certain that ulceration exists; this drug binds to the ulcer site and has sustained local protective effects. Sucralfate is dosed at 0.5–1.0 gm orally 4 times/day. Another drug to consider if ulceration exists or is strongly suspected is misoprostol (Cytotec). Misoprostol is both antisecretory and cytoprotective and has been shown to be quite effective in ulcer management in dogs and humans. Misoprostol is dosed at 2–4 µg/kg orally 3 times/day.

6. Is treatment for acetaminophen toxicosis different from that described for aspirin?
Yes. Methemoglobinemia must be aggressively treated. N-acetylcysteine (Mucomyst) is given at 140 mg/kg initially, followed by 70 mg/kg every 6 hours for 5–7 treatments. N-acetylcysteine is generally administered orally in a 5% dextrose solution but may be given intravenously to patients unable to receive oral therapy. Vitamin C can also be given in addition to N-acetylcysteine to reverse methemoglobinemia, especially in cats. Vitamin C is dosed at 200 mg/cat 3 times a day, intravenously, subcutaneously, or orally. In cats, a single dose of methylene blue at 1.5 mg/kg intravenously has been used to reverse methemoglobinemia successfully and rapidly. Repeated doses are not recommended, however, because they may actually cause methemoglobinemia.

Fluids and electrolytes should be given as needed to replace losses. While blood transfusions may be necessary in patients with severe methemoglobinemia, massive red blood cell destruction, or hepatic necrosis from hepatocyte destruction.

Gastric irritation or ulceration should be treated as described for aspirin toxicosis.

7. What kind of follow-up care is important?
For aspirin, monitor electrolytes, liver enzymes, and renal function. Anemia from bone marrow suppression is a poor prognostic indicator.

In acetaminophen toxicosis, continual monitoring of methemoglobinemia is vital for effective management, especially in cats. Also, monitor liver enzymes, especially in dogs.

8. How should toxicities from other over-the-counter NSAIDs be treated?
Ibuprofen essentially causes the same symptoms as aspirin and should be treated as such. Acetophenetidin (phenacetin) is contained in some over-the-counter analgesics and sinus remedies. Acetophenetidin is metabolized into acetaminophen and should be treated and managed like acetaminophen toxicosis.

BIBLIOGRAPHY

1. Johnston SA, Leib MS, Forrester SD, Marini M: The effect of misoprostol on aspirin-induced gastroduodenal lesions in dogs. J Vet Intern Med 9:32–38, 1995.
2. Jones RD, Baynes RE, Nimitz CT: Nonsteroidal anti-inflammatory drug toxicosis in dogs and cats: 240 cases (1989–1990). J Am Vet Med Assoc 201:475–477, 1992.
3. Murtaugh RJ, Matz ME, Labato MA, Boudrieau RJ: Use of synthetic prostaglandin E1 (misoprostol) for prevention of aspirin-induced gastroduodenal ulceration in arthritic dogs. J Am Vet Med Assoc 202:251–256, 1993.
4. Oehme FW: Aspirin and acetaminophen. Current Veterinary Therapy IX. Philadelphia, W.B. Saunders, 1986, pp 188–190.
5. Rose BD: Clinical Physiology of Acid-Base and Electrolyte Disorders, 4th ed. New York, McGraw-Hill, 1994, pp 565–567.

XIV. Emergency Procedures

Section Editor: Robert J. Murtaugh, D.V.M.

109. TEMPORARY TRACHEOSTOMY

Steven Mensack, V.M.D.

1. What are the indications for performing a temporary tracheostomy?

An emergent tracheostomy is indicated in animals with upper airway compromise secondary to laryngeal or tracheal foreign body, laryngeal paralysis, laryngeal crushing injuries, and proximal tracheal tears or avulsions. Additional indications include:

- Long-term (> 12 hours) mechanical ventilation
- Surgical intervention to the larynx or proximal trachea that renders endotracheal intubation impossible and postoperative maintenance of a patent airway is necessary.
- Conditions requiring facilitated removal of lower airway secretions when the cough reflex is abolished, as in comatose patients and cases of smoke inhalation
- Conditions in which large amounts of secretions are produced, as in patients that have undergone lung lobe resection

2. What types of tracheostomy tube are available?

Tracheostomy tubes are available as single-cannula tubes, with or without an inflatable cuff, in sizes ranging from internal diameters of 2.5–10 mm. For tracheostomy tubes with internal diameters of 7–9 mm, a disposable inner cannula is also manufactured. The inner cannula decreases the internal diameter of the tube by 2 mm. One such unit is the Blue Line tracheostomy tube manufactured by Smith Industries Medical System, Keene, NH.

3. What are the indications for the different types of tubes?

Cuffed tracheostomy tubes are indicated when the patient is scheduled for anesthesia, is comatose and thus at increased risk of aspiration pneumonia, or will be placed on ventilatory support. The cuff should be a high-volume, low-pressure cuff. An uncuffed tracheostomy tube should be used for most other situations in which a tracheostomy is indicated. Alternatively, the cuffed tracheostomy tube may be placed without inflating the cuff. The uncuffed tracheostomy tube allows air to move around the tube, making tube obstruction less of a life-threatening situation.

A double-cannula tracheostomy tube is preferred when the diameter of the patient's trachea is large enough. The double-cannula tube allows removal of the inner cannula for cleaning while the outer cannula maintains airway patency. Unfortunately, the sizes required for use in small-breed dogs and cats are available only in single-cannula tubes.

4. If a commercial tracheostomy tube is not available, what are the alternatives?

A modified tracheostomy tube can be made from an endotracheal tube. The breathing circuit adapter is removed from the end of the endotracheal tube. The body of the tube is split longitudinally, preserving the cuff-inflation mechanism. The tube should be split so that approximately 4–7 cm of endotracheal tube remains intact at the distal end. Thus 2 cm of intact tube lie within the trachea, and 2 cm of intact tube lie outside the skin incision in small dogs and cats. In larger-breed dogs, a longer segment of endotracheal tube is left intact so that 4 cm of the tube are inserted into the trachea. The adapter is replaced in the endotracheal tube, and holes are made in both flanges to facilitate securing the tube to the patient. Once in place, the tube is secured with gauze or umbilical tape passed through these holes. Red-rubber endotracheal tubes should be avoided in making a modified tracheostomy tube because they may be more irritating to the tracheal mucosa than other materials.

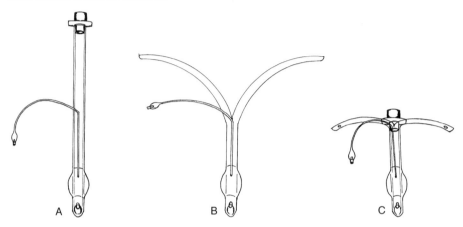

Procedure for modifying an endotracheal tube for use as a tracheostomy tube. *A*, The adapter is removed from a standard endotracheal tube. *B*, The tube is split longitudinally, preserving the inflation mechanism. *C*, The adapter is replaced and holes put in the flanges.

5. Is special equipment required to perform a temporary tracheostomy?
No. An ideal tracheostomy pack includes the following:
- 4 towels/drapes
- 4 towel clamps
- 1 scalpel handle
- 1 no. 10 Bard-Parker scalpel blade
- 1 no. 11 or no. 15 Bard-Parker scalpel blade
- 2 mosquito forceps
- 1 pair of Metzenbaum scissors

- 1 rat-tooth tissue forceps
- 2 Allis tissue forceps
- 1 small Weitlander retractor
- 1 large Weitlander retractor
- 1 needle holder
- Gauze sponges

6. How is tracheostomy performed?
1. The patient is placed in dorsal recumbency after induction of general anesthesia, when possible. The neck is extended, and the thoracic limbs are pulled caudally and secured lateral to the thorax. The ventral cervical region is clipped of hair and prepared in a sterile fashion (time permitting). In an immediate life-threatening situation, the ventral cervical region is clipped and infiltrated with lidocaine.

2. A longitudinal midline incision is made from the larynx to about the eighth tracheal ring. The paired strap muscles (sternohyoideus and sternothyroideus) are bluntly separated at the midline to expose the trachea. Retracting these muscles with a Weitlander retractor helps to protect neurovascular structures and provides better tracheal exposure.

3. A stab incision is made in the annular ligament between the fourth and fifth tracheal rings. The incision is extended laterally in both directions to encompass approximately 50% of the tracheal circumference. The recurrent laryngeal nerve lies in close proximity to the trachea and should be identified before the tracheal incision is extended laterally.

4. Long stay sutures of silk or nylon are placed around 1–2 tracheal rings immediately cranial and caudal to the tracheal incision to facilitate isolation of the stoma for tube placement and replacement.

5. A tracheostomy tube of the appropriate size is inserted into the stoma. The tube is secured by tying pieces of gauze or umbilical tape from the phalanges of the tube around the dorsal aspect

of the neck. The most rostral and caudal ends of the skin incision are closed with sutures. The skin incision around the tracheostomy tube is left open to allow air to pass.

7. What is the proper size of the tracheostomy tube?

A tracheostomy tube should be between ⅔ and ¾ of the tracheal diameter. This size aids in the prevention of respiratory arrest by allowing inspired air to move continuously around an un-cuffed or uninflated cuffed tube if it becomes occluded. This tube size also minimizes the occurrence of iatrogenic tracheal trauma and decreases the incidence of postintubation stenosis.

8. What complications may occur during placement of a tracheostomy tube? How can they be avoided?

Complications encountered in placing a tracheostomy tube include damage to neurovascular structures around the trachea, airway obstruction, and subcutaneous emphysema. Damage to peritracheal neurovascular structures can be avoided by familiarity with regional anatomy before surgery, good surgical technique, and maximal tracheal exposure. The incidence of airway obstruction can be decreased by choosing a tracheostomy tube of the proper size. Even with appropriately sized tubes, kinking or occlusion of the distal end of the tube may occur during insertion. It is important to recognize such occurrences rapidly and to adjust or replace the tube as needed. A small degree of subcutaneous emphysema usually occurs but can be minimized by leaving the skin and soft tissue around the tube open so that air leaking from the tracheal incision can escape the tissues.

9. Once the tracheostomy tube is placed, what steps are necessary to maintain it?

Proper care of the patient and tracheostomy tube includes humidification of inspired gas, suctioning of respiratory secretions, periodic replacement of the tracheostomy tube, and proper wound management.

1. **Humidification.** Humidification helps to maintain the normal tracheal defense mechanisms and facilitates the removal of respiratory secretions. Humidification of inspired gas is best accomplished by the use of a commercial humidifier or nebulizer (PulmoAide, DeVilbiss Co., Somerset, PA). If the patient is receiving supplemental oxygen, the gas can be run through the humidifier before reaching the patient. If the patient is breathing room air, placement in a chamber with a humidifier or nebulizer for 15 minutes every 4–6 hours helps to keep the airways moist. If neither of these devices is available, instilling 0.1 ml/kg sterile saline (1 ml minimum, 5 ml maximum) into the tracheostomy tube every 1–2 hours helps to maintain upper airway hydration.

2. **Suctioning.** Routine suctioning of respiratory secretions from the trachea and tracheostomy tube helps to prevent airway obstruction while the tube is in place. Suctioning should be performed with sterile technique. The patient is preoxygenated with 100% oxygen for several breaths before suctioning. A sterile suction catheter is inserted without vacuum down the tracheostomy tube into the trachea. A light intermittent vacuum is applied as the catheter is rotated and removed. The vacuum should not be applied for longer than 10–15 seconds; longer applications have been associated with severe hypoxemia. Suctioning should be done as needed, depending on the amount of respiratory secretions produced. It may be required as often as every 15 minutes initially and should be done at least 4 times daily. Complications of suctioning include hypoxemia, vomiting, retching, gagging, cardiac arrhythmias, and tracheal mucosal damage.

3. **Tube replacement.** The tracheostomy tube should be replaced at least once every 24 hours or more frequently if occlusion from respiratory secretions occurs. In tubes with a double cannula, the inner cannula may be removed while the outer cannula is suctioned, as described above. A sterile inner cannula can then be inserted. In the single-cannula tracheostomy tube, the patient is preoxygenated with 100% oxygen, the stay sutures are grasped, and the old tube is removed. A sterile tracheostomy tube can then be placed.

4. **Wound management.** The wound should be cleaned daily with sterile saline and gauze or cotton-tipped applicators. Antiseptic solutions may irritate the exposed tracheal mucosa and should be avoided.

10. Should the tracheostomy tube cuff be periodically deflated?

If the tracheostomy tube cuff has been inflated for ventilatory support or the patient is comatose, the cuff should remain inflated throughout the time that the tube is in place. Periodically deflating the cuff has not been proved to reduce cuff-induced tracheal damage. At the same time, periodically deflating the cuff may lead to complications. Patients that have a tracheostomy tube in place because of inability to protect the airway may develop aspiration pneumonia while the cuff is deflated. Patients on ventilatory support cannot maintain proper airway pressure while the cuff is deflated, leading to ineffective ventilation.

11. What complications may occur while the tracheostomy tube is in place? How can they be avoided?

Obstruction, nosocomial infections, and dislodgment of the tracheostomy tube are the most commonly reported complications. Obstruction can be avoided by carefully monitoring the patient for signs of dyspnea, stridor, or anxiety, which may indicate that the lumen of the tube is becoming obstructed. Proper humidification, frequent suctioning of respiratory secretions, and appropriate tube changes help to minimize this risk. The incidence of nosocomial infection can be lessened by following proper tube care guidelines, including use of sterile technique whenever the tracheostomy tube is handled, daily wound care, removal of respiratory secretions by suctioning, and appropriate tube placement. Prophylactic antibiotics are not indicated; their use may increase the risk of infection by selecting for antibiotic-resistant bacteria. Tracheostomy tube dislodgment can be avoided by carefully securing the proper-length tube with gauze or umbilical tape and checking frequently to ensure that it is secure.

12. When should the tracheostomy tube be removed?

The tracheostomy tube may be removed once a patent proximal upper airway is reestablished or ventilatory support is no longer needed. The tube should be removed in a stepwise fashion to evaluate airway patency. Tracheostomy tubes of sequentially smaller diameter are inserted, and the patient is observed for respiratory distress or stridorous breathing. When a tube of less than one-half the tracheal diameter is in place, the lumen of the tube may be occluded; again, the patient is observed for distress or stridor. If the patient is breathing comfortably while the lumen is occluded, the tube may be removed and the patient monitored. If at any time during the tube removal process signs of respiratory compromise are observed, a tube large enough for comfortable breathing is inserted. Tube removal may be reattempted in 12–24 hours.

13. Should the tracheostomy incision be surgically closed?

No. The tracheostomy incision should be allowed to heal by second intention. Surgical closure may lead to subcutaneous emphysema and infection. The healing wound should be cleaned at least once daily with sterile saline until a bed of granulation tissue forms.

CONTROVERSY

14. What is the best method for incision of the trachea?

Four methods are available for making an incision in the trachea: transverse, longitudinal/vertical, transverse flap, and longitudinal flap. Few studies describe the complications encountered with each of these methods in animals. The parameters compared in limited studies include ease of changing the tracheostomy tube, necrosis of tracheal mucosa around the stoma, and degree of postextubation tracheal stenosis. The studies found that the flap techniques facilitate replacement of tracheostomy tubes. The flap techniques require only a single stay suture to open the stoma, leaving one hand free to insert the tube. Some degree of necrosis of the tracheal mucosa adjacent to the tracheal opening has been reported with all techniques. With the longitudinal and transverse techniques, mucosal necrosis is due to the semirigid nature of the trachea, which causes pressure against the tube. The flap techniques were designed to decrease this problem. However, the longitudinal flap technique has the disadvantage of destruction or deformation of the created tracheal flap due to repeated traction on the flap during tube changes. No studies of the degree of tracheal mucosal necrosis with the transverse flap technique have been undertaken. Finally, multiple studies have shown no significant differences in the degree of tracheal stenosis after the tracheostomy tube is removed and the incision is allowed to heal by second intention. The degree of stenosis after temporary tracheostomy has been reported to be 18–25% of the tracheal diameter. This degree of stenosis has not been associated with clinically apparent compromise of respiratory ability.

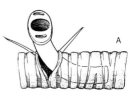

Three methods of creating a temporary tracheostomy. *A,* Transverse tracheotomy. *B,* Longitudinal tracheal flap. *C,* Vertical/longitudinal tracheotomy. (From Slatter D: Textbook of Small Animal Surgery, 2nd ed. Philadelphia, W.B. Saunders, 1993, with permission.)

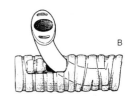

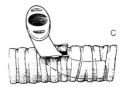

BIBLIOGRAPHY

1. Caywood DD: The larynx, trachea, and thyroid and parathyroid glands. In Harvey CE, Newton CD, Schwartz A (eds): Small Animal Surgery. Philadelphia, J.B. Lippincott, 1990, pp 197–199.
2. Fingland RB: Temporary tracheostomy. In Bonagura JD (ed): Current Veterinary Therapy XII. Philadelphia, W.B. Saunders 1995, pp 179–184.
3. Gibbons G: Respiratory emergencies. In Murtaugh RJ, Kaplan PM (eds): Veterinary Emergency and Critical Care Medicine. St. Louis, Mosby, 1992, p 416.
4. Hedlund CS: Tracheostomies in the management of canine and feline upper respiratory disease. Vet Clin North Am Small Animal Pract 24:873–886, 1994.
5. Huber ML, Henderson RA, et al: Tracheal healing after short and intermediate duration transverse flap tracheostomy in the dog. Proc Am Coll Vet Surg 27, 1996.
6. Macintire DK, Henderson RA, et al: Transverse flap tracheostomy: A technique for temporary tracheostomy of intermediate duration. J Vet Emerg Crit Care 5:25–31, 1995.
7. Nelson AW: Lower respiratory system. In Slatter D (ed): Textbook of Small Animal Surgery, 2nd ed. Philadelphia, W.B. Saunders, 1993, pp 791–794.
8. Powaser MM, et al: The effectiveness of hourly cuff monitoring in minimizing tracheal damage. Heart Lung 5:734, 1976.
9. Westgate HD, Roux KL: Tracheal stenosis following tracheostomy: Incidence and predisposing factors. Anesth Analg 49:393, 1970.
10. Wheeler SJ: Care of respiratory patients. In Slatter D (ed): Textbook of Small Animal Surgery, 2nd ed. Philadelphia, W.B. Saunders, 1993, pp 808–811.

110. THORACIC DRAINAGE

Nancy S. Taylor, D.V.M.

1. Who was the first physician to recommend placement of a thoracic drain?

Hippocrates was the first physician to describe placement of a metal tube in the pleural space to drain "bad humors."

2. What is the purpose of thoracocentesis and chest tube drainage?

These techniques can be used as diagnostic and therapeutic interventions.

3. What are the main indications for thoracic drainage?

- To alleviate signs caused by free air or fluid in the chest cavity
- To obtain fluid for cytologic and microbiologic evaluations

4. How does air accumulate in the thoracic cavity?

A pneumothorax, or accumulation of free air between the chest wall and lung, may be caused by numerous factors. Pneumothorax may be partial, or the entire lung may collapse. When a lung is ruptured or torn, a one-way valve mechanism leads to progressive lung collapse. During inspiration, negative intrapleural pressure causes the edges of the laceration on the surfaces of the lungs to pull apart, pulling air into the pleural space. During expiration, positive intrapleural pressure closes the hole and compresses the leaking surface.

Causes of Pneumothorax

Rupture of lung parenchyma	Rupture of pneumomediastinum into pleural space
Trauma	Rupture of bronchus
Rib fracture	Bronchiectasis
Surgery	Foreign body
Thoracocentesis	Tumor
Pneumonia	Trauma
Foreign body	
Positive pressure ventilation	Perforation of chest wall
Rupture of pulmonary cyst, bulla, or bleb	Rupture of esophagus
	Trauma
Rupture of trachea	Foreign body
Parasites	Neoplasia
Trauma	Parasites
Foreign body	

From Murtaugh RJ, Kaplan PM (eds): Veterinary Emergency and Critical Care. St. Louis, Mosby, 1992, with permission.

5. What are the different types of pneumothorax?

- A **closed pneumothorax** results from a tear in the visceral pleura.
- An **open pneumothorax** results from a tear in the chest wall.
- A **spontaneous pneumothorax** is a closed pneumothorax that occurs unexpectedly after rupture of a pulmonary bulla or bleb.
- A **traumatic pneumothorax** results from direct trauma to the lung or from a broken rib that lacerates the lung.
- A **tension pneumothorax**, which causes severe compromise of respiratory function, occurs when air continues to leak through the one-way valve mechanism after complete

lung collapse. The result is a progressive increase in intrapleural pressure that exceeds atmospheric pressure. This effect causes the mediastinum to shift toward the opposite side of the chest with resultant compression of the opposite lung. In addition, the vena cava becomes compressed, decreasing venous return and cardiac output. If the mediastinum is not intact, both lungs collapse because of the increased intrathoracic pressure. Although any pneumothorax compromises respiratory function, a tension pneumothorax is especially life-threatening. It must be relieved immediately, or the animal will die.

6. Does the character of a pleural effusion affect the approach to chest drainage?

Yes. **Transudates** are caused when fluid is passively transferred into the pleural space because of an imbalance among intravascular, intrapleural, and oncotic fluid pressures. This type of effusion is seen in congestive heart failure, pericardial disease, hepatic failure, and nephrotic syndrome. The protein levels are low in transudates. If the underlying problem is corrected the effusion dissipates. If the fluid is drained but the underlying problem is not corrected, the effusion recurs. It makes sense to drain large amounts of fluid in patients with congestive heart failure to relieve respiratory distress, but the benefits of chest drainage must be weighed against the risk of stress from the procedure.

Exudates are fluids with high protein content that are actively secreted into the pleural space in association with tumors, inflammation, viral or bacterial infections, and disrupted lymphatic drainage (chylous effusions). Exudates are treated by drainage procedures. Recurrence of the effusion is common unless the cause is addressed.

Hemorrhagic effusions also may be drained. However, draining blood due to trauma or coagulopathy is still a controversial procedure. The accumulation of blood may increase intrapleural pressure enough to provide tamponade for cessation of bleeding, but a substantial hemorrhagic pleural effusion may cause a significant decrease in pulmonary function. It is generally recommended that blood be removed if it is causing a significant decrease in pulmonary function and respiratory compromise. The quantity of blood removed should be only the amount needed to relieve respiratory distress.

Purulent effusions should be drained with a chest tube because the viscosity of the fluid limits removal via needle thoracocentesis. Chest tube drainage also promotes resolution of the inflammatory response and removes bacterial toxins.

7. What do you need for a needle-based thoracocentesis?

- Clippers
- Materials for a sterile scrub
- 19–22 gauge butterfly needle with extension tubing coupled to it
- Three-way stopcock
- 12-cc or larger syringe
- Assistant

8. How is thoracocentesis performed?

1. Minimal restraint of the animal is usually required. Placing the animal in lateral recumbency is best for removal of a pneumothorax. Standing, sitting, or sternal position is best for tapping fluid.

2. An area of the chest wall at intercostal space 7–8 should be clipped and aseptically prepared. The spot for the needle insertion is dorsal on the chest wall for a pneumothorax and lower on the chest for removal of pleural effusions, depending on the positioning of the animal.

3. The butterfly apparatus is attached to the stopcock, which is attached to the syringe. The butterfly needle is introduced into the thoracic cavity at the cranial edge of rib 7 or 8 to avoid laceration of intercostal vessels. The fluid or air accumulation is then aspirated into the syringe. Sometimes it is best to have the assistant manage the syringe and stopcock while you maneuver the needle. When the needle is in the pleural space, it is best to orient it parallel with the chest wall (wrapped around the rib) with the bevel facing the pleural surface of the chest wall to minimize potential laceration of the lung as it reexpands. The use of a 3-way stopcock allows evacuation of the syringe without having to withdraw the needle.

4. Fluid should be saved in an EDTA tube for cytologic evaluation. Aerobic and anaerobic samples for bacterial culture and isolation also should be obtained. Sometimes redirection of the needle, repositioning of the animal, or multiple insertions are necessary to ensure complete evacuation of any nonconfluent pockets of air or fluid.

9. What are the complications of thoracocentesis?

Iatrogenic lung laceration and pneumothorax may result from needle thoracocentesis. If excessive restraint is used, dyspnea and respiratory compromise may worsen. It may be prudent to sedate the animal with butorphanol (0.2–0.4 mg/kg IV) to decrease anxiety and the need for excessive restraint. Infection is usually a rare complication.

10. When is a chest tube inserted?

A chest tube is indicated when a pyothorax is present or when the patient requires frequent chest taps to alleviate reaccumulation of air or fluid in the chest. In addition, chest tubes are frequently placed after thoracic surgery to ensure complete evacuation of intraoperative air or postoperative fluid accumulation.

11. What items are needed to place a chest tube?

Clippers and materials for preparing the skin for a sterile procedure are required. In addition, a sterile commercial chest tube (Argyle Trocar Catheter, Sherwood Medical, St. Louis) or a red-rubber catheter is needed. The size of the chest drain depends on the size of the animal: 14–16 French can be used in cats and very small dogs, 18–22 French in small dogs, 22–28 French for medium-to-large dogs, and 28–36 French for large dogs. It is best to cut additional holes near the end of the chest tube before insertion, which should be done in a sterile manner. Ensure that none of the holes will be outside the thoracic cavity after insertion. If you are using a commercial chest tube, place the last hole on the radiopaque line to facilitate radiographic determination of chest tube placement.

General anesthesia is preferred for placement of a sterile chest tube; however, if the patient's condition is critical, necessitating rapid intervention, local infiltration with 2% lidocaine may be used in the chest wall.

A full surgical kit is necessary, including cap, mask, sterile drape and gloves, scalpel blade and handle, needle driver, curved and straight hemostats, and gauze sponges. A stopcock, bubble tubing (Argyle, Sherwood Medical, St. Louis), nonabsorbable suture material, large catheter tip syringe, 22-gauge wire, bandage scissors, and bandage material are also required.

12. What is the procedure for placing a chest tube?

If the patient's condition permits, induce anesthesia with the animal in lateral recumbency. Then clip and surgically prepare the skin over the lateral thorax from the fifth to the ninth intercostal spaces. With 2% lidocaine, locally infiltrate the skin, subcutaneous tissue, intercostal muscles, and pleura at mid-thorax over the sixth or seventh intercostal space. Don cap, mask, sterile gown, and gloves, and place sterile drapes.

Commercial chest tube. An assistant should grasp the skin along the entire lateral chest wall just caudal to the elbow and pull it forward. A small skin incision should be made at the mid-thorax over the sixth or seventh intercostal space. Preplace a pursestring suture around this incision, and estimate the length of the tube to be inserted. Next, with the chest tube tip resting on the chest wall in the incision, maintain a good hold of the chest tube and trocar a few centimeters above the surface of the chest wall, and pop the commercial chest tube through the pleura by delivering a firm blow to the top of the trocar with the heel of your hand. The trocar should not extend beyond the tip of the chest tube once you have entered the pleural space to avoid damage to the lung, heart, or vessels. After you have advanced the partially retracted trocar and tube unit a few centimeters into the chest cavity, advance the chest tube the premeasured distance from the trocar at a 45° angle into the chest cavity. Angle the tube in a cranial ventral direction for pleural effusions or in a cranial dorsal direction for a pneumothorax.

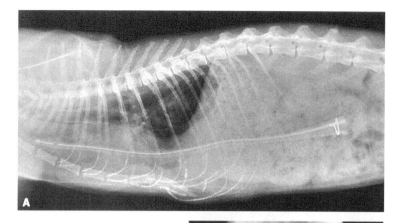

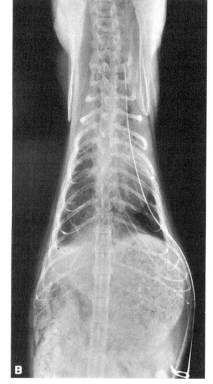

Proper placement of a chest tube for a cat with pyothorax. *A*, Lateral chest radiograph. *B*, Ventrodorsal chest radiograph.

Next, remove the trocar and clamp the chest tube before the trocar is fully withdrawn from the tube to minimize the amount of air entering the pleural cavity. A 60-cc syringe or 3-way stopcock with bubble tubing attachment is placed into the exposed end of the chest tube, and the skin is allowed to fall back into its normal position. The skin fold forms a tunnel around the tube and acts as an occlusive dressing to prevent air from entering the pleural space. The preplaced pursestring suture through the skin edges is tied around the exit point of the chest tube through the skin. A butterfly bandage around the tube is sutured to the skin, or a Chinese finger trap (see Smeak reference in bibliography) is placed to secure the tube to the body wall.

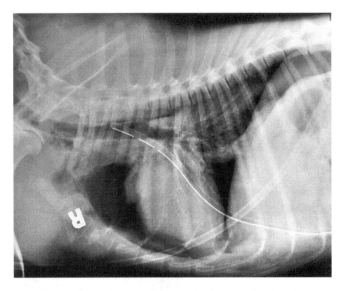

Lateral chest radiograph showing proper placement of a chest tube in a dog with pneumothorax.

Red-rubber chest tube. If a commercial chest tube is not available, a red-rubber tube may be used. Prepare and hold the skin as described previously, and make your incision. Using a closed curved hemostat, force a hole into the thoracic cavity, keeping close to the cranial edge of the seventh or eighth rib. Spread the jaws of the hemostat, and leave the spread hemostat in place. Take the tip of the red-rubber tube in the jaws of a second hemostat, and advance it so that the tip of the hemostat enters the thoracic cavity. Open the second hemostat, and advance the tube into the thoracic cavity as described. Remove both hemostats, and let the skin return to its former position. The skin opening and tube are secured as described above.

The external end of the chest tube is connected to the suction apparatus or a Heimlich valve (Heimlich Chest Drain Valve, Bard-Parker, Rutherford, NJ). A triple antibiotic dressing is placed over the skin incision, and a bandage is placed securely but nonconstrictingly around the thorax, incorporating the chest tube. Make a small loose coil in the excess drainage tubing, and secure it to the outside of chest bandage with tape. This procedure helps to prevent dislodgment of the chest tube. It is important to avoid kinks in the chest tube, connection tubing, and drainage tubing because the kinks will impede drainage and possibly allow pressure to build up in the pleural cavity.

All connections should be wired securely to prevent accidental disconnection. If continuous suction or the Heimlich valve is not used and only intermittent aspiration is required, a 3-way stopcock with the bubble tube connector is placed at the end of the chest tube and secured in place by cerclage wire.

12. How does a chest tube drainage system work?

Most drainage systems work on the principle of gravity and positive expiratory pressure. A three-way bottle system consists of two bottles for collection of drainage in the presence of a water seal and a third bottle that controls suction applied from an external source and serves as an air vent. The level of fluid in the suction control bottle determines the amount of suction provided to facilitate drainage from the pleural space.

Commercial chest tube drainage systems (Hemovac, Snyder Labs, Dover, OH) are based on the three-bottle system. The first chamber is the collection chamber. Any air aspirated from the patient moves into the second chamber, which is the water seal. The water seal usually contains about 2 cm of water. The incoming air bubbles upward through the water, which acts as a one-way valve to prevent backflow of air through the system. The air then exits the water seal chamber and enters the third, or suction control, chamber. The suction chamber allows regulation of the amount of negative pressure that can be applied to the pleural space. Normally the chamber is filled with 20 cm of sterile water. When the negative pressure generated by the suction applied to the third chamber exceeds 20 cm of water, air from the atmosphere enters through a vent and begins to bubble through the water, relieving excessive pressure. The drainage unit should remain below the patient to promote gravity drainage and to prevent fluid and air from reentering the chest cavity by backflow.

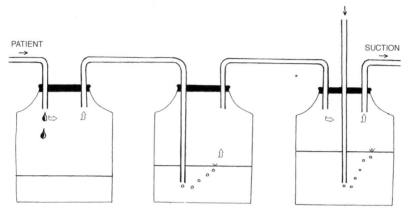

Three-bottle chest tube drainage system.

13. Should I use a collection system or perform intermittent aspiration from the tube?

A continuous-suction drainage collection system is used to facilitate constant drainage of a pyothorax. This approach is often beneficial because of the thickness of the material and aids in minimizing fluid accumulation in the chest, which creates ongoing local and systemic inflammatory responses. Unrelenting pneumothorax and any conditions in which large amounts of fluid reaccumulate will benefit from continuous-suction drainage. Usually these systems are used only with dogs because of the amounts of fluid or air being drained, apparatus size, and amount of required tubing. Such factors make use in cats cumbersome.

14. What is a Heimlich valve?

A Heimlich valve is a small, plastic one-way valve that is connected to the chest tube (Heimlich Chest Drain Valve, Bard-Parker, Rutherford, NJ). It has a collapsible rubber tube inside a chamber that acts as a one-way valve. Air escapes from the pleural space during expiration when intrathoracic pressure exceeds atmospheric pressure. Heimlich valves do not work well for drainage of pleural fluid. Fluid passing through the tube may not allow the valve to close completely because of accumulation of proteinaceous fluid, which clots or adheres to the sides of the valve, preventing drainage or allowing air to enter the pleural cavity.

15. What should I watch for in patients with a chest tube and continuous suction?

Check for air leaks by monitoring bubbling in the water seal bottle. The absence of bubbling indicates that the evacuation of air is complete and that the pressure of the expanded lung has sealed the chest tube openings. Intermittent bubbling during inspiration indicates normal function and continuing pneumothorax. Continuous bubbling on inspiration and expiration indicates an air leak in the system. In this case, if you clamp the tube near the patient and the bubbling stops, the leak most likely is in the tube. The tube may have become dislodged, or there may be a leak around the tube at the site of insertion. If bubbling continues after the initial check, the leak is somewhere between the clamp and chamber. Continue to move the clamp down the tubing toward the drainage unit, checking the water with each move. If you find a point at which the continuous bubbling stops, the clamp is between the leak and the drainage unit, and the defective tubing needs to be changed.

If the leak persists when you clamp the end of the tubing, the drainage systems are leaking and need to be replaced. Observe the patient for subcutaneous emphysema. If it develops, reassessment of the insertion site for dislodgment of the tube is necessary.

16. Should I regularly milk the tubes?

Good luck. Milk rarely comes from the tube. Milking or stripping the chest tube or drainage tubing to maintain patency is not necessary. Recent studies suggest that stripping a chest tube may harm the patient by producing negative pressures as high as 400 cm H_2O in the pleural space.

17. Should I clamp the chest tubes when I move the patient?

No. Clamping a chest tube may cause air from a pneumothorax to accumulate in the thoracic cavity and create enough pressure to cause a tension pneumothorax, which may be life-threatening. In general, clamping for more than a moment is indicated only for assessing how a patient will tolerate removal of the tube. If an animal must be moved, disconnect the drainage system from suction and move the entire system with the patient. If the chest tube or connection tubing becomes disconnected between the patient and drainage system, submerge the end of the chest tube connection in a container with 2 cm of sterile saline until it can be reconnected. The saline acts as a water seal without building up excessive pressure in the thoracic cavity.

18. What happens if the chest tube is pulled out by mistake?

Quickly apply a dry sterile dressing. If the lung still has a leak that causes ongoing pneumothorax, be careful not to apply an occlusive dressing, which may result in development of a tension pneumothorax. If there is no ongoing air leak, apply an occlusive dressing. An emergency thoracocentesis may be performed to evacuate ingress of air as a result of an open chest wound in the latter cases or before replacement of the chest tube in the former case.

19. When is the chest tube removed? How?

Chest tube removal is indicated when the patient's respiratory condition improves, radiographs demonstrate reexpansion of the lungs, fluid drainage is less than 10 ml/kg day, and no air leak is noted in the drainage system.

Before removing the chest tube, continuous suction should be turned off for a trial period of a few hours to ensure that the lung will remain inflated and no respiratory distress is noted. Before pulling the chest tube, administration of an analgesic agent is recommended (butorphanol, 0.2–0.4 mg/kg IV). If chest tube withdrawal is indicated, remove the bandage, cut the suture(s), and pull the chest tube out in one swift, continuous motion. The insertion site may be closed with sutures if necessary, and an occlusive dressing should be placed. The patient is monitored closely for the next 24 hours for signs of recurrent pleural disease.

20. What complications are associated with chest tubes?

Improper positioning, bleeding of an inadvertently lacerated intercostal vessel, intercostal nerve damage, injury to the diaphragm and thoracic or abdominal organs, infection, and pain may be complications after insertion of chest tubes.

21. How can I control pain due to the chest tube?

In medium- to large-breed dogs, bupivacaine (1.5 mg/kg diluted in 20–25 cc of sterile saline) may be introduced into the chest tube, followed by 10–15 cc sterile saline flush to deliver local anesthetic to the parietal pleura. This procedure may be repeated every 6 hours if needed. For cats and small dogs, 1.1 mg/kg of bupivacaine diluted in 10–15 cc of sterile saline every 6 hours may be used. Butorphanol, 0.2–0.4 mg/kg given intravenously every 6 hours, may be administered in cats and dogs to provide analgesia and to reduce anxiety associated with placement and maintenance of a chest tube.

22. Should I irrigate the chest tube?

In general, no. Irrigation of the chest tube involves risk of introducing nosocomial bacteria into the thoracic cavity. An exception is to provide pain relief, as described above. If a chest tube becomes clogged with blood or purulent material, it is best to change the chest tube.

23. Is antibiotic administration required for patients with chest tubes?

In general, no. However, a decrease in complications such as pneumonia or pyothorax has been observed when prophylactic antibiotics were administered for chest tube placement in human patients with traumatic hemothorax.

BIBLIOGRAPHY

1. Carroll P: Chest tubes made easy. RN 12:46–55, 1995.
2. Crow SE, Walshaw SO: Manual of Clinical Procedures in the Dog and Cat. Philadelphia, J.B. Lippincott, 1987.
3. Fishman NH: Thoracic Drainage: A Manual of Procedures. Chicago, Year Book, 1983.
4. Harvey CE, Newton CD, Schwartz A: Small Animal Surgery. Philadelphia, J.B. Lippincott, 1990.
5. Iberti TJ, Stern PM: Chest tube thoracostomy. Crit Care Clin 8:879–895, 1992.
6. Murtaugh RJ, Kaplan PM: Veterinary Emergency and Critical Care Medicine. St. Louis, Mosby, 1992.
7. O'Hanlon-Nichols T: Commonly asked questions about chest tubes. Am J Nutr 5:60–64, 1996.
8. Smeak DD: The Chinese finger trap suture technique for fastening tubes and catheters. J Am Animal Hosp Assoc 26:215–218, 1990.

111. PERICARDIOCENTESIS

Jean M. Betkowski, V.M.D.

1. When is pericardiocentesis indicated?

Animals with pericardial effusion or pericardial effusion with cardiac tamponade are in need of pericardiocentesis for diagnostic and therapeutic purposes. Cardiac tamponade, a state of cardiogenic shock caused by pericardial effusion, occurs when intrapericardial pressure exceeds pressure in the right atrium, and at times the right ventricle, during diastole. With elevated intrapericardial pressure, the central venous pressure (CVP) must increase to maintain adequate cardiac output. Clinical manifestations of CVP elevation are distended jugular veins, jugular pulses, ascites, and pulsus paradoxus. Pulsus paradoxus is manifested by femoral pulses that are palpably weaker during inspiration than during expiration. This variation in pulse pressures is caused by increased venous return to the right heart coupled with decreased venous return to the left heart with inspiration. Cardiac tamponade may occur with either a large or small amount of fluid accumulation. If fluid accumulates rapidly, a small amount of intrapericardial fluid may cause a substantial increase in intrapericardial pressure. If intrapericardial fluid accumulates slowly, the pericardial sac stretches, and large volumes of fluid may need to be present before cardiac tamponade occurs. In the latter case, animals may present for other manifestations of pericardial effusion before reaching the stage of cardiac tamponade.

2. What diagnostic studies should be considered to confirm the need for pericardiocentesis?

If the animal has stable cardiopulmonary function and suspected or confirmed pericardial effusion, full cardiac evaluation is recommended before pericardiocentesis. A **complete physical examination** of the cardiovascular system, including examination of the jugular veins, palpation of the femoral pulses, and careful auscultation of the thorax, provides useful clues. The jugular veins may be distended, or jugular pulses may reach past the thoracic inlet when the neck is extended. The femoral pulses may be weak or vary in intensity with respiration. The heart sounds may be muffled in conjunction with a tachycardic heart rhythm.

An **electrocardiogram** (EKG) may show characteristic features of sinus tachycardia, electrical alternans, and low-voltage complexes. Electrical alternans is defined by beat-to-beat variations in the height of the R wave and is caused by the rocking back and forth of the heart within the pericardial sac. The low-voltage complexes are caused by the attenuation of electric current through the intrapericardial fluid (and pleural fluid, if present). CVP also may be measured; elevations above 10 cm H_2O are supportive of significant pericardial effusion.

Thoracic radiographs are strongly suggestive of pericardial effusion if a large globoid cardiac silhouette with preservation of cranial and caudal waist is observed. The caudal vena cava also is distended.

Echocardiograms provide direct evidence of pericardial effusion and cardiac tamponade. Ideally, echocardiographic examination is performed before pericardiocentesis to maximize sensitivity in demonstrating an underlying cause, such as neoplasm or ruptured left atrium. Such findings may be less obvious on echocardiograms after the fluid has been removed.

CT or MRI scan may be used after the patient is stabilized with pericardiocentesis to examine for intrapericardial neoplasia or foreign body as well as to evaluate the thickness of the pericardial sac.

3. What are the proper approaches to treatment before or in conjunction with pericardiocentesis?

Fluid administration before pericardiocentesis may not be necessary if the patient is hemodynamically stable. If the patient is in shock, the increased preload provided by intravenous fluid administration at 1–3 times maintenance rate may be helpful for stabilization. EKG may reveal arrhythmias or electrical alternans. Significant ventricular arrhythmias (> 25–30% of beats) may require specific therapy, such as intravenous lidocaine (20 mg/kg IV bolus, repeated up to 3 times). Oxygen administration also may be useful. Diuretics generally are not indicated because they reduce preload to the right heart, which compromises right heart filling and further depresses cardiac output.

4. What type of sedation and analgesia may be used?

Most animals with pericardial effusion that warrants pericardiocentesis do not require sedation. If the animal is fractious or active and alert, small doses of sedation may be prudent to prevent iatrogenic injury to the heart or lungs during the procedure. The combinations of intravenously administered sedatives that may be used include ketamine (11 mg/kg) and diazepam (0.02 mg/kg), acepromazine (0.025 mg/kg) and butorphanol (0.02 mg/kg) or buprenorphine (0.0075 mg/kg), or diazepam and butorphanol. Drugs should be titrated to effect because compromised animals may not require full doses. Local infiltration with 2 ml of 2% lidocaine from skin surface to pleura should be used in the area of the puncture to prevent discomfort in all patients.

5. What equipment is necessary to perform pericardiocentesis?

A large-bore catheter is used for the pericardiocentesis, and continuous EKG monitoring is maintained throughout the procedure. In dogs, a 14- or 16-gauge, 5¼-inch over-the-needle catheter (Abbocath Laboratories, North Chicago, IL) is used most frequently. Full evacuation of the pericardial sac may be enhanced by adding 1–3 side holes at the distal end of the catheter with a scalpel blade (be careful not to leave burrs on the cut edges). In cats, an 18- or 19-gauge butterfly catheter may be used for pericardiocentesis.

A 3–6-ml syringe is attached to the catheter after insertion through the chest wall, and negative pressure is applied as puncture of the pericardial sac is attempted. The initial sample drawn with the syringe is placed in a red top or activated clotting time tube to observe for evidence of clot formation. Clot formation most likely indicates that a cardiac chamber or an intrapericardial tumor has been punctured. After this initial assessment to ensure proper placement of the catheter, the needle stylet is removed and intravenous extension tubing is connected to the catheter. The tubing is connected to a three-way stopcock and a larger syringe (12 cc for cats, 60 cc for dogs) for ease in evacuation of the pericardial effusion. In large-breed dogs, an adequate container for fluid collection should be at hand; pericardiocentesis may yield from 500 ml to over 1 liter of fluid. Both red top and EDTA collection tubes should be available for sample collection for possible cytologic and microbiologic analysis.

6. How is pericardiocentesis performed?

1. The animal is placed in left lateral recumbency. An area of the right chest wall is clipped from the sternum to the mid-thorax and from the ninth to third intercostal spaces. The area is aseptically prepared with an antiseptic solution. The area of insertion of the catheter is infiltrated with 1–2 ml of 2% lidocaine.

2. A small stab incision is made in the skin to facilitate insertion of a large-bore catheter. The exact point of catheter insertion may be based on palpation of the apex beat or use of the echocardiogram and thoracic radiographs to judge proximity of the pericardium to the chest wall and the best trajectory for needle insertion. In general, the catheter is inserted in the fifth or sixth intercostal space at the level of the costochondral junction.

3. The catheter is inserted through the chest wall and angled dorsocranially toward the opposite shoulder. After penetration of the chest wall, the catheter is gently advanced while negative pressure is applied to the attached syringe. If hemorrhagic fluid is obtained, the possibility of cardiac puncture should be considered (see question 5).

4. After this determination is made, the catheter is advanced well into the pericardial sac and as much fluid as possible is removed. Withdrawal of fluid may be facilitated by changing the position of the animal and by slowly withdrawing or advancing the catheter to tap isolated pockets of effusion. Echocardiographic guidance to identify pockets also may be useful at this point.

Complete removal of fluid is recommended so that reaccumulation can be monitored accurately by ultrasound. Complete removal of pericardial effusion is unnecessary to return the heart to normal function. Partial removal of effusion, even small amounts in some instances, usually causes the intrapericardial pressure to drop sharply and relieves cardiac tamponade. Puncture of the pericardial sac sometimes results in drainage of pericardial fluid into the pleural space rather than through the catheter. This effect still decreases intrapericardial pressure, although complete drainage of the pericardial sac is generally not achieved.

7. What parameters should be monitored during and after pericardiocentesis?

The most important monitoring tool is continuous EKG. EKG detects premature ventricular contractions (PVCs), which may occur during the procedure as the catheter contacts the heart or after the procedure as a result of primary disease or reperfusion injury to the myocardium. When PVCs occur during the procedure, the catheter should be repositioned to avoid potential ongoing mechanical irritation to the myocardium. As the fluid is removed and pressure decreases in the pericardial sac, EKG manifestations of pericardial effusion should resolve. Heart rate decreases, R waves may increase in size, and electrical alternans, if present, disappears. CVP values also return to normal once the intrapericardial pressure decreases. Return to normal may be delayed if right heart failure and large-volume ascites or pleural effusion are present. Continuous EKG monitoring for 24 hours after pericardiocentesis is ideal because of the potential life-threatening cardiac arrhythmias. Appropriate antiarrhythmic therapy, such as intravenous lidocaine (20 mg/kg, repeated up to 3 times and followed by constant-rate infusion at 40–80 µg/kg/min if necessary), is indicated if ventricular tachycardia is observed. Monitoring CVP values or jugular pulses in the hours after the procedure is a useful way of assessing reaccumulation of pericardial fluid. A repeat echocardiogram the following day is a more sensitive test for the presence of smaller fluid volumes in the pericardial sac. A two-week recheck echocardiogram is also recommended to assess the long-term success of pericardiocentesis. The recheck allows the examiner to identify underlying causes, such as a neoplasm that may have grown in the intervening period.

8. What tests should be performed on the pericardial fluid?

Although cytologic evaluation of pericardial fluid is often unrewarding, it is recommended, especially if the fluid does not have the typical nonclotting, hemorrhagic appearance. Samples should be collected and handled for potential bacterial and fungal culture. The need for submission of samples for microbiologic culture should be based on the results of rapid cytologic examination. Recently, pH analysis of pericardial fluid in dogs has been shown to be of diagnostic value. A pH < 7.0 is consistent with an inflammatory process, whereas a pH > 7.0 suggests neoplastic disease. The pH of the fluid may be determined with a blood gas analyzer or urine dipstick reagent strip.

9. What are the most common complications of pericardiocentesis?

Complications of pericardiocentesis requiring intervention are relatively uncommon. Ventricular arrhythmias are common but often require no specific treatment. Postpericardiocentesis hemorrhage occurs occasionally, especially if a right atrial hemangiosarcoma is present and punctured during the procedure. A coronary artery may be lacerated inadvertently, but the approach from the right side makes this less likely because the descending coronary artery lies on the left side of the heart. Recurrence of pericardial effusion is common and may take place within hours to weeks.

10. What treatment is required after pericardiocentesis?

If the animal remains hypovolemic after pericardiocentesis, appropriate replacement and maintenance fluids should be administered intravenously. Most often fluid administration is not indicated because of natural diuresis due to restored cardiac output and mobilization of ascitic fluid. Diuretics should not be administered unless a large volume of ascites or pleural effusion compromises respiratory function.

Antiinflammatory agents have been used to prevent recurrence of idiopathic pericarditis. Prednisone, 1 mg/kg orally every 12 hours, tapered over 2–3 weeks, has been advocated after initial pericardiocentesis. Dexamethasone, 1 mg/kg subcutaneously every 24 hours, also may be used. No studies have confirmed the efficacy of corticosteroid therapy for idiopathic pericarditis. Recently, azathioprine, 1 mg/kg orally once daily for 3 months, has demonstrated promise in preventing recurrence of idiopathic pericardial effusion. Pericardectomy may prove curative if fluid reaccumulates. If a hemangiosarcoma is present on the right atrial appendage, surgical removal is possible, although micrometastases have most likely occurred and long-term survival is poor. Pericardectomy, along with surgical debulking of a chemodectoma, may prevent recurrence of clinical signs for months. Intrapericardial infusion of chemotherapeutic agents, such as cisplatin (70 mg/m^2) or Adriamycin (30 mg/m^2), or antiinflammatory agents, such as dexamethasone (0.2 mg/kg), has been attempted on an experimental basis. Anecdotally, the response to intracavitary cisplatin has been favorable, but no controlled studies have been performed. Antiinflammatory agents have been less promising.

BIBLIOGRAPHY

1. Bjorling DE, Keene BW: Canine pericardial disease. Compan Animal Pract 19:9–15, 1989.
2. Bussadori C: Idiopathic haemorrhagic pericarditis: Update on clinical evaluation. In Proceedings of the 13th American College of Veterinary Internal Medicine Forum, 1995, pp 225–227.
3. Edwards NJ: The diagnostic value of pericardial fluid pH determination. J Am Animal Hosp Assoc 32:63–66, 1996.
4. Jones CL: Pericardial effusion in the dog. Comp Cont Educ 1:680–685, 1979.
5. Lombard CW: Pericardial disease. Vet Clin North Am Small Animal Pract 13:337–353, 1983.
6. Miller MW, Fossum TW: Pericardial disease. In Bonagura JD (ed): Kirk's Current Veterinary Therapy XII. Philadelphia, W.B. Saunders, 1996, pp 725–731.
7. Miller MW, Sisson DD: Pericardial disorders. In Ettinger SJ, Feldman EC: (eds): Textbook of Veterinary Internal Medicine, 4th ed. Philadelphia, W.B. Saunders, 1995, pp 1032–1045.

112. EMERGENCY VENOUS ACCESS

Lisa L. Powell, D.V.M.

1. List two common emergency situations in which venous access is necessary.
• Shock
• Cardiopulmonary arrest

2. Is it difficult to obtain vascular access to a peripheral vein in hypovolemic states?
It may be difficult to place intravenous catheters in hypovolemic and hypotensive patients. Peripheral veins are often constricted because of the adrenergic response after an event that stimulates the hypovolemic or hypotensive state. Venous access also may be complicated in small patients, pediatric patients, small exotic veterinary patients, edematous patients, and obese patients. In most situations, an intravenous catheter can be placed with conventional methods.

3. If conventional methods fail, what other ways are available to obtain venous access?
Alternate methods of obtaining venous access include facilitation incisions, venous cutdown procedures, and intraosseous catheterization.

4. Is chemical sedation necessary for placement of an intraosseous catheter or venous cutdown?
Because most patients are critically ill, chemical restraint usually is not necessary for placement of an intraosseous catheter or venous cutdown. Local infusion of 2% lidocaine is usually sufficient.

5. What is a facilitation incision?
A facilitation incision is a full-thickness skin incision over the vein into which catheterization is attempted. Time permitting, the area is aseptically prepared, and lidocaine is infused. A no.-11 blade or the bevel of an 18-gauge needle is used to make a small, full-thickness skin incision in the area of catheterization. The catheter can then be advanced through the incision and into the more easily visualized vein. This method decreases skin tension and friction against the catheter and allows better catheter control.

6. How is venous cutdown performed?
Two different types of venous cutdown procedures can be performed: minicutdown and full cutdown. The **minicutdown** is similar to facilitation incision, but the incision is extended so that the superficial surface of the vein is visualized. The vessel is incised with the bevel of a 20-gauge needle, and the catheter is advanced into the vein.

The **full cutdown** must be performed under sterile conditions. After infusion of lidocaine into the area, a 2.5–5-cm incision is made through the skin parallel and to one side of the vessel. The vessel is dissected free of the surrounding tissues and clamped proximally and distally with either vascular clamps or sutures. A venotomy is made between the clamps, and a catheter is advanced through the venotomy site toward the proximal clamp. The clamps are removed, sutures are placed around the catheter and vein proximal and distal to the insertion site to secure the catheter into the vein, the area is flushed with sterile saline, and the skin is closed with sutures around the catheter. The full cutdown is used when a long-term intravenous catheter is needed or in emergency settings when other venous access methods have failed.

7. What are the major contraindications for doing a cutdown?
Relative contraindications for performing venous cutdown include significant coagulopathy, such as disseminated intravascular coagulation (DIC); systemic infection; metabolic disease;

immune-mediated thrombocytopenia and thrombocytopenia secondary to DIC, hemorrhage, or infectious disease (e.g., Rocky Mountain spotted fever, ehrlichiosis, Lyme disease); factor deficiencies such as von Willebrand's disease; and toxicities such as warfarin ingestion. If a catheter must be placed via cutdown in such situations, efforts must be made to control hemorrhage at the placement site (i.e., use of direct pressure). The facilitation incision, minicutdown, or intraosseous methods are preferred if conventional methods have failed.

8. What complications are associated with venous cutdown?

Possible complications associated with the cutdown procedure include hemorrhage at the catheter placement site, which can be avoided if hemorrhage is controlled during the placement procedure, and infection, which can be avoided if sterile methods are used when the catheter is initially placed. Sterile bandage material should be used to cover the catheter site for further protection against contamination and infection.

9. What sites are most commonly used for placement of an intraosseous catheter?

The most common sites for placement of an intraosseous catheter include the intertrochanteric fossa of the femur, wing of the ilium, tibial tuberosity, medial surface of the proximal tibia just distal to the tibial tuberosity, and greater tubercule of the humerus.

10. How do you place an intraosseous catheter?

In placing an intraosseous catheter, the following materials are needed:
- 1% lidocaine for local anesthesia
- No. 11 scalpel blade
- Needles: 16–20-gauge bone marrow needle (dogs, cats)
  18–22-gauge spinal needle (cats, young dogs)
  18–25-gauge hypodermic needle (neonates)
  12- and 15-gauge commercial intraosseous catheter
- 12-ml syringe
- Heparinized saline (3 ml)
- Antiseptic ointment

The site must be clipped and aseptically prepared. The skin and periosteum are infused with 2% lidocaine solution. The scalpel blade is used to make a stab incision down to the periosteum. The needle is then passed through the stab incision and into the cortex of the bone. The needle is seated in the cortex by applying light pressure and turning the needle back and forth at about 30° turns. A sudden decrease in resistance usually occurs once the marrow has been entered. The needle is advanced to the hub if possible. Placement is checked by moving the limb and noting that the needle moves solidly with the limb when it is flexed and extended; the needle will wobble if it is not seated in the bone. The 12-cc syringe is used to aspirate marrow, further verifying placement within the marrow cavity. The needle is flushed with heparinized saline. Little resistance should be encountered in flushing the needle. If resistance is felt, turning the needle 90–120° may help to move the bevel away from the inner cortex. A tape strip should be placed at the junction of the needle and skin. Sutures are placed through the tape strip and then through the periosteum or surrounding skin. Antiseptic ointment on gauze is applied over the entrance site, and the whole needle apparatus is covered with bandage to prevent movement and breakage of the needle and to protect against contamination of the site. A common bandage method consists of figure-eight placement of cast padding around the catheter, then coverage with a small amount of stretch gauze and Vetwrap or elasticon for the outer layer.

11. What are the indications for use of intraosseous catheters?

Intraosseous catheterization is an excellent method for gaining venous access in small patients, pediatric patients, and severely hypotensive and hypovolemic patients. Intraosseous administration of fluids and medications achieves the same blood levels as administration into peripheral veins. Patients in cardiopulmonary arrest often benefit from intraosseous catheterization for two reasons: (1) most peripheral veins are collapsed, and (2) gaining venous access is often impossible.

12. What are the major contraindications to placing an intraosseous catheter?
Contraindications to placement of an intraosseous catheter include bone disease at the insertion site (e.g., fractures, neoplasia, osteomyelitis), abscesses over the placement area, skin and wound infections, and sepsis. In treating septic patients, the potential for causing osteomyelitis (i.e., providing a nidus for hematogenous spread of bloodborne pathogens) must be weighed against increased mortality due to inadequate fluid resuscitation.

13. What complications are associated with placing an intraosseous catheter?
The most common complication associated with intraosseous catheterization is infection. Other complications include extravasation of fluids into surrounding tissues if the catheter pierces both bone cortices and, rarely, bone fractures. The risk of infection increases with the amount of time the catheter remains in the bone.

14. Which medications can be delivered through an intraosseous catheter?
Many drugs have been shown to be effective when administered through the intraosseous catheter, including:

Aminophylline	Dexamethasone	Epinephrine
Atropine	Diazepam	Insulin
Calcium gluconate	Digitalis	Morphine
Sodium bicarbonate	Diphenhydramine	Thiopental
Cefoxitin	Dobutamine	Dextrose

15. What about administration of plasma, blood products, hypertonic saline, hetastarch, and dextrans through an intraosseous catheter?
Plasma, blood products, hypertonic saline, and synthetic colloids can be administered safely through an intraosseous catheter. The maximal rate of infusion is slower than that achievable with a large-bore venous catheter, but resuscitation may be successful when the intraosseous route is used.

16. Do you need to change the dose of medications, colloids, blood products, or crystalloids when they are administered through an intraosseous catheter?
Using an intraosseous catheter is comparable to using an intravenous line. Therefore, the dose of medications, colloids, blood products, and crystalloids administered through an intraosseous catheter is the same as the intravenous dose.

17. How long can intraosseous catheters remain safely in a patient?
An intraosseous catheter can remain in place safely for 72 hours as long as aseptic technique is used for placement and bandaging is adequate.

18. Overall, what is the safest and most effective method of catheter placement if conventional methods fail in the emergency setting?
In an emergency situation, venous access may be the one procedure necessary to save the patient's life; it also may the most difficult and, in some instances, a seemingly impossible procedure to perform. With alternative methods for catheter placement such as venous cutdowns and intraosseous catheterizations, aseptic technique should be used. If there is no time for aseptic preparation of the catheter site, a conventional venous catheter should replace the emergent catheter when resuscitation and stabilization are achieved.

BIBLIOGRAPHY
1. Hansen B: Treatment of shock. ACVECC Proceedings, San Antonio, TX, 1995, pp 21–24.
2. Otto C, McCall-Kaufman G, Crowe DT: Intraosseous infusion of fluids and therapeutics. Comp Vet Cont Educ 11:421–430, 1989.
3. Poundstone M: Intraosseous infusion of fluids in small animals. Vet Tech 13:407–410, 1992.
4. Okrasinski EB, Krahwinkel DJ: Treatment of dogs in hemorrhagic shock by intraosseous infusion of hypertonic saline and dextrans. Vet Surg 21:20–24, 1992.

113. URETHRAL CATHETERIZATION

Steven Mensack, V.M.D., and Orna Kristal, D.V.M.

1. What are the indications for urethral catheterization?

Single or intermittent catheterization is most frequently used to relieve urethral obstruction or to obtain urine directly from the bladder for diagnostic purposes when cystocentesis is not possible. Other indications include instillation of contrast media for radiographic study of the bladder or urethra, retrieval of urocystoliths for analysis, prostatic washes, and removal of urine in animals that are unable to void normally because of recumbency, neurologic dysfunction of the bladder, and pain.

An **indwelling urinary catheter** is indicated for measuring urine output, maintaining urethral patency after relief of urethral obstruction (especially when the obstruction is associated with significant inflammation and persistence of debris in the urinary tract), continued emptying of a hypotonic bladder, and collection of urine in recumbent animals. It also is used in selected cases after surgery involving the urinary bladder, urethra, and prostate.

2. What are the relative contraindications for urethral catheterization?

Urethral catheters should be avoided in patients that are immunocompromised (e.g., viral infections such as parvovirus, pancytopenia, chemotherapy) or septic, when urinary catheterization is not easily achieved without significant risk of urethral or bladder trauma (urethral or bladder neoplasia), and when the presence of a urethral catheter may adversely affect the outcome of a surgical intervention (prepubic urethrostomy).

3. Which catheter types are most commonly used?

Urinary catheters vary in size, composition, and design. They are sized according to outer diameter, using the French (Fr) system. One French unit equals $\frac{1}{3}$ mm. The inner diameter of the catheter is affected by design and material. Catheters may be either self-retaining or non–self-retaining.

The **Foley catheter** is the most commonly used self-retaining catheter. It has a balloon at the tip that can be inflated with sterile saline through an inflation channel incorporated into the catheter wall. Inflation of the balloon when the tip of the catheter is in the bladder prevents removal of the catheter from the bladder lumen. Foley catheters are composed of Latex with a Teflon coating or silicone; this composition makes the catheter flexible and inert. Foley catheters are highly flexible and less traumatic than many stiff, non–self-retaining catheters. The Foley catheter is used mainly as an indwelling catheter in larger female dogs; the narrow and long urethra of male dogs requires a stiffer, longer catheter. The 8-Fr or larger size of the Foley catheter precludes its use in cats and small dogs.

The most commonly used non–self-retaining catheters are straight urethral catheters with a single lumen and one or more openings at the distal end. Materials used in these catheters include metal, polypropylene, and polyvinyl chloride (red rubber). Non–self-retaining catheters may be secured by use of tape and/or sutures. **Metal catheters** for female dogs are available in a single size. They are sometimes used for a single catheterization because their rigidity facilitates catheterization. However, metal catheters are more traumatic to the urinary tract and therefore not highly recommended. **Polypropylene catheters** are relatively stiff, have a closed end, and are available with various internal diameters but only a single length (22 inches). They are commonly used in male and female dogs. **Tomcat catheters**, also made of polypropylene, are available only in one diameter (3.5 Fr) with either a closed or open end. Their main use is for the relief of urethral obstruction in male cats. Polypropylene catheters are not ideal for use as indwelling catheters because the stiffness may cause urethral and bladder trauma. **Polyvinyl** chloride (red-rubber) catheters are available in multiple diameters and two lengths. Most of these catheters are 16 inches in length. The 8-Fr size is also available in a 22-inch length. Red-rubber catheters are more flexible and less traumatic than polypropylene catheters. Studies also have shown that they are less irritating to the urethral mucosa than the polypropylene type. These properties make the red-rubber catheter more suitable for use as indwelling catheters in both genders of dogs and cats.

4. How do you decide the proper size of urethral catheter to use?

Urethral catheters are available in sizes ranging from 3.5–14 Fr. In dogs, the proper size is based on body weight. A 3.5–5 Fr catheter should be used for male dogs weighing less than 12 kg, an 8-Fr catheter for male dogs weighing 12–35 kg, and a 10- or 12-Fr catheter for male dogs weighing more than 35 kg. A 5-Fr catheter should be used for female dogs weighing less than 5 kg, an 8-Fr catheter for female dogs weighing 5–25 kg, and a 10–14-Fr catheter for female dogs weighing more than 25 kg. A 3.5-Fr catheter should be used for most cats. Occasionally, a 5-Fr catheter may be used for urethral catheterization in larger cats.

Recommended Sizes and Types of Urethral Catheters for Use in Dogs and Cats

ANIMAL	CATHETER TYPE	CATHETER SIZE (FRENCH)
Cat	Tomcat (polypropylene) or polyvinyl chloride	3.5
Male dog		
Weight ≤ 12 kg	Polypropylene or polyvinyl chloride	3.5–5
Weight 12–35 kg	Polypropylene or polyvinyl chloride	8
Weight ≥ 35 kg	Polypropylene or polyvinyl chloride	10–12
Female dog		
Weight ≤ 5 kg	Polypropylene or polyvinyl chloride	5
Weight 5–25 kg	Polypropylene, polyvinyl chloride, or Foley	8
Weight ≥ 25 kg	Polypropylene, polyvinyl chloride, or Foley	10–14

5. How is urethral catheterization performed in male dogs?

In general, two people are required to catheterize a male dog. The dog is placed in lateral recumbency.

1. The first person retracts the prepucial sheath to expose the glans penis, which is gently cleansed with a 1% povidone-iodine solution.

2. The second person dons sterile gloves and obtains a catheter of appropriate length and diameter. The distance to which the catheter is to be inserted is estimated by measuring the length from the tip of the prepuce to the perineum and half the distance back to the prepuce. The distal 3-5 cm of the catheter is lubricated with a sterile lubricant (K-Y Jelly, Johnson & Johnson). As an alternative to wearing sterile gloves, two slits can be cut into the packaging of the catheter about 3–5 cm apart near the distal end of the catheter. The end of the packaging is removed, and the 3–5-cm section is broken away from the rest of the packaging. This segment acts as a sterile handle for introducing the catheter.

3. The tip of the catheter is introduced into the distal urethral orifice and passed slowly into the bladder. Resistance may be encountered as the catheter passes over the ischial arch. Passing over the ischial arch may be facilitated by rotating the catheter and pushing on the perineum below the anus. Excessive force should be avoided because it may lead to urethral mucosa damage and potential rupture of the urethra.

4. If no urine is obtained after passing the catheter a sufficient distance to be within the bladder, an attempt should be made to aspirate urine with a sterile syringe. Compression of the urinary bladder at this point should not be attempted because it may damage the bladder. If no urine is obtained, the catheter should be withdrawn and/or advanced a short distance; aspiration for urine should be repeated before gentle removal and a second attempt at catheterization.

5. If catheterization is used to obtain a urine specimen or to decompress the bladder, the catheter is gently removed after completion of the procedure.

6. If the catheter is to remain in place as part of a closed collection system, it should be the soft, red-rubber type. To secure the catheter to the patient, phalanges made of 1-inch waterproof adhesive should be placed in a butterfly fashion on the catheter as it exits the prepuce. The phalanges are secured to the paraprepucial area with nonabsorbable sutures. Alternatively, the catheter may be secured to the paraprepucial area with nonansorbable sutures in a Chinese fingerknot technique. The collection system is then attached to the urinary catheter. A piece of tape or bandage may be placed circumferentially around the catheter and cranial abdomen of the patient to help prevent the catheter from kinking and to prevent the patient from removing the catheter. An Elizabethan collar should be used if the patient is able to reach the catheter.

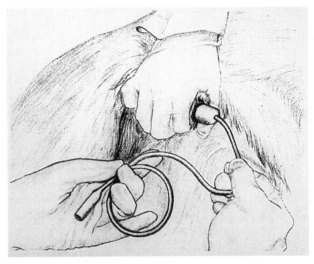

Placement of urethral catheter in male dogs. (From Crow SE, Walshaw SO: Urethral catheterization. In Manual of Clinical Procedures in the Dog and Cat. Philadelphia, J.B. Lippincott, 1987, pp 110–127, with permission.)

6. How is urethral catheterization performed in female dogs?

Urethral catheterization in female dogs requires two people.

1. The first person restrains the dog in a standing position. If this is not possible, lateral or sternal recumbency with the hind limbs hanging over the edge of a table is an acceptable alternative. A towel or other padding should be placed under the dog at the edge of the table if the sternal recumbency position is used. The dog's tail is pulled to the side to expose the vulva. The vulva and perivulvar region are gently cleansed with 1% povidone-iodine solution.

2. The second person dons sterile surgical gloves in preparation for urethral catheterization. A topical anesthetic, such as ophthalmic anesthetic drops (Ophthaine 0.5%, Solvay), 2% lidocaine liquid, or 2% viscous lidocaine, may be instilled into the vagina to decrease discomfort associated with catheter placement.

3. A sterile vaginal speculum or sterile otoscopic speculum is lubricated with sterile lubricant (K-Y Jelly, Johnson & Johnson) and inserted into the vagina. The speculum is directed dorsally to avoid the clitoral fossa and then ventrally to visualize the urethral papilla. The urethral papilla appears as a slit or dimple, usually located at the caudal pelvic brim.

4. A catheter of appropriate type and diameter is chosen, and the end is lubricated with sterile lubricant. The catheter is inserted into the urethra under direct visualization and advanced into the bladder. This distance is normally 8–14 cm (the length of the female dog's urethra). Excessive force should not be used because it may lead to urethral mucosa damage and rupture of the urethra.

5. If no urine is obtained after the catheter is passed a sufficient distance to be within the bladder, aspiration of urine may be attempted with a sterile syringe. If urine still is not obtained, the catheter is advanced and/or withdrawn a short distance, and aspiration is repeated. Compression of the urinary bladder should not be attempted at this point because it may damage the bladder. If urine is not obtained, the catheter is gently removed and catheterization is reattempted.

6. Once the urine sample is taken or the bladder decompressed, the catheter is gently removed. If the catheter is to remain in place for continuous drainage it is secured to the dog, as described below, and a closed urine collection system is attached.

Alternatively, a urinary catheter can be placed in female dogs using a tactile technique:

1. The dog is positioned and prepared as with the visual technique. Topical anesthetic may be introduced as previously described.

2. The person placing the catheter dons sterile gloves and chooses a catheter of appropriate diameter and type. The catheter is lubricated.

3. The index finger of the nondominant hand (left hand for the right-handed person) is lubricated and inserted into the vagina. The urethral papilla is palpated.

4. The catheter is passed ventral to the finger, which is used to guide the catheter gently into the urethra. If the catheter can be palpated beyond the tip of the index finger, it is not in the urethra. In this case, the catheter should be withdrawn a short distance and redirected ventrally (beneath the finger) into the urethral orifice.

5. Once the catheter tip is in the urethra, the catheter is advanced as described previously.

In female dogs, an indwelling catheter may be secured by several methods:

1. If a Foley catheter is used, the balloon is inflated with sterile saline. If resistance is met during inflation, the balloon may be within the urethra. The balloon should be deflated, and the catheter is advanced a short distance before reinflating the balloon. The amount of saline necessary for inflation is usually listed on the balloon inflation mechanism as well as the packaging.

2. If the dog is too small for a Foley catheter, a red-rubber catheter is recommended. The catheter is secured to the dog by waterproof adhesive tape phalanges placed around the urinary catheter in a butterfly fashion as it exits the vulva. The catheter is sutured through the tape phalanges to the perivulvar area with nonabsorbable suture. An Elizabethan collar is placed on the dog if it is able to reach the catheter.

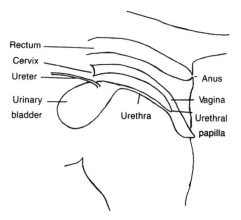

Lower urinary tract of female dogs. (From Phillip S: Urine collection in cats and dogs. Part II: Urinary catheterization. Vet Tech 11:1, 1990, with permission.)

7. How is urethral catheterization performed in male cats?

Two people are required to place a urethral catheter in male cats. Sedation or short-term anesthesia is usually necessary.

1. The first person holds the patient in lateral recumbency while pulling the hind limbs cranially and the tail laterally or dorsally. The area around the prepuce is clipped and cleansed with 1% povidone-iodine solution.

2. The second person dons sterile gloves. The end of a 3.5-Fr polypropylene tomcat catheter or 3.5-Fr (5-Fr in larger cats) red-rubber catheter is lubricated with sterile lubricant (K-Y Jelly, Johnson & Johnson). Closed-end tomcat catheters are preferred because the tip is less traumatic to the urethral mucosa.

3. The penis is extruded from the prepucial sheath by placing the thumb and index finger of the nondominant hand on either side of the prepuce, with the palm resting on the cat's spine at the tail base. Pressure is exerted in a cranial direction to extrude the penis.

4. The tip of the catheter is introduced into the urethral orifice, and the catheter is gently advanced into the bladder. Gentle traction with the thumb and forefinger on the prepuce in a caudoventral direction helps to straighten the urethra and allows the catheter to pass smoothly over the ischial arch into the bladder.

5. If difficulty is encountered in advancing the catheter (secondary to urethral obstruction or deviation), the catheter may be flushed gently with sterile saline to straighten the urethra, to dislodge an obstruction, and to allow advancement into the bladder. Excessive force should not be used because it may lead to urethral mucosa damage and potential rupture of the urethra.

6. If the catheter is to remain in place as part of a closed urine collection system, the indwelling catheter, which should be made of polyvinyl chloride, is secured to the cat. If a polypropylene catheter was initially used to remove an obstruction, it should be replaced. Flushing the polypropylene catheter with sterile saline during removal helps to flush grit in the urethra back into the bladder and distends the urethra for reinsertion of a polyvinyl chloride catheter. Freezing the polyvinyl chloride catheter before lubrication and insertion into the urethra stiffens the catheter and facilitates passage.

7. To secure the catheter, phalanges made of 1-inch waterproof adhesive tape are placed on the catheter in a butterfly fashion as it exits the prepuce. The phalanges are secured to the perineal region of the cat with nonabsorbable sutures. The collection system is attached to the catheter, which is then taped to the tail to relieve tension on the catheter and sutures and to prevent premature removal of the catheter by the patient. An Elizabethan collar should be used if the cat is able to reach the catheter.

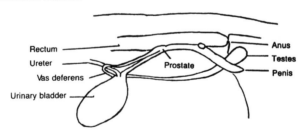

Lower urinary tract of male cats. (From Phillip S: Urine collection in cats and dogs. Part II: Urinary catheterization. Vet Tech 11:1, 1990, with permission.)

8. How is urethral catheterization performed in female cats?

Urethral catheterization in female cats requires two people. Sedation or short-term anesthesia is usually necessary.

1. The first person restrains the cat in lateral recumbency and pulls the tail laterally or dorsally. The perivulvar region is gently cleansed with 1% povidone-iodine solution. Topical anesthetics, such as ophthalmic anesthetic drops (Ophthine, Solvay), 2% lidocaine liquid, or 2% viscous lidocaine, may be instilled into the vagina to lessen discomfort associated with catheter placement.

2. The second person dons sterile gloves. The end of a 3.5-Fr polypropylene tomcat catheter or 3.5-Fr red-rubber catheter is lubricated with sterile lubricant (K-Y Jelly, Johnson & Johnson).

3. The vulvar lips are pulled caudally with one hand while the catheter is advanced along the ventral vaginal wall until it slides into the urethral orifice. A thin wire stylet inserted into the lumen of the catheter may facilitate passage. Excessive force should not be used because it may lead to urethral mucosa damage and rupture of the urethra.

4. If urine is not obtained once the catheter has been advanced a sufficient distance to be within the bladder, aspiration of urine with a sterile syringe may be attempted. Compression of the bladder is not recommended because it may damage the bladder. If no urine is obtained, the catheter should be withdrawn and/or advanced a short distance, and aspiration of urine should be reattempted before gentle removal and a second attempt at catheterization.

5. Once a urine sample is obtained or the bladder is decompressed, the catheter is gently removed. If the catheter is to remain in place as part of a closed urine collection system, it should be made of polyvinyl chloride and secured to the patient. The catheter is secured by placing 1-inch waterproof adhesive tape phalanges around the catheter in a butterfly fashion as it exits the vulva. The catheter is sutured to the perivulvar region through the tape phalanges with nonabsorbable sutures. The collection system is attached to the catheter. An Elizabethan collar should be placed if the patient can reach the catheter.

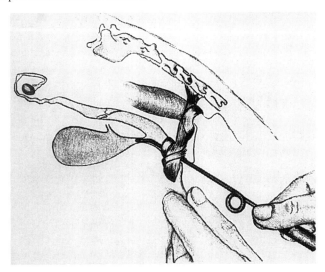

Placement of urethral catheter in female cats. (From Crow SE, Walshaw SO: Urethral catheterization. In Manual of Clinical Procedures in the Dog and Cat. Philadelphia, J.B. Lippincott, 1987, pp 110–127, with permission.)

9. If the catheter is left in place for continuous urine collection, what are the guidelines for catheter and collection system care?

When a urinary catheter is left in place, certain guidelines should be followed to lessen the incidence of trauma and infection. Once the catheter is secured to the patient, a closed urine collection system is attached. The closed system usually consists of sterile intravenous tubing attached to an empty sterile intravenous fluid bag. Alternatively, commercial urine collection systems (Dover Urinary Drainage Bag, Sherwood Medical) are available. They allow drainage of urine from the collection bag without disconnection. Many commercial systems are adapted to fit the Foley catheter.

The closed urine collection system should be handled in an aseptic manner. Once the catheter is connected to the sterile tubing, the connection should not be disrupted unless the catheter becomes obstructed. If it does, the tubing should be disconnected aseptically, and the catheter should be flushed with sterile saline. The catheter should be removed if it becomes nonfunctional or if bladder catheterization is no longer needed. The urine collection bag should be kept below the level of the patient to prevent urine reflux into the bladder; urine reflux increases the chance of bacterial colonization of the bladder. The urine collection bag also should be kept off the floor to reduce the chance of contamination of the system and colonization of the bladder with hospital pathogens. Addition of povidone-iodine or hydrogen peroxide to the urine collection bag has not been shown to prevent bacterial contamination of the system or subsequent bacterial colonization of the bladder. Any patient with an indwelling urinary catheter and the ability to reach the catheter should be fitted with an Elizabethan collar.

10. When should an indwelling urinary catheter be removed?

An indwelling urinary catheter should remain in place for the shortest time necessary. Urinary catheters should be removed under the following three circumstances:

1. **If it becomes nonfunctional.** Before removal the catheter and system should be checked for kinks. If no kinks are noted, the catheter should be flushed gently with sterile saline. If urine flow cannot be reestablished after these procedures, the catheter should be removed and examined for an explanation of malfunction. A new sterile urinary catheter may be inserted and connected to a new sterile collection system, if indicated.

2. **If bladder or urethral trauma or systemic signs of infection are observed.** If systemic signs of infection (pyuria, fever, and leukocytosis) are present, catheter removal and microbiologic cultures of both urine and catheter are recommended. Recatheterization of the urethra should be avoided unless absolutely necessary.

3. **If the condition that prompted catheterization resolves.** After removal of an indwelling catheter, the patient should be monitored carefully to ensure adequate passage of urine (volume and stream) when voiding.

11. Should antibiotics be administered during indwelling urethral catheterization?

No. Multiple studies in dogs of both sexes and male cats have shown that antibiotic administration while an indwelling urinary catheter is in place provides no protection against urethral and urinary bladder bacterial colonization. Bacterial colonization of the bladder occurred within 4 days of catheter placement despite antibiotic administration. Several studies also showed that if antibiotics were given while the animal was catheterized, the bacteria developed resistance. Antibiotics administered after catheter removal should be based on results of microbiologic culture and antibiotic sensitivity testing of urine samples.

CONTROVERSIES

12. What are the effects of urethral catheterization on urinalysis and microbiologic testing of urine specimens?

Several studies have addressed this issue in male and female dogs and male cats. Urinalysis results may be altered by obtaining samples via urethral catheter rather than cystocentesis. Reported differences include the presence of blood and increased protein concentration on urinalysis of catheterized samples from the bladder. Examination of comparative urine sediments revealed an increased presence of red blood cells (caused by urethral and/or bladder trauma), white blood cells, and bacteria (from urine contamination in the urethra and/or vagina) in samples obtained by catheterization. Results in dogs have shown that contamination of specimens is more likely in females than males. The results of urinalyses taken by urethral catheterization should be interpreted with caution.

Results of microbiologic culture should be reviewed critically if the specimen was obtained by urethral catheterization. Several studies have shown that cultures may be negative even though bacteria are present in the urine sediment of catheterized samples. This may be attributed to low bacterial colony counts (a minimum of 10^5 bacteria/ml is necessary to differentiate infection from contamination); large amounts of amorphous debris, which may mimic the presence of bacteria; or presence of anaerobic bacteria. Other studies have shown that microbiologic cultures obtained by catheterization are falsely positive compared with results of urine samples obtained by cystocentesis in the same animal.

13. What ancillary methods may be used to dislodge urethral obstructions?

Hydropulsion, the most commonly used method to remove obstructions of the urethra, involves injecting sterile saline through the catheter into the urethra in an attempt to flush the obstructing object back into the bladder. Gentle pressure is applied to the syringe to create a steady stream of saline. Alternatively, short pulsatile jets of saline may be used in an attempt to dislodge the obstruction. In male dogs and cats, digital occlusion of the urethra distal to the obstruction during hydropulsion may increase retrograde pressure and distend the urethra sufficiently to dislodge the obstruction. If tremendous resistance is met during injection of saline, hydropulsion should be discontinued because it may cause urethral mucosal damage and potentially rupture the urethra.

In male cats, several other types of catheters and adjuncts to catheterization have been used successfully to relieve urethral obstructions. Open-end tomcat polypropylene catheters, small over-the-needle intravenous catheters with the stylet removed, and metal lacrimal catheters have been used with hydropulsion to dislodge urethral obstructions. These types of catheters may cause significant urethral trauma and should be used with caution and only when attempts with a closed-end polypropylene tomcat catheter have failed.

Walpole's solution is a highly acidic flush that aids in the dissolution of mucocrystalline plugs. If an obstruction cannot be relieved by the above methods, a small amount of Walpole's solution may be instilled through the catheter, followed several minutes later by additional attempts at hydropulsion. This solution is highly irritating to the tissues and should not be instilled directly into the bladder. If all attempts at relief of urethral obstruction are unsuccessful, surgical intervention (urethrostomy, cystotomy, or temporary tube cystostomy) is indicated.

BIBLIOGRAPHY

1. Barsanti JA, Blue J, Edmunds J: Urinary tract infection due to indwelling bladder catheters in dogs and cats. J Am Vet Med Assoc 187:384–388, 1985.
2. Barsanti JA, Shotts EB, et al: Effect of therapy on susceptibility to urinary tract infection in male cats with indwelling urethral catheters. J Vet Intern Med 6(2):64–70, 1992.
3. Comer KM, Ling GV: Results of urinalysis and bacterial culture of canine urine obtained by antepubic cystocentesis, catheterization, and the midstream voided methods. J Am Vet Med Assoc 179:891–895, 1981.
4. Crow SE, Walshaw SO: Urethral catheterization. In Manual of Clinical Procedures in the Dog and Cat. Philadelphia, J.B. Lippincott, 1987, pp 110–127.
5. Kirk RW, Bistner SI, Ford RB: Urine collection. In Handbook of Veterinary Procedures and Emergency Treatment, 6th ed. Philadelphia, W.B. Saunders, 1995, pp 483–489.
6. Lees GE, Osborne CA: Urinary tract infections associated with the use and misuse of urinary catheters. Vet Clin North Am Small Animal Pract 9:713–727, 1979.
7. Lees GE, Simpson RB, Green RA: Results of analyses and bacterial cultures of urine specimens obtained from clinically normal cats by three methods. J Am Vet Med Assoc 184:449–454, 1984.
8. Lees GE: Use and misuse of indwelling urethral catheters. Vet Clin North Am Small Animal Pract 26:499–505, 1996.
9. Phillip S: Urine collection in cats and dogs. Part II: Urinary catheterization. Vet Tech 11(1):21–32, 1990.
10. Stone EA, Barsanti JA: Surgical materials, instruments, and urinary catheters. In Urological Surgery of the Dog and Cat. Philadelphia, Lea & Febiger, 1992, pp 83–90.

114. ABDOMINAL PARACENTESIS

Orna Kristal, D.V.M.

1. What is abdominal paracentesis?
Needle or catheter puncture of the abdominal cavity to remove variable amounts of fluid for diagnostic and/or therapeutic purposes.

2. What are the indications for abdominal paracentesis?
• Peritonitis
• Obvious or suspected blunt abdominal trauma
• Penetrating abdominal wall trauma (especially if peritoneal penetration is unknown)
• Acute abdomen
• Suspected postoperative gastrointestinal dehiscence
• Peritoneal fluid accumulation
• Evaluation of trauma patients with multiple injuries
• Evaluation of patients with hypovolemic or hemorrhagic shock and unsatisfactory response to shock therapy
• Removal of excessive quantity of ascitic fluid

3. How is abdominal paracentesis performed?
Abdominal paracentesis in dogs and cats may be performed with a simple needle, over-the-needle intravenous catheter, or peritoneal dialysis catheter. Preparation of the patient and site for paracentesis is essentially the same with all methods. The urinary bladder should be emptied by allowing the animal to void, manual expression, or catheterization to avoid accidental cystocentesis. The animal is restrained in left lateral recumbency to minimize risk of puncturing the spleen. A standing position in large dogs is also acceptable for needle paracentesis. The ventral midline area is clipped and aseptically prepared for needle or catheter insertion 1–2 cm caudal to the umbilicus. Use of this site avoids the falciform fat, which readily blocks the needle barrel.

Needle paracentesis. The use of local anesthesia is usually not necessary. A 1-inch, 18–20 gauge needle is inserted in the ventral midline or slightly lateral to it (see figure at top of next page). Insertion through obvious scars should be avoided because of the possibility of adhesion of underlying abdominal viscera. After needle insertion, the fluid is collected from the hub of the needle into an EDTA tube and a serum (red-top) tube for analysis, and the needle is removed. This technique of open-needle abdominocentesis is reportedly more sensitive than aspiration with a syringe. If a syringe is attached, only mild negative pressure should be applied; otherwise the needle may be occluded with omentum or other abdominal contents.

Over-the-needle intravenous catheter paracentesis. The paracentesis site is infiltrated with 1% lidocaine down to and including the linea alba. A 2.5-inch, 14-gauge, styleted intravenous catheter is used. Once the peritoneum is penetrated, the catheter is advanced into the abdominal cavity, and the stylet is removed. The addition of side holes to the catheter and application of abdominal compression may enhance fluid collection.

Peritoneal dialysis catheter paracentesis. The dialysis catheter (Diacath, Travenol Laboratories, Deerfield, IL) may be introduced into the abdominal cavity by using the trocar supplied with the catheter. The patient is placed in left lateral recumbency and prepared as described above. A small skin incision is made, and the catheter-trocar unit is inserted through the linea alba with a controlled rotational movement. Once the peritoneum is penetrated, the point of the trocar is pulled back into the catheter, and the whole unit is advanced a short distance into the abdomen. The catheter is then threaded caudally over the trocar until all of the catheter holes are within the abdominal cavity. Then the trocar is removed, allowing fluid collection.

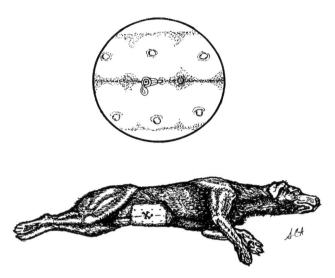

Needle paracentesis. The needle is inserted in the ventral midline 1–2 cm caudal to the umbilicus. The fluid sample is collected from the hub of the needle into the appropriate tubes.

4. What is a "minilap" procedure?

The minilaparotomy procedure is an alternative method of peritoneal dialysis catheter paracentesis. It has a lower risk for laceration or puncture of abdominal viscera and is more suitable for small patients. The patient is placed in dorsal recumbency, and a small incision is made through the skin, subcutaneous tissue, and linea alba. Strict hemostasis is necessary to avoid bleeding into the peritoneal cavity, which may create false-positive results. The catheter, without use of the trocar, is then inserted caudally, and a fluid sample is aspirated with a syringe. After a sample is obtained, the catheter is removed and the skin incision is sutured. If a sample cannot be obtained with either technique of peritoneal dialysis catheter paracentesis, the animal is rolled gently from side to side, and reaspiration is attempted. The catheter may be sutured in place if repeated sampling, drainage, or peritoneal lavage is indicated.

5. What are the advantages and disadvantages of the three techniques for paracentesis?

Needle paracentesis is rapid, inexpensive, and easy to perform; it requires minimal equipment and restraint. The risk of puncturing bowel is low because the mobile loops of gut simply move away from the needle. Patient restraint is important while the needle is in the abdomen because movement increases the risk of lacerating abdominal viscera. The main disadvantage of needle paracentesis is that it is not sensitive to small amounts of intraperitoneal fluid. A single-hole needle is also easily occluded by the omentum. Kolata has shown that at least 5.2–6.6 ml/kg body weight (BW) of fluid must be present in the abdominal cavity of dogs to obtain positive results in 78% of cases. Other investigators report 47–52% accuracy with needle paracentesis.

A 14-gauge **over-the-needle intravenous catheter** with added side holes has the same advantages as needle paracentesis. In addition, there is less chance of lacerating abdominal organs. This technique is more sensitive because of additional length and presence of side holes. The plastic catheter, however, may easily kink and occlude.

Paracentesis with a dialysis catheter is the most sensitive method of the three and can detect the presence of 1–4.4 ml/kg BW of abdominal fluid. Other investigators found that this technique accurately detects presence of abdominal fluid in 41–83% of cases. The great reliability of this method can be attributed to the large internal diameter (11 French), length of the catheter, and multiple fenestrations. The fenestrations make complete occlusion of the catheter by the omentum and bowel unlikely and provide a large surface area for fluid contact. These qualities make the dialysis catheter more efficient in recovering large volumes of abdominal fluid and most suitable for use in abdominal lavage techniques. Disadvantages include expense, time, and effort requirements, increased discomfort to the patient, and use of a surgical approach with sedation and local anesthetic. In addition, if the trocar is used, accidental puncture of abdominal organs is possible.

6. Is it possible to get false-positive results with abdominocentesis ?

Yes. False-positive results may be obtained with iatrogenic hemorrhage or penetration of an abdominal organ (e.g., spleen, bowel, bladder). Collection of blood that clots usually indicates that the needle has entered a blood vessel or organ. This finding can be confirmed microscopically by identifying the presence of platelets and the absence of erythrophagocytosis. When the reliability of the results is in doubt, paracentesis at a different site is indicated. Truly positive findings are repeatable.

7. How should one proceed if the results of needle paracentesis are negative?

A tap should be considered positive when a minimal amount of nonclotting fluid is obtained, sometimes filling only the hub of the needle. False-negative results are significantly more common than false-positive results, particularly with simple needle paracentesis. The main causes for false-negative results are a small amount of peritoneal fluid, occlusion of the needle by the omentum, and retroperitoneal injuries. In cases of a suspected false-negative result, all or some of the following steps may be taken to enhance the chance of obtaining a positive result:

1. **Repositioning** of the needle should be attempted (i.e., rotating the needle and/or changing the angle of insertion).

2. **Gentle aspiration** with a syringe and, if unsuccessful, injection of a small quantity of sterile saline to alleviate positional occlusion of the needle hole by the omentum.

3. Paracentesis may be attempted at several sites. In **four-quadrant abdominocentesis**, four separate needle paracenteses are performed. Paracentesis is undertaken in the center of each anatomic quadrant of the abdomen (cranial right, cranial left, caudal right, and caudal left).

4. Paracentesis with a 14-gauge intravenous catheter and **added side holes** or with a peritoneal dialysis catheter.

5. **Diagnostic peritoneal lavage** (DPL) is the most reliable method for early detection of intraabdominal injury or disease. It accurately detects abdominal fluid in 94–100% of cases, regardless of the amount present. A 14-gauge intravenous catheter or, preferably, a peritoneal dialysis catheter is placed as previously described. The catheter insertion is followed by instillation of 22 ml/kg BW of warm lactated Ringer's solution or 0.9% saline, rapidly infused via an intravenous administration set into the abdominal cavity. The animal is gently rolled from side to side to distribute and mix the fluid; then a representative sample of 10–20 ml is collected for analysis. It is not necessary to collect all of the infused lavage fluid. If no fluid is collected after the lavage, another 22 ml/kg BW may be infused and the collection attempt repeated.

8. How should the fluid sample be handled?

When possible, a sample of 2–3 ml should be collected into an EDTA tube for analysis of total cell counts, total protein concentration, and cytologic examination. Another sample of 3–10 ml should be collected into one or two serum (red-top) tubes, which can be used for biochemical analysis and bacteriologic culture. The fluid should be examined as soon as possible, especially if the sample was obtained by DPL because the salt solution in the lavage results in cell lysis within 30 minutes. If immediate analysis is not possible, air-dried smears should be made soon after fluid collection, and the remainder of the fluid should be refrigerated (maximum of 24–36 hours) until further examination is possible. A culture sample should be transferred to a transport medium or culture broth and handled appropriately. Fluid specimens with low turbidity warrant centrifugation and examination of sediment smears.

9. What tests should be performed on the fluid sample?

Fluid analysis should include assessment of color and turbidity, specific gravity, hematocrit, and white cell count, along with cytologic examination of air-dried smears. Biochemical tests for total protein, creatinine, and bilirubin concentrations or amylase, alanine aminotransferase, and alkaline phosphatase activities may be selected, depending on the suspected abdominal disease. Aerobic and anaerobic cultures should be submitted if fluid cytology and clinical signs suggest bacterial infection. In many cases, the definitive cause of fluid accumulation can be discovered. Even when the specific cause cannot be determined, this analysis may indicate the direction of further investigation. A point to remember is that long-standing effusions nearly always incite some degree of peritoneal reaction, resulting in secondary sterile inflammation that may modify fluid characteristics.

Interpretation of Abdominal Paracentesis Fluid Data

CHARACTERISTIC	TRANSUDATE	MODIFIED TRANSUDATE	EXUDATE	HEMORRHAGIC EXUDATE
Physical appearance	Clear to straw	Serous to serosanguineous	Amber to red	Pink to red
Specific gravity	< 1.018	1.018–1.025	> 1.025	> 1.025
Total protein	< 2.5 gm/dl	2.5–7.5 gm/dl	> 3 gm/dl	> 3 gm/dl
Nucleated cells	< 1000/µl	1000–7000/µl	> 7000/µl	> 7000/µl
Cell composition	Macrophages Mesothelial cells Neutrophils	Macrophages Mesothelial cells Neutrophils Small lymphocytes (occasionally) Red blood cells with or without neoplastic cells	Neutrophils predominate with inflammation Macrophages Mesothelial cells Small lymphocytes Red blood cells with or without neoplastic cells	Red blood cells and white blood cells with or without mesothelial cells or neoplastic cells
Cause	Hypoproteinemia Neoplasia Obstructed intestinal lymph drainage Prehepatic and hepatic portal hypertension Uroperitoneum	Neoplasia Congestive heart failure Posthepatic and hepatic portal hypertension Feline infectious peritonitis Chyle/pseudochyle (ruptured lymph vessel, lymphosarcoma, lymphangiectasia)	Infectious peritonitis Pancreatic peritonitis Bile peritonitis Urine peritonitis Neoplasia Feline infectious peritonitis Chyle/pseudochyle with or without secondary inflammation	Bleeding disorders Neoplasia Trauma Torsion of spleen or stomach

Interpretation of Chemical Analysis of Abdominal Paracentesis Fluid

TEST	INTERPRETATION
Bilirubin	Values greater than serum concentration indicate leakage of bile from the hepatobiliary tree or proximal GI tract. Not valid in jaundiced animals.
Amylase	Values greater than serum concentration indicate pancreatitis or intestinal ischemia.
Creatinine	Values greater than serum concentration indicate leakage of urine into abdominal cavity.
Alanine aminotransferase (ALT)	Values greater than serum concentration indicate direct liver trauma or inflammation.
Akaline phosphatase (SAP)	Values greater than serum concentration indicate small bowel ischemia or perforation.

10. Which abdominal paracentesis findings indicate the need for exploratory laparotomy?

1. Hemoperitoneum that is not responsive to volume replacement.

2. If DPL is performed, a packed cell volume (PCV) of lavage fluid greater than 5% indicates that significant intraabdominal bleeding has occurred. This warrants repeat lavage sampling at 20–30-minute intervals. If the PCV progressively increases, surgical intervention is indicated.

3. A high white cell count with a high number of degenerative neutrophils indicates suppurative peritonitis. Exploration should be performed.

4. Intracelluar bacteria in neutrophils from the fluid sample indicate infectious peritonitis (the finding of extracellular bacteria exclusively needs to be interpreted with caution because the bacterial origin may be from the stain).

5. Vegetable fibers in the fluid sample indicate bowel perforation.

6. Creatinine concentration in the fluid sample greater than serum concentration indicates urinary tract injury and uroperitoneum.

7. Concentrations of bilirubin in the fluid sample greater than concentrations in serum indicate hepatobiliary or proximal gastrointestinal tract injury and leakage of bile.

8. The results of peritoneal fluid analysis should be evaluated in conjunction with clinical manifestations. Overzealous interpretation of findings may result in unnecessary surgery.

11. When is drainage of large quantities of abdominal fluid indicated?

Therapeutic abdominal fluid drainage by paracentesis is not routinely done for several reasons:

1. Visible ascites is a secondary sign of disease. Consequently, the correct approach to ascites is to determine the nature of the primary disease (e.g., heart disease, renal disease, neoplasia) and to attempt treatment. The removal of abdominal fluid without addressing the primary problem results in rapid reaccumulation of fluid.

2. In some cases, depending on the primary disease, gradual and controlled removal of abdominal fluid may be achieved medically with the use of sodium-restricted diets, diuretics, aldosterone-inhibiting drugs, and angiotensin-converting enzyme inhibitors.

3. The risks of rapid removal of large quantities of abdominal fluid include development of hypovolemic shock from rapid reaccumulation of ascites, protein depletion, and iatrogenic infections.

Therapeutic removal of ascitic fluid is recommended only when the volume is large enough to result in respiratory distress due to compression of the diaphragm or abdominal discomfort. Although no documented evidence indicates that rapid withdrawal of peritoneal fluid results in the development of circulatory shock, it is recommended that fluid be withdrawn slowly with provision of intravenous fluid support. The removal of large volumes of peritoneal fluid also may be indicated for enhancement of the ability to perform percutaneous abdominal organ biopsy, laparoscopy, or abdominal radiography.

12. What are the possible complications of abdominocentesis?

The prevalence of complications of abdominocentesis is low if the exact procedural protocol is followed. The main complication of needle paracentesis is laceration of abdominal organs. This risk is increased if the animal is struggling. The complications of catheter paracentesis are visceral perforation, iatrogenic or spreading infection from a localized lesion, and iatrogenic hemorrhage. With DPL, subcutaneous hematoma and subcutaneous leakage of lavage fluid have been reported.

13. What are the contraindications to abdominal paracentesis?

The only conditions in which abdominal paracentesis is generally not recommended unless absolutely necessary are coagulopathy and thrombocytopenia, both of which may increase bleeding tendency. Needle or catheter puncture of the abdominal wall (with the risk of lacerating a visceral organ or blood vessel) may induce or exacerbate serious bleeding. In such cases, the decision whether to perform abdominocentesis should be made on a case-by-case basis after weighing the risk against the benefit. In addition, paracentesis with or without lavage must be used cautiously in patients with dyspnea, organomegaly, suspected body wall adhesions, or suspected diaphragmatic hernia.

14. What are the general recommendations for use of the different techniques of abdominal paracentesis?

Needle paracentesis should be attempted first because it is rapid, inexpensive, and relatively safe. It usually is sufficient in patients with obvious abdominal effusion. Catheter paracentesis with or without lavage is recommended in cases with a high index of suspicion of intraperitoneal injury or disease requiring surgery, but in which other methods of diagnosis (including needle paracentesis) provide inconclusive results.

BIBLIOGRAPHY

1. Cowell RL, Tyler RD, Meinkoth JH: Abdominal and thoracic fluid. In Cowell RL, Tyler Rd (eds): Diagnostic Cytology of the Dog and Cat. Goleta, CA, American Veterinary Publications, 1989, pp 151–166.
2. Crowe DT Jr, Crane SW: Diagnostic abdominal paracentesis and lavage in the evaluation of abdominal injuries in dogs and cats: Clinical and experimental investigations. J Am Vet Med Assoc 168:700–705, 1976.
3. Crowe DT Jr: Diagnostic abdominal paracentesis technique: Clinical evaluation in 129 dogs and cats. J Am Animal Hosp Assoc 20:223–230, 1984.
4. Crowe DT Jr: Abdominocentesis and diagnostic peritoneal lavage in small animals. Mod Vet Pract 65:877–882, 1984.
5. Davenport DJ, Martin RA: Acute abdomen. In Murtaugh RJ, Kaplan PM (eds): Veterinary Emergency and Critical Care Medicine. St. Louis, Mosby, 1992, pp 153–162.
6. Ettinger SJ, Barrett KA: Ascites, peritonitis, and other causes of abdominal distention. In Ettinger SL, Feldman EC (eds): Textbook of Veterinary Internal Medicine. Philadelphia, W.B. Saunders, 1995, pp 64–71.
7. Hunt CA: Diagnostic peritoneal paracentesis and lavage. Comp Cont Educ Pract Vet 2:449–453, 1980.
8. Kolata RJ: Diagnostic abdominal paracentesis and lavage: Experimental and clinical evaluations in the dog. J Am Vet Med Assoc 168:697–699, 1976.
9. Larkin HA: Veterinary cytology—collection and examination of body cavity fluids in animals. Irish Vet J 47:211–219, 1994.
10. Osborne CA, Perman V, Low DG: Clinical and laboratory evaluation of abnormal body fluid accumulations. Part 1: Techniques of paracentesis. Proc Annu Meet Am Animal Hosp Assoc 40:610– 612, 1973.
11. Paddleford RR, Harvey RC: Critical care surgical techniques. Vet Clin North Am 19:1091–1094, 1989.
12. Scott RC, Wilkins RJ, Greene RW: Abdominal paracentesis and cystocentesis. Vet Clin North Am 4:413–417, 1974.

115. CEREBROSPINAL FLUID COLLECTION AND ASSESSMENT

John J. McDonnell, D.V.M., M.S.

1. Why perform a cerebrospinal fluid (CSF) tap?

Certain central nervous system (CNS) conditions, particularly infectious and inflammatory brain diseases, may alter the CSF. Analysis of CSF often determines the category or specific cause of CNS disease.

2. What sites can be used to obtain CSF?

• The cisterna magna (CM) at the atlantooccipital junction is the site of choice for collecting CSF in dogs and cats.
• The lumbar cistern (LC) at the L4–L5 or L5–L6 vertebral level is a less satisfactory site.

3. What equipment do I need to perform a CSF tap?

1. For most dogs and cats, a $1\frac{1}{2} \times 22$-gauge spinal needle with stylet is adequate. For large and giant breeds, a $2\frac{1}{2} \times 22$-gauge spinal needle with stylet is recommended. Collection of CSF

from lumbar puncture typically requires a slightly longer spinal needle in comparison with collection from the CM. The distance between the skin and the subarachnoid space of the CM in cats and various sized dogs is specified in the table below.

2. An EDTA, clot (red-top), and/or plastic test tube is needed for sample collection and transportation. The submission of samples for cell count and cytologic evaluation in EDTA, clot, or plastic tubes is often at the discretion of the laboratory analyzing the sample.

3. Access to an in-house or commercial clinical pathology laboratory that can rapidly analyze the sample (within 60 minutes of collection) is an important requirement.

Distance between the Skin and Subarachnoid Space at the Cisterna Magna as a Function of Weight

WEIGHT (KG)	DISTANCE (CM)
Cats or dogs < 4.5	0.5–1.25
Dogs 4.5–9.1	1.8
Dogs 22.7–50.9	3.8
Dogs > 50.9	5.0

4. What are the landmarks for collection of CSF from the cisterna magna?

A right-handed person should use the left hand to locate the landmarks. Use the thumb and middle finger to palpate the cranial aspects of the wings of the atlas (C1). The index finger palpates and locates the occipital protuberance of the skull and axis (C2). The site for entry of the spinal needle is the intersection of a line joining the cranial borders of the wings of the atlas with a line from the occipital protuberance to the spinous process of the axis.

5. How is CSF collected?

1. The animal is placed under general inhalant anesthesia. Dissociative agents such as ketamine or teletimine (Telazol) should be avoided because they increase the risk of seizures.

2. An endotracheal tube should be used to ensure a patent airway during the procedure. The endotracheal tube may become occluded if neck flexion is excessive during sample collection.

3. The skin over the cisterna magna is clipped and surgically prepared from the ears caudally to the dorsal spinous process of the axis.

4. For a right-handed person, the animal is placed in right lateral recumbency. An assistant holds the patient's head with the neck flexed at a 90° angle to the upper cervical vertebrae. Ensure that the spine, head, and nose are aligned and parallel to the table surface.

5. The collector should kneel so that the atlantooccipital area is at eye level. After determination of the proper entry site, visualize an imaginary line from the point of entry to the patient's nose, and follow the imaginary line during puncture.

6. The spinal needle should be handled with sterile gloves. The skin is pierced in a controlled manner to prevent the needle from being driven too deeply once the initial skin resistance is overcome. In particularly thick- or tough-skinned dogs and cats, an 18-gauge needle is used initially to puncture the skin and to facilitate advancement of the spinal needle.

7. The spinal needle (with stylet in place) is advanced very slowly. A "pop" is typically felt as the needle penetrates the subarachnoid space into the cisterna magna.

8. At this point, remove the stylet and check for the flow of CSF from the hub of the needle. Use the left hand to stabilize the needle and hub while removing the stylet with the right hand to prevent iatrogenic injury to the spinal cord or brainstem.

9. If no CSF is observed after initial withdrawal of the stylet, replace the stylet, advance the needle a few millimeters at a time, and repeat the procedure of observation for flow of CSF after each advancement (see table in question 3 for typical distances between skin and cisterna magna).

10. Once CSF is flowing, collect the samples by dripping the CSF into the collection tubes held 3–5 mm below the hub of the spinal needle.

6. If the CSF is flowing slowly, may I aspirate with a syringe?

No. Aspirating CSF with a syringe increases the risk of contaminating the sample with blood. This approach also increases the risk of iatrogenic injury to the spinal cord and caudal brainstem. Be patient. In many animals with inflammatory brain disease it may take 3–5 minutes to collect 1 ml of CSF. If the flow of CSF is slow, the assistant may occlude the jugular veins to increase the intracranial pressure, which in turn increases CSF flow.

7. No CSF was visible as I advanced the spinal needle. What should I do now?

If you have advanced past the usual depth of the cisterna magna, withdraw the needle slowly and check for CSF flow every millimeter. Also check to be sure that the needle is not occluded.

8. The CSF sample looks like fresh blood. What should I do?

If the sample clots in a red-top tube, it is probably blood from the vertebral venous plexus. Withdraw the needle, and begin again with a clean spinal needle. If you are unsuccessful in obtaining a CSF sample in three attempts, abandon the procedure. Trauma to the spinal cord from needle penetration or iatrogenically induced bleeding into the subarachonid space is a potentially serious complication of repeated attempts to collect CSF.

9. This procedure sound risky and dangerous. How can I practice the technique?

Use a fresh cadaver to gain competence and confidence in the collection of CSF. A fresh cadaver is necessary because cerebrospinal pressure and consequent ability to collect CSF are greatly diminished within 10–20 minutes after death.

10. Can I collect CSF from the lumbar area?

Yes, but the lumbar cistern is more difficult to enter and yields smaller volumes of CSF. In obese animals it is difficult to palpate the point of entry. In many middle-aged and older animals, it is extremely difficult to enter the lumbar cistern because of mineralization of the interarcuate ligament and subsequent narrowing of the intervertebral canal. The preferred volume for CSF analysis (1 ml) is rarely collected from the lumbar cistern. In addition, this approach commonly yields a higher rate of blood contamination of CSF samples.

11. What is the procedure for lumbar cistern collection?

1. Palpate the point of entry by locating the dorsal spinous process of L6, which lies between the wings of the ilium.

2. Site preparation and other general approaches described in question 5 hold true for CSF collection from the lumbar cistern.

3. As an assistant flexes the lumbar spine of the patient, direct a spinal needle (typically 1½–3 inches × 22 gauge) perpendicular to the spine and slightly to one side of the spinous process of L6 to penetrate the interarcuate ligament between L5–L6.

4. After insertion through the skin, the needle contacts bone. At this point, direct the needle cranially or caudally to locate the interarcuate depression of L5–L6.

5. The needle is forced through the interarcuate ligament of L5–L6 and into the dorsal subarachnoid space.

6. This approach often results in piercing of the spinal cord and needle stoppage on the ventral floor of the vertebral canal. In this case, withdraw the needle slowly to enter the ventral subarachnoid space. Needle penetration of the spinal cord at the L5–L6 level is not usually associated with residual neurologic signs.

7. If hemorrhage is evident when the stylet is removed, wait for a few drops to flow and/or pull the needle back slightly to determine whether the CSF will clear. If the fluid does not clear within 8–10 drops, withdraw the needle and begin the procedure with a clean needle.

12. How much CSF can be safely obtained from dogs and cats?

One milliliter is the volume required to perform most tests. This amount generally can be obtained safely from dogs and cats that weigh at least 4 kg. If the animal weighs more than 9 kg and a sample is desired for either microbiologic culture or infectious disease titers, 2 ml of CSF can be withdrawn safely. In collecting for culture and/or titers, remember to collect the sample in either transport media or sterile clot (red-top) tube.

13. What if I am able to collect only 0.5 ml of CSF?

The collection of less than 0.5 ml of CSF limits the number of tests that can be performed. The most useful diagnostic tests, in order of decreasing importance, are white blood cell (WBC) and red blood cell (RBC) counts, cytologic examination, and determination of protein concentration.

14. What are the normal values for various CSF parameters in dogs and cats?

As with all reference values, those determined for CSF parameters vary from laboratory to laboratory. Representative normal values are listed in the table below.

Normal Values of Canine CSF Obtained from the Cisterna Magna and Lumbar Cistern

CELL COUNTS	CISTERNA MAGNA	LUMBAR CISTERN
White blood cells	0–5 cells/µl	0–8 cells/µl
Differential cell counts		
Neutrophils	0–9%	NA
Lymphocytes	0–27%	NA
Monocytes	69–100%	NA
Macrophages	0–3%	NA
Eosinophils	< 1%	NA
Total protein	5–25 mg/dl	25–45 mg/dl

NA = not available.

15. Why do I have to analyze the sample within 60 minutes of collection?

CSF is low in protein and nucleated cell count. This combination may cause the cells to degenerate or lyse after 30–60 minutes. A delay in analysis alters the nucleated cell count and cytologic evaluation. If access to a laboratory is not readily available, concentrating techniques may be used: (1) cytospin, (2) centrifuging and slide preparation of CSF sediment, (3) millipore filtration, or (4) well-slide sedimentation preparation (see references at the end of this chapter). Clinicians should talk to laboratory personnel before CSF collection to determine preferences in sample handling and slide preparation.

16. How are concentrated cells analyzed?

Slide preparations of cells should be air-dried rapidly by waving the slides vigorously for 2 minutes, followed by alcohol fixation for 1 minute. The prepared slides may be sent for analysis by an experienced cytopathologist. For in-house analysis, stain the slides with Diff-Quick Differential Stain Set (American Scientific Products), Wright's stain, or Giemsa stain. Because it is difficult to differentiate between monocytoid and lymphoid cells in CSF, results must be interpreted with care.

17. Can I do the other CSF analysis in the clinic?

Red blood cell and white blood cell counts in CSF can be determined with a hemocytometer. One chamber of the hemocytometer is filled with unstained CSF. The white and red blood cells in all nine squares of the chamber are counted. The total number of white and red blood cells is multiplied by 1.1 to obtain the number of cells per microliter. Red and white blood cells can be differentiated with a little experience (WBCs are larger, more granular, and more refractile than RBCs).

18. How can I measure the protein concentration of the CSF sample?

The protein concentration is much lower in CSF than in plasma; it is measured in mg/dl vs. gm/dl. Because CSF protein concentration is similar to urine protein concentration, a urine dipstick may be used to estimate the CSF protein concentration. Dogs and cats normally have less than 30 mg/dl protein in CSF; most animals test negative or have trace amounts (< 30 mg/dl) with a urine dipstick (e.g., Multistix, Bayer, Miles, Diagnostic Division, Elkhart, IN). CSF protein concentration should be confirmed by submitting the sample to a reference laboratory.

19. Is there a way to store CSF so that analysis is not flawed?

Refrigeration of CSF in a plastic vial may slow cellular degradation. Because normal values for refrigerated samples are not published, results must be interpreted cautiously. Protein concentration in CSF is not altered by refrigeration. CSF that is to be submitted for infectious disease titers should be refrigerated until analysis is performed. Samples to be submitted for microbiologic culture should be inoculated into appropriate culture media.

20. Can I still use the sample if it is contaminated with RBCs?

If the sample has < 5000 RBC/µl, various formulas have been created to correct the WBC count and protein concentration. In dogs, for every 500 RBC/µl, subtract 1 WBC/µl. In cats, 1 WBC/µl is subtracted for every 100 RBC/µl. Protein concentration is corrected by subtracting 1 mg/dl total CSF protein for every 1000 RBC/µl. If > 10,000 RBC/µl are in the sample, the collection procedure should be repeated in 24–48 hours.

21. What diseases can be diagnosed with a CSF sample?

CSF collection and analysis are most useful in diagnosing infectious and inflammatory brain or spinal cord diseases. The general nature of the disease process can be determined in most cases, and the specific cause is evident in some diseases. Fungal and bacterial organisms occasionally are observed on analysis of a CSF sample. Feline infectious peritonitis (FIP) causes a tremendous protein and cellular response. FIP meningitis or encephalomeningitis is typically seen in young cats less than 3 years old. Bacterial, viral, rickettsial, and fungal diseases can be diagnosed by appropriate serologic, microbiologic, or ultrastructural test procedures. Many infectious diseases demonstrate multisystemic clinical signs and can be diagnosed via cytologic or histopathologic analysis of specimens obtained from other sites or from serologic tests of blood, negating the need for a CSF tap.

The table below lists selected diseases with a typical pattern of CSF abnormalities. However, because these parameters demonstrate substantial overlap with various diseases, be conservative in interpreting results.

Selected Diseases with Typical Patterns of CSF Abnormalities

DISEASE	WBC COUNT	PROTEIN (MG/DL)	CYTOLOGIC FEATURES
Neoplasia (except meningioma)	N or ↑	↑, ↑↑	N, M, Ma, L
Meningioma	↑, ↑↑, ↑↑↑	↑, ↑↑	N, Ma, L
Bacterial meningitis	↑↑, ↑↑↑	↑↑, ↑↑↑	N (org)
Fungal meningitis	↑, ↑↑	↑↑, ↑↑↑	N, L, E, M, Ma (org)
Protozoan meningitis	↑, ↑↑	↑↑, ↑↑↑	L, E, M, Ma
Aseptic meningitis (young dogs)	↑↑, ↑↑↑	↑↑, ↑↑↑	N, L
Viral encephalitis	N or ↑↑	N or ↑↑	M, L, Ma
FIP encephalitis	↑↑, ↑↑↑	↑↑, ↑↑↑	M, L, Ma
Rickettsial diseases	↑, ↑↑	↑, ↑↑	M, L, N
Granulomatous meningoencephalitis	↑↑, ↑↑↑	↑↑, ↑↑↑	M, L, Ma

FIP = feline infectious peritonitis. For WBC count: N = normal value, ↑ = mild pleocytosis (10–50 cells/µl); ↑↑ = moderate pleocytosis (50–100 cells/µl); ↑↑↑ = marked pleocytosis (> 100 cells/µl). For protein concentration: ↑ = mild increase (10–50 mg/dl); ↑↑ = moderate increase (50–200 mg/dl); ↑↑↑ = marked increase (> 200 mg/dl). Cytologic findings: N = neutrophils, L = lymphocytes, M = monocytes, Ma = macrophages, E = eosinophils, org = organisms (occasionally the causative organism can be identified on cytologic evaluation).

Except for infectious diseases, CSF analysis rarely gives a definitive diagnosis. Although CSF bathes the central nervous system, a disease process must involve the subarachnoid space or ventricular system to alter values in CSF. For instance, most CNS tumors do not exfoliate cells into the CSF and do not cause an increase in CSF cell count. CNS tumors may alter the blood–brain barrier and increase the CSF protein concentration. Meningiomas are often in close contact with the subarachnoid space; an increase in WBCs (predominantly neutrophils) in the CSF can be seen with necrosis of these tumors.

22. Can the CSF analysis be normal when brain disease is present?

Yes, depending on the location of the disease process and the course of the illness. The influence of the location of the disease process is discussed in question 21. In addition, if a CSF tap is performed early in the course of a disease that may later involve the subarachnoid space, a normal CSF tap is possible.

23. What factors should be considered before doing a spinal tap?

A spinal tap is an invasive diagnostic procedure that is not without risks. A spinal tap requires general anesthesia, and animals should be stable (airway, breathing, circulation) before the procedure is done. All ancillary and less invasive tests for the differential diagnosis should be performed and interpreted before a spinal tap is done. The potential consequences of a spinal tap include subarachnoid bleeding, spinal cord trauma, and respiratory arrest or death from brain herniation. These consequences are quite serious, and the potential benefits of the diagnostic information should be weighed against the risks.

24. When should I definitely *not* do a spinal tap?

1. If anesthesia is contraindicated, CSF should not be obtained.

2. Myelography causes an inflammatory reaction in the subarachnoid space for at least 48 hours after the procedure. Analysis of CSF will be abnormal in this time frame, making interpretation of the sample difficult or impossible. CSF collection should precede myelography in animals with spinal cord disease.

3. A CSF tap should not be performed on an animal with a recent history of head trauma or with suspected or confirmed cervical vertebral fractures or luxations.

4. Any animal with signs of increased intracranial pressure, such as altered consciousness (stupor, coma), propulsive walking, head pressing, or papilledema on fundic examination, should be treated for increased intracranial pressure before consideration of a CSF tap. Brain imaging (computed tomography or magnetic resonance imaging) also should be performed.

5. CSF should not be tapped in animals with brain herniation. Brain herniation may be recognized by a rapidly deteriorating state of consciousness, change in pupils from small and reactive to fixed and dilated, loss or slowing of the oculocephalic reflex, development of decerebrate or decorticate rigidity, and pathologic breathing (Cheyne-Stokes or apneustic breathing).

25. Can I give corticosteroids or mannitol to lower intracranial pressure before collecting CSF?

If you are concerned enough about intracranial pressure to intervene with drugs, the animal is not likely to be stable enough to undergo a CSF tap. Administration of corticosteroids and mannitol may alter the results obtained from a CSF tap.

BIBLIOGRAPHY

1. Bailey CS, Higgins RJ: Comparison of total white blood cell count and total protein count of lumbar and cisternal cerebrospinal fluid of healthy dogs. Am J Vet Res 46:1162–1165, 1985.
2. Braun KG: Clinical Syndromes in Veterinary Neurology. St. Louis, Mosby, 1994.
3. Christopher MM, Perman V, Hardy RM: Reassessment of cytologic values in canine cerebrospinal fluid by use of cytocentrifugation. J Am Vet Med Assoc 192:1726–1729, 1988.
4. Jacobs RM, Cochrane SM, Lumsden JH, Norris AM: Relationship of cerebrospinal fluid protein concentration determined by dye-binding and urinary dipstick methodologies. Can Vet J 31:587–588, 1990.

5. Rand JS: The analysis of cerebrospinal fluid in cats. In Bonagura JD (ed): Kirk's Current Veterinary Therapy XII. Philadelphia, W.B. Saunders, 1995, pp 1121–1127.
6. Tipold A: Diagnosis of inflammatory and infectious diseases of the central nervous system in dogs: A retrospective study. J Vet Intern Med 9:304–314, 1995.
7. Wilson JW, Steven JB: Effects of blood contamination on cerebrospinal fluid analysis. J Am Vet Med Assoc 171:256–258, 1977.

116. INVASIVE BLOOD PRESSURE MONITORING

Carolyn M. Selavka, M.S., V.M.D., and Elizabeth Rozanski, D.V.M.

SYSTEMIC ARTERIAL BLOOD PRESSURE

1. What is systemic arterial blood pressure?

The term **systemic arterial blood pressure (SABP)** refers to the amount of force exerted on the walls of the large arteries by the action of the contracting heart. SABP is the product of cardiac output and systemic vascular resistance. The description of SABP is generally divided into three components:

1. **Systolic arterial pressure (SAP)**, which is the pressure generated by cardiac contraction (or systole);

2. **Mean arterial pressure (MAP)**, which is the average pressure across the vessel during the cardiac cycle and is the main determinant of adequate organ perfusion; and

3. **Diastolic arterial pressure (DAP)**, which represents the lowest pressure in the arteries during the period of cardiac filling (diastole).

2. Why is measurement of SABP important?

Abnormalities in SABP are common in animals with acute conditions (e.g., trauma, sepsis, anesthesia) or chronic diseases (renal failure). In critically ill animals, SABP is maintained within a normal range by compensatory mechanisms until severe compromise occurs. Serial determination of SABP, coupled with other routine monitoring, helps to detect patients at risk for decompensation at a point when resuscitation is possible. In addition, SABP monitoring is indicated during anesthesia and administration of medications known to affect blood pressure (e.g, dopamine, vasodilators).

3. What is normal SABP?

	Systolic	Diastolic	Mean
Dogs	100–160 mmHg	80–120 mmHg	90–120 mmHg
Cats	120–150 mmHg	70–130 mmHg	100–150 mmHg

Mean SABP can be approximated by the formula:

$$MAP = \frac{SAP - DAP}{3} + DAP$$

4. Define hypotension.

A mean SABP < 60 mmHg represents hypotension and results in inadequate perfusion of renal, coronary, and cerebral vascular beds. The causes of hypotension include hypovolemia, sepsis, and cardiogenic shock. The clinical signs of hypotension are nonspecific and include cerebral depression, weak pulses, and tachycardia. Rapid identification and appropriate corrective measures are required to prevent irreversible organ damage or death.

5. Define hypertension.

Hypertension is defined as a repeatable SABP > 200/110 mmHg (systolic/diastolic) or a mean SABP > 130 mmHg (mean: 133 mmHg) in animals at rest. Because "white-coat " hypertension has been shown to occur in small animal patients, readings must be reproducible and ideally coupled with appropriate clinical signs. Hypertension results from increased cardiac output or increased systemic vascular resistance and may occur as a primary disease or be related to various conditions, including cardiac disease, hyperthyroidism, renal failure, hyperadrenocorticism, pheochromocytoma, and pain. Untreated hypertension may result in retinal detachment, encephalopathy, vascular accidents, and organ failures.

6. How is SABP measured?

SABP may be measured directly or indirectly. Direct SABP measurement involves placement of a catheter or needle into an artery and connecting the catheter to a pressure transducer. It is considered the gold standard in determination of SABP. Indirect SABP measurements are made with oscillometric or Doppler ultrasound techniques over a peripheral artery (see chapter 117).

7. How do you monitor direct SABP measurement?

SABP may be continuously measured by placing a catheter in the dorsal metatarsal artery. Catheters are generally easily placed in any animal with palpable pulses that weighs more than 5 kg. The arterial catheter is placed either percutaneously or via surgical cutdown. Percutaneous catheter placement is done by clipping the hair and sterile preparation of the insertion site over the dorsal metatarsal artery. The artery runs in the groove between the second and third metatarsal bones. The pulse should be palpable before an attempt to place the catheter is made. Typically, a 22-gauge, 1½-inch over-the-needle catheter is placed, although in small dogs a 24-gauge catheter may be placed instead. The catheter is inserted at a 30–45° angle directly over the pulse until arterial blood is observed freely flowing through the catheter. The catheter is then advanced, the stylet removed, and the catheter secured with standard intravenous catheter techniques.

The differences in placement of an arterial catheter compared with a venous catheter include higher risk of catheter "burring" during placement, increased difficulty in feeding the catheter despite proper insertion, and increased problems with maintaining catheter patency. Arterial catheters should be flushed with a heparinized solution every 4 hours and require an occasional resecuring of catheter placement.

The measurement of the SABP after placement of an arterial catheter involves use of a pressure transducer and monitor. Many commercially available EKG machines also have adaptation for pressure measurements. In general, the pressure transducer is connected to the monitor, and the transducer should be at the approximate level of the patient's heart. Sterile plastic tubing filled with heparinized saline is connected via stopcocks to the pressure transducer at one end and to the patient at the other. An attempt must be made to ensure that no air bubbles are present in the tubing; otherwise, the trace may be dampened. Use of stiffer tubing provides less alteration in pressure waves.

Before measurement, the system is zeroed first by making sure that there is no pressure across the transducer (i.e., close the stopcock to the patient) and then by zeroing the transducer as directed by the manufacturer. Typically this procedure involves holding the zero button until zero is displayed on the screen. The stopcock to the patient is then reopened, and the generated pressure trace is observed.

Pressure waves appearing as a steep upstroke with a dicrotic notch indicate reliable measurement. If the pressure wave appears dampened, flush the arterial catheter. If the patient moves during measurement, zero the transducer again. Overall, the first few arterial catheters that a clinician places can be frustrating, but soon the benefits far outweigh the occasional inconveniences.

8. What are the advantages and disadvantages of direct SABP measurement?

Direct SABP monitoring is the gold standard to which indirect methods are compared. The readings are considered more accurate, and the technique enables constant monitoring.

The continuous access to arterial blood sampling is also of benefit when serial blood gas samples are required to monitor the patient's status.

Disadvantages include the advanced technical skills required to place and maintain arterial catheters. The invasive nature of arterial catheter placement predisposes the patient to infections or vessel thrombosis, and bleeding from the cannulation site is a concern if the line becomes dislodged or damaged.

CENTRAL VENOUS PRESSURE

9. What is central venous pressure?

Central venous pressure (CVP) is the pressure exerted on the cranial venal cava or right atrium; CVP reflects intravascular volume, cardiac function, and venous compliance. Following the patient's CVP trends may give a close approximation of circulation efficiency. The CVP is not wholly a measure of circulating blood volume; it is a measure of the ability of the heart to accept and pump blood brought to it.

10. How is CVP measured?

CVP can be measured accurately only by direct methods. An intravenous catheter is introduced into an external jugular vein and advanced so that the tip of the catheter rests in the cranial vena cava near the right atrium. A three-way stopcock is connected via intravenous extension tubing to the catheter, fluid administration set, and manometer. The manometer must be vertically positioned on the wall of the patient's cage, with the zero level aligned to approximate the position of the catheter tip and right atrium. This level can be approximated with the patient in sternal recumbency at a point 2–3 inches above the sternum at the fourth intercostal space. If the patient is in lateral recumbency, the zero point is parallel to the sternum at the fourth sternebrae. CVP is measured by filling the manometer with isotonic crystalloid fluid solution and turning the stopcock off in the direction of the fluid port. This procedure allows the pressure of the fluid column in the manometer and the blood in the catheter (vena cava) to reach equilibrium. The reading on the manometer at the equilibrium point is equivalent to the patient's cranial vena caval pressure.

11. What are normal CVP values?

Dogs   0–10 cm H_2O
Cats   0–5 cm H_2O

Single measurements of CVP do not necessarily reflect hemodynamic status. Serial measurements and interpretation of the trends as they correlate with treatment regimen are generally more informative about blood volume, cardiovascular function, and vascular tone.

12. When should CVP be monitored?

The measurement of CVP allows titration of fluid therapy in animals with poor perfusion, circulatory failure, lung disease with pulmonary hypertension, decreases in systemic vascular resistance, leaky capillaries, cardiac compromise, or questionable renal function.

13. What are critical point CVP values?

CVP reading (cm H_2O)	Interpretation
< 0	Patient needs fluids. If signs of vasoconstriction or hypotension exist, recommend bolus to reach 5–10 cm H_2O.
0–10	Normal range.
10–15	Venous return is more than adequate; recommend conservative fluid therapy.
> 15	Fluid therapy should cease; cardiac compromise is likely. Persistently high CVP values in conjunction with vasoconstriction or hypotension are suggestive of heart failure.

BIBLIOGRAPHY

1. Haskins SC: Monitoring the critically ill patient. Vet Clin North Am Small Animal Pract 19:10–59, 1989.
2. Kittleson MD, Oliver NB: Measurement of systemic arterial blood pressure. Vet Clin North Am Small Animal Pract 13:321–335, 1983.
3. Kirk RW, Bistner SI, Ford R (eds): Handbook of Veterinary Procedures and Emergency Treatment, 5th ed. Philadelphia, W.B. Saunders.
4. Murtaugh RJ, Kaplan PM (eds): Veterinary Emergency and Critical Care Medicine. St. Louis, Mosby, 1992.
5. Podell M: Use of blood pressure monitors. In Kirk RW (ed): Current Veterinary Therapy XI. Philadelphia, W.B. Saunders, 1992.

117. NONINVASIVE BLOOD PRESSURE MONITORING

Erika Zsombor Murray, D.V.M.

1. Who first recorded mean blood pressure in an unanesthetized horse?

In *Statistical Essays* (1733), the Rev. Stephen Hales includes the following account:

In December I laid a common field gate on the ground, on which a white mare was cast on her right side, and in that posture bound fast to the gate . . . . Then laying bare the left Carotid Artery, I fixed to it towards the Heart the Brass Pipe, and to that the Wind Pipe of a Goose; to the other End of which a Glass Tube was fixed which was twelve Feet nine Inches long. . . . The blood rose to the Tube in the same manner as in the Case of The two former Horses, till it reached to nine Feet six Inches Height.

2. What methods of indirect blood pressure monitoring are available?

• **Ultrasound** (Doppler Flow Detector, Park Electronics)

An inflatable cuff is used to occlude blood flow proximal to a transducer. The Doppler technique detects red blood cell or arterial wall movement beneath the ultrasonic piezo-electric probe as the cuff is released. The point at which the Korotkoff sounds are first heard is the systolic arterial pressure (SAP). The diastolic arterial pressure (DAP) corresponds to the point at which the sounds change from a short pulsatile to a more continuous sound.

• **Oscillometer** (Dinemap, Critikon)

A cuff containing an air bladder is used to occlude blood flow. Pressure oscillations within the air bladder reflect the pulse pressure within the artery beneath. As the cuff is deflated, a microprocessor samples pressure oscillations and calculates SAP, DAP, and mean arterial pressure (MAP).

• **Photoplethysmography** (Finapres, Choeda)

This method measures arterial volume by attenuation of infrared radiation. Arterial volume is assumed to be a constant; thus, measured cuff pressure equals intraarterial pressure.

3. How is a Doppler-based device used to determine indirect blood pressure?

Clip the hair immediately proximal to the metacarpal or metatarsal pad. Ultrasonic jelly is applied to the concave surface of the Doppler probe, which is then placed on the hairless patch. The amplifier is turned on, and the probe is moved until the sound of blood flow within the artery is clearly heard. Fasten the probe in place with tape. A cuff is wrapped securely around the ante-brachium between the cubital and carpal joints or mid-tibia if a hind limb is used. A general rule is to use the infant-size blood pressure cuff for dogs weighing more than 15 kg and the newborn cuff for dogs weighing less than 15 kg and cats. Otherwise, limb circumference should be measured to determine the ideal cuff length and width. After the sphygmomanometer is attached, the cuff is inflated to 200–250 mmHg. The valve on the manometer is gradually opened to release the pressure within the cuff. Systolic blood pressure is the point at which the Korotkoff sounds first reappear. Diastolic pressure is determined when the sounds change from a pulsatile to a continuous sound.

4. How is an oscillometric device used to obtain a measure of blood pressure?

Place the cuff over the cranial tibial artery on the lateral aspect of the tibia. Inflate the cuff to a pressure of 30–40 mmHg higher than needed to obliterate the pulse (normally to 200 mmHg). The microprocessor samples pressure oscillations at this constant pressure and at each 5–10-mmHg pressure decrement as the cuff is gradually deflated. The pressure at which the oscillation amplitude increases and decreases rapidly identifies the systolic and diastolic pressures, respectively.

5. What are the best locations for Doppler and oscillometric probe placement in dogs?

Artery	Location
Superficial palmar	Proximal to metacarpal pad
Superficial plantar	Proximal to metatarsal pad
Lingual	Ventral aspect of the tongue
Brachial	Medial aspect of the humerus
Common carotid	Lateral aspect of the hock
Femoral	Medial aspect of the thigh
Cranial tibial	Lateral aspect of the tibia
Aorta	Flank region
Ophthalmic arterial plexus	Cornea (use plenty of ultrasound jelly)

6. What are the best locations for blood pressure measurement in cats?

Oscillometric technique	Tail
	Cranial tibial artery
Doppler technique	Tail
	Hind limb (cranial tibial artery)
	Palmar or plantar arteries

7. When using the oscillometric or Doppler method of indirect blood pressure measurement, how does one calculate the ideal cuff size for a given animal?

- Cuff width/limb circumference = 0.40

   or

- Optimal cuff bladder width = 40–50% of circumference of extremity

   and

- Optimal cuff length = 150% of limb circumference

8. How is error introduced into indirect blood pressure measurements?

If one uses a cuff that is too large or applies a cuff too tightly, artifactually low blood pressure readings are obtained. Alternatively, if the cuff is undersized or applied too loosely, blood pressure readings are artifactually high.

9. What do indirect blood pressure techniques measure? How do they relate to direct blood pressure measurement?

Only direct blood pressure monitoring techniques measure blood pressure. Indirect techniques measure some variable related to blood flow. If we assume that vascular resistance or compliance remains at a constant value, it is possible to make inferences about blood pressure from indirect monitoring techniques.

Blood flow × vascular resistance = pressure difference between two ends of a vessel

Arterial blood pressure (bp) = cardiac output (CO) × vascular compliance × blood volume

10. What does palpation of peripheral pulses assess? What does it indicate about blood pressure?

Peripheral pulse characteristics reflect the pulse difference, i.e., systolic arterial pressure (SAP) minus diastolic arterial pressure (DAP). As long as the pulse difference is greater than 30 mmHg, a strong pulse is palpable. Thus, a strong pulse may be just as easily detected in a hypotensive patient as in a normotensive or hypertensive patient. Similarly, because digital palpation of pulse quality reflects stroke volume, pulses may be weak in hypovolemic patients, even though many of them are normotensive, as a result of compensatory increases in systemic vascular resistance.

11. When should indirect blood pressure monitoring be considered?

Indirect blood pressure monitoring is indicated for animals with unstable or potentially unstable cardiovascular status (e.g., patients with traumatic injuries, pancreatitis, renal disease, gastric dilatation-volvulus [GDV], hyperthyroidism). Indirect blood pressure measurement is indicated for patients undergoing general anesthesia. Indirect techniques also may be useful during minor surgical procedures when a technician is unavailable to monitor anesthesia. The strengthening of Doppler sounds or increases in blood pressure readings with oscillometric techniques may indicate that the anesthetic plane is too light. Diminished Doppler sound intensity or decreases in blood pressure readings may indicate that the anesthetic plane is too deep. In addition, a Doppler probe may be placed on the corneal surface during cardiopulmonary resuscitation (CPR) to monitor blood flow generated by resuscitation efforts.

12. What are normal values for canine and feline arterial blood pressures as measured by direct methods?

Normal Arterial Blood Pressures

	CANINE	FELINE
Systolic arterial pressure (mmHg)	100–160	120–180
Diastolic arterial pressure (mmHg)	80–120	70–130
Mean arterial pressure (mmHg)	90–120	100–150

13. What indirect blood pressure readings are suggestive of hypertension?

Canine: > 200/110 mmHg
Feline: > 190/140 mmHg

14. What diseases or situations may result in hypertension?

Disease	*Mechanism*
Renal disease	Increases stroke volume and total peripheral resistance
Hyperadrenocorticism	Increase stroke volume and total peripheral resistance
Pheochromocytoma	Increases heart rate and total peripheral resistance
Hyperaldosteronism	Increases stroke volume and total peripheral resistance
Head trauma	Increases total peripheral resistance
Hyperparathyroidism	Increases total peripheral resistance
Pain, fear (increased sympathetic tone)	Increases total peripheral resistance and heart rate

15. What diseases or situations may cause hypotension?

Disease	Mechanism
Hypovolemia	Decreases venous return, causing decreased cardiac output (CO)
Anesthesia	Decreases heart rate, total peripheral resistance, and CO
Dilated cardiomyopathy	Decreases CO by decreasing contractility
Cardiac tamponade	Decreases CO by decreasing cardiac filling
Valvular heart disease	Decreases CO by regurgitation of blood through mitral valve
Gastric dilatation-volvulus	Decreases CO by decreasing venous return
Endotoxemia	Decreases total peripheral resistance, causes myocardial depression
Thrombus (hypercoagulable states)	Obstruction of blood flow artifactually lowers readings
Hyperkalemia	Decreases heart rate and CO, causes myocardial depression
Acidosis	Decreases CO, causes myocardial depression

16. Explain why pulse pressures and systolic and diastolic arterial blood pressures may vary from one pulse to the next.

Sinus arrhythmia may cause variations in pulse pressure due to variation in the amount of time between heartbeats. A longer time between heartbeats results in increased cardiac filling, whereas a shorter time results in decreased cardiac filling. In this instance, take an average of several readings to determine SAP and DAP.

17. How is MAP calculated from readings generated by the Doppler method of indirect blood pressure monitoring?

$$MAP = \frac{SAP - DAP}{3} + DAP$$

18. Of what clinical significance is MAP?

Adequate MAP establishes a perfusion pressure for the major organs. An MAP of 60 mmHg is required to ensure adequate minimal blood flow to kidneys, brain, and liver. In addition, a minimal diastolic pressure of 40 mmHg is needed to ensure adequate coronary arterial blood flow.

19. Which method of indirect blood pressure monitoring is considered to be the most accurate?

In general, both Doppler and oscillometric methods are reliable, but Doppler is more accurate in most cases. Inaccuracies are easily introduced in the oscillometric method if an inappropriate cuff size is selected. This error is easy to make in trying to assess blood pressure in cats and small dogs.

20. Which clinical situations may hamper the use of the oscillometric method of indirect blood pressure monitoring?

The oscillometric method uses oscillations produced in an air-filled cuff encircling the limb to reflect pulsatile blood flow. Hypotension, vasoconstriction from cold ambient temperatures, shivering, and movement by the patient can introduce inaccuracies or make the measurements difficult to perform.

21. What is the sensitivity of the Doppler method compared with direct blood pressure measurement?

In a study in which shock was induced by phlebotomy, the SAP values obtained via direct and Doppler methods correlated well. The Doppler method measured DAP accurately in 70% of dogs, but DAP was difficult to measure accurately in cats. The study also determined that

Doppler-derived measurements of SAP, DAP, and MAP were slightly lower than the values obtained with direct blood pressure monitoring techniques (by 10 mmHg ± 3 mmHg).

BIBLIOGRAPHY

1. Binns SH, et al: Doppler ultrasonographic, oscillometric sphygmomanometric, and photoplethysmographic techniques of noninvasive blood pressure measurement in anesthetized cats. J Vet Intern Med 9:405–414, 1995.
2. Coulter DB, et al: Blood pressures obtained by indirect measurement in conscious dogs. J Am Vet Med Assoc 184:1375–1378, 1984.
3. Grandy JL: Evaluation of the Doppler ultrasonic method of measuring systolic arterial blood pressure in cats. Am J Vet Res 53:1166–1169, 1992.
4. Kirk RW, Bonagura JD (eds): Current Veterinary Therapy XII (Small Animal Practice). Philadelphia, W.B. Saunders, 1995.
5. Littman MP, Drobatz KJ: Hypertensive and hypotensive disorders. In Ettinger's Textbook of Veterinary Internal Medicine, 4th ed. Philadelphia, W.B. Saunders, 1995, pp 93–100.
6. Lumb, Jones: Veterinary Anesthesia, 3rd ed. Baltimore, Williams & Wilkins, 1996.
7. Murtaugh RJ, Kaplan: Veterinary Emergency and Critical Care Medicine. St. Louis, Mosby, 1992.
8. Remilland R, et al: Variance of indirect blood pressure measurements and prevalence of hypertension in clinically normal dogs. Am J Vet Res 52:561–565, 1991.
9. Weiser MG, et al: Blood pressure measurement in the dog. J Am Vet Med Assoc 171:364–368, 1977.

118. ENTERAL NUTRITION

Karin Allenspach, D.M.V., and Jeffrey Proulx D.V.M,

1. What metabolic events are associated with uncomplicated short-term starvation?

In animals without injury or illness, several metabolic adaptations may result from lack of nutrient intake. Initially, during the postabsorptive phase, the insulin-to-glucagon ratio decreases, allowing an increase in hepatic glycogenolysis to support euglycemia. With continued nutrient restriction, glycogen stores are depleted within 12–24 hours. At this point, glucocorticoid levels begin to rise to support metabolic adaptations. Glucocorticoids facilitate protein catabolism with consequent release of free amino acids from muscular tissue. The amino acids serve as substrate for gluconeogenesis by the liver and kidney. In addition, plasma catecholamines in conjunction with glucocorticoids activate hormone-sensitive lipase within adipocytes to release free fatty acids. With prolonged starvation, the lipolytic effect is most pronounced; it allows sparing of protein stores with increased utilization of free fatty acids for energy supply and formation of ketone bodies by the liver. Organs with obligate glucose utilization, such as central nervous system tissue, adapt to using ketone bodies for up to 50% of energy needs. A balance is maintained between protein and fat catabolism to prevent large fluctuations in blood pH and to preserve the structural integrity of tissues.

2. What metabolic events are associated with stressed starvation during disease processes?

The magnitude of the metabolic aberration is proportional to the severity of the illness or injury and associated tissue damage. During stressed starvation, an elevated metabolic rate and catabolism may be observed and peak at approximately 72 hours after injury. Fatty acids are the primary source of energy during stressed starvation, but protein metabolism becomes more pronounced in the hypermetabolism associated with injury and severe illness. Much of this response results from the release of inflammatory cytokines, such as tumor necrosis factor and interleukins, that augment the effects of increased glucocorticoids and catecholamines associated with stress. Despite institution of adequate nutritional support, muscular wasting and negative nitrogen balance often ensue. The induced protein catabolism depletes the body of functional protein, thereby impairing wound healing and immune function. The figure below illustrates the general hormonal influences on hypermetabolism after illness or injury.

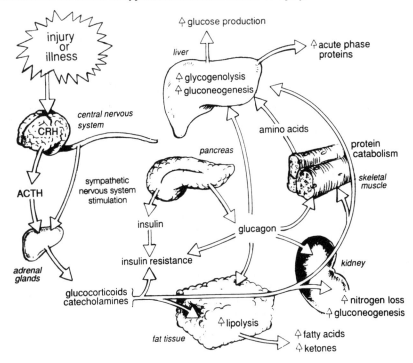

Hormonal influences on hypermetabolism after illness or injury. CRH = corticotropin-releasing hormone, ACTH = adrenocorticotropic hormone. (From Chandler ML, Greco DS, Fettman MJ: Hypermetabolism in illness and injury. Comp Cont Educ Pract Vet 14:1284–1290, 1992, with permission.)

3. What are the clinical consequences of malnutrition? What are the benefits of nutritional support?

If nutritional support is not initiated in anorectic, injured, or ill patients, severe complications develop. Gastrointestinal atrophy is observed within 72 hours after major trauma, resulting in decreased ability to absorb nutrients and increased risk of bacterial translocation. Increased protein catabolism in response to illness or injury depletes the body of structural and functional protein stores, thereby affecting wound healing and immune and cellular function on a local scale; it also decreases cardiac and respiratory function on a global scale. Studies in humans and guinea pigs demonstrate that early enteral feeding decreases the hypermetabolism and catabolism associated with severe acute illness and injury, helps to maintain intestinal function, and may prevent bacterial translocation from the intestines. Clinical studies of humans have demonstrated that early enteral nutrition reduces intra- and postoperative morbidity and mortality and decreases length of hospitalization.

4. What types of patients are candidates for nutritional support?

The general guidelines for the use of enteral nutritional support include loss or expected loss of more than 10% of body weight, anorexia for 3 or more days, trauma, surgery or severe systemic inflammatory disease, and increased nutrient losses through vomiting, diarrhea, draining wounds, or burns associated with hypoalbuminemia. In addition, increased demands due to the catabolic response associated with fever, infection, and neoplasia may require initiation of nutritional support early in the course of disease.

5. How is the caloric requirement of a patient calculated?

The basal energy requirement (BER) is calculated for a patient resting quietly in a thermoneutral environment and a postabsorptive state. The following formulas are used:

Dogs < 2 kg: BER = $70 \times$ weight $(kg)^{0.75}$
          > 2 kg: BER = $30 \times$ weight $(kg) + 70$ or $70 \times$ weight $(kg)^{0.75}$
Cats < 2 kg: BER = $70 \times$ weight $(kg)^{0.75}$
          Adult: BER = $60 \times$ weight (kg) or $70 \times$ weight $(kg)^{0.75}$

6. What methods are available for providing enteral nutritional support?

Methods of enteral nutritional support include natural appetite stimulants, pharmacologic appetite stimulants, force feeding, nasoesophageal and nasogastric tube feeding, pharyngostomy and esophagostomy tube feeding, gastrostomy tube feeding, and jejunostomy tube feeding.

7. How can the appetite be stimulated?

Natural methods of appetite stimulation include heating foods, hand feeding, cleaning of the nostrils, and offering a variety of appropriate foods. These methods are inexpensive and should be the initial effort in providing enteral nutrition in anorectic animals that are able to prehend food. Often, these techniques are time-consuming and provide suboptimal nutrient intake.

Pharmacologic methods may be used for short-term appetite stimulation. Diazepam, 0.1–0.2 mg/kg, may be administered intravenously, intramuscularly or orally once or twice daily to a maximal daily dose of 5 mg. Unfortunately, there are recent reports of an idiosyncratic reaction causing fulminant hepatic failure in feline patients given oral diazepam. Oxazepam, 0.2–0.4 mg/kg orally once daily, and cyproheptadine, 2–4 mg orally once or twice daily, have proved useful in providing an immediate increase in appetite. The disadvantages of appetite stimulation through medication include inconsistent results and potential side effects of sedation and dysphoria.

8. What are the advantages and disadvantages of nasoesophageal and nasogastric tube feeding?

Nasoesophageal and nasogastric tube feeding is often used for short-to-medium duration nutritional support (up to 14 days). It is an easy and effective method of providing nutritional support in patients with general illness or oral cavity disease that also have a functional gastrointestinal tract. It is inexpensive, and no special equipment or general anesthesia is required. Tube placement should be verified by radiography. Tube feeding can be accomplished with bolus or continuous infusion.

Contraindications include vomiting, functional or mechanical gastrointestinal obstruction, upper airway obstruction, pneumonia, cardiac disease, facial trauma, and esophageal disease. In animals with decreased mental status or consciousness, the risk of aspiration pneumonia must be carefully evaluated. Disadvantages may include patient discomfort, risk of epistaxis, vomiting, rhinitis, dacrocystitis, and reflux esophagitis. Liquid diets are necessary to prevent plug formation within the feeding tube; hospitalization may or may not be required.

9. What are the indications and risks for pharyngostomy or esophagostomy tube feeding?

The indications for pharyngostomy or esophagostomy tube placement include inability to prehend food in patients with mandibular and maxillary fractures, upper airway obstruction, or upper airway infection. Associated risks include aspiration pneumonia, reflux esophagitis, and vomiting of the tube. Esophagostomy tubes are well tolerated by most patients, although general anesthesia is required for tube placement.

10. What are the indications for gastrostomy tube placement?

Gastrostomy tube placement is the method of choice for medium- to long-term enteral nutritional support. The placement of gastrostomy tubes bypasses the oral cavity, pharynx, and esophagus. Gastrostomy tubes are generally well tolerated in anorectic and ill animals. Methods of placement include blind percutaneous, endoscopic, or surgical placement. Contraindications to tube placement include persistent vomiting or functional or mechanical gastrointestinal obstruction. The risk of aspiration is still present in animals with decreased mental status secondary to gastroesophageal reflux. To allow adequate adhesion formation at the ostomy site, gastrostomy tubes must be left in place for at least 5 days before removal is attempted. Malnourished and hypoalbuminemic patients may require longer periods because delayed wound healing is common. The disadvantages include the necessity of general anesthesia for tube placement, infection at the stoma site, and possibly tube migration with ostomy site dehiscence and peritonitis.

11. What are the indications for jejunostomy tube placement?
Jejunostomy tubes should be placed during abdominal surgery for conditions in which feeding via oral or gastrostomy tube may or will be precluded. Jejunostomy tubes and feedings are to be considered in animals with major dysfunction or disease of the proximal gastrointestinal tract, including pancreatitis or gastric disease. The disadvantages include the need for surgical placement, risk of ostomy site infection, dehiscence, and peritonitis. Jejunostomy tubes must remain in place for 10 days before removal is attempted.

12. What types of enteral diets are available? What diet properties must be considered?
Several types of liquid enteral nutrition formulations are available in human medicine, whereas canine and feline CliniCare and RenalCare (PetAg, Inc.) are the only specific veterinary diets available. Formulation selection should be based on knowledge of patient needs, including degree of malnutrition, caloric and protein requirements, and digestive and absorptive capabilities, as well as method of enteral feeding. The disease process also may be relevant to the type of enteral nutrition. In general, enteral diets for humans, with modifications, may be used initially for enteral nutritional support in dogs and cats. However, enteral veterinary diets are balanced for canine and feline patients and should be used whenever possible.

13. How do enteral diets supply protein requirements? What patient factors should be considered in choosing the appropriate product?
Dietary protein requirements are supplied in enteral nutrition products as free amino acids, protein hydrolysates (di-, tri-, and oligopeptides), or intact protein. The concentration varies from less than 10% to more than 20% and is often expressed as a function of percent calories provided. Hydrolysates are freely absorbed by enterocytes in a non–energy-dependent fashion (faster than free amino acids). Intact proteins depend on gastric acid secretion and pancreatic exocrine function. Most enteral products are composed of proteins with a high biologic value. In general, veterinary patients require greater amounts of protein than human patients. Modular formulations such as amino acid powders (Promod, Ross Laboratories) may be used to supplement enteral products formulated for people.

Patient factors that dictate enteral formula selection may include renal or liver insufficiency, which necessitates high-quality, low-protein formulations and decreased concentrations of aromatic amino acids. Patients in highly catabolic states (e.g., burns, sepsis) require higher protein supplementation. Branched-chain amino acids, such as leucine, isoleucine, and valine, are the preferred energy source for gluconeogenesis and may be beneficial in highly catabolic states. Feline patients needing enteral nutritional support with commercial products for humans require taurine supplementation at 500 mg/1000 kcal.

Many enteral products are now supplemented with glutamine and arginine. Both of these amino acids have been found to be conditionally essential in stress catabolic states (see question 21). Glutamine and arginine are important in maintaining the structural and functional integrity of the intestinal mucosa as well as supporting gut-associated immune function.

14. How do enteral diets supply carbohydrates and fiber?
Carbohydrates are provided in enteral products as polysaccharides, disaccharides, and monosaccharides and should supply approximately 60% of daily calories. Monosaccharides add sweetness and increase the relative osmolarity of the product. Fiber is provided in some enteral

formulations for humans. The recommended human dosage is 10–13 gm/1000 calories. Most enteral products supply fiber as soy polysaccharide, which contains cellulose and hemicellulose. Dietary fiber undergoes fermentation by colonic anaerobes, resulting in production of short-chain fatty acids such as butyrate, acetic, and propionic acids. These acids provide an energy source for clonocytes, increase bacterial mass, stimulate sodium and water reabsorption, and may prevent nutrition-associated diarrhea (see question 22).

15. How do enteral diets supply lipids, vitamins, and minerals?

Lipid components used in enteral feeding products typically contain the long-chain fatty acids, including the essential fatty acids, linoleic (w-6) and linolenic (w-3), which should be 1–2% and 0.2–0.3% of total calories, respectively. Excessive supplementation of essential fatty acids may cause immunosuppression due to induced changes in arachidonic acid metabolism. Medium-chain triglycerides are absorbed directly into enterocytes, do not depend on brush-border enzyme activity or active transport processes, and do not require digestion by pancreatic enzymes. Diets containing medium-chain fatty acids are ideal for initiating nutritional support in patients that have not had oral or enteral alimentation for several days and in patients with maldigestion or malabsorption syndromes. Medium-chain triglycerides do not depend on the carnitine transport system necessary for transport of long-chain fatty acids into mitochondria for oxidation. Medium-chain triglycerides should not be used in diabetic ketoacidotic patients because they are especially ketogenic.

Vitamins and minerals in general are supplied in adequate quantities in both human and veterinary enteral nutritional formulations.

16. Discuss the relevance of osmolarity in enteral formulations.

Enteral formulations vary considerably in osmolarity and caloric density. In most veterinary patients, enteral products delivered directly in to the small intestine via jejunostomy or nasojejunostomy tube should be isosmotic (290–310 mOsm) to limit local fluid fluxes, nausea, cramping, vomiting, and possibly diarrhea. Hyperosmolar liquid diets delivered into the esophagus or stomach are often well tolerated, although patients that have not eaten or received enteral nutritional support in 2–3 days may initially require isosmolar formulations.

17. How is enteral nutrition instituted? Is continuous or bolus feeding indicated?

All patients entering an intensive care unit should be assessed for the potential benefit of nutritional support. Patients with trauma, sepsis, or systemic inflammatory syndromes should be supported early with nutrition (< 8 hours after admission). If the gastrointestinal tract is fully or partly functional, tube placement should be considered on admission to the hospital. After consideration for diet type based on disease process and route of enteral feeding, diets should be introduced slowly to provide assessment of gastrointestinal function, which includes absorptive capacity and motility. Isosmolar solutions in frequent small volumes or as a constant-rate infusion are best for beginning enteral nutritional support. Most clinical studies have shown no significant difference in administering a liquid enteral diet as a constant-rate infusion or as boluses, although cycled continuous infusion has been shown to be more physiologic (8–12 hours with a constant-rate infusion followed by 12–16 hours of rest) in humans. A graduated increase in calories or fluid volumes should parallel the prior onset of anorexia. In some patients with acute disease, full enteral nutrition may be instituted within 2 days, whereas a chronically malnourished patient may require slower introduction. Parameters used to assess the appropriate increase in nutritional support include measurement of residual volumes of diet in the stomach and presence of nausea, bloating, or vomiting.

Jejunostomy tube feeding needs to be performed frequently and in small volumes. The diet should be isosmolar and similar to the ingesta expelled from the stomach during normal feeding. Canine and feline patients tolerate the RenalCare and CliniCare (PetAg, Inc.) polymeric diets well; elemental diets are not generally necessary for feeding via jejunostomy tubes. The clinician should consider adding blue food coloring (blue dye no. 1) to enteral products. This addition may prevent inadvertent intravenous administration of enteral products and allow identification of airway aspiration if blue fluid is identified on tracheal suctioning.

18. What is microenteral nutrition?

Microenteral nutrition is provided by administering small volumes (0.5 ml/kg/hr) of electrolyte and glucose solution (e.g., lactated Ringer's solution with 2.5% dextrose). Enteral fluid administration may allow maintenance of gastrointestinal integrity and facilitate introduction to enteral nutrition. Microenteral nutrition may be used regardless of the disease process, including patients with pancreatitis or gastric surgery. The fluid may be administered intermittently (every 1–2 hours) or as a constant-rate infusion. Periodic gastric suctioning should be performed in conjunction with microenteral feeding to ascertain gastric residual volumes.

19. What purpose may nasogastric or nasoesophageal tubes have other than nutritional support?

Nasogastric tubes may be used for intermittent or continuous suctioning to remove gastric gas or fluid accumulations. This use may alleviate distention-induced nausea as well as reduce the risk of aspiration in patients with decreased level of consciousness. Continuous decompression is also useful in postoperative patients with gastric torsion because bloating may recur and inhibit recovery of normal gastrointestinal function and motility. The volume of fluid recovered from suction techniques gives an indication of forward motility and whether it is appropriate to initiate or continue administration of enteral products. Caution must be used in suctioning large volumes, because metabolic alkalosis may result from loss of hydrochloric acid. Venous blood gases are useful in assessing this concern.

Nasoesophageal tubes are useful in patients with megaesophagus. Intermittent suctioning decreases the likelihood of aspiration by clearing fluid and ingesta accumulation and may be especially advantageous in patients with concurrent pneumonia because coughing increases intrathoracic pressure, mobilizes settled esophageal contents, and increases potential for aspiration on subsequent breaths.

20. Discuss the four most common complications of enteral nutritional support.

Aspiration. Aspiration may occur in any patient that is depressed or recumbent, lacks airway control, or has pharyngeal or esophageal dysfunction. The risk is heightened in patients that actively regurgitate or vomit. Problems or risks may be greater in patients that are fed with nasoesophageal or gastric tubes. Aspiration also may occur with esophageal or gastric tubes that are incorrectly placed or with tubes that have become displaced. The risk of aspiration may be decreased by placement of jejunostomy tubes, concomitant use of antiemetics and antinausea medications, or frequent gastric or esophageal decompression by suctioning. Administration of promotility medications such as cisapride, metoclopramide, and erythromycin also decreases the risk of aspiration. Sinusitis is rarely seen as a sequela to placement of nasal tubes.

Diarrhea. Diarrhea may occur in many circumstances of enteral feeding. Diets with high osmolarity may draw fluid into the gastrointestinal tract in amounts sufficient to overwhelm absorptive capacity. Concurrent use of antibiotics and antacids may alter preexisting bacterial populations or cause bacterial growth in the distal colon, initiating secretory diarrhea. In many enteral formulations, the lack of dietary fiber decreases intraluminal colonic production of short-chain fatty acids, thereby decreasing the ability of the colon to reabsorb sodium and water. Patients with severe illness or injury often have multisystemic organ involvement with derangements in blood flow, oxygen delivery, and interstitial fluid dynamics (edema), which may result in malabsorption, maldigestion, and altered intestinal motility. Such changes often predispose to diarrhea. A potentially dangerous source of infectious diarrhea includes delivery of contaminated enteral products in aged or mishandled formulas.

Tube placement complications. Inappropriate nasoesophageal or nasogastric tube placement may lead to aspiration of enteral products or damage to airways from inadvertent placement in the trachea. Gastrostomy and jejunostomy tube placement has the risk of stoma site dehiscence and infection or leakage of nutrients and ingesta, which leads to local infection, peritonitis, and sepsis. All ostomy and tube placement sites should be inspected daily, gently cleansed with dilute povidone-iodine solution, and covered with sterile gauze and antibiotic ointment. Nasal tube placement should not be attempted in patients with increased intracranial pressure because induced sneezing may acutely increase intracranial pressure.

Nausea and vomiting. The introduction of diets in a rapid fashion or use of diets high in osmolarity may cause irritation to the stomach or intestine, resulting in cramping, nausea, and vomiting. Gastric or intestinal distention due to lack of forward motility may lead to similar problems.

21. What is the importance of glutamine in enteral nutritional support?

In normal animals, glutamine is the most abundant free amino acid, representing a major intermediary amino acid for interorgan nitrogen transport and substrate for gluconeogenesis in the liver. Glutamine is also important as a precursor for nucleotide synthesis, as a substrate for renal ammoniagenesis in acidotic states, and as a primary respiratory fuel for rapidly dividing cells such as lymphocytes, endothelial cells, fibroblasts, renal tubular cells, and enterocytes. Glutamine has been shown to be essential for maintenance and integrity of gastrointestinal mucosal structure and function, prevention of bacterial translocation, and maintenance of local immune function. In critically ill patients, glutamine is considered a conditionally essential amino acid because plasma glutamine levels decline markedly and significantly in the stressed states. Although no specific dosage of glutamine has been established in veterinary patients, a dosage of 0.5 gm/kg has been adapted from studies in humans. Enteral formulations may be supplemented with glutamine powder (Glutamine, Cambridge Nutraceuticals) or supplied by many newer immune-enhancing enteral feeding products (ImmunAid, McGaw, Inc.).

22. What is the importance of fiber in enteral nutritional support?

Dietary fiber is composed of minimally digested (10–15%) insoluble fibers, such as cellulose, hemicellulose, and lignin, and soluble fibers, such as pectin, gum, and mucilages, most of which are digested (90–99%). Dietary fibers are fermented by colonic anaerobes to produce short-chain fatty acids, including acetate, propionate, and butyrate. These fatty acids are actively and passively absorbed by colonocytes and indirectly stimulate the reabsorption of electrolytes and water. In addition, short-chain fatty acids have a trophic influence and serve as a preferential fuel for colonocytes. Experimental studies in humans have demonstrated a decrease in colonic bacterial translocation with high fiber diets. The concurrent hydrogen ion production associated with fermentation of fiber traps ammonia by forming ammonium ion and therefore increases fecal nitrogen content. This quality is useful in patients with renal and liver failure that need enteral nutritional support. Controlled clinical studies in humans are lacking, and variable results have been seen with the limited studies currently available. In general, enteral feeding-associated diarrhea has been decreased in patients that are fed enteral formulations supplemented with fiber. Enteral nutrition products supplemented with fiber mainly contain soy polysaccharide (20% cellulose and 80% hemicellulose). The available veterinary enteral formulations do not contain fiber.

BIBLIOGRAPHY

1. Bowling TE: Enteral-feeding-related diarrhea: Proposed causes and possible solutions. Proc Nutr Soc 54:579–590, 1995.
2. Crowe DT: Nutritional support for the hospitalized patient: An introduction to tube feeding. Comp Cont Educ Pract Vet 12:1711–1721, 1990.
3. Heyland D, Cook DJ, Winder B, et al: Enteral nutrition in the critically ill patient: A prospective surgery. Crit Care Med 23:1055–1060, 1995.
4. O'Leary MJ, Coakley JH: Nutritional and immunonutrition. Br J Anaesth 77:118–127, 1996.
5. Rodman DP, Gaskins SE: Optimizing enteral nutrition. Am Fam Physician 53:2535–2542, 1996.
6. Souba WW: Nutritional support. N Engl J Med 336:41–48, 1997.
7. Souba WW, Klimberg VS, Plumley DA, et al: The role of glutamine in maintaining a healthy gut and supporting the metabolic response to injury and infection. J Surg Res 48:383–391, 1990.
8. Walton RS, Wingfield WE, Ogilvie GK, et al: Energy expenditure in 104 postoperative and traumatically injured dogs with indirect calorimetry. J Vet Emerg Crit Care 6:71–79, 1976.
9. Zaloga GP (ed): Nutrition in Critical Care. St. Louis, Mosby, 1994.

119. MECHANICAL VENTILATION

Elizabeth Rozanski, D.V.M., and Therese O'Toole, D.V.M.

1. When is mechanical ventilation indicated?

Mechanical ventilation is indicated in (1) an animal that cannot maintain a $PaO_2 > 50$ mmHg despite supplementary oxygen (via face mask, nasal oxygen, or oxygen cage) or (2) an animal that cannot maintain a $PaCO_2 < 50$ mmHg despite reversal of respiratory depressant drugs or thoracocentesis (as clinically indicated). This is commonly referred to as the 50/50 rule. Other indications for mechanical ventilation include (1) clinical deterioration to the point that respiratory failure appears imminent and (2) cardiopulmonary arrest.

2. What options are available for mechanical ventilation?

Options for artificial ventilation can be as simple as an Ambu bag attached to an endotracheal tube or as complex as a computerized ventilator designed for long-term care. In general, a ventilator designed for long-term respiratory support provides better control of ventilatory variables (e.g., oxygen level, humidity, tidal volume, inspiratory pressures) than a manually operated ventilator.

3. What types of ventilation are commonly used in veterinary medicine?

In **volume-limited ventilation**, the ventilator delivers a set volume of air to the patient, regardless of the pressure required to do so. Generally, alarms are set to detect sudden increases in airway pressure, which usually signal an obstruction. In **pressure-limited ventilation**, the ventilator delivers air to a preset inspiratory pressure, regardless of the volume. Because of the tendency for decreasing tidal volume as airway obstruction or decreased lung compliance develops, $PaCO_2$ as well as tidal volume (via spirometry) must be monitored more closely. Some evidence suggests that pressure-limited ventilation may be more desirable in small animals (< 10 lbs).

4. What modes of ventilation are commonly used?

In the **assist-control** mode, the ventilator is set to give a specific number of breaths per minute. The ventilator delivers the breath when the patient generates negative inspiratory pressure or, if the patient is not breathing, at a preset rate. If the patient is breathing rapidly (i.e., panting), hyperventilation may result. In this case, another mode of ventilation may be used.

In the **synchronous intermittent mandatory ventilation (SIMV)** mode, the machine delivers a set number of breaths per minute. The breaths may be initiated by negative inspiratory pressure, but if the patient breathes faster than the set rate, the machine will not deliver another breath. This mode is useful in weaning, because the number of breaths delivered by the ventilator may be slowly decreased.

Spontaneous ventilation is also possible with many ventilators; the ventilator functions similarly to an anesthesia machine. This mode of ventilation is not commonly used in veterinary medicine but may be useful if set concentrations of oxygen are to be given to an animal or during continued monitoring after weaning from ventilatory support.

5. Should a patient be orally intubated, or is a tracheostomy recommended?

The choice for type of airway depends on both the underlying disease and clinician preference. The advantages of an oral airway include speed, familiarity, and decreased tissue trauma. The disadvantages include the need for significant amounts of sedation and immobility. The advantages of a tracheostomy include less sedation and immobility as well as the potential for oral intake of food and water. The disadvantages include a surgical procedure in a possibly immunosuppressed patient and the potential need for more careful monitoring than in an anesthetized patient (because of the potential for tracheal tube occlusion or dislodgment). In general, if a patient is to be ventilated for more than 36–48 hours, it is reasonable to consider tracheostomy.

6. What are useful protocols for sedation and anesthesia?

The ideal drug creates minimal cardiovascular depression and is easily titratable and economical. Obviously no such drug exists. In many dogs, pentobarbital (2–16 mg/kg IV every 4–6 hours) has been used successfully. The principal advantage of pentobarbital is long duration of action; it is also relatively inexpensive. The disadvantages of pentobarbital include a lengthy recovery phase and lack of reversal agents. Other commonly used drugs include a combination of oxymorphone (0.05–0.1 mg/kg IV as needed) and diazepam (0.25–0.5 mg/kg IV as needed). The opiates are generally cardiovascular-sparing but require frequent dosing and are expensive. Other protocols include continuous-rate infusions (to effect) of fentanyl or propofol. Occasionally, paralytics such as atracurium (0.2 mg/kg IV) are used to facilitate mechanical ventilation. It is important to use paralytics in conjunction with sufficient analgesic agents.

7. What is PEEP?

Positive end-expiratory pressure (PEEP) may improve oxygenation in patients that are hypoxemic despite a high concentration of inspired oxygen and a normal-to-low $PaCO_2$. PEEP prevents complete expiration and thus increases functional residual capacity, prevents early closure of small airways, and increases alveolar size and recruitment, thereby aiding in matching of ventilation and perfusion. Of importance, PEEP also decreases venous return to the heart and potentially decreases cardiac output.

8. What are the potential problems caused by mechanical ventilation?

Mechanical ventilation is not risk-free. The primary clinical problems are barotrauma and infection. **Barotrauma** results from excessive positive pressure in certain areas of the lung, causing rupture and formation of pneumothorax (or pneumomediastinum). One of the most common causes of desaturation in a previously stable ventilator patient is development of a significant pneumothorax. A pneumothorax should be anticipated in animals with significant lung disease. Clients and staff should be counseled not to consider it a major setback.

Infection is another significant problem in ventilated patients. Infections often spread to the lungs from the contamination of the upper airway and oropharynx because the normal upper airway defense mechanisms are bypassed. In addition, ventilated patients are often immunosuppressed and immobile, which also increases risk of infection. Every effort should be made to be as clean and sterile as possible. Cultures of the airway should be performed regularly (every 24–48 hours) and used in combination with clinical signs to direct antimicrobial therapy.

Other potential concerns with mechanical ventilation include decreased venous return, oxygen toxicity, upper airway damage or irritation, and musculoskeletal problems associated with prolonged recumbency.

9. What is the prognosis for ventilated animals?

The underlying prognosis for ventilated patients depends largely on the underlying disease. For example, a 15-year-old dog with recurrent aspiration pneumonia secondary to megaesophagus with rapidly progressive respiratory failure has a grave prognosis, whereas a young dog with a traumatic flail chest and pulmonary contusions may have a fair prognosis. In the author's experience, a survival rate greater than 30–40% with good quality of life should be the goal.

BIBLIOGRAPHY

1. King LG, Hendricks JC: Use of positive-pressure ventilation in dogs and cats: 41 cases (1990–1992). J Am Vet Med Assoc 204:1045–1052, 1994.
2. Parent C, King LG, Walker LM, et al: Clinical and clinicopathologic findings in dogs with acute respiratory distress syndrome: 19 cases (1985–1993). J Am Vet Med Assoc 9:1419–1427, 1996.
3. Parent C, King LG, Van Winkle TJ, et al: Respiratory function and treatment in dogs with acute respiratory distress syndrome: 19 cases (1985–1993). J Am Vet Med Assoc 208:1428–1433, 1996.
4. Pasco PJ: Oxygen and ventilatory support for the critical patient. Semin Vet Med Surg (Small Animals) 3:202–209, 1988.

5. Van Pelt DR, Wingfield WE, Wheeler SL, et al: Oxygen-tension based indices as predictors of survival in critically ill dogs: Clinical observations and review. J Vet Emerg Crit Care 1:19–25, 1991.
6. Van Pelt DR, Wingfield WE, Hackett TB, et al: Application of airway pressure therapy in veterinary critical care. J Vet Emerg Crit Care 3:63–70, 1994.

120. INITIAL OPHTHALMIC EVALUATION

Cynthia C. Powell, M.S., D.V.M., Dip. ACVO,
and Steven M. Roberts, M.S., D.V.M., Dip. AVCO

1. What is an ocular emergency?

An ocular emergency is any condition or event that threatens or causes visual impairment, blindness, loss of globe integrity, or serious loss of periocular tissue integrity and function. Ocular emergencies are not life-threatening but require rapid diagnosis and appropriate management to maximize the chance of preserving or restoring ocular function. Ocular emergencies may be associated with life-threatening emergencies that require immediate management.

2. Which types of ocular conditions represent a true emergency?

Many ocular problems present as an acutely painful and red eye. Such cases must be evaluated to determine their urgency and need for immediate treatment. Although the following list is not all-inclusive, it is a good starting point to categorize most general practice ocular emergencies:

- Blunt trauma
- Corneal ulceration
- Eyelid laceration
- Glaucoma (acute)
- Globe perforation or laceration
- Ocular foreign body
- Ocular hemorrhage
- Ocular proptosis
- Sudden blindness
- Uveitis

3. What is the first step after the patient arrives?

A history of the current problem should be quickly collected. Determine whether the patient has a previous history of ocular disease, trauma, chemical ocular irritation, drug use that may cause reactions, or indications of systemic disease. Many eye problems are related to systemic disease or trauma; do not forget that more than the obvious may be going on. Begin by performing a thorough physical examination, making sure that no systemic disease or life-threatening conditions require immediate attention; then proceed with the eye examination.

4. Describe appropriate overall procedures in approaching an acute emergency.

Ocular disorders are often misdiagnosed, partially diagnosed, undiagnosed, or diagnosed and inappropriately emphasized. To a large degree, such mistakes can be minimized by performing a sequential stepwise examination to incorporate all ocular regions. It is more important to be thorough and accurate than to implement immediate but inappropriate or incorrect treatment. Delaying treatment a few minutes usually does not adversely alter outcome but may improve chances of successful overall treatment.

5. What ophthalmic equipment should be available?

- Bright light source
- Culture swabs
- Fluorescein stain strips
- Magnification aid (e.g., head loupe or slit-lamp)
- Microscope slides
- Mydriatic agent
- Schirmer tear test strips
- Spatula for cytology specimens
- Tonometer (e.g., Schiotz)
- Topical anesthetic

6. What restraint techniques should be used?

The pros and cons of chemical and physical restraint should be considered for each case. Excessive physical restraint may dramatically increase intraocular pressure by increasing central venous pressure or skeletal muscle and tissue tension on the globe. If the globe structure is weakened, ocular rupture may result. In high-risk patients, in whom general sedation and anesthesia are not advisable, topical and/or regional anesthesia may be adequate. Dogs often become submissive if muzzled, and cats become more complacent if placed in a cat bag.

7. How is the examination best performed?

First, determine whether a microbial culture of the cornea or conjunctival surface is needed. Next, determine whether a Schirmer test is indicated. The balance of the examination is performed in a logical progression from the outside to the inside. A prepared eye examination form is helpful to decrease the chance of accidental omissions in gathering information (see figure below).

Ophthalmology History and Examination Form

Date: _____ History: _____

Temp.:   Pulse: Chest Ascultation: Resp. Rate: Muc. membranes: Weight:

Right Eye Nm Ab   **Left Eye** Nm Ab

- Visual Function
- PLR
  - direct
  - indirect
- Orbit
- Eyelids
- Nict. Membrane
- Nasolacrimal Sys.
  - STT/60s
  - STTa/60s
  - Excretory
- Conjunctiva (culture / cytology)
- Episclera & Sclera
- Cornea (fluorescein stain)
- Anterior Chamber IOP

Schiotz, PTG, Tonopen
- Iris

Gonioscopy:
- Lens
- Ciliary Body
- Vitreous
- Fundus ERG:

Right Eye (OD)   Left Eye (OS)

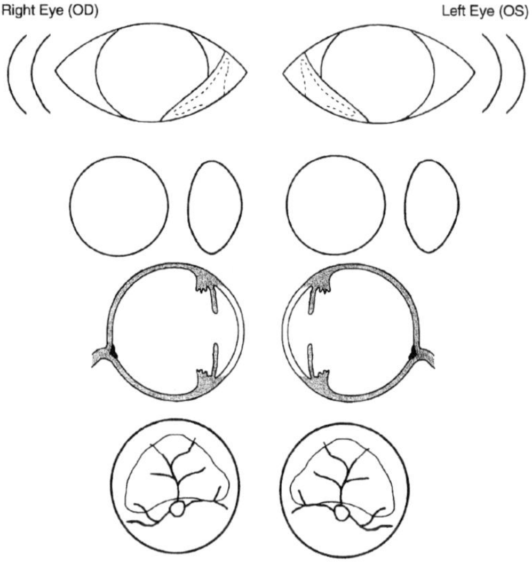

Temp. Problem List	Initial Plan	Treatment

Clinician(s): [Resident / Faculty] _____

Compare the abnormal with the normal eye, if possible. Avoid pressure on the globe until the possibility of perforation has been excluded. After pupillary light reflexes (PLR) have been evaluated, a short-acting mydriatic (e.g,. tropicamide) may be instilled for pupil dilation. Mydriatic use is contraindicated if glaucoma is suspected.

8. If an injured eye appears dry, what should be done?

Ocular trauma or patient sedation may result in a decreased blink reflex and tear film production rate. Ocular lubrication may be achieved with artificial tears or antibiotic eye drops. Topical agents should be avoided until after measuring the Schirmer test or collecting microbial culture material. Ointment should be avoided if the globe is perforated or suspected to be perforated.

9. What are the major indications of a ruptured globe?

Uveal prolapse and collapse of the anterior chamber often accompany rupture of the globe, especially if the rupture is corneal or near the limbus. Prolapsed uveal tissue appears dark in color and may be covered by a layer of fibrin. If the rupture is large, the globe is soft (hypotonic). Aqueous humor may be observed leaking from the perforation site. Other signs include severe ocular pain, aqueous flare, hyphema, miosis, irregular pupil shapes, iritis, retinal or vitreal hemorrhage, and retinal detachment.

10. When are culture and cytology specimens indicated?

If septic, unusually purulent, or bizarre tissue reactions are suspected, collect a specimen for culture, microbial sensitivity testing, and cytologic evaluation. Deep corneal ulcers, especially those with white infiltrates or smooth, melted-appearing edges should be suspected of infection. Such ulcers first should be swabbed for culture, followed by application of a topical anesthetic, and then scraped to obtain a cytology specimen. Aqueous humor may be evaluated for evidence of purulent inflammation, sepsis, neoplastic cells, free photoreceptor disk segments (indicating retinal detachment), and lens material (indicating lens rupture).

11. How rapidly should treatment be started? What first-line treatments are safe?

Rapid treatment is important, but a delay in implementation of minutes to hours will not seriously alter most ocular emergencies. It is more important to be sure of the animal's entire state than to risk inappropriate or contraindicated treatment. Because inflammation and potential infection are paramount concerns, rapid administration of intravenous antibiotics (e.g., first-generation cephalosporins) and corticosteroids (e.g., methylprednisolone sodium succinate or dexamethasone) is usually safe. If ocular tissues have not suffered wounds or lacerations, the antibiotic use may be unnecessary.

BIBLIOGRAPHY

1. Gelatt KN: Ophthalmic examination and diagnostic procedures. In Gelatt KN (ed): Veterinary Ophthalmology. Philadelphia, Lea & Febiger, 1991, pp 195–236.
2. Severin GA: Severin's Ophthalmology Notes. Ft. Collins, FL, Design Point Communications, 1996, pp 1–62.

Appendix: Emergency Drugs

Drug	Formulation	Indications	Dosage	Actions
Acepromazine (ProAce)	10 mg/ml	Preanesthesia, sedation	0.062–0.025 mg/kg parenteral (maximal IV dose = 3mg/dog or 1 mg/cat)	Sedative
Aminophylline	25 mg/ml; 100 mg tablet	Asthma, pulmonary edema	Dogs: 10 mg/kg every 8 hr orally, IM, or IV	Coronary and bronchial dilator, diuretic
Amlodipine	2.5 mg tablet	Supraventricular tachycardia, hypertrophic cardiomyopathy, systemic hypertension	Cats: 0.625 mg/cat ($1/4$ tablet) once daily orally	Calcium channel blocker
Antivenin	10 ml vial	Rattlesnake envenomation	1–5 vials every 2 hr IV	Antivenom antidote
Atenolol	25 mg tablet	Systemic hypertension, cardiac arrhythmia	Dogs: 0.5–1 mg/kg twice daily orally Cats: 6.25 mg/cat daily orally	Beta$_1$ antagonist
Atropine sulfate	0.5 mg/dl	Sinus bradycardia, AV nodal block, ventricular asystole	0.04 mg/kg IV 0.1 mg/kg IT	Parasympatholytic
Bretylium tosylate	50 mg/ml	Ventricular tachycardia, ventricular fibrillation	10 mg/kg IV 1–2 mg/min CRI	Chemical defibrillator, ventricular anti-arrhythmic
Butorphanol (Torbugesic, Torbutrol)	10 mg/ml	Analgesia	Dogs: 0.1 mg/kg IV; 0.1–0.4 mg/kg every 6–12 hr SQ or IM	Centrally acting analgesic, narcotic agonist-antagonist
Calcium chloride	10% solution	Hyperkalemia, hypocalcemia, calcium channel blocker toxicity, hypermagnesemia	1–2 ml IV to effect; observe EKG closely	Positive inotrope
Captopril (Capoten)	Tablet: 12.5, 25, 50, 100 mg	Arterial and venous vasodilation	Dogs: 0.5–2 mg/kg orally 2–3 times/day Cats: 0.5–1.5 mg/kg orally 2–3 times/day	Angiotensin-converting enzyme (ACE) inhibitor
Charcoal, activated	1 lb bag; suspension, 200 mg/ml, 240 ml bottle	Absorption of toxin	2–8 gm/kg orally (repeat as necessary)	Absorbent for any orally ingested toxin
Chlorpheniramine (Aller-Chlor, Chlortrimeton)	4 mg tablet	Antihistamine	Dogs: 4–8 mg 2–3 times/day Cats: 2–4 mg 1–2 times/day	Antihistamine
Cimetidine (Tagamet)	Injection: 150 mg/ml Oral: 60 mg/ml solution, 200 and 300 mg tablets	To block release of gastric HCl	Dogs: 4 mg/kg every 6 hr orally or IV Cats: 2.5 mg/kg twice daily orally	H$_2$ receptor-blocking agent
Desmopressin (DDAVP)	0.01% solution	von Willebrand's disease; antidiuretic hormone derivative	Dogs: 1 µg/kg SQ	Increases release of factor VIII in von Willebrand's disease
Desoxycorticosterone	25 mg/ml pivalate salt	Hypoadrenocorticism	Dogs: 25–75 mg pivalate every 4 wk	Mineralocorticoid
Dexamethasone sodium phosphate	4 mg/ml	Shock	2–4 mg/kg IV	Glucocorticoid

Table continued on next page.

Drug	Formulation	Indications	Dosage	Actions
Dextromethorphan	3 mg/ml syrup with guaifenesin 20 mg/ml (Robitussin DM)	Cough	Dogs: 1–5 ml as needed	Antitussive
Diazepam (Valium)	Injection: 5 mg/ml	Seizures, convulsions, appetite stimulation	Dogs: 1 mg/kg IV or rectally to effect Cats: 0.75 mg/kg IV; as appetite stimulant: 0.05–0.1 mg/kg IV	Benzodiazepine; anticonvulsant, ataractic
Digoxin (Cardoxin, Lanoxin)	Tablet: 0.125, 0.25, 0.5 mg Injection: 0.25 mg/ml Elixir: 0.05, 0.15 mg/ml Capsule: 0.05, 0.1, 0.2 mg	Supraventricular tachyarrhythmias, myocardial failure	Dogs: 0.22 mg/M² twice daily oral tablets, 0.18 mg/M² twice daily elixir; **or** 0.005–0.01 mg/kg twice daily (do not exceed 0.25 mg twice daily) Cats: Use 0.125 mg tablet; 4–7 lb, ¼ tab every 48 hr; 7–13 lb, ¼ tab daily; > 13 lb, ¼ tab twice daily. With Lasix, 0.007 mg/kg every 48 hr	Positive inotrope, decreased conduction through AV node
Diltiazem (Cardiazem)	Tablet: 30 mg; 60 mg extended release (Dilacor XR)	Supraventricular tachycardia, hypertrophic cardiomyopathy	Dogs: 0.5–1.5 mg/kg 3 times/day orally Cats: 1.75 mg/kg 3 times/day orally; 60 mg extended release once daily	Calcium channel blocker
Diphenhydramine (Benadryl)	Injection: 50 mg/ml	Antihistamine	Dogs: 2–4 mg/kg every 6–8 hr IV or IM	Antihistamine
Dobutamine (Dobutrex)	12.5 mg/dl	Myocardial failure	5–20 μg/kg/min CRI	Synthetic catecholamine, positive inotrope
Dopamine (Intropin)	40 mg/ml	Low cardiac output, low renal or mesenteric blood flow	3–5 μg/kg/min CRI to increase renal blood flow 5–10 μg/kg min CRI to increase cardiac output and blood pressure	Dopaminergic, beta₁ agonist, norepinephrine precursor
Doxapram (Dopram-V)	20 mg/ml	Central respiratory stimulation	Dogs, cats: 1–5 mg/kg IV	Central respiratory stimulant
Edrophonium chloride	10 mg/ml	Diagnostic aid for myasthenia gravis	Dogs: 1–2 mg IM or IV	Anticholinesterase
Electrical therapy (defibrillation)	1–400 joules	Electrical defibrillation	1–2 joules/kg	Simultaneous myocardial depolarization
Enalapril (Enacard, Vasotec)	2.5, 10 mg tablets	Arterial and venous vasodilation; congestive heart failure	Dogs: 0.25–0.5 mg/kg 1–2 times/day orally Cats: 0.25–0.5 mg/kg every 12–24 hr orally	Vasodilator
Epinephrine	1:1000 solution	Ventricular fibrillation, ventricular asystole, electromechanical dissociation	0.1 mg/kg IV 0.2–0.4 mg/kg IT	Alpha and beta agonist

Table continued on next page.

Drug	Formulation	Indications	Dosage	Actions
Fentanyl (Sublimaze)	Injection: 0.05 mg/ml Transdermal: 2.5, 5 mg patch	Analgesia	Dogs: 4 µg/kg IV; 2–4 µg/kg/hr CRI; 10–40 lb, 2.5 mg patch; > 40 lb, 5.0 mg patch	Narcotic analgesic
Furosemide (Lasix)	Tablet: 12.5, 20, 40, 50, 80 mg Injection: 10, 50 mg/ml Oral solution: 10 mg/ml	Pulmonary edema, congestive heart failure, hypertension, anuria, oliguria	Dogs: 2–4 mg/kg every other day to 3 times/day orally, IM, IV Cats: 1–2 mg/kg every other day to twice daily, orally, IM, IV	Loop diuretic
Heparin sodium	1000 U/ml	Anticoagulation, disseminated intravascular coagulation	300 U/kg IV bolus, 600 U/kg/day CRI	Acts on coagulation factors in both intrinsic and extrinsic pathways
Hydralazine (Apresoline)	10 mg tablet	Arterial vasodilation, congestive heart failure	Dogs: 0.5–2.0 mg/kg 2-3 times/day	Arterial vasodilator
Insulin	100 U/ml regular, Lente, NPH, Ultra-Lente	Diabetes mellitus, hyperkalemia	0.5–1 U/kg SQ	Hormone
Isoproterenol (Isuprel)	Injection: 0.2 mg/ml	Severe atropine-resistant bradycardia	0.0025 mg/kg CRI; 0.1–0.2 mg every 6 hr IM or SQ	Beta adrenergic agonist
Lidocaine (Xylocaine)	Injection: 20 mg/ml (2%)	Ventricular arrhythmias	Dogs: 2–8 mg/kg IV bolus followed by 50–100 µg/kg/min CRI	Ventricular antiarrhythmic
Lisinopril (Zestril)	20 mg tablet	ACE inhibition, vasodilation	Dogs: 0.25–0.5 mg/kg once daily orally	ACE inhibitor
Magnesium chloride	Injection: 200 mg/ml	Unresponsive ventricular dysrhythmias, chemical defibrillation, severe hypotension	0.15–0.3 mEq/kg IV given over 2–10 min; 0.75–1.0 mEq/kg/day	Electrolyte, chemical defibrillator
Mannitol	25% solution	Diuresis, cerebral edema	0.25–1 gm/kg IV	Osmotic diuretic
Meclizine	25 mg tablet	Antiemetic for vestibular disease	Dogs: 4 mg/kg once daily Cats: 2 mg/kg once daily	Antihistamine
Meperidine (Demerol)	50 mg/ml	Analgesia	Dogs, cats: 11 mg/kg IM	Analgesic
Methylprednisolone sodium succinate (Solu-Medrol)	500 mg vial	Spinal trauma	Dogs: 30 mg/kg IV	Glucocorticoid
Metoclopramide (Reglan)	Injection: 5 mg/ml Oral: 10 mg tablet, 1 mg/ml solution	Gastric motility stimulation, vomiting, nausea	Dogs: 1–2 mg/kg/day CRI IV Dogs, cats: 0.2–0.4 mg/kg 3 times/day orally	Gastrointestinal stimulant, antiemetic
Misoprostol (Cytotec)	100 µg tablet	Prevention of gastric ulceration, reduction of cyclosporin-induced nephrotoxicity, treatment of NSAID-induced GI ulceration	Dogs: 2–4 µg/kg 3–4 times/day orally	Synthetic prostaglandin E_1 analog

Table continued on next page.

Drug	Formulation	Indications	Dosage	Actions
Morphine sulfate	Injection: 0.5 mg/ml or 15 mg/ml	Analgesia, vasodilation, pulmonary edema, sedation	Dogs: 0.5–2 mg/kg IM, SQ; 0.05–0.1 mg/kg for pulmonary edema Cats: 0.1 mg/kg IM,SQ	Narcotic analgesic
Naloxone	Injection: 400 µg/ml	Narcotic antagonism, electromechanical dissociation (EMD) in cardiac arrest	Dogs: 15 µg/kg IV; 30 µg/kg IV for EMD	Narcotic antagonist
Nitroglycerin (Nitro-BID, Nitrol)	2% ointment	Venodilation for congestive heart failure	Dogs: 0.25 inch/kg cutaneously 3–4 times/day Cats: $\frac{1}{8}$ to $\frac{1}{4}$ inch cutaneously 3–4 times/day	Venodilator
Nitroprusside (Nipride)	200 µg/ml	Congestive heart failure, pulmonary edema	1–5 µg/kg/min CRI	Venous and arterial vasodilator
Oxymorphone (Numorphan)	1.5 mg/ml	Narcotic analgesia	Dogs: 0.11–0.22 mg/kg IM, SQ, IV (maximal dose = 4.5 mg/dog) Cats: 0.06 mg/kg every 4 hr SQ	Narcotic analgesic
Pentobarbital, sodium	65 mg/ml; 400 mg/ml	Sedation, convulsions, seizures, IV anesthesia, euthanasia	Dogs, cats: 25–30 mg/kg IV for anesthesia; 3–15 mg/kg given slowly IV for anticonvulsant	Barbiturate
Phenobarbital	Injection: 130 mg/ml Tablet: 15, 30, 60, and 100 mg	Sedation, convulsions, seizures	Dogs, cats: 2–4 mg/kg twice daily orally; 6–20 mg/kg IV loading dose	Barbiturate
Potassium bromide	250 mg/ml	Convulsions, seizures	Dogs: 10–30 mg/kg orally twice daily May want to provide loading dose of sodium bromide (350–520 mg/kg)	Anticonvulsant
Prednisone (Deltasone)	Tablet: 5, 20 mg; 1 mg/ml oral solution	Corticosteroid therapy, hypoadrenocorticism, inflammatory disease, immune-mediated diseases	Dogs, cats: 0.5–2.2 mg/kg/day orally	Glucocorticoid
Procainamide (Procan SR, Pronestyl)	Capsule: 250, 375, 500 mg Tablet: 250, 375, 500 mg SR tablet: 250, 500, 750, 1000 mg Injection: 100, 500 mg/ml	Ventricular arrhythmia, supraventricular arrhythmias	Dogs: 8–30 mg/kg IM, orally 4 times/day (SR = 3 times/day); 2 mg/kg IV over 3–5 min to total dose of 15 mg/kg; 20–50 µg/kg/min CRI	Antiarrhythmic
Propofol (Diprivan)	10 mg/ml	Short-duration anesthesia	Dogs: 4–6 mg/kg IV to effect Cats: 6–8 mg/kg IV to effect	Short-acting hypnotic
Propranolol (Inderal)	Tablet: 10, 20, 40, 60, 80, 90 mg Injection: 1 mg/ml	Atrial and ventricular arrhythmias, hypertrophic cardiomyopathy, hypertension, myocardial infarction, thyrotoxicosis	Dogs: 0.2–1.0 mg/kg orally 3 times/day; 0.02–0.06 mg/kg IV Cats: < 4.5 kg, 2.5–5 mg orally 2 or 3 times/day; > 4.5 kg: 5 mg orally 2 or 3 times/day; 0.02–0.06 mg/kg IV	Beta adrenergic blocker

Table continued on next page.

Drug	Formulation	Indications	Dosage	Actions
Ranitidine (Zantac)	Injection: 25 mg/ml Tablet: 15 mg/ml Syrup: 150 mg	To decrease gastric acid secretion, as in patients with gastric ulcers	Dogs: 2 mg/kg 2–3 times/day orally, IV, SQ Cats: 3.5 mg/kg twice daily orally; 2.5 mg/kg twice daily IV	H_2 receptor-blocking agent
Sodium bicarbonate	1 mEq/ml	Severe metabolic acidosis	0.5–2 mEq/kg IV	Alkalinizing agent
Sucralfate (Carafate)	1 gm tablet	Duodenal ulcer	Dogs: 0.5– 1 gm 3 times/day orally	Reacts with gastric HCl to form pastelike complex that binds to proteinaceous exudates around ulcers
Theophylline (Theo-Dur)	Tablet: 100, 200, 300, 450 mg Capsule: 50, 75, 125, 200 mg	Asthma, chronic obstructive lung disease	Dogs: 9 mg/kg orally 2–3 times/day; Theo-Dur, 20 mg/kg orally twice daily Cats: 4 mg/kg orally 2–3 times/day; Theo-Dur, 25 mg/kg orally at night	Bronchodilator
Thiacetarsamide, sodium	Injection: 10 mg/ml	Adult dirofilariasis	Dogs: 2.2 mg/kg twice daily IV for 2 days	Organic arsenical compound
Verapamil (Calan, Isoptin)	Injection: 2.5 mg/ml	Supraventricular tachycardias, calcium overdose	0.05–0.15 mg/kg IV slowly over 15 min; 2–10 µg/kg/min CRI	Calcium channel blocker
Vitamin K (Phytonadione)	Injection: 10 mg/ml	Warfarin antidote	Dogs, cats: 1 mg/kg IM or orally; 2.5–5 mg/kg for long-acting rodenticide toxicity	Promotes coagulation
Xylazine (Rompun, AnaSed, Tranquived)	Injection: 20 or 100 mg/ml	Sedation, analgesia; emesis in cats	Dogs: 1 mg/kg IM or IV Cats: 0.44 mg/kg IV	Sedative, anesthetic
Yohimbine (Yobine)	Injection: 2 mg/dl	To reverse effects of xyalzine or amatraz	Dogs, cats: 0.1–0.5 mg/kg IV	Alpha$_2$ antagonist

IV = intravenously, IM = intramuscularly, SQ = subcutaneously, IT = intratracheally, CRI = constant-rate infusion, NSAID = nonsteroidal antiinflammatory drug, EMD = electromechanical dissociation, ACE = angiotensin-converting enzyme, AV = atrioventricular, NPH = neutral protamine Hagedorn [insulin].

INDEX

Page numbers in **boldface type** indicate complete chapters.